GLIAL CELLS: THEIR ROLE IN BEHAVIOUR

GLIAL CELLS:
THEIR ROLE IN BEHAVIOUR

Edited by
PETER R. LAMING
Queen's University of Belfast

with

EVA SYKOVÁ
*Charles University, Prague, and the
Institute of Experimental Medicine,
Academy of Sciences of the Czech
Republic*

ANDREAS REICHENBACH
Leipzig University

GLENN I. HATTON
University of California, Riverside

HERBERT BAUER
University of Vienna

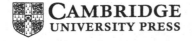

CAMBRIDGE
UNIVERSITY PRESS

CAMBRIDGE UNIVERSITY PRESS
Cambridge, New York, Melbourne, Madrid, Cape Town, Singapore,
São Paulo, Delhi, Dubai, Tokyo, Mexico City

Cambridge University Press
The Edinburgh Building, Cambridge CB2 8RU, UK

Published in the United States of America by Cambridge University Press, New York

www.cambridge.org
Information on this title: www.cambridge.org/9780521183826

© Cambridge University Press 1998

First published 1998
First paperback edition 2010

A catalogue record for this publication is available from the British Library

Library of Congress Cataloguing in Publication data

Glial cells: their role in behaviour / edited by Peter R. Laming,
    with Eva Syková . . . [et al.].
        p.   cm.
    Includes bibliographical references and index.
    ISBN 0-521-57368-8 (hb)
    1. Neuroglia.   2. Neuropsychology.   1. Laming, P. R.
    [DNLM: 1. Neuroglia—physiology.   2. Behavior—physiology.
    3. Cell Communication—physiology.   WL 102 G55873 1998]
    QP363.2.G586   1998
    611′. 0188—dc21
    DNLM/DLC
    for Library of Congress   98-10902
                                                            CIP

ISBN 978-0-521-57368-9 Hardback
ISBN 978-0-521-18382-6 Paperback

Contents

Contributors

Dr N. Joan Abbott
Biomedical Sciences Division, Physiology Group, King's College London, Strand, London WC2R 2CS, UK

Dr Chiye Aoki
Center for Neural Science, New York University, New York, NY 10003, USA

Professor Herbert Bauer
Institute for Psychology, University of Vienna, Leibiggasse 5, 1010 Vienna, Austria

Professor Niels Birbaumer
Institut für Medizinische Psychologie, Gontenstrasse 29, D-72074 Tübingen, Germany

Dr Joanna B. Bobak
Department of Anatomy, West Virginia University School of Medicine, 4052 HSN, Morgantown, WV 26506, USA

Dr Jonathan Coles
INSERM, U394, Rue Camille Saint-Saëns, 33077 Bordeaux Cedex, France

Dr Joachim W. Deitmer
Abteilung für Allgemeine Zoologie, Universität Kaiserslautern, Postfach 3049, D-67653 Kaiserslautern, Germany

Dr Ralf Dringen
Physiologisch-chemisches Institut der Universität, Hoppe-Seyler-Str 4, D-72076 Tübingen, Germany

Dr Elisabeth Hansson
Institute of Neurobiology and Institute of Clinical Neuroscience, Department of Neurology, University of Göteborg, Göteborg, Sweden

Professor Glenn I Hatton
Department of Neuroscience, University of California at Riverside, Riverside, CA 92521, USA

Dr Nicholas Hawrylak
Division of Physical Therapy, West Virginia University School of Medicine, 4052 HSN, Morgantown, WV 26506, USA

Professor Uwe Heinemann
Institute of Physiology, Department of Neurophysiology, Charité, Humboldt University, Tucholskystr. 3, D-10117 Berlin, Germany

Professor Leif Hertz
Department of Pharmacology, University of Saskatchewan, Saskatoon, Saskatchewan S7N 0W0, Canada

Dr Tuula O. Jalonen
University of Tampere, Medical School, Building B (Bio), Medisiinarinkatu 3, PO Box 607, 33101 Tampere, Finland

Professor Harold K. Kimelberg
Division of Neurosurgery, Albany Medical College, Albany, NY 10003, USA

Dr Jeffery D. Kocsis
Neuroscience Research Center, VA Medical Center, West Haven, Connecticut 06516, USA

Dr Peter R. Laming
School of Biology and Biochemistry, The Queen's University of Belfast, Medical Biology Centre, 97 Lisburn Road, Belfast BT9 7BL, UK

Dr Pierre Magistretti
Institute of Physiology, University of Lausanne, CH-1005 Lausanne, Switzerland

Professor Ken McCarthy
Department of Pharmacology, University of North Carolina, Chapel Hill, NC 27599, USA

Dr Christian M. Müller
Max-Planck Institute for Developmental Biology, Spemannstr. 35/1, D-72076 Tübingen, Germany

Professor Kim T. Ng
Department of Psychology, Monash University, Clayton, Victoria 3168, Australia

Professor Charles Nicholson
Department of Physiology and Biophysics, New York University Medical Center, First Avenue, NY 10016, USA

Dr Alister U. Nicol
Department of Zoology, University of Cambridge, Downing Street, Cambridge CB2 3EJ, UK

Dr Brona O'Dowd
Vision, Touch and Hearing Research Centre, University of Queensland, Brisbane, Queensland 4072, Australia

Professor Ciaran Regan
Department of Pharmacology, University College Dublin, Foster Avenue, Blackrock, Co. Dublin, Ireland

Dr Winfried Reichelt
Paul-Flechsig Institute for Brain Research, Department of Neurophysiology, Leipzig University, Jahnallee 59, D-04109 Leipzig, Germany

Professor Andreas Reichenbach
Paul-Flechsig Institute for Brain Research, Department of Neurophysiology, Leipzig University, Jahnallee 59, D-04109 Leipzig, Germany

Dr Stephen R. Robinson
Vision, Touch and Hearing Research Centre, University of Queensland, Brisbane, Queensland 4072, Australia

Professor Lars Rönnbäck
Institute of Neurobiology and Institute of Clinical Neuroscience, Department of Neurology, University of Göteborg, Göteborg, Sweden

Professor Betty I. Roots
Department of Zoology, University of Toronto, Toronto, Canada

Professor Frank Rösler
Department of Psychology, Philipps University, D-35032 Marburg, Germany

Dr John V. Roughan
Comparative Biology Centre, University of Newcastle, Framlington Place, Newcastle-upon-Tyne NE2 4HH, UK

Dr Adrienne K. Salm
Department of Anatomy, West Virginia University School of Medicine, 4052 HSN, Morgantown, WV 26506, USA

Professor Arne Schousboe
Department of Biological Sciences, Pharma Biotec Research Centre, Royal Danish School of Pharmacy, 2 Universitetsparken, DK-2100 Copenhagen, Denmark

Dr Serguei N. Skatchkov
Institute of Neurobiology, 201 Boulevard del Valle, San Juan, PR 00901, USA

Professor Eva Syková
Institute of Experimental Medicine, Academy of Sciences of the Czech Republic, Videnskà 1083, 142 20 Prague 4, Czech Republic

Professor Wolfgang Walz
Department of Physiology, University of Saskatchewan, 107 Wiggins Road, Saskatoon, Saskatchewan S7N 5E5, Canada

Professor Stephen G. Waxman
Department of Neurology, School of Medicine, PO Box 208018, Yale University, New Haven, Connecticut 06520-8018, USA

Preface

This book has been inspired by the perception of its editors and authors that there is an urgent need for the neuroscience and behavioural neuroscience communities to familiarise themselves and, more critically, their students with the new knowledge of how neurons and glia may interact with each other to provide a behavioural outcome.

In the first two-thirds of this century, the neuron doctrine reigned supreme in neuroscience research and in explanations of how behaviour was triggered and coordinated. Curiosity, combined with the belief that the other major cellular component of the brain, the glia, must make *some* useful contribution, has led to increasing interest in glial–neuronal interactions. The growing interest and understanding of the intimate involvement of glia in neuronal function has been facilitated by new techniques in cellular and molecular biology, biochemistry and physiology. The increasing body of knowledge of glial function has demonstrated the dangers of either studying neuronal *or* glial functions *alone* when attempting to explain brain activities and the consequent behaviour.

One of the results of the historical emphasis on neuronal regulation of brain function has been to incur reluctance in many practising neuroscientists to consider the new knowledge of glial functions either in their own research, or perhaps more importantly, in their teaching. We hope that this volume will provide both information and stimulation for neuroscientists at all stages in their careers to study and research how *all the cells* that comprise the central nervous system interact to receive, process and respond to environmental information in order to elicit appropriate adaptive behaviour.

List of Abbreviations

4-AP4	aminopyridene
5-HT	5-hydroxytryptamine (serotonin)
AAT	aspartate aminotransferase
ACh	acetylcholine
ACTH	adrenocorticotrophic hormone
$ACTH_{1-24}$	a fragment of adrenocorticotropic hormone involving the first 24 amino acids
ADC	apparent diffusion coefficient
ADP	adenosine diphosphate
AMP	adenosine monophosphate
AMPA	α-amino, 3-hydroxy, 5-methyl, 4-isoxazole proprionic acid (glutamate receptor)
AP5	2-amino-5-phosphonopentanoate
ATP	adenosine triphosphate
β-AR	beta-adrenergic receptor
BBB	blood–brain barrier
BrdU	bromodeoxyuridine
CA	carbonic anhydrase
CA1	hippocampal region 1
CA3	hippocampal region 3
cAMP	cyclic adenosine monophosphate
Ca^{2+}	calcium ion
CCD	charge coupled device
cGMP	cyclic guanosine monophosphate
Cl^-	chloride ions
CNS	central nervous system
CNV	contingent negative variation
CNQX	6-cyano-7-nitroquinoxaline-2,3-dione
CO_2	carbon dioxide
CRABP	cellular retinoic acid binding protein

CREB	cyclic AMP-response element-binding protein
CSF	cerebrospinal fluid
DC	direct current
DIA	depolarisation-induced alkalinisation
DNA	deoxyribonucleic acid
DNP	2,4-dinitrophenol
DNQX	6,7-dinitroquinoxaline-2,3-dione
EAA	excitatory amino acid
ECS	extracellular space
EPSP	excitatory postsynaptic potential
ERG	electroretinogram
FA	fluoracetate
GABA	gamma-aminobutyric acid
GABA-T	GABA transaminase
GABA$_A$	GABA receptor subtype A
GAD	glutamate decarboxylase
GFAP	glial fibrillary acidic protein
GFAP(+)	glial fibrillary acidic protein (positive)
GLAST	L-glutamate/L-aspartate transporter
GLDH	glutamate dehydrogenase
GLT-1	glutamate transporter 1
Glu	glutamate
GluR2	glutamate receptor subtype 2
GnRH	gonadotropin releasing hormone
GS	glutamine synthetase
HCO$_3^-$	bicarbonate
HNS	hypothalamo-neurohypophysial system
Hvc	vocal control nucleus (birds)
INL	inner nuclear layer of retina
IO	iodoacetate
IOI	integrative optical imaging
IP	inositol phosphate
IPL	inner plexiform layer of retina
IPSP	inhibitory postsynaptic potential
ISM	ion-sensitive microelectrode
ITM	intermediate-term memory
K$^+$	potassium ion
[K$^+$]$_e$	extracellular potassium concentration
[K$^+$]$_i$	intracellular potassium concentration
KA	kainic acid/kainate glutamate receptors
Lac2	galactoside
LGN	lateral geniculate nucleus
LHRH	luteinising hormone releasing hormone

LTD	long-term depression
LTM	long-term memory
LTP	long-term potentiation
MARCKS	myristoylated alanine-rich C kinase substrate
MCPG	methyl-4-carboxyphenylglycine
MeA	methylanthranilate
MFB	medial forebrain bundle
mGluR	metabotrophic glutamate receptor
MK-801	dizocilpine maleate (NMDA receptor antagonist)
MNC	magnocellular neuroendocrine cell
mRNA	messenger ribonucleic acid
MRS/MRI	magnetic resonance scanning/imaging
MSO	methionine sulphoximine
Na^+	sodium ions
Na^+/K^+-ATPase	sodium/potassium adenosine triphosphatase
Na^+/K^+ pump	sodium/potassium pump
Na^+/HCO_3^-	sodium bicarbonate cotransporter
NCAM	neural cell adhesion molecule
NMDA	*N*-methyl-D-aspartate glutamate receptors
NMR	nuclear magnetic resonance
NO	nitric oxide
NSP	non-seizure-prone
OPL	outer plexiform layer
p(x)–p(y)	postnatal days x–y
PAG	phosphate-activated glutaminase
PCR	polymerase chain reaction
PET	positron emission topography
pH	hydrogen ion concentration measure
PKC	phosphokinase C
PMA	phorbol-12-myristate-13-acetate
PSA-NCAM	polysialic acid-linked neural cell adhesion molecule
PSP	postsynaptic potential
Quis	quisqualate glutamate receptor
RVD	regulatory volume decrease
S-100-β-protein	a glial marker protein
SAC	stretch-activated channels
SAS	subarachnoid space
SB	spatial buffering
SCN	suprachiasmatic nucleus
SON	supraoptic nucleus
son-VGL	ventral glial limitans subjacent to the supraoptic nucleus
SP	seizure-prone
SPS	sustained or slow potential shift

SRS	subretinal space
STM	short-term memory
t-ACPD	*trans*-1-amino-1,3-cyclopentane dicarboxylic acid (metabotrophic glutamate agonist)
TCA	tricarboxylic acid
TMA	tetramethylammonium
TTX	tetradotoxin
VGL	ventral glial limitans
VLSI	very large scale integrated circuitry

1

Changing Concepts on the Role of Glia

PETER R. LAMING

Summary

Although the contribution of neurons to brain function and behaviour has been the subject of intense research throughout this century, that of their partner cells, the glia, was sadly neglected until the last three decades. There is now a growing new perspective of brain function which recognises that neurons are not simply the generators of spiking messages as was once thought, but can also communicate by more subtle graded potentials. More importantly, there is a new insight that glial cells are not just homeostats, providing a stable environment for neurons, but that they also communicate with each other and with neurons in a manner that is cooperative, yielding many of the changes in nervous system function that leads to adaptive behaviour of the whole organism.

Early in development, glial cells are intimately involved in regulating neuronal growth, differentiation and the development of appropriate connections. This interaction in terms of plasticity continues into adult life, as glia respond to the ionic and neurotransmitter contents of the neuronal microenvironment at their apposed perisynaptic and perinodal processes, but also via their gap–junction connectivity with each other and their highly conductive interfaces with blood vessels and cerebrospinal fluid. Their involvement in regulating, or modulating, extracellular potassium is reflected in slow potential shifts with definable links with behaviours ranging through sleep to wakefulness, with motivation, learning and possibly higher cognitive functions in humans. Along with potassium fluxes, those of hydrogen (pH) and calcium are likely ionic candidates for signalling between neurons and glia. It has become apparent that ensheathing glia are involved in the properties of the ensheathed neuron not only by affecting its ability to conduct action potentials.

The intimate interface of glia with the vascular supply for energy substrates and removal of metabolites places these cells in a potentially regulatory position for control of brain function, which is amplified by their unique possession of key enzymes for energy storage and supply, pH regulation and that of the excitatory neurotransmitter, glutamate. Involvement of many of these enzymes has been implicated in sensory function and learning.

The apparently complex morphological association of glial processes with neurons and other brain structures is not a static one. These cells change their associations in a variety of situations where behaviour also changes dynamically, including responses to dehydration, onset of lactation and parturition, in parallel with the circadian cycle, in response to steroid hormones, and with exposure of the animal to an enriched environment. It is these interactions between neurons and glia and these associations between glial functions and behaviours that make it imperative that we explore the role that glia play in the evocation of behaviour.

1.1 Historical Perspective

At the beginning of this century, it had become evident that peripheral and central nervous system (CNS) tissue contained cells that were electrically excitable. These cells, the neurons, were believed to form the basis for integration of information within the brain by communicating at synapses (Sherrington 1906). This 'neuron doctrine' was strongly supported by Ramon y Cajal (1909, 1911) from his histological studies. It stressed the individuality of neurons, their electrical excitability and the belief that they were the functional units of the brain, the integrative powers of which lead to behaviour and ultimately consciousness.

During the first half of this century, research on the mechanisms that underlie the excitability of nerve cells continued apace, culminating in the explicit model of Hodgkin and Huxley (1952) for the generation of the action potential. This research reinforced the 'neuron doctrine' in that it was now redefined to imply that individual neurons carried information by action potentials, transmitted and integrated with that from other cells by synapses. Although graded potentials were described (Eccles 1953), they received little credence as a conduction mechanism, even over short distances.

The nervous system, however, is also composed of neuroglial or 'glue' cells which have only recently attracted much attention. To many, this lack of interest in cells that in primates may comprise some 50% of the mass of the brain may seem surprising, especially as they were first identified by Virchow in 1856! The clearest descriptions, however, had to wait until the beginning of this century with the revolution in neuroanatomy led by Golgi, Ramon y Cajal, Del Rio Hortega and Penfield amongst others (see Somjen, 1993). They described glia primarily by their lack of an axon and speculated on their possible function; Golgi thought that they may have a nutritive function for neurons, while Ramon y Cajal preferred to think of them as neuron insulators. As we shall see, both of them were right, but at about the same time another discovery was reported which seemed at the time to be totally unrelated. This was the description by Caton (1875) of a sustained cortical 'current voltage', which we now describe as a slow potential shift, probably reflecting ionic currents through glia and extracellular fluid (ECF).

It is sobering to think that it was not until the middle of this century that interest was reawakened in both the cell biology and the physiology of glia. The advances, especially in the last 10–20 years have been spectacular, but more recently, the previously heretical suggestion that glia play a role in nervous activity, and therefore behaviour, has begun to gain respectability. Pioneers in this area were Galambos (1961), Hertz (1965) and Roitbak (1965, 1988), followed more recently by Laming (1989a,b), Bevan (1990), Barres (1991) and Smith (1992). This chapter will critically assess the 'neuron doctrine' and suggest what glial functions are most involved in neuronal activity and behavioural change, concentrating on areas not reviewed extensively in other chapters.

1.2 What is a Neuron?

There is no such thing as a conventional neuron, yet we usually describe a motor neuron as being 'typical' to our students. The soma of such a cell radiates dendritic processes, which with the soma, receive incoming information from synapses of other neurons. A single long process, the axon, arises from the axon hillock, where action potentials are usually generated and thence propagated along the axon to its terminals. At the axon terminals, depolarisation causes the release of transmitter from the presynaptic membrane, which in turn affects the activity of the (postsynaptic) dendrite or soma of another neuron, or in this particular case, muscle cell. A 'conventional' view of such a cell is depicted in Fig. 1.1A, with the axon wrapped in a series of sheaths of myelin derived from Schwann glial cells in the peripheral nervous system or oligodendroglia in the CNS. Many neurons in the brain bear little resemblance to that described here, some having vast dendritic arborisations, often with a small axon, others being small internuncial neurons from which direct recordings have only infrequently been made. Although the 'conventional' neuron is considered to generate spikes in the axon, with graded potentials in the dendritic trees, spikes can occur in dendrites, some neurons have no axon, yet spike, (amacrine cells) and some more 'typical' neurons do not spike, like retinal bipolar cells or interneurons in the olfactory bulb. In order to assess the contributions non-spiking cells may make to information processing it is necessary to identify what is critical to the spiking activity of a neuron.

1.2.1 The Resting Potential

All cells, neurons included, are bounded by a membrane whose function is to contain and protect the metabolic life processes of the internal organelles and the biochemistry of cellular metabolism and *selectively* to allow ingress and egress of inorganic ions and small organic molecules. Inside the cell, larger molecules (e.g. proteins) are manufactured and retained, most being negatively charged. The cell membrane is fairly freely permeable to K^+ which enters the cell due to the

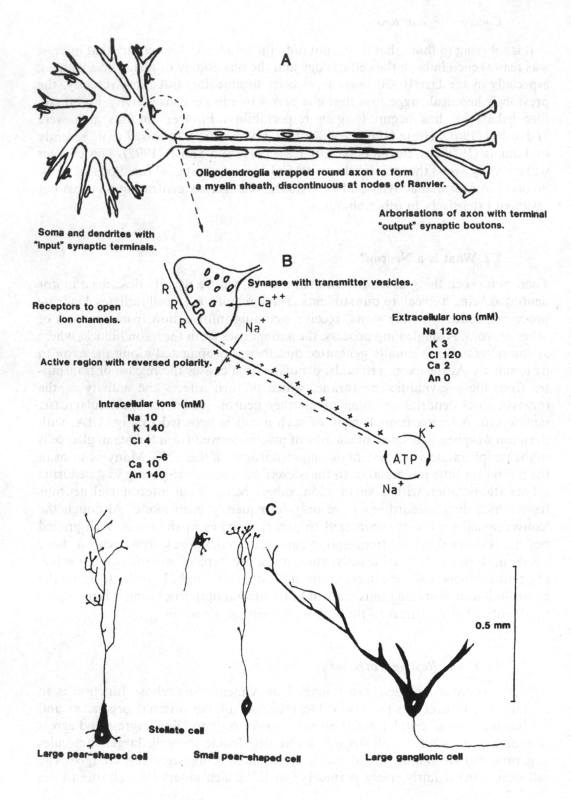

A

Oligodendroglia wrapped round axon to form a myelin sheath, discontinuous at nodes of Ranvier.

Soma and dendrites with "input" synaptic terminals.

Arborisations of axon with terminal "output" synaptic boutons.

B

Synapse with transmitter vesicles.

Receptors to open ion channels.

Ca^{++}

Na$^+$

Active region with reversed polarity.

Extracellular ions (mM)
Na 120
K 3
Cl 120
Ca 2
An 0

Intracellular ions (mM)
Na 10
K 140
Cl 4
Ca 10^{-6}
An 140

K$^+$

ATP

Na$^+$

C

0.5 mm

Stellate cell

Large pear-shaped cell

Small pear-shaped cell

Large ganglionic cell

activity of an energy-using 'sodium pump' which actively removes Na^+ ions out of the cell, linked to K^+ ingress. This sets up an outward diffusion gradient for K^+, counteracted by the negativity produced by the large intracellular anions.

The effects of the unequal distribution of ions across the membrane is that there develops a potential difference of some 70–80 mV, inside negative in relation to outside (Fig. 1.1B). This voltage can, in most neurons, be shown to be largely due to the unequal distribution of K^+, the prime diffusible ion in the resting condition of the neuron. Ionic conductances for other ions may, however, also contribute both to the resting potential and the potential changes which occur during neuronal responses. Apart from K^+ ions, numerous channels are known for Na^+, Cl^- and Ca^{2+}. The resting membrane potential is thus critically determined by the population of intracellular non-diffusible anions, the number of open ion channels for diffusible ions and most importantly in the context of this book, the extracellular concentration of the diffusible ion species, primarily potassium.

1.2.2 *Current Conduction*

Ions, and therefore current, can in the appropriate circumstances, pass through the membrane via channels selective for the particular ion species. Channels may open due to a configurational change in their structure which may be brought about by a variety of agencies. These may be mechanical distortion of the membrane (touch and acoustic receptors), chemical changes within the cell due to an external energy source (photoreceptors), chemicals present at the exterior of the cell (olfactory receptors), or specific biochemical messengers to which the cell is sensitive (neurotransmitters – see below) or changes in the electrical potential across the cell membrane itself. Many neurons may have different types of ion channels, each responsive to one specific agent, other channels responding less specifically. There are, for example, an increasing number of K^+ channels recog-

---

Fig. 1.1. The 'typical' neuron (A) is most akin to a spiking spinal motor neuron, the axon of which is invested in the plasma membranes of a Schwann cell, rich in myelin. In the central nervous system, oligodendroglia provide this myelin sheath. Inputs arrive via axonal terminals at synapses on dendrites or the soma (B), where depolarisation causes Ca^{2+} ingress and release of transmitter from vesicles, 'docked' on the presynaptic membrane, into the synaptic cleft. The transmitter then diffuses to specific receptors on the postsynaptic membrane which, either directly or via second messengers, causes ion channels (e.g. Na^+) to open and depolarises the postsynaptic membrane. If sufficient, this depolarisation may, after integration with other inputs, produce an action potential or 'spike'. The wide range of neuronal morphologies, however (e.g. C, from the anuran tectum), may include many neurons which need not generate spikes to relay information.

nised, responding to a variety of chemical messengers. Some channels appear to be rectifying, i.e. they only allow their selected ion species to pass in one direction.

The resting neuron already has a high conductance for potassium, giving it a resting potential of some -70 to -80 mV inside. This polarised condition may be increased if conductance to Cl^- is enhanced and decreased if that to Na^+ is increased (hyperpolarisation and depolarisation, respectively). If we take the conventional case of a local increase in Na^+ conductance, Na^+ flows into the cell down its chemical gradient and the internal negative electrical gradient caused by the unequal distribution of all the major ion species. This causes current to flow in the cell cytoplasm (i.e. along the axon away from the depolarised region and out through the membrane at distant regions). The current thus flows decrementally and passively away from the source of depolarisation. If the distance is great, then the signal (the local depolarisation) will dissipate and be lost. If it is in the order of 10s of microns, however, as with many CNS interneurons, then this electronic spread of current may be sufficient and adequate to trigger events in other cells. This is an important consideration in regions (like the CNS) where small neurons are often densely packed. There is considerable evidence that many neurons may indeed communicate in this way, without spikes, both in their dendritic trees and axons (Shepherd 1981). There is an advantage in this form of information conduction in that the temporal pattern of the depolarisation may faithfully represent that of the initiating input. The disadvantage is that over distance the amplitude decay may be sufficient to make the signal 'unreadable'. Thus, most well studied, relatively large neurons, are excitable, i.e. there is a voltage gated conductance increase for an ion species when depolarisation of some 20% of the resting potential obtains. This explosively increased conductance, normally to Na^+, initiates a 'spike' or action potential. The current flow to adjacent, still polarised regions, also reaches the voltage threshold for spike generation so the spike is propagated along the axon without decrement.

The rapid ionic exchanges which occur during a single spike transmission hardly affect the ionic concentrations across the membrane because of the short spike duration, but bursts of spikes cause a requirement for a high energy expenditure for operation of the Na^+/K^+-ATPase pump. This accounts in large part for the high metabolic demand of the brain. The main advantage of spikes is perceived as being that of encoding information by a frequency code which is non-decremental. Thus spiking is a requisite for long distance communication, like that from peripheral sensory organs to the brain or from brain to effectors, like muscles, ultimately the agents of behaviour. The amplitude of spikes is such that they may also allow information transfer at well above the electrical noise level of the rest of the tissue (Perkel and Bullock 1981).

In CNS tissue as a whole, it is probable that the input to dendrites of a neuron is a graded potential which is usually conducted electrotonically either to the body of the cell or to other dendrites. On reaching the soma, inputs, be they depolarising (excitatory) or hyperpolarising (often inhibitory), integrate and pass along the axon either as a graded potential or as a frequency code of spikes. In order to increase the rate of conduction, of spiking neurons at least, the axon is often invested in a lipoprotein sheath of myelin, interrupted at intervals (nodes of Ranvier) to expose 'bare' axon. Sodium channels are concentrated at the nodes and so depolarisation of the axon and generation of the action potential occurs sequentially from node to node. Towards the axonal terminals, the myelin sheath is thinner or even absent and the propagated spike may continue to travel with no loss of amplitude or may decline to a graded potential which decrements towards the presynaptic terminal.

1.2.3 Synaptic Transmission

Neurons communicate with each other via synapses which can be categorised as electrical or chemical. At electrical synapses, the pre- and postsynaptic membranes of the cells are in close apposition. Current flow between the cells is via gap junctions. Often current can flow in either direction, i.e. the synapse is not rectifying. Attenuation of the potential may be quite large at an electrical synapse if the postsynaptic cell is large. This attenuation may be sufficient to block transmission of an action potential across the electrical synapse, due to current sinking. However, electrical synapses may be important for rapid conduction between cell processes of matched size, e.g. dendro–dendritic synapses.

In chemical synapses, depolarisation of the axon terminal causes opening of Ca^{2+} channels. Calcium ions enter the presynaptic terminal down the electrical and chemical gradients and cause transmitter-containing vesicles docked on the presynaptic membrane to fuse with that membrane and release their contents into the synaptic cleft. The transmitter release is related to the degree of depolarisation of the presynaptic terminal. This transmitter diffuses to the postsynaptic membrane, where it binds to specific receptors which directly or via second messengers cause ion channels to open and the membrane either to depolarise (cation, usually Na^+ channels) or hyperpolarise (Cl^-, K^+ channels). The transmitter must then be deactivated by enzymic breakdown or sequestration to terminate its effects. The length of time for which the transmitter exerts its effects will depend on the speed of inactivation, the distance across and the volume of the synaptic cleft and the availability of uptake sites in the region. The amount of transmitter released depends on the degree of depolarisation of the presynaptic terminal, so partial depolarisation prior to the arrival, say, of an action potential may actually reduce the amount of transmitter released. This is one mechanism of presynaptic inhibition. One of the major features of chemical synaptic transmission is that it may amplify a signal by the presynaptic release sensitivity to voltage change, the postsynaptic receptor availability and the mechanisms of channel opening on the postsynaptic membrane.

The above summary description of neuronal cellular function is intended to stress the following features.

1 Neurons are biological devices which integrate many depolarising and hyperpolarising electrical inputs to produce an output to other elements of the system. Outputs may be excitatory or inhibitory or both.
2 Voltage signals in neurons are the product of membrane conductance's for several ion species.
3 Amplification of outputs or inputs may occur at synapses by increased transmitter release or receptor density, respectively, and at any region of the cell where voltage gated ion channels are present in sufficient quantity to elicit an action potential.
4 The evolutionary requirement for gain by spiking is largely a product of a 'leaky' high resistance cable and a noisy environment.
5 The nature and amplitude of membrane currents and therefore the way neurons integrate and transmit information is dependent on the relationship between the intra- and extracellular concentrations of ions, the extracellular presence of neuro-active substances and the energy supply.

The above summary account of neuronal function is intended to both remind non-neuroscientists of the conventional wisdom and to broaden that view to include non-spiking conduction by neurons, electrical synapses and the importance of the extracellular environment. There may be many neurons which use both graded potentials and action potentials in communication (Perkel and Bullock 1981).

1.3 What are Glia?

There are three main functional classes of macroglial cell in the nervous system, the ependymoglia, astrocytes and myelinating glia. Their number and degree of differentiation increase both with phylogeny (Chapter 2) and during development (Chapter 3).

Ependymoglia include radial glia that span the neural tube during development, tanycytes that form the ventricular cerebrospinal fluid (CSF) interface, and the radial (Müller) glial cells of the retina. Astrocytes are found throughout the central nervous system, with diverse morphologies and probably diverse functional capabilities. They are regionally radially oriented (Colombo et al. 1995), though as their name suggests, they have an abundance of cellular processes. Myelin forming cells include oligodendroglia in the CNS and Schwann cells in the peripheral nervous system (PNS). They have the characteristic of ensheathing axonal processes, the sheaths being interrupted by nodes of Ranvier. All these types of glial (or 'glue') cells have long been considered to be the passive supportive cells for neurons. Until recently, the only accepted useful function attributed to glia was the insulative function of myelin which reduces current loss at the internode and also increases the speed of conduction. The original view was that this was a passive phenomenon, similar to the function of plastic ensheathment of an electrical cable (but see Chapters 8, 9).

Electron microscope studies of brain tissue have revealed much of the morphological relationships between glial cells and other structures and cells in the CNS. Both ependymal glia and astrocytes have processes which contact those of other glial cells, often forming, via gap junctions, a continuum or functional syncytium for transport of ions and small organic molecules. Other processes invest capillaries (pericapillary), synapses (perisynaptic), nodes of Ranvier (perinodal), or abut the CSF interfaces of the ventricles and subarachnoid space (diagramatically represented in Fig. 1.2).

Thus, the most active regions of neurons (synapses and nodes) are largely surrounded by astrocytic or ependymal processes, whilst the relatively inactive internodal regions are enveloped in sheaths of oligodendroglial or Schwann cell membranes. Furthermore, the other glial processes envelop the non-neural interfaces of the brain, the blood vessels and the CSF reservoirs. This organisation raises many new questions about glial functions, some of which are beginning to be answered. These are:

1 Does the ensheathment of blood vessels imply that all metabolic substrates and metabolites have to pass through glia?
2 Does the separation of brain from CSF and blood by glia indicate a regulated interface?
3 Does the presence of a perinodal envelopment have implications for ionic fluxes and signal conduction?
4 Do perisynaptic envelopes affect synaptic transmission?

These questions and more derive simply from the morphological apposition of astrocytic and ependymal glial processes, but many more derive from studies of their physiology and biochemistry. Much of this research has been performed on cultured cells, so its applicability to the in vivo brain remains to be validated.

Before we try to answer the question of what neurons and glia do with respect to the evocation of behaviour, let us try to examine what is meant by behaviour and then assess the likelihood of glial/neuronal involvement.

1.4 What is Behaviour?

Behaviour can be described by a catalogue of the muscular contractions that an animal performs. When studying nerve–muscle relations, this tells us that it is neurons that control the force and duration of muscular contractions, the contribution of ensheathing or myelinating glia being limited to maintaining the optimal conduction properties of the motor output. Given that motor fibres have differing sizes, degrees of myelination and conduction velocities, however,

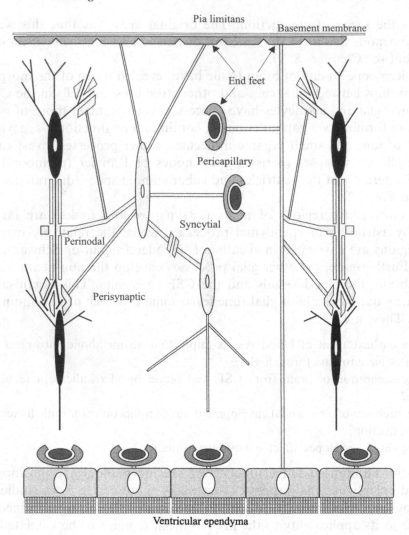

Fig. 1.2. Cartoon of an astrocyte-like cell (left) and a radial glial cell (right) with their possible interrelationships with other cellular elements in the brain. Perisynaptic processes of the glial cells (stippled) embrace synapses of neurons (black). Pericapillary and perinodal processes invest blood vessels and nodes of Ranvier, respectively. Astrocytes electrically connect with each other as a functional syncytium via gap junctions. Glial cells may have end feet, highly conductive for potassium, forming part of the brain–CSF and brain–blood interfaces. Ventricular glial processes may be ciliated or invested in microvilli, presumably for absorptive purposes.

there exists the possibility that the effectiveness of conduction might be modified by Schwann cells in response to demand for muscular activity.

Normally, however, we describe behaviour in a more generalistic way, such as walking, flying, etc., each of which includes the activities of large numbers of motor commands, often integrated by reflexes at spinal, brainstem and higher levels. Again, the sequence of motor activities seems to be mediated entirely by neural influences, though these can be modified by experience, and the likelihood of them occurring seems to be modulated by the sensory environment and the internal state of the animal. These 'states' include sleep, wakefulness and arousal, where the activity of much of the brain ranges from being suppressed to being enhanced. In conditions of motivation like hunger, thirst, or sexual appetite, populations of cells seem to change their levels of activity in response to internal 'stimuli' like circulating glucose, plasma osmotic pressure and/or circulating hormone levels.

If we examine the sensory input to the brain and its possibility of being affected by non-neural processes, the purely neural origin of activity to a given stimulus is not so clear. Many sensory organs include non-neural supportive epithelial cells which may modify neuronal responsiveness. Often the sensory receptor has little resemblance to a neuron and responds to environmental change with a graded depolarisation, or in the retina, hyperpolarisation. Some of these cells may have an origin more akin to glia than neurons (Reichenbach and Robinson 1995a). There is growing evidence for changing sensory and regional brain activity, with changes in behavioural state or with modification of behavioural responses during learning. Because the output of the brain and the transmission of sensory input to the brain are considered entirely neural and recordable as action potentials, the assumption has been made that integration of sensory information and internal information must also be by this process. Evidence in favour of purely neural integration may derive from spinal reflex activity, where a spiking sensory neuron makes direct contact with a spiking motor neuron. Here there would seem to be no possibility of non-neural involvement, but are these reflexes always predictable? They are not, as for instance, pain-detecting neuronal responses can be modified by other mechanoreceptor spinal neurons, descending projections and potentially by the associated glia. Indeed, any recording of neuronal activity in the CNS is often beset by (unpublished) 'spontaneous' changes or 'background' noise. Neuroscientists go to great lengths to average out this variability from the results of the particular function they are examining, though at times it may be an integral, though non-neural part of that function.

What is evident is that glia are unlikely to carry *specific* information as their connectivity is diffuse and multidirectional. They may, however, affect local operations of neurons at synapses in response to the neuron itself or may affect populations in response to external or internal signals.

As in the spinal cord so also in the brain are functions, to some extent, localised. This is evident for localisation of sensory processing regions and regions concerned with motivational states. Even within a region like the visual or somatosensory cortex, the part of the environment represented is organised in columns. Thus, to enhance responsiveness to a particular information source, as during attention, a particular population of cells should be facilitated. The same argument applies for changes due to motivation, though the brain region involved may be more extensive, or to sleep where most neural activity is suppressed. Conventionally, neuronal projections between networks of cells have been postulated as mechanisms to control population responsivity, but a more parsimonious explanation would be by regulation of the environment of these neurons. Glia are uniquely placed to perform in this way, as they are syncitially organised to influence a relatively large volume of tissue (i.e. number of neurons, but see Chapter 7) and their points of apposition are those on neurons which are most crucially sensitive. More importantly, they are often coupled to form groups or columns of interconnected cells. This is especially evident in the retina (Chapter 4) for radial glia in non-mammalian vertebrates and may apply to radially oriented glia in the mammalian cortex (Colombo et al. 1995). This organisation not only places glia in a conventionally accepted position to maintain homeostatically the stability of the neuronal microenvironment so that neurons can get on with the job of responding predictably, but also suggests a more dynamic role. Just as hormones maintain homeostasis within limits and are also modulators of brain activity and behaviour, so too does glial regulation of the neuronal microenvironment operate within broad limits which allows for modulation of neuronal responsiveness.

1.5 Glial Involvement in Neuronal Function

1.5.1 The Neuronal Ionic Microenvironment

Apart from synaptic interactions, a common conception of the neuron is of a device divorced from the extracellular milieu, which is assumed constant. Yet, as has been stressed here, it is the relationship between intra- and extracellular concentrations of ion species that gives rise to the resting membrane potential and will affect the magnitude of current flow along the neuron whether this be electrotonic or a propagated spike (see Chapter 7). There is now considerable evidence that extracellular potassium concentration ($[K^+]_e$) may fluctuate from its 'normal' level of ca. 3.5 mM to up to 9+ mM in conditions of high neuronal activity (Syková 1983, 1992b). If the resting potential of a neuron was entirely dependent on K^+ distribution and was ca. −80 mV inside relative to outside a 4 mM $[K^+]_e$ would give a $[K^+]_i$ of ca. 96 mM. If $[K^+]_e$ should change to 8 mM the resting potential would decline to −75 mV, 17% below its initial level and perhaps close to levels required for voltage-gated conductances to be initiated. It is known that moderate elevation of $[K^+]_e$ reduces neuronal excitation thresholds and may even induce spikes, though sustained elevations reduce neuronal excitability (Somjen et al. 1986). Elevated $[K^+]_e$ at the synapse has been long suggested to reduce transmitter release by a form of presynaptic inhibition, though many experimental studies find an increased synaptic release of transmitter with elevation of $[K^+]_e$ (Vyklický 1978; Syková 1983).

What distinguishes glia from neurons, considering that we have now extended our definition of neurons to neural cells which do not have explosive voltage-dependent conductances? Glia cell membranes are, like those of neurons, polarised with a 'resting potential' (ca. 90 mV) almost entirely due to potassium distribution. Changes in the $[K^+]_e$ due to release on neuronal activity causes depolarisation of the glial membrane. Electrotonic current flow then occurs through glia and the extracellular space, and can be recorded extracellularly as a sustained or slow potential shift (SPS) (Chapter 10). Near the source of neuronal excitation the K^+ potential reflects glial depolarisation and the SPS in mammalian cortex (Roitbak et al. 1987) and in the frog brain (Roitbak et al. 1992; Chapter 12). Astrocytes and ependymoglia are electrotonically connected via gap junctions forming a functional syncytium (Gutnick, Connors and Ransom 1981; Coles and Orkand 1983), yet estimates of 200–400 μm are the limits of current spread suggested from dye-coupling experiments (Gutnick, Connors and Ransom 1981) or theoretical considerations (Gardner-Medwin 1983c). Although this represents a considerable volume of tissue and therefore a large neuronal population whose environment will have been subjected to elevated $[K^+]_e$, it is far smaller than the spread of SPS responses recorded from immobilised animals whose neuronal activity was also recorded (Chapter 12).

Based on our original perceptions of glia as homoeostatic regulators it has been demonstrated that the 'syncytial' organisation of glia could act spatially to buffer local $[K^+]_e$ rises by removing K^+ from the site of release and thus reduce the impact of the rise on the local neuron (Gardner-Medwin 1983c). Three factors would suggest that this might not be the only function of K^+ redistribution by glia. First, glia are radially organised in cortical structures, in a manner which parallels the neuronal information processing pathway. Thus, K^+ redistribution will probably be to functionally related areas. Secondly, the redistribution may be more rapid than the neuronally conducted information, as there is no synaptic delay. This may be why 'preemptive' SPSs to visual stimuli may be recorded in deep layers of the toad tectum before the visual unit responses in that region (Laming and Ewert 1984; Chapter 12). The third reason why the relocation of K^+ is not likely to be to 'functionally irrelevant' regions is related to the morphology of astrocytic and radial glial processes. These processes envelop nodes of Ranvier (perinodal) or synapses (perisynaptic) so that, within brain tissue, much of the redistributed K^+ would be to sensitive nodal or synaptic regions which would be partially depolarised as a consequence. Indeed, because of the intimacy of astrocyte processes with these regions, it is likely that our measures of $[K^+]_e$ rise achieved with invasive introduction of large glass micropipettes are gross underestimates. The even more highly conductive perivascular and pial end-feet may act to siphon K^+ between nervous and non-nervous tissue.

The above arguments obtain for passive electrotonic redistribution of K^+. However, the ionic conductance for K^+ is not entirely passive, as elevated K^+ causes active uptake of K^+ by glia (Walz and Hinks 1986). It would thus seem that glia, especially astrocytes, can regulate $[K^+]_e$ within bounds that still allow sufficient flexibility for neuromodulation.

Some glial K^+ channels are inwardly rectifying (Barres 1991) and this, with the possible triggering of glial Na^+/K^+ pump activity by elevated $[K^+]_e$ (Ballanyi 1995), has suggested to Barres (1991) that glia may accumulate K^+ in response to neuronal activity. With Cl^- ingress also, this would increase glial volume, with possibly related decreases in extracellular space (ECS) and with profound effects on neuronal activity (Chapter 7).

A wide variety of behaviours are associated with a DC voltage change lasting for periods of 100s of milliseconds to tens of seconds (a SPS) recorded intra-cranially (Chapter 12) or epicranially (Chapter 13). In those cases of intracranial recording where it was possible to record $[K^+]_e$, this was highly correlated with the SPS, suggesting a glial role in its generation. Although it has not yet been possible to determine the precise relationship between intra- and epicranially recorded SPS responses, it is likely that glial 'spatial buffering' currents also con-tribute to these (Chapter 13).

The movement of potassium between neurons, ECS and glia acts as a signal, communicating the activity of neurons to glia, with a response which is not only electrical but also a metabolic promoter (see later). The main differences between glia and 'excitable' neurons in terms of ionic conductances appears to be in the number of, and threshold for opening of, voltage-gated ion channels. Apart from K^+ channels, voltage-gated channels for Na^+ and Cl^- (Bevan et al. 1985) and Ca^{2+} (MacVicar 1985) have been demonstrated for astrocytes in primary culture. Sodium channels on astrocytes, although of the neuronal type, are present in insufficient densities to allow generation of action potentials, and their function may be to provide an additional source of channels for neurons (Sontheimer and Ritchie 1995). Voltage-gated depolarisations to all these ions are unlikely to occur in vivo when the functional syncytium is intact and a large shunting conductance exists (Ransom and Carlini 1986). When the 'syncytium' is compromised by gap junction closure which also causes astrocytic swelling, however, these voltage-gated conductances may be important.

Apart from potassium, other ions may also act as intercellular signals. Of these, the most recognised candidates are Ca^{2+} and protons.

Calcium levels in the extracellular environment are lower than those of K^+ at about 1–2 mM. The effect of changes in extracellular calcium levels are more complex than for potassium. Low $[Ca^{2+}]_e$ would obviously affect synaptic release of transmitter as its uptake is required for vesicle fusion with the presynaptic membrane. Nevertheless, low $[Ca^{2+}]_e$ is associated with increased neuronal excit-ability. In pathological cases, $[Ca^{2+}]_e$ declines prior to the development of seizures (Pumain et al. 1985) which may, in part, be a cause of seizure initiation. The increase in neural excitation with low $[Ca^{2+}]_e$ is probably due to shifting of the activation of Na^+ channels to less depolarised values (Chao et al. 1994b), allowing greater ion influx on depolarisation or even spontaneous depolarisation in pathological conditions.

Calcium has been described as important for transmitter release at synapses, but it also offers a mechanism for neuron to glial signalling, as use of calcium-sensitive dyes have illustrated waves of increased $[Ca^{2+}]_i$ propagating through the astrocytic syncytium, especially in response to glutamate (see Smith 1992, for a review). These Ca^{2+} waves could have a wide range of effects on astrocytes which could then affect neuronal function. These include: modulation of Ca-dependent K^+ channels, regulation of $[Ca^{2+}]_e$, and regulation of internal metabolism of energy substrates and neurotransmitters for neurons (see Smith 1992 and Chapters 5, 6).

The oxidation of carbohydrates by CNS cells, to provide energy, results in the formation of bicarbonate and H^+, under the influence of carbonic anhydrase, located within the cytoplasm or cell membrane of glial cells (Deitmer 1995). In order to maintain the slightly alkaline intracellular environment necessary for survival, glial cells actively regulate pH by ion exchangers and transporters. The movement of protons resulting from metabolic acidification is thus crucially buffered by bicarbonate, but involves ionic movement which results in membrane potential shifts, which may contribute to SPSs and affect the spatial buffering of K^+ (Chapter 10).

1.5.2 Neurotransmitter Regulation

Apart from possessing voltage-gated ionic conductances, albeit with high thresholds, there is a growing body of evidence for an active role of glia in response to neurotransmitters and neuroactive peptides (Chapter 6). Glutamate, especially, will be discussed here because it is the neurotransmitter about which most is known and it also has effects on ionic distribution in the microenvironment. Glutamate is the most ubiquitously distributed and prevalent amino acid in the brain, where it is not only a metabolic substrate but is an excitatory neurotransmitter. Of the types of glutamate receptors recognised in neurons by glutamate analogs, glial depolarisation is only induced by kainic acid (KA) and quisqualate (Quis) in cell cultures, not by N-methyl-D-aspartate (NMDA), though activity of the latter has been determined for glia in cerebellar slices (Müller et al. 1993). Glutamate is actively co-transported into glia with two Na^+ ions, thus depolarising the cell (Bowman and Kimelberg 1984). There are also glutamate receptors on glial cells which open channels permeable to both Na^+ and K^+, and possibly Ca^{2+} (Teichberg 1991).

Depolarisation of glia by glutamate will cause instead of K^+ uptake, K^+ release into the neuronal microenvironment as well as uptake of Ca^{2+} from that environment. If the extracellular Ca^{2+} falls sufficiently, neurons may become more excitable (Somjen 1984). The released K^+ will also contribute to neuronal depolarisation. High $[Ca^{2+}]_i$ may cause closure of interglial gap junctions and, consequently, a loss of the ability of the syncytium to redistribute ions, metabolic substrates and metabolites.

Apart from glia and neurons being directly involved in responding to glutamate, there is also a coupling of NMDA receptor activation by glutamate with nitric oxide (NO) release, leading to an increase in cyclic guanosine monophosphate (cGMP) levels (Garthwaite 1991). More recently, the release of NO in the brain has been demonstrated to be involved in several physiological mechanisms in the CNS. In particular, NO formation has been shown to occur within hippocampus during long-term potentiation (LTP) a process underlying learning and memory (Garthwaite 1991). The NO synthase inhibitor, L-nitro arginine, impairs memory formation in mice (Libri, Giglio and Nisticò 1993). Recently, also the NO agonist, sodium nitroprusside, has been implicated in stimulating consolidation of long-term memory in chicks (Rickard, Ng and Gibbs 1994). Glia have been implicated not just because they act as the brain reservoir for arginine, the NO substrate, but also because they, as well as neurons, contain NO synthase, the enzyme responsible for NO production (Mollace et al. 1990).

Both neurons and glia can synthesise and release arachidonic acid (Dumuis, Pin and Oomargari 1989; Dumuis et al. 1990), which induces a long-term enhancement of synaptic transmission in the hippocampus (Williams et al. 1989) similar, if not identical, to long-term potentiation (LTP).

The new data showing that glia actively respond to glutamate suggests a modulatory role for glia which would extend to some extent throughout the normal range of current flow in the functional syncytium. Thus, a significant population of neurons may be affected. Neuronal activation at a few synapses causing glutamate release and a $[K^+]_e$ rise will contribute to effects in the surrounding tissue due to depolarisation of the syncytium and Ca^{2+} removal from the environment. The interaction of glutamate uptake by glia, K^+ release or uptake and Ca^{2+} uptake, and the effects of these processes on neuromodulation, are not the only ways in which the syncytium may affect neuronal activity (Teichberg 1991), but they are sufficient to demonstrate that glia may have a significant role in neuromodulation.

1.5.3 Developmental Organisation

Early in the development of a vertebrate embryo there appears in the dorsal midline a thickening of the ectoderm (skin) termed the neural plate. This thickening increases and forms a groove as the constituent cells become more columnar (pseudo-stratified columnar epithelium). Initially in the mid-region of the embryo, progressing both to anterior and posterior, this groove joins dorsally to form a tube. This neural tube is the basic structure of the vertebrate nervous system. The inner surface of the tube is the ventricular interface, the outer surface the pial meningeal interface with cerebrospinal fluid surrounded by arachnoid and dural meninges and the skeleton (cranium and spinal vertebrae). The neural tube is a single layer of cells, some of which are already destined to become glia (glioblasts), others to become neurons (neuroblasts). Some glioblasts, which connect the ventricular and pial surfaces, differentiate into radial glia which maintain these connections throughout development, and in lower vertebrates, throughout life. These cells, or their terminal processes form the junctions between CSF and the brain. If they spatially buffer K^+ between CSF and brain, as do retinal Müller cells in the eye (Newman 1986a) to the vitreous humor, then one function of CSF may be to act as a reservoir for K^+ and Na^+, its primary cation constituents.

With the establishment of radial glia, neuroblasts divide and the daughter cells migrate by amoeboid movement along the radial glia. Mechanical, electrical and chemical signals dictate the distance of migration and probably the subsequent differentiation which defines the morphological type of the neuron. Subsequent divisions of neuroblasts produce cells which migrate through the earlier population and form an outer layer.

This continues until there may be several layers or laminae of cells which by this time are becoming electrically active and are receiving inputs from the external world and are sending signals through processes which have grown out of the central nervous system (CNS) to target organs like muscles and glands. Just as within the CNS, these outgrowths are targeted by chemical and electrical signals and by mechanical signals provided by elongate glial cells. Many of these later differentiate to form Schwann cells. Our basic nervous system thus consists of a tube with inputs and outputs, with layers of neuronal cells, oriented and connected radially. The layers of cell bodies alternate, therefore, with layers of processes giving the laminar appearance, e.g. of the cerebral cortex of mammals or the optic tectum of vertebrates as a whole. The glia differentiate within the brain tissue into more adult forms of astrocytes and oligodendroglia and in mammals the radial glial cells often dedifferentiate to form new astrocyte precursors. In the adult there are several forms of astrocytes characterised by the possession of fibrous protein (fibrous) or not (protoplasmic) or their binding properties to, e.g. tetanus toxin (non-binding, type 1; binding, type 2; Raff et al. 1983). Since regional differences in astrocytic morphology and functions within the brain have been found, it is likely that many more 'types' will emerge. What is crucial, is the finding that glial cells are intimately and necessarily involved in the guidance of neurons during development, a guidance system that involves collaboration in mechanical, chemotactic, electrical and chemotrophic signalling between neurons and glia (see Chapter 3).

1.5.4 Morphologically Dynamic Glial–Neuronal Relationships

When we look at sections of brains or electron photomicrographs, we are looking at a permanent preparation which is static, and also because we believe that the brain must be stable in order to function, we forget that in real life things might be different!! This appears to be the case with astrocytes in the brain which are morphologically dynamic.

Of particular interest with respect to plastic morphology are the 'perisynaptic' astrocytic processes. These enclose synapses, and part of the process may even be inserted into the synaptic cleft, reducing the area of synaptic apposition and therefore the area available both for transmitter release and uptake. These potential obstructions to neurotransmission have been found to move in different physiological (and behavioural) circumstances (Chapter 14).

One circumstance in which large behavioural changes are associated with changes in physiology is during parturition and lactation when magnocellular neurons of the supraoptic nucleus (SON) of the hypothalamus secrete oxytocin to be delivered to the neurohypophysis, where it is released into the circulation to cause contraction of uterine muscle in parturition or to cause milk release during lactation (Theodosis and Poulain 1993). Electron microscope evidence indicates that, in the SON, during conditions of high hormone demand, there is a dramatic reduction in the number of fine glial processes which are normally interposed between magnocellular neuroendocrine cell somata. This retraction of astrocytic processes not only allows an increase in synapse size, but is also associated with the formation of novel multiple synapses which probably form by increase in the available apposition area by retraction of the glial processes and/or the enlargement of the presynaptic terminal. This is reversed on the cessation of the stimulus. At the light microscopic level, it is seen that staining for glial fibrillary acid protein (GFAP, a glial marker) was less in lactating rats than for controls in SON, while it was similar in other brain regions. The peak staining density was also less (Salm, Smithson and Hatton 1985; Chapter 14). It will be of interest in the future, to determine if the process retraction is a cause of, or is a response to, increased hormone production.

Pituicytes, modified astrocytes of the posterior pituitary, normally engulf the secretory terminals of the supraoptic neurons and the basal lamina of the perivascular space, but retract under stimulation conditions to allow closer neuronal contact to the blood vessels. This retraction of astrocytic processes in times of behavioural changes is not limited to the oxytocinergic system, it also occurs during dehydration in the biochemically related vasopressin system (Chapter 14).

Retraction of astrocytic processes is not the only possible morphological change. In situations of dehydration, astrocytic process orientation changes from being radial in the SON with respect to the ventricles, to being parallel to the ventricular surface (Chapter 14).

There is also evidence that astrocytes respond to steroid hormones, as castration of males causes retraction of astrocytic processes in slices of the hippocampal CA1 region (Del Cerro, Garcia-Estrada and Garcia-Segura 1995), which is reversed by testosterone administration. The functional significance of this steroid-mediated plasticity of glia in the hippocampus is unknown, but if it involves gating of synapses as previously described, then the effects could be dramatic, as the hippocampus is necessary for spatial learning which may be involved in male territorial behaviour.

Garcia-Segura et al. (1995) have also demonstrated effects of the female sex hormone, oestradiol, on astrocytes, this time specific to cells derived from the hypothalamus. The changes in shape of these astrocytes is under the influence of neural cell adhesion molecule (NCAM) sialylation as enzymes against the sialic residue stopped the process formation. Similar changes in NCAM sialylation may occur during synaptic remodelling during learning (Chapter 15).

Astrocytic morphological changes are not apparently restricted to times when hormones are being secreted. There is a region of the brain lying just dorsal to the optic tract where optic fibres cross to the other side of the brain, the supra chiasmatic nucleus, which is involved in the circadian rhythm of activity of the brain and also of behaviour. In this region also, Lavialle and Serviere (1995) have found a rhythm of GFAP expression which is also circadian. Furthermore, if the animal is placed in constant darkness, both the behavioural and the GFAP rhythm persist.

Modifications of astrocytic morphology are not restricted to the hypothalamus and hippocampus or to intrasynaptic events. Astrocytic ensheathment of the whole of the synapse can increase during and possibly in response to, neuronal activity. Thus rats presented with an enriched visual environment, compared to controls, show an increase in astrocytic synaptic contact, especially in layer 4 of the visual cortex. This response occurs within days of experience of the new environment (Jones and Greenough 1996).

Russian workers have described morphological responses to experience also in oligodendroglia (Roitbak 1988). High levels of activity in central neurons causes growth of the myelinating oligodendroglial cell so that the myelination extends further towards the axonal terminal boutons. This extends the travel distance for the axonal action potential, before it decays into a graded potential. The attenuation of the graded potential is thus reduced, and so a greater terminal depolarisation and transmitter release is achieved. A facilitated synapse is the result.

1.5.5 Glial Involvement in Neural Metabolism

The brain has an enormous requirement for energy, primarily derived from glucose uptake from the circulation. Ependymal glia form a major component of the blood–brain and brain–CSF boundaries and pericapillary astrocytic processes form the other interface between the supply of metabolic substrates and the nervous tissue. These vital substrates are therefore taken up by the glial syncytium to be transferred to neurons. The glia therefore offer a potential barrier or control interface for the availability of metabolic substrates for neurons and the removal of the waste products of metabolism. In general though, we shall see that glia operate in a far more cooperative way with neurons, not only to provide them with what they need, but to adapt that supply to the ongoing circumstances (Chapter 5).

Neurons depend on some biochemical reactions which can only occur in glia, due to their unique production of key enzymes not available to neurons. The three enzymes most clearly identified in this category are pyruvate carboxylase, glutamine synthetase and carbonic anhydrase.

Pyruvate carboxylase catalyses the fusion of carbon dioxide with pyruvate to produce the four-carbon oxaloacetate. This is not only the starting point for the tricarboxylic acid cycle but also of gluconeogenesis, where glucose is synthesised from two molecules of oxaloacetate with a corresponding decarboxylation. This astrocytic glucose can then be polymerised to form glycogen, found almost exclusively in astrocytes as the energy reserves for the brain. The reverse reactions, to provide energy for cellular metabolism, via glycogenolysis and glycolysis also occur in astrocytes, at least as far as lactate or pyruvate. This is then released for utilisation by neurons, while the energy released from the previous catalytic steps is used by the glial cells (Chapter 5). It is transmitters and ions released from active neurons, that stimulates this metabolic activity and thus neuronal 'refuelling'. By active participation in the energy supply for neurons, glia have been implicated in the learning process (Chapter 15). An alternative fate for oxaloacetate is in the formation of α-ketoglutarate which by an aminotransferase reaction can form glutamate, the most ubiquitously distributed excitatory amino acid transmitter in the brain.

Another enzyme which is exclusive to astrocytes is glutamine synthetase, which facilitates the conversion of neuroactive glutamate to glutamine. The traditional story is that glutamate is released from active neurons and taken up by glia to be inactivated. The glutamine may then be returned to neurons for its re-use. This occurs, but the glia by their synthesis, de novo, of glutamate and by their ability to regulate glutamine supply, are in the position of regulating all the available glutamate for neural transmission. This has been shown for retinal transmission in the rabbit (Pow and Robinson 1994 and Chapter 5).

1.6. Implications of Glial–Neuronal Interactions for Neuroscience

1.6.1 Neural Network Research

The data summarised here suggest that modelling CNS activity, especially in terms of spikes, may not be an adequate representation of brain computational functions, nor does it emulate the 'best features' of the process of biological evolution. New models using networks of analog integrators (artificial neurons) and very large scale integrated circuitry could model neuronal membrane potential changes and ionic conductances (e.g. Mahowald and Douglas 1991). It is suggested that it is unnecessary and perhaps detrimental to base these 'artificial neurons' on the physiology of spiking cells in the CNS, especially as these may be rare and the biological requirements for spiking do not apply to electrical circuitry. Modulation of the 'level of activity' or gain in a particular network, (or sub-network) may then be achieved by simulating changes in membrane potential consequential to ionic changes in the extracellular environment of neurons as mediated by glia (Laming 1993).

This modulation might be possible by changing the gain of all artificial neuronal components of a particular sub-network so the activity of this network took priority over that of others, thus changing the 'behaviour' of the total system. Internal events like a clock or external cues could be used to trigger such 'behavioural' changes and therefore produce in an artificial system some of the adaptive complexity of the behaviour of a living entity.

1.6.2 Behavioural Neuroscience

The information summarised here demonstrates that our old view of the brain as being full of spiking neurons which are solely responsible for behaviour, was wrong. Apart from contributions from non-spiking neurons, it is becoming progressively more apparent that glia are major partners in determining the brain's operations, whether these be sensory, integrative or the motor output. We have only reviewed a few aspects, but at least we now know that glial cells are morphologically dynamic and are intimately involved in development and learning. They are vital for, and may regulate, the energy supply of neurons, the supply of many neurotransmitter substrates and the extracellular ionic environment. By any of these mechanisms they are in a position to determine the activity of whole populations of neurons.

Much of the evidence provided in the past decades to demonstrate the regional presence of transmitters, hormones, or metabolic activity within the brain assumed that these were produced by, or responded to by, neurons. The same applies to enzymes for synthesis and metabolism of neuroactive agents and energy substrates. These assumptions are now open to question and much of the old data will have to be re-examined in the light of the new realisations of the involvement of glia in brain function. In the future, new data should try to determine the interactions of glia and neurons in the processing of information and decision making that leads to behaviour. The next few years should then provide much new evidence for how glia contribute to behaviour and should herald a revolution in neuroscience where, at last, we consider the function of *all* the cells of the brain.

Acknowledgements

The author would like to thank Andreas Reichenbach for constructive criticism of the manuscript.

2
The Phylogeny of Glial–Neuronal Relationships and Behaviour

BETTY I. ROOTS and PETER R. LAMING

Summary

Glial cells and neurons have had an intimate association since the evolutionary dawn of a central nervous system. The early centralisation and cephalisation of the nervous system was associated with the formation of neural circuits for the regulation of simple behavioural sequences, vital for survival. Early glial cells may have had the function of partial separation of these circuits to prevent 'cross talk'.

As brains evolved, enabling more complex behavioural activities and thus environmental exploitation, constraints on brain size were encountered, especially in the invertebrates, as a consequence of the design of their skeletal and vascular systems.

Limits on brain size in the invertebrates did not restrict the evolution of complex behaviours, though these are coordinated by relatively few neurons in a sophisticated circuitry, seeming to lack flexibility. Glial cells become progressively more involved in the compartmentalisation of this circuitry and maintaining a constant environment for it to operate reliably and effectively as environmental circumstances dictate. Thus, complex adaptive behaviour evolved in small brains.

In the vertebrates and cephalopod molluscs, brain size was a minor constraint and so both neuronal and glial numbers could increase to allow alternative pathways for information processing, integration and response execution. In vertebrates, myelination compartmentalised neurons in tracts and improved their performance to optimise brain mass in relation to function.

Astrocytes become more numerous and increasingly differentiated with vertebrate phylogeny, as does the intimacy of their relationship with neurons. They maintain tropic functions, though these may be modulatory rather than purely homeostatic. The perisynaptic morphological dynamism of astrocytic processes may facilitate synaptic connectional plasticity, already enhanced by the profligacy of possible connections enabled in brains evolving without constraints on size. The flexibility of these large systems of neurons and glia has endowed the vertebrate brain with the ability to modify patterns of behaviour to be truly adaptable in a variety of environmental circumstances.

2.1 Introduction

With the evolution of the metazoa upwards of some 600 million years ago came the origins of communication systems within animals for integration of tissue and organ functions and interaction of the organism with its environment. Since that time, the major evolutionary advances have been the increasing size and/or differentiation of the nervous system to improve adaptedness or adaptability of behaviour. It is evident that extant animals, whether unicellular or multicellular, are adapted to their particular niche, a trait that has ensured their survival to the present. What has allowed animals to emerge from the original aquatic environment or successfully to exploit that environment more fully has been the evolution of a variety of new differentiated systems for structural support, locomotion, gaseous exchange and circulation. These required the parallel evolution of intra-organismic communication systems and a growing ability to organise behaviour in relation to environmental events.

Complex behaviour is expressed by animals in many different phyla, and is associated with possession of a sophisticated nervous system. It seems, however, that many animals with complex behaviour may organise this with relatively small brains. Thus, insects with very small brains exhibit a wide variety of complex, adaptive behavioural activities. Many of these behaviours seem to be stereotyped and stimulus bound and therefore inflexible. In a predictable world, such an evolutionary outcome is economical and extremely successful. In flying animals, where weight must be minimised, it may have been imperative (Table 2.1). Another evolutionary outcome for nervous systems and behaviour has been to make behaviour adaptable, so that flexible responses could be made to environmental circumstances, depending on the perceived needs of the individual. This type of behaviour seems to have required the evolution of large brains with much internal processing capability as shown by vertebrates and cephalopod molluscs (Table 2.2). Most animals, however, express both stereotyped and adaptable behaviours, though in differing degrees. What is evident is that the increase in sophistication of behaviour and nervous system development and differentiation is also associated with the increased prevalence of glial cells in the brain. It is the aim of this chapter to consider relationships between behavioural capabilities of animals and the presence, anatomical disposition, properties and functions of glia in their nervous systems.

2.2 Outline of the Phylogenetic Relationships of Animals

Classically, the phylogenetic relationships of animals were deduced from studies of the fossil record, comparative anatomy and embryology. The advent of ribosomal ribose nucleic acid (RNA) and deoxyribose nucleic acid (DNA) sequencing led to the hope that an unequivocal phylogenetic tree could be determined. This has not been realised and it has become apparent that the interpretation of molecular data

Table 2.1. *A phylogeny of adaptive behaviours (X = presence, Coel = Coelenterates, Helm = Platyhelminths, Moll Annel = Gastropod molluscs and annelids, Arthro = Arthropods, Ceph Moll = Cephalopod molluscs, Fish = Fish, Amph = Amphibians, Rept = Reptiles, Bird = Birds, Mamm = Mammals)*

	Coel	Helm	Moll Annel	Ceph Moll	Arthro	Fish	Amph	Rept	Bird	Mamm
Parental care				X	X	X	X	X	X	X
Territoriality				X	X	X	X	X	X	X
Nest building				X	X	X	X	X	X	X
Behavioural thermoregulation						X	X	X	X	X
Courtship			?	X	X	X	X	X	X	X
Patterns of behaviour			?	X	X	X	X	X	X	X
Visual discrimination			X	X	X	X	X	X	X	X
Acoustic discrimination			?	?	X	X	X	X	X	X
Tactile discrimination		X	X	X	X	X	X	X	X	X
Olfactory discrimination		?	?	X	X	X	X	X	X	X
Tube/burrow making		X	X	X	X	X	X	X	X	X
Active feeding	X	X	X	X	X	X	X	X	X	X
Taxes and kineses	?	X	X	X	X	X	X	X	X	X
Directional movement	?	X	X	X	X	X	X	X	X	X
Reflexes	X	X	X	X	X	X	X	X	X	X

Table 2.2. *A phylogeny of adaptable (plastic) behaviours (X = present, abbreviations as in Table 2.1)*

	Coel	Helm	Moll Annel	Arthro	Ceph Moll	Fish	Amph	Rept	Bird	Mamm
Language										X
Conceptualisation									?	X
Play									?	X
Tool using					?				X	X
Problem solving				?					X	X
Emotional communication				X	X	X	X	X	X	X
Learning 'set'				?	?	?	X	X	X	X
Spatial learning			X	X	X	X	X	X	X	X
Discrimination learning		X	X	X	X	X	X	X	X	X
Classical conditioning			X	X	X	X	X	X	X	X
Habituation	?	X	X	X	X	X	X	X	X	X
Sensory adaptation	X	X	X	X	X	X	X	X	X	X
Phylum/class	Coel	Helm	Moll Annel	Arthro	Ceph Moll	Fish	Amph	Rept	Bird	Mamm

Distinctions between spatial and discrimination learning may be spurious.

is as difficult as that of morphological data (Field et al. 1988, 1989; Raff et al. 1989; Hillis and Moritz 1990). The use of cladistic analysis has been valuable in establishing the branching points of the phylogenetic tree and a comprehensive phylogeny has been developed by Nielsen (1995). Issues such as whether or not the coelom has evolved more than once, the evolution of mesoderm, and the fate of the blastopore continue to be matters for discussion, and many aspects of phylogenetic relationships are as yet unresolved. Nevertheless, there is general agreement on the main lines of evolution. What follows is based on Nielsen's analysis.

It is now believed that multicellular organisms evolved only once from a protist ancestor. After the emergence of Porifera (sponges), Cnidaria (sea anemones, jellyfishes) and the Bilateria stock, there was divergence into protostomes ('first mouth', in which the blastopore becomes the mouth and a second opening breaks through to become the anus) and deuterostomes ('second mouth', in which the blastopore becomes the anus and a second opening becomes the mouth, although there are some deviations from this pattern of development) (Fig. 2.1). The origin of the Ctenophora (sea gooseberries, comb jellies) is not yet firmly established. The principal phyla evolved during Cambrian times and there was rapid radiation from the Bilateria stock. Primitive deuterostome stock gave rise to the echinoderms and the chordates. The radially symmetrical echinoderms (sea urchins, star fishes and sea cucumbers) may appear to be very different from the bilaterally symmetrical chordates but they have many features in common, including some in the nervous system. Moreover, the larval stages are bilaterally symmetrical and are most similar to deuterostomes.

The Enteropneusts (acorn worms) separated early from the main chordate line, which subsequently gave rise to the Urochordata (sea squirts and salps), the Cephalochordata (the lancelet), and the Vertebrata. The vertebrate line gave rise to the Agnatha (lampreys and hagfishes), and to the stock from which the Chondrichthyes (cartilaginous fishes, including the elasmobranchs, sharks and rays, and the holocephalans, rat fishes) and the Osteichthyes (bony fishes) evolved. The Osteichthyes gave rise to the Actinopterygii (the spiny finned fishes) and the Sarcopterygii (the fleshy finned fishes). Sturgeons arose early from the Actinopterygian ancestral stock followed by lungfish and the gars. Evolution in the Actinopterygii culminated in the Teleostei, the enormously successful and varied modern bony fishes.

The lungfishes, coelacanths and the tetrapods evolved from the Sarcopterygii. The amphibians were the first tetrapods, followed by reptiles, birds and mammals.

The invertebrate phyla which are of interest in considering glial-neuronal relationships radiated from the protostome stock. Platyhelminthes (flatworms) diverged early, followed by the other phyla. Living classes of Mollusca include the Gastropoda (slugs and snails), Bivalvia (mussels and oysters) and Cephalopoda (squids and octopi). There are three classes in the Annelida: the Polychaeta (bristleworms), the Oligochaeta (earthworms and freshwater ringed worms) and the Hirudinea (leeches). It is now generally agreed that the

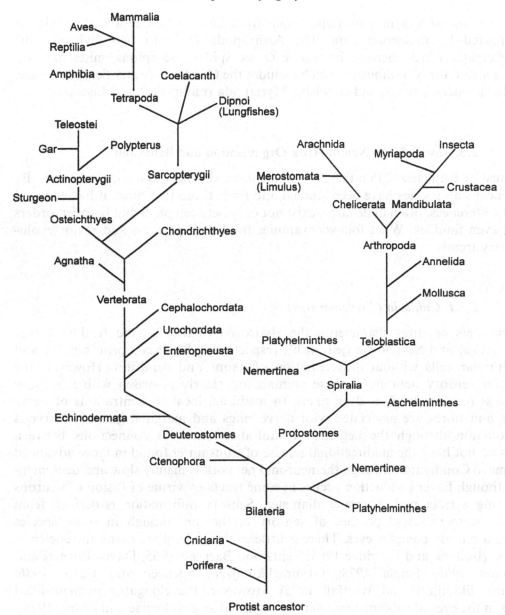

Fig. 2.1. Phylogenetic relationships of animals.

Arthropoda have a monophyletic origin from an annelid-like ancestor. This is supported by molecular data. The Arthropoda fall into two divisions, the Chelicerata, which includes horseshoe crabs, spiders, scorpions, mites and sea spiders, and the Mandibulata, which includes the Crustacea (water fleas, woodlice, crabs, lobsters, prawns and crayfish), Myriapoda (millipedes) and Insecta.

2.3. Invertebrate Neuron–Glia Organisation and Behaviour

It must be emphasized that there is a tremendous diversity in the invertebrates. By no means all species have been studied and from those that have, it has emerged that differences, often quite large, exist not only between phyla but between orders and even families. What follows examines the broad patterns and major evolutionary trends.

2.3.1 Cnidaria (Coelenterates)

Nerve nets or rings characterise the Hydrozoa (hydroids), the Anthozoa (sea anemones) and Scyphozoa (jelly fish), respectively. These comprise bipolar and multipolar cells without differentiation of axons and dendrites. However, the bipolar sensory neurons of these animals are clearly polarised with a sensory process (or 'dendrite') and an axon. In medusae, local concentrations of nerve cells and fibres are associated with nerve rings and marginal ganglia. Nervous conduction through the net can be multidirectional, as connections between cells do not have the unidirectional release of transmitter found in more advanced animals. Conduction through the neuronal network is mainly slow and decremental, though faster conduction occurs in some tracts by virtue of fusion of neurons forming a tract with a greater diameter. Sensory information is derived from ocelli, statocysts and patches of sensory epithelium, though in some species there are fairly complex eyes. There is little evidence for glia among the coelenterates. (Bullock and Horridge 1965; Lentz and Barrnett 1965; Davis, Burnett and Haynes 1968; Singla 1978; Grimmelikhuijzen, Spencer and Carré 1986; Grimmelikhuijzen and Westfall 1995). However, the elongated pigment-filled cells in the eyes of cubomedusae may be regarded as glia (Pearse and Pearse 1978).

The behavioural repertoire is small, comprising slow locomotion and fast contraction reflexes in Anthozoa (sea anemones), startle reactions in Hydrozoa (siphonophores) and rhythmic swimming movements in the Scyphozoa (jelly fish). Movement seems to be regulated by intrinsic mechanisms, though it is affected by sensory experience and by internal states, like those resulting from food deprivation. In some species, periods of quiescent behaviour occur. Mechanical or electrical stimulation of the column of Anthozoa produces summation of neural responses (Ross and Pantin 1940) and progressively stronger muscular avoidance responses. Prolonged light mechanical stimulation can incur adaptation, however.

Feeding and food rejection can both be elicited by strong stimulation of the column in anthozoa, or by weak stimulation of the oral disc. The feeding process is coordinated, involving sequential movements of tentacles, oral disc and column on contact with food items. Feedback from food products is required to maintain feeding behaviour. These products, simulated by application of glutathione, (Lenhoff and Schneiderman 1959) may be released after penetration of prey by the threads of the independent effectors, the nematocysts.

Coelenterates show slow adaptive behaviour with a simple nervous system, that utilises through conduction rather than conventional synapses and is unaided by glia.

2.3.2 *Platyhelminthes*

The nerve net seen in coelenterates has become condensed to form two to five pairs of nerve cords, which are connected by commissures in a ladder-like fashion. An anterior concentration of neurons, a 'brain' is present in most but not all species. Two nerve plexuses, one subepidermal, the other submuscular appear to coordinate movement in most flatworms. Neurons are differentiated with many bipolar and multipolar cells with definable axons and dendrites, as well as unipolar cells. In the better developed nervous systems of the polyclad flatworms, the brain is comparatively large and distinct. In these, an important invertebrate feature is established, i.e. an outer rind of cells and inner core of fibres in the large cords and ganglia. Photoreceptors are found all over the body but planarians also have eye cups on the head. This cephalisation is most developed in land forms (Koopowitz and Chien 1975; Rieger et al. 1991; Elvin and Koopowitz 1994; Reuter and Gustafsson 1995). Glial cells are relatively few in number and poorly differentiated. They have been reported in some free-living flatworms and in the liver fluke, *Fasciola hepatica*. Spindle-shaped glial cells are found along nerve tracts, between nerve cells and in the peripheral plexuses. These may have an insulating function. In some species multiple lamellae are found around neurons or their axons and invaginations have been reported (Morita and Best 1966; Rohde 1970; Reuter, Wikgen and Palmberg 1980; Rohde and Webb 1986; Golubev 1988; Sukhdeo, Sukhdeo and Mettrick 1988).

The phylum shows a great range of nervous system development, though many species show little advance on the coelenterate nerve net, with only a slight preponderance of longitudinal fibres and little cephalisation. Locomotion in this very varied phylum is by ciliary action, muscular waves, looping or swimming. Behavioural activity is faster than in Coelenterates and is directional, with the head incorporating the majority of the sense organs and associated 'brain' to the fore. The possession of a more sophisticated sensory apparatus allows these animals to show orientated taxes and kineses in response to light and gravity. They also show twisting responses to stimuli and a righting response to being over-turned (Bullock and Horridge 1965). Flatworms will habituate and thus cease to respond to a repeated non-threatening stimulus, and many workers have demon-strated that they may be conditioned to light and mechanical stimuli. The central nervous system may not be necessary for this latter capability (Corning and Kelly 1973). Parasitic platyhelminthes may have rudimentary organs in many respects but have well-developed nervous systems to behave appropriately within their hosts, e.g. *Fasciola*, showing adaptive behaviours like migration in the host gut (Sukhdeo, Sukhdeo and Mettrick 1988). The development of more rapid and coordinated responses in flatworms may have required some separation of neural circuits by glial cells.

2.3.3 Annelida

The central nervous system consists of paired ventral nerve cords which usually have ganglia in each segment. Ganglia are largest in the head region, where sense organs are concentrated, although development of sense organs is not markedly greater than in the more advanced Platyhelminthes. The 'brain' comprises the cerebral ganglion which innervates the head region with the suboesophageal gang-lion, the largest and most anterior segmental ganglion. The cerebral ganglia are well developed with the typical invertebrate structure of a rind of cell bodies of neurons and glia and a core of medullary neuropil consisting of axons, dendrites, nerve tracts, glial processes and some glial cell bodies. All synapses are found in the neuropil. Glial cells are well developed and in the oligochaetes and polychaetes three types may be distinguished: supportive, migratory and those forming myelin-like sheaths around giant fibres in the nerve cords. The invagination of neurons by glia (trophospongium) is well developed and may represent a tropic function of glia for neurons. Differentiation of glial cells is not complete, however, as inter-mediate forms are often found. In leeches (Hirudinea) several kinds of glial cells, some of which are stellate, are found. Particularly notable are the packet glial cells that encompass groups of neurons (for reviews, see Roots 1978, 1986, 1995). Physiological studies on leech packet glial cells and their neurons established the role of glia in regulating the microenvironment of neurons (Nicholls and Kuffler 1964, 1965; Kuffler and Nicholls 1964; Wuttke 1990; Saubermann, Castiglia and Foster 1992), which clearly has significance for behaviour (see Chapter 7). Giant glial cells in the leech are associated with the ganglionic neuronal somata where they are involved in pH regulation which may involve glial–neuronal signalling (Deitmer and Schneider 1995 and Chapter 11). Glia comprise 51% by volume in the leech central nervous system (Kai-Kai and Pentreath 1981).

In the Annelida a new feature of nervous systems is established, the compart-mentalisation of the central nervous system by glial cells. A framework of glial cell processes forms more or less distinct partitions between the rind and the core and between small masses of cells and processes. Glomeruli, knots of 'tighter weave' than surrounding neuropil, occur, which are probably bounded by glia if they are like similar structures in insects. The significance of this glial compartmentation of neuropil may be to allow discrete neuronal circuitry to produce defined patterns of behaviour.

The multilayered glial sheaths round axons increases conduction velocity, which is important for protective escape behaviour and startle responses. The evolution of a coelom and metameric segmentation has been accompanied by the appearance of discrete groups of muscles associated with locomotory appendages and more specialised mouthparts for feeding on a variety of food sources. In oligo-chaetes, locomotion is by peristaltic and antiperistaltic creeping, in polychaetes by 'rowing' with parapodia and in leeches by a looping walk. In the earthworm, *Lumbricus*, locomotory peristaltic waves are generated by segmental reflexes in response to tension caused by contraction of the adjoining segment. Thus, a 'decerebrate' earthworm can still crawl, burrow, feed and enter coitus, though in a less coordinated manner than formerly. Righting reflexes are also still present, as is the ability to be conditioned to light, mechanical stimuli or an electric shock. In leeches also the more complex looping locomotion is performed without the cerebral ganglion (Bullock and Horridge 1965). Aquatic species of annelid, especially the polychaetes and leeches, are proficient swimmers and those with advanced mouthparts are adept at food capture and manipulation. The errant polychaetes have the largest and most partitioned brains of all the annelids and these animals are often active predators. Some, like the palolo worm of the Pacific, aggregate prior to spawning in response to the phase of the lunar cycle, inducing neurosecretory changes, which induce the behaviour. Other species with less developed nervous systems are nevertheless capable of constructing burrows or protective tubes of sedimentary material. Like platyhelminthes, annelids can be conditioned, but also show more active and complex behaviour patterns. In part, this may be because of greater compartmentalisation of more complex neural circuitry by greater numbers of glia.

2.3.4 Arthropoda

The arthropods (primarily crustacea and insecta) are the largest and most diverse phylum of the metazoa. They have developed a much more pronounced cephalisation and more highly developed sense organs than the annelids, e.g. compound eye and statocysts. The brain has three main regions, proto, deuto and tritocerebrum, to which are ascribed fairly discrete sensory and motor functions. Glomeruli are highly developed in arthropods (Fig. 2.2), and have been particularly well studied in insects (Oland and Tolbert 1989; Tolbert and Oland 1989; Oland, Krull and Tolbert 1995). The structure of the ganglia is a rind of cell bodies

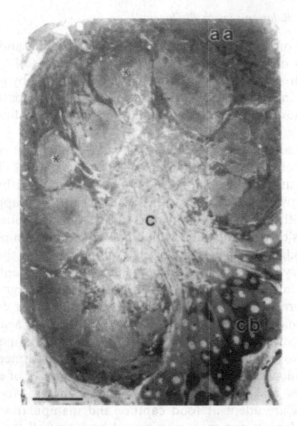

A

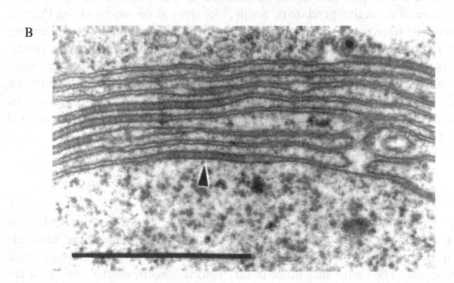

B

Fig. 2.2. Glomerular structure in the antennal lobe of an insect, *Manduca sexta*. (A) 1 μm toluidine blue-stained cross-section of the antennal lobe showing a ring of spheroidal glomeruli (*) surrounding the central neuropil (c). Each glomerulus is bordered by darkly staining glial cells.

with a neuropil core as in annelids, but differentiation in the nervous system is much more apparent. The highest centres are believed to be the globuli, masses composed of small tightly packed unipolar globuli cells. Globuli are particularly concentrated in the optic neuropil and mushroom bodies of insects. Glial cells are differentiated into at least three types in the various arthropod groups and the trophospongium is well developed (Hámori and Horridge 1966b; Sohal, Sharma and Couch 1972; Obenchain 1974; Fahrenbach 1976; Radojcic and Pentreath 1979; Saint Marie, Carlson and Chi 1984; Carlson 1987; Meyer, Reddy and Edwards 1987). In the retina of the male bee (drone) they constitute 57% by volume (Coles and Tsacopoulos 1979), where they act as metabolic substrate providers for neurons (Chapter 5).

Separation of neuronal elements by glia is well developed. Some glial cells have thin diaphanous sheet-like processes similar to velate astrocytes, e.g. in *Limulus* brain and the optic lamina of lobster where the processes separate neurons. In the neuropil, groups of 'en passant' synapses are separated as are other neuronal processes to prevent synaptic contact. Tight junctions partition the neuropil into high resistance sectors. Globuli are compartmentalised by glial processes separating groups of cells. The separation of discrete elements of neuropil, initiated in the platyhelminths, enables development of complex adaptive behaviours although these are stereotyped. This limits selection of information to what is relevant, e.g. bees are limited to recording of a few highly specific features, discriminating shapes by the flicker frequencies that are generated by their outline as the bee flies over them. They can thus be trained to fly to an interrupted outline (a star rather than a circle) but not vice versa (von Frisch 1954). In insects, glia of the perineurium form a blood–brain barrier, which in phytophagous species protects the brain from high blood levels of K^+ ions related to high potassium levels in the diet (Hoyle 1953; Lane 1972; Treherne and Pichon 1972).

Amongst the arthropods, well-developed multilayered, myelin-like sheaths around axons are found only in the decapod crustacea. As in annelida, these sheaths are associated with rapid startle reactions such as the retraction of eye stalks and rapid locomotory responses (see Roots 1993, 1995 for reviews).

Another feature of nervous system evolution, namely stratification, is first seen in arthropods. It is especially apparent in the optic lobes of insects and crustacea. Glial sheaths isolate the columnar synaptic region of optic cartridges of the retina above, from the other parts of the optic lobe below. Units of the compound eyes

Sensory axons (aa) from receptors on the antenna reach the lobe via the antennal nerve; cb, cell bodies of antennal-lobe neurons. Scale-bar = 100 μm. (From Oland, Tolbert and Mossman 1988, with permission.) (B) Electron micrograph through a portion of the glial border. Glial cell processes are readily identified by their ribosomal and glycogen content. Processes are interconnected by multiple scalariform-like junctions, one indicated by the arrow. Scale bar = 1 μm. (From Tolbert and Hildebrand 1981, with permission.)

are also separated by glia. Isolation of these various components is needed for colour vision and navigation (Hámori and Horridge 1966a; Saint Marie and Carlson 1983). The evolution of an exoskeletal structure and jointed limbs paralleled the increased differentiation of the nervous system and was also associated with the development of complex patterns of behaviour. Many of these appear to be stereotyped and require relatively few neurons, necessitated by the limits on body size imposed by the exoskeleton. The arthropods have all the survival-requirement behaviours that were found in the annelids, but the acquisition of limbs has increased their behavioural complexity.

Startle and escape responses are more elaborate, like the escape tail flip of lobsters and shrimps and the sideways scuttle of crabs. In the insects, jumping and flight responses are similarly more elaborate. In addition to escape, arthropods also make defensive or even offensive reactions to threat. Thus, crabs and lobsters will raise their chelipeds (pincers) towards a real or potential aggressor or predator. This is especially the case when the animal is protecting a resource like food, a mate, a crevice or burrow or a territory. Similarly, insects have evolved a multitude of defensive and offensive behaviours to protect individual, or in the case of social insects, genotypical, interests. Antipredator devices include camouflage behaviour associated with either natural blending colouration or morphology or with acquisition of a harvested 'coat' of natural debris as in spider crabs.

The diversity of mouthparts and food sources available to the arthropods has also been associated with a wide variety of foraging and feeding behaviours. This ranges from the relatively simple use of chelipeds in addition to mouthparts in crustacea, to the elaborate hunting strategies of predatory wasps which seek, attack and paralyse prey, carry it to their nest, and then masticate it to a pulp to ingest or feed to larvae (Kemper and Dohring 1967). Few animals have to pursue such a complex behavioural programme to obtain a meal. Examples of behavioural diversity in feeding, especially in the insects, are legion, but the point to be emphasised here is that this behaviour requires extensive sensory–motor integration capability and a series of generators of behavioural sequences.

Reproductive behaviour in the arthropods often involves courtship behaviour, especially in the terrestrial species, in which fertilisation is internal. Sexual communication can be acoustic (crickets, grasshoppers, cicadas), visual (butterflies, fireflies), olfactory (moths) or tactile. More often, it is a combination of these which results in copulation. Often the adult lifespan is extremely brief and copulation, especially for the male, is the raison d'etre for the development of a complex behavioural repertoire. This is often the case with hymenoptera (bees, ants, wasps), butterflies and mantises. In the latter case, the devouring of the male's head (and brain) by the female may enhance copulatory efforts by removing central inhibition!

Arthropods are often territorial, in that they will defend an area of the environment that contains a valuable resource from conspecifics and even individuals of other species. This is true for many crustacea and insects, but is most pronounced in the Hymenoptera, which will aggressively defend a nest and its resources. In relation to nervous system evolution, this is a major step, as it indicates the development of a spatial memory which may only have been rudimentary in the annelida.

The Hymenoptera and especially the social species are the most behaviourally advanced of the arthropods. They have highly developed manipulative skills, common amongst arthropods, but have developed them to the extent of constructing complex nests in which food is stored and progeny are reared by closely related individuals. Precise information between individuals is communicated by tactile, visual, acoustic and chemical signals to describe food source, content and location, maintain colony cohesion and define the role of individuals in the duty rota. Apart from habituation, classical conditioning and associative conditioning are normal components of the life of social insects which learn the location of a food source and the position of the colony, and can rapidly relearn these if they are experimentally relocated. It is the complex sequences of adaptive behaviour of the social insects which gives the impression that the phylum as a whole is extremely advanced, yet the majority of species do not display such complex behavioural activities.

2.3.5 *Mollusca*

Of the eight classes of living mollusca, only two, the gastropoda and cephalopoda, are of interest from the point of view of this chapter.

2.3.5.1 *Gastropoda*

Condensation and cephalisation are manifested with a pair of cerebral ganglia and a varying number of other ganglia joined by connectives and commissures. Differentiation of glia is well developed with three types recognised in *Archachatina marginata* (Amoroso et al. 1964) and as many as five in *Helix pomatia* (Reinecke 1975). In the buccal ganglia of *Planorbis corneus*, glial cells outnumber neurons (approximately 4:3) but occupy only 43% of the volume (Pentreath et al. 1985). A trophospongium is present. In gastropod molluscs, the cerebral ganglion has become the controlling centre for behaviour. There is in many species a sense of 'home' (limpets) to which animals will repeatedly return after foraging. Experiments on gastropods have illustrated an ability to be conditioned and to learn a simple T maze. They also show quite complex courtship behaviour in comparison with annelids, but their nervous system and behavioural repertoire are simpler than the arthropods.

2.3.5.2 *Cephalopoda*

Cephalisation is advanced. The brain consists of a compact mass ringing the oesophagus. It has 30 distinct lobes associated with different functions. Most prominent are the optic lobes, which comprise half the tissue of the brain. Glial cells are numerous and differentiated into many types, some resembling vertebrate protoplasmic and fibrous astrocytes. There is a trophospongium, but neither glomeruli of the type found in insects nor multiple layered wrappings of axons are present. Nevertheless, the neuropil is far more organised than in any other invertebrate. Neurons are not confined to the rind but islets of nerve cells are found scattered throughout the neuropil. Multipolar neurons are common in these islands. The cephalopods have highly developed sense organs with an eye comparable to that of vertebrates and optic lobes showing a high degree of stratification (Young 1971). The sense of touch is also highly developed in these animals. They have the largest brain, both in absolute terms and in relation to body size, of any invertebrate, rivalling that of the vertebrates, with a total number of neurons in *Octopus* estimated to be 168×10^6. Their behaviour is equally complex. Apart from all the behavioural capabilities described for annelids and other molluscs, cephalopods have been shown through extensive research to be capable of both tactile and visual discrimination learning to avoid a punishing shock or obtain a food reward (Young 1961; Wells 1962). They seem to express emotive behaviour during decision-making as to whether to flee or attack. This is often evidenced by hesitation combined with pigment redistribution on the skin. Some species show territorial behaviour, indicating a spatial memory, and many demonstrate complex courtship behaviour, also involving pigment redistribution.

Complex behaviour, involving flexibility of response (i.e. adaptable) requires many separate channels which may be limited by available space in the nervous system. Cephalopods have many channels and a large brain. They have achieved this by variation in the diameter of axons which range from 1 µm to 1 mm (> 1000 times). Velocity, however, only increases by the square root of diameter; therefore there is a need for a great increase in diameter for high velocity. This is limited by space, solved in the vertebrates by myelin sheaths, nodes of Ranvier and saltatory conduction. Vertebrate fibres of 20 µm diameter conduct at twice the rate of 1 mm fibres in squid (Young 1967).

2.3.6 Summary of the Invertebrates

Several trends are evident in the evolution of nervous systems, notably condensation and cephalisation, compartmentalisation and stratification. Glia which differentiate into several types contribute to the latter two and probably to the well developed adaptive behaviours of the higher invertebrates possessing small brains. The eye and nervous system of cephalopods, and their flexibility in terms of adaptability of behaviour, represent a remarkable example of convergent evolution with vertebrates.

With the possible exception of the cephalopods, the brain of which shows many features of that of vertebrates, much of invertebrate behaviour is stereotyped and stimulus-bound. This is true even of the complex behaviour patterns of the social insects. Plasticity in terms of learning is evidenced in the more advanced forms, especially in relation to spatial memory of territory and food sources. Behaviour is largely triggered by homeostatic requirements and external events and in the absence of these stimuli, there appears to be little activity. There is little evidence for a state comparable to vertebrate sleep in the invertebrates.

2.4 Vertebrates

Many of the trends manifest in the evolution of invertebrate nervous systems are found in vertebrate brain evolution to an enhanced degree, especially the contribution of glia to plasticity. Cephalisation is advanced with well-developed visual, auditory and olfactory organs concentrated in the head. In addition, a major event in vertebrate evolution was the tremendous increase in brain size, particularly in the forebrain, culminating in the enormous cerebral hemispheres of primates.

In the central nervous system as a whole, macroglial cells outnumber neurons and account for 50% of brain volume, a figure similar to that for advanced invertebrates. There is, however, local variation and in the cerebellum, for example, there are five to six neurons per glial cell (Ghandour, Vincendon and Gombos 1980). Radial glia predominate in brains with relatively thin walls, e.g. teleosts, whereas non-ependymal glia are more prevalent in thick walled brains (Wicht, Derouiche and Korf 1994). The glia : neuron ratio increases up the phylogenetic scale of vertebrates. It also increases with axon length, brain weight and brain wall thickness (Reichenbach 1989). These differences are related to the trophic needs of neurons, to compartmentalisation and to the degree of myelination. Differentiation of glia is well developed and is greatest in higher vertebrates. Multipolar neurons predominate and numerous synaptic contacts are found on the soma as well as on dendritic processes. Stratification is unsurpassed with a separation of grey and white matter and layers within grey matter. Glomeruli are prevalent and other forms of compartmentalisation are being increasingly identified. Myelin sheaths are well developed in all but the Agnatha, with a remarkably similar morphology across the groups (Roots 1984).

2.4.1 Teleosts

Although ependymal-type glia predominate, oligodendrocytes remarkably similar in structure to those in mammals occur (Kruger and Maxwell 1967). Biochemically, however, these cells are not as fully differentiated as in mammals, and they show characteristics of Schwann cells as well as oligodendrocytes. The myelin membranes produced by the oligodendrocytes differ in that they contain a 36 kDa protein unique to the central nervous system (CNS) of teleosts, in other respects they are similar to those produced by Schwann cells (Jeserich, Stratmann and Strelau 1995).

The optic tectum, which is the main integrative centre, is highly stratified. There are five principal layers which may be subdivided according to degree of differentiation in the various species (Leghissa 1955). In the optic tectum, astroglial envelopes are associated with synaptic structures, especially round dendritic spines. Differentiation of glia is not complete and there are many cells intermediate between astrocytes and oligodendrocytes (Lara et al. 1989).

In terms of numbers of species, the teleosts are the largest class of the vertebrates with diverse specialisations for particular habitats. As a class, however, some generalisations about their brains and behavioural capabilities can be made. The brain comprises the five major regions common to all vertebrates: telencephalon, diencephalon, mesencephalon, cerebellum and medulla. All regions demonstrate slow potential shifts, probably representing glial potassium sensitivity in response to an arousing novel stimulus (Chapters 10, 12). Most sensory integration takes place in the midbrain though the telencephalon has been implicated in aggressive and reproductive behaviour, habituation and instrumental conditioning (see Laming 1981a for reviews). Fish have extremely well-developed olfactory, mechanical, acoustic and visual sensitivities, as well as specialisations such as electroreception. Like the more advanced invertebrates, they perform complex sequences of behaviour associated with courtship, territoriality, nest building and parental behaviour. These have been described for a number of species since the pioneering work of Tinbergen (1954) on the reproductive behaviour of the stickleback. Apart from intricate reproductive displays, teleosts also show a variety of gregarious behaviours, such as schooling and may maintain territories, requiring a high degree of spatial learning. Experimentally, they have been shown to habituate and be capable of being classically, instrumentally and associatively conditioned (Flood and Overmier 1981).

Although many of the behaviours of teleosts seem quantitatively to mirror those of the most advanced invertebrates, there is a qualitative difference, in that there is a greater degree of variation in response to a given environmental situation. This may reflect the plasticity of behaviour associated with a relatively large brain with increased diversity of synaptic connectivity. A primitive form of sleep-like state, in which sensory thresholds are raised during inactivity, makes its first appearance in fish (Peyrethon 1968).

2.4.2 Amphibia

The extant amphibia are a relatively small class of vertebrates which in many cases show regression of brain and behavioural complexity in comparison with the teleosts. The brain size is similar in relation to the size of the animals, but the cerebellum is much reduced. Visual and acoustic senses are well developed and understood, but other senses may be less well developed than in fishes. As in teleosts, the optic tectum is the main integrative centre and in anurans (frogs and toads) has a similar multilayered structure (Potter 1969, 1971). Visual information processing pathways in the tectum have a radial organisation, parallelling that of the radial glia. Slow potential shifts to visual stimuli correlate with extracellular potassium and are of presumed glial origin, though their dependence on local neuronal activity varies with experience and motivational state (Chapter 12). In urodeles (salamanders and newts) the tectum is relatively simple and lacks the multiple lamination (Herrick 1942).

Glia are somewhat more differentiated and there is a greater proportion of astrocytes than in teleosts. In anurans these cells combine the features of ependymal cells and astrocytes (Naujoks-Manteuffel and Roth 1995). As in teleosts, sheet-like profiles envelop specific types of synapses (Korte and Rosenbluth 1981). An evolutionary advance is, however, shown by oligodendrocytes which are fully differentiated from Schwann cells. Thus, central and peripheral myelin generated by these cells respectively, is different. Proteolipid protein (PLP) is present in central myelin and the myelin is more compact. PLP made its appearance in the ancestors common to the tetrapods and the coelacanth. Modern amphibia appear to be an offshoot from the main line. There is no evidence that there is any enhancement of the behavioural repertoire in amphibia, though a well-defined sensory processing system for prey catching activity exists which comprises interactions of sensory processing systems within the optic tectum and the pretectal thalamus. These are responsible for the relatively stereotyped sequence of behaviours which starts with prey recognition and leads to prey capture in these animals (see Ewert 1989 for a review). Similarly, male anuran amphibia produce vocalisations to attract mates which are recognised by conspecifics and used in mate selection. Spatial learning is evidenced by the development of transient territories and by the ability of displaced animals to return after displacement. Habituation to a repeated visual stimulus readily occurs and animals can be classically conditioned. Prey catching behaviour can be modified by experience, so that animals associate either a new visual or an olfactory experience with feeding. In a few species there is parental care, usually by the male. The degree of plasticity of behaviour is in general more limited than that of extant teleosts. In many species, prolonged periods of inactivity occur in which animals are unresponsive. This 'sleep'-like behaviour is associated with little electrical activity in the midbrain tectum (Laming, personal observation).

2.4.3 *Reptiles and Birds*

Differentiation of glia in birds is virtually as complete as it is for mammals. In reptiles, however, there is a greater prevalence of intermediate forms (see Roots

1986; Font et al. 1995). In birds, the optic tectum continues to be an important integrative centre and shows greater laminar differentiation with fifteen primary tectal layers. Differentiation of oligodendrocytes and the composition of myelin is basically the same as in mammals. The protein DM20 (produced by the PLP gene by alternative splicing), which appears first in the coelacanths, is present in reptiles, birds and mammals.

The reptiles are truly terrestrial and have adapted well morphologically, physiologically and behaviourally to that environment. They are mostly predatory animals, with well-developed visual, olfactory and vibration sensitivity. In most species acoustic senses are less well developed, though some, like geckos, use acoustic signals in territorial disputes. Territorial behaviour and the use of visual, tactile and olfactory cues in courtship is common and some species, like crocodilians, make nests and invest in some degree of parental care. Spatial learning is implied by this territoriality and lizards have been classically conditioned, have learnt discriminant tasks and have been instrumentally conditioned when heat has been provided as a reward (Brattstrom 1978).

In birds, which may be regarded as homeothermic, feathered, flying reptiles in many respects, a relatively enormous brain has evolved. Unlike the mammals which have exploited the emergence of the advanced reptile's isocortex, birds have massively enlarged striatum or basal ganglia. These regions are traditionally associated with stereotyped behaviour patterns and it has not unnaturally been assumed that the enlargement of these regions in birds has allowed complex behaviours without the added weight which would preclude flight. It would be interesting to see if the compartmentalisation of the striatum by glia is enhanced in birds compared to mammals. It is certainly true that birds have a considerable repertoire of behavioural patterns associated with very well-developed visual and auditory systems. Many species are territorial and display both visually and acoustically, often with complex songs which are largely learnt. In many birds considerable manipulative skills are utilised in nest building (weaver birds, bower birds). These are often also a signal for attracting a mate.

All species show some degree of parental care and may teach by example. The degree of sensory motor integration required for flight must be considerable. It is probable that many of the behaviour sequences required are largely preprogrammed, but birds also have a considerable flexibility as to how and in what circumstances they are expressed. This is evidenced by the imprinting which occurs in the young of nidifugous birds in which, during a restricted developmental period, they learn to recognise their parent and optimal food sources (Hinde 1962). Learning of taste aversions is rapid in young chicks and requires provision of energy substrates for neurons by glia (see Chapter 15). Similarly, young birds learn from conspecifics the intricate components of their song, which is often unique and aids in individual recognition. Birds reared in isolation have rudimentary songs in comparison (Johnston 1988). In laboratory situations, birds have been shown to exhibit classical, association, discriminant and instrumental conditioning. In spatial learning, they probably rival any other species of animal in their ability to memorise routes for navigation and to return to their natal region, and subsequently the same nest site annually after journeys of many thousands of miles. Some birds have been shown to use 'tools' (sticks for extracting prey, rocks for breaking shells). Birds show a similar form of sleep to that of mammals.

2.4.4 Mammals

In comparison to birds, mammals have little restriction on brain size, yet instead of developing a simple mass of new brain tissue, increase in size has been achieved by expansion of the sheet of isocortex (neocortex) which comes to overlie the rest of the telencephalon. The development of this sheet causes a correspondingly massive increase in the number of cells and the area of the glia overlying it at the brain pial surface. Associated with this enormous increase in size is greater anatomical complexity and more elaborate architectonics. The cortical sheet is intricately folded, greatly increasing its surface area, more than 1100 cm^2 per hemisphere in humans. It is layered and it is postulated that the earliest mammals had a six-layered isocortex with 10–20 functional subdivisions.

During the course of evolution of the placental mammals, additional division into sublayers has occurred (Northcutt and Kaas 1995).The layers themselves show an elaborate columnar organisation. During development, glia provide the scaffolding which underlies the architecture of radially arranged columns intersected by horizontal layers of neurons. These radial columns are particularly prominent in primates. Physiological and metabolic studies indicate that functional modules are associated with these columns in the adult (Goldman-Rakic 1984). Recently (Colombo et al. 1995), a new type of astrocyte has been described in adult monkeys which has long processes traversing several cortical laminae. It is tempting to relate these to the functional modules and adaptive radial spatial buffering of potassium (Chapter 12). Differentiation of oligodendrocytes is complete and myelin sheaths with nodes of Ranvier are fully developed (Roots 1984).

Compartmentation of the kind seen in other animals is abundant. Glomeruli have been described in species across the orders of mammals (Guillery 1969; Sotelo, Llinás and Baker 1974; Gwyn, Nicholson and Flumerfelt 1977; Peters, Palay and Webster 1991). There is considerable evidence that astrocytes are involved in the remodelling of synaptic connections (Theodosis and Poulain 1993) and thus have a role in brain plasticity essential for the modification of behaviour (Chapter 14).

The behavioural repertoire of the least evolved mammals, which have a smooth cortical surface, is comparable to that of birds in that they display courtship and parental behaviour and usually make a nest for the rearing of their young. Depending on the species, visual, tactile, auditory, and olfactory senses are well developed and are used in differing degrees in intra- and interspecies communication. The degree of sophistication of the incoming sensory information allows intermodality integration to be used to assess the relevance of environmental changes and respond accordingly. As a result, less of the behaviour of mammals appears to be stereotyped and responses seem to be more flexible. Learning plays an ongoing role in modifying behaviour. This is probably best exemplified by the evolution of play, in which young animals, often with their parents and siblings, learn behaviours relevant for survival in adult life. Often exploratory behaviour is part of this developmental stage. In the higher mammals play and exploration persist into adulthood. Apart from the learning capabilities ascribed to birds, more advanced mammals (primates) show considerable manipulative skills and use tools which may be modified for a particular purpose. Primates are also capable of solving problems by deductive reasoning, suggesting that they may be able to conceptualise a situation.

With the advent of a soft exterior skin, especially of the face, mammals have developed the ability to convey information about emotional state more effectively than other vertebrates. This is in addition to acoustic and more overt visual displays. In the many species which live in social groups this is important in the maintenance of a dominance hierarchy, which is often dynamic. More precise intraspecific communication has been achieved by vocalisations, especially in the cetacea. This, of course, reaches its nadir in the development of language in man, which allows the intercommunication of the benefits of combined experience of previous and present individuals. More specifically, it allows the transmission of concepts, like the contribution that glial cells may make to the operation of the conceptual entity itself.

2.4.5 *Summary of the Vertebrates*

The vertebrate brain was a new design, not constrained significantly in size because of the design of the skeletal system of the animal. Even in fish and amphibia, it is comparatively large and incorporates the multi-channel inputs and outputs required for flexibility of response. The inactivity of invertebrates, lacking sensory input, has been replaced by a progressively more definable state of sleep. With the development of the isocortex and glia specialised for insulation, metabolic regulation, ionic conductance and involvement in synaptic efficacy, came the ability to make behaviour adaptable to the needs of the individual in the pertaining environmental circumstances.

2.5 Conclusions

During the course of evolution, there have been a number of developments in neuron–glia relationships which have significance for the role of glia in behaviour. One big change from invertebrates to vertebrates was in the way in which neurons and glia are morphologically apposed. In the invertebrates (with the possible exception of the Cephalopoda), increased surface contact between neurons and glia is achieved by invagination of neuronal somata by glial processes. This is related to the absence or paucity of a blood supply to invertebrate ganglia and is largely trophic in function. In the vertebrates, with a good blood supply, neurons branch outwards. The development of extensive dendrites provides a greater surface for synaptic contacts. The removal of the glial trophospongium allows synaptic contacts on the neuronal soma. As we have seen, vertebrate nervous systems have a greater capacity for integration, learning and storing temporal sequences of experience leading to more modifiable behaviour. The different relationship between neurons and glia opened the way for a greater diversity and flexibility of synaptic connectivity. In vertebrates, the greater the stratification of structures and the more complex the architecture of the nervous system, the more complex is the animal's behaviour. Glia play a role not only in the construction of this architecture during development but are responsible, at least in part, for its maintenance.

Greater precision and organisation of behavioural activities is made possible by the specialisation and separation of pathways, and by compartmentalisation at a microscopic level. The separation of groups of synapses, processes or cells by glial processes in glomeruli occurs in all phyla except the cnidaria and platyhelminthes. A prime function of such compartmentalisation may be to enable 'packages' of behavioural sequences to be organised, serve to contain humoral exchanges within the compartment and mediate the transfer of ions to different regions of the compartment. Glial communication by spatial buffering, especially of K^+, may be facilitated from compartment to compartment via common parts of the same glial cell or through gap junctions. Many glial cells have neurotransmitter receptors and enzymes for transmitter metabolism. Compartmentalisation may be related to the local metabolism of transmitters which may also modify the buffering of potassium and other ions (Chapters 6, 7, 10).

There is evidence for a role for glia in the plasticity of vertebrate behaviour by virtue of their participation in the formation and dissolution of synapses. Dynamic synaptic morphology is likely to be a requirement for the modification of behavioural responses (Chapter 14).

The development and perfection of insulation of axons by glial processes, myelin-like and myelin sheaths were crucial for the evolution of varied and complex behaviour such as that exhibited by mammals. Not only is the conduction velocity of action potentials increased with economy of space and energy but variation in the thickness of the sheath enables fine tuning of conduction velocity and precision in the timing sequence of signals, vital for complex behaviour (see Chapter 9). Chemical differences in the composition of myelin appear to be related to its degree of compaction, which in turn is related to axonal conduction velocity (Roots 1993).

In both invertebrates and vertebrates, glial cells have a trophic function for neurons. Control of the metabolic substrates for neurons may be equated with the regulation or modulation of behavioural states (Chapter 5). There is increasing evidence also for a role for glia in the electrical activity of the nervous system (see Mennerick and Zorumski 1994 and Chapters 9–12 in this book).

Clearly, the increase in differentiation and relative quantity of glia to neurons which has accompanied the evolution of adaptive and adaptable behaviours is an indicant of their functional importance. Some ideas about evolutionary trends have been presented here, but a more detailed knowledge of the ways in which glia are involved in operation of nervous systems and behaviour is an essential task for future research.

Acknowledgements

The contribution by BIR was supported by Grant No. A6025 from the Natural Sciences and Engineering Research Council of Canada.

3

Glial Cells in Brain Development and Plasticity

CHRISTIAN M. MÜLLER

Summary

The functioning of the brain is critically linked to brain architecture at different levels, e.g. accuracy of local circuitries, regional compartmentalisation, long range axonal connectivities, and the presence of functional topographies within areas. The mature appearance of brain tissue and the establishment of neuronal connectivities is achieved during development and is governed by genetic instruction and activity-dependent adaptation of axonal projections. The latter mechanisms gain increasing importance in highly evolved organisms. In this overview, evidence for a crucial role of glial cells in different phases of brain development is presented. These include the guidance of neuronal migration, their role in the differentiation of neuronal phenotypes, axonal outgrowth, and the parcellation of specific brain areas into functional units. Possible mechanisms by which glial cells can influence synaptic interactions between nerve cells, including those related to behavioural modification by experience, are also addressed. Glial mechanisms in brain development and function, as well as neuronal mechanisms, cannot be considered as separable phenomena, but appear to be highly interdependent. A more detailed analysis of the ways by which neurons and glial cells communicate and interact, in vivo, will therefore be necessary in future to determine mechanisms by which the brain functions.

3.1 Introduction

3.1.1 Brain Function and Brain Architecture

Progress in brain research over the last decades has allowed us to get a first glimpse at how this fascinating organ processes information and ultimately controls the behaviour of individuals. One important breakthrough in the understanding of the brain came with the descriptions of its functional parcellation. Specific brain regions could be linked to particular functions, e.g. Broca's area to language production, the hippocampus to certain aspects of learning and memory.

Furthermore, individual brain regions are shown to comprise functional modules; for example, ocular-dominance stripes in the visual cortex are important for depth vision, somatosensory 'barrels' dealing with information of individual body parts, or olfactory 'glomeruli' subserving the recognition of smells. Such modules are integrated into topographic maps that represent important aspects of the information processed in a given brain region. Such maps often reflect special behavioural adaptations of an organism, like the map for echo-delays in the bat's auditory cortex.

There is accumulating evidence that brain function is closely dependent on brain architecture at different morphological levels. The location of synapses on different parts of the neuronal surface, for example, determines the impact of incoming synaptic transmission. Such different locations are often selectively innervated by different classes of afferent neurons, suggesting a very elaborated 'plan' of brain architecture. Another widespread feature of brain architecture is the presence of multilayered structures comprising individual, repetitive functional units, e.g. cortical columns. Every location within a functional map thereby contains one functional unit which may interact with neighbouring units by horizontal, associative projections. The very regular repetition of such units and the functional coherence of neuronal response characteristics within such columns calls for some means to guarantee accurate morphogenesis and interconnectivity. Disturbances in the development of such basic architectonics of the brain, as seen in several mutants, sometimes result in severe behavioural deficits. Studies on the development of circuitries have shown that in highly evolved organisms interconnectivities are not determined by genetic instruction alone, but are gradually refined during development (for review, see Gierer and Müller 1995). Therefore, mechanisms of the development of brain architecture appear to be fundamental for the functioning of the brain. As outlined below, glial cells can be shown to participate significantly in developmental processes during different phases of the elaboration of brain architecture.

3.1.2 Brain Architecture and Brain Development

Development of the brain roughly proceeds in three important steps. First, neurons and glial cells are generated at distinct locations, usually the ventricular zone. While macroglial cells can continuously be generated throughout life, the vast majority of neurons become postmitotic and largely determined after their final division. Therefore it is of considerable importance that neurons migrate to the appropriate locations in the brain where they fulfil their function. The second phase of brain development includes the outgrowth of dendrites and axons from immature neurons, the development of neuronal specificities, and the establishment of axonal and synaptic connections. These two phases of development are predominantly governed by genetic instruction. In the final step of brain development, neuronal connectivities are refined in an activity-dependent manner. Beside the refinement of local and long-range axonal connections, this phase includes the final allocation of the brain into distinct areas and the establishment of functional subdivisions within areas. During evolution, the last phase gained increasing importance, probably due to the necessity of very complex but accurate functional architectures, and also due to the necessity of a highly adaptable brain architecture. The latter appears to have a direct link to the behaviour of organisms, as the functioning of the brain has to cope with an increased diversity in the phenotype of individuals and allows for adaptability of individuals to diverse environmental conditions. The latter is ultimately linked to the phenomena of learning and memory, which become increasingly important with the evolution of complex social interactions but also with the evolution of organisms which can successfully adapt to many different environments.

3.1.3 Brain Development and Glial Cells

Towards the end of the last century, glial cells were already considered to be important for brain development but also for mechanisms underlying learning, memory, and even conscious experience (Soury 1899). Similar hypotheses can be found throughout the literature of this century. However, experimental proof for such claims has been, and for many aspects of glial function is still, rare. Over the last decades, glial cells have attracted increasing interest due to the development of new techniques which allowed the study of these cells in more detail. Especially important have been the development of specific markers to allow the identification of glial cells, modern culturing techniques, and the application of intracellular recording techniques. Two findings can be considered central for changing concepts on glial participation in brain development and function. Culturing techniques revealed that neuronal survival, differentiation, and maturation are considerably supported by cocultured glial cells, especially by astrocytes (e.g. Banker 1980). Secondly, intracellular recording techniques revealed that glial cells express a variety of receptors for neurotransmitters and neuromodulators. Meanwhile, it became clear that glial cells are capable of responding to neuronal signals with electrical, as well as biochemical responses. Even signal propagation has been observed in astroglial cells (Cornell-Bell and Finkbeiner 1991), and the propagating signals in astrocytes influence neuronal activity (Nedergaard 1994; Hassinger et al. 1995). Thus, brain development and function can be considered to be the result of a highly interactive and concerted action of neurons and glial cells. In the following paragraphs, experimental evidence for glial participation in the developmental processes introduced above will be presented.

3.2 Neuronal Migration

Among the first cells generated and differentiating in the developing brain are radial glial cells. These cells express several characteristics of astrocytes, e.g. the expression of the cell markers vimentin, glial fibrillary acidic protein (GFAP), and S-100 (Engel and Müller 1989). In higher mammals, radial glia can transform to stellate astrocytes in later development (Voigt 1989). The soma of radial glial cells first resides in the ventricular zone, while an apical process spans the entire thickness of the neural tube and contacts the pial surface. Light and electron microscopic studies, especially by Pasco Rakic and his collaborators have shown that the apical process of radial glia serves as a substrate for migrating neurons (Rakic 1971a,b). These observations led to the hypothesis that the arrangement of radial glial fibres may be a scaffold for the vertical organisation of laminated structures, like cerebellum, tectum, and cortex. Recent studies using the retroviral infection of neuronal cell clones have stressed and extended this hypothesis (Kornack and Rakic 1995; Reid, Liang and Walsh 1995). Injection of a low concentration of retroviruses which were genetically modified to carry the *Escherichia coli* gene coding for β-galactosidase (lacZ) into the embryonic brain, leads to the infection of only a few precursor cells. As the viral genome is transferred to the progeny of the infected cell, it is possible to identify and map cell populations originating from a common precursor at subsequent developmental stages by visualising the lacZ enzyme expression. By using this technique, it was shown that clonally related cells originating from successive steps of asymmetric cell divisions (generating one postmitotic cell per division) often migrate along a common radial glial process and thereby integrate into a common cortical column. Such a mechanism of guidance (Fig. 3.1) may guarantee that neurons in a given cortical column share a cell fate which may be defined by the location in the ventricular wall during early development. A clonal relation of cells within a cortical column may help to establish vertical connectivities by the presence of common recognition molecules. In addition, cell clones may also migrate to diverse horizontally spaced locations in a given cortical layer. The latter distribution of cells is thought to be based on symmetric divisions, generating a population of 'cousin' cells which disperse horizontally in the ventricular zone before they migrate along different radial glial fibers (Kornack and Rakic 1995). Thus, clonal relations could also be implicated in some aspects of the horizontal interconnectivity of layered structures.

The mechanisms of the underlying neuron–glia recognition and interaction have been analysed by in vitro studies. Coculturing embryonic neurons and radial glia leads to rapid adhesion of neurons to glial fibres and subsequent migration (for review see Hatten 1990). Adhesion and migration is also possible on glass fibers coated with radial glial membranes (Fishman and Hatten 1993). Antibodies raised against astrotactin, a surface molecule expressed by migrating neurons, reduce the interaction of neurons and radial glia, as well as with membrane-coated glass fibres. These data suggest that astrotactin interacts with an as-yet unidentified

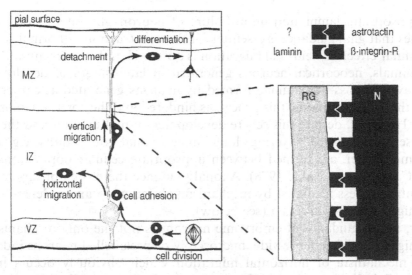

Fig. 3.1. Guidance of neuronal migration in neocortex by radial glial cells. Neuronal precursor cells divide in the ventricular zone and the postmitotic cells adhere to radial glial processes. Migration mainly occurs via an interaction of the neuronal surface molecule astrotactin with an unknown partner on radial glial processes. An interaction of laminin and the β-integrin receptor may also participate in radial migration. Horizontal migration is observed in about 10% of neurons and does not involve radial glial cells. Migrating neurons detach after reaching the superficial layers of the cortex and differentiate in an 'inside-out' fashion. (Based on Rakic 1971a,b; O'Rourke et al. 1995; Fishman and Hatten 1993.)

partner on radial glial fibres. Distinct polypeptides present during the time of neuronal migration may serve as recognition molecules (Cameron and Rakic 1994). Also, laminin, expressed on radial glia and interacting with the neuronal β-integrin receptor, appears to participate in neuronal migration (Fishman and Hatten 1993). The importance of this recognition between neurons and radial glia becomes clear in mouse mutants. In weaver mutants, cerebellar granule cells fail to adhere to radial glial cells and to migrate to their appropriate layer. This failure results in an ectopical location of granule cells which subsequently die (Hatten, Liem and Mason 1986). However, the cell death does not seem to be causally related to the failure of migration, as weaver granule cells also die when transferred to tissue culture under conditions where wildtype cells readily survive (Willinger, Margolis and Sidman 1981). By combining radial glial fibres and embryonic neurons from wildtype animals and weaver mutants, in vitro, it became clear that the defective migration resides in neurons and not radial glia. Thus, neurons from mutant mice fail to adhere and migrate on wildtype radial glial cells and wildtype neurons readily migrate along radial glia from mutant animals. The defect in appropriate lamination upon failure of neuron–glia interaction clearly demonstrates that glial guidance is essential for the construction of normal cortical layers. A similar effect on neuronal migration is observed in the reeler mutation. In wildtype animals, neocortical neurons generated in later stages of development normally have to cross the laminae formed by neurons generated at earlier time periods. In the mouse mutants, this process is hindered and the cortical lamination is inverted. However, despite this severe developmental malfunction and the consequent absence of cortical layering, long range axonal connections, e.g. those from thalamic nuclei, are formed between appropriate cellular populations (for review see Caviness and Rakic 1978). Axonal guidance therefore appears to be a developmental process mediated by mechanisms different to and independent of neuronal migration and targeting (see below).

However, radial guidance of embryonic neurons is not the only mechanism of neuronal migration. Time lapse videomicroscopy of prelabelled neurons indicates a separate mechanism of horizontal migration which obviously occurs in the absence of radial glial processes (O'Rourke et al. 1995). The underlying mechanisms have yet to be elucidated. Migrating neural crest cells appear to follow pathways which are characterised by the expression of matrix molecules. Tenascin-C is one such molecule expressed by astroglial cells (for review see Faissner 1993). Therefore, it appears likely that glial cells also participate in this form of non-radial migration.

The mechanism of radial glia guidance is not restricted to early developmental stages, but can be repeated in adulthood in selected species and structures. One such example is the vocal control nucleus, Hvc, in the canary forebrain, a nucleus of utmost importance for the control of bird song. Male canaries acquire a new song repertoire early each year; this process of song acquisition is paralleled by extensive morphological changes in Hvc, including the generation and insertion of new neurons into the local network and the connectivities to other nuclei of the vocal control pathway (Alvarez-Byulla, Kirn and Nottebohm 1990). Interestingly, prior to song acquisition, radial glial cells become evident, the processes of which span the region of neuronogenesis and the song nucleus (Alvarez-Buylla, Buskirk and Nottebohm 1987). In vitro data suggest that these glial fibres underly the migration of newly formed neurons and may thereby participate in the changing song repertoire.

3.2.1 Neuronal Phenotype

After migration of immature neurons to their final destination in the brain, several steps of neuronal maturation take place. These include the differentiation of neuronal phenotype and the establishment of both dendritic and axonal neuronal processes. While part of the phenotype is predetermined, morphological features are malleable to environmental, especially astroglial influences. In a series of in vitro studies Alain Prochiantz and coworkers have analysed the influence of the astroglial environment on developing neurons (Denis-Donini, Glowinski and Prochiantz 1984; Chamak et al. 1987; Rousselet et al. 1990). It became apparent that neurons cultured on a layer of astrocytes obtained from their natural environment ('homotopic co-cultures') developed a different phenotype than if cultured on astrocytes originating from a different brain region ('heterotopic co-cultures'). Similar data could be obtained by culturing the neurons in the presence of medium which had been conditioned by the different astroglial populations. This finding indicates that soluble factors released from astrocytes influence neuronal development. To date, it is unclear which factors are responsible for these effects. Studies on cerebellar granule cells have suggested that astroglial-derived fibroblast growth factor is essential for neurite outgrowth (Hatten et al. 1988).

3.2.2 Axon Guidance (Fig. 3.2)

Axons can grow over considerable distances to reach their target region. There is abundant evidence showing that axonal targeting does not rely on intrinsic programmes, but is guided by external influences. One of the earliest indications for a guidance mechanism came from behavioural studies on frogs by Roger Sperry. After transection of the optic nerve, retinal ganglion cells regenerate their axons which ultimately reach the optic tectum and again allow visually guided behaviour. If the eye was rotated by 180 degrees coincidently with the optic nerve transection, then a peculiar behaviour of the animals was observed after regeneration was completed. When prey was presented in front of the animal, catching behaviour was directed towards the back of the animal (Sperry 1948). These data were in line with the hypothesis that retinal axons reinnervated the same targets in the tectum to that during initial development and that the eye rotation did not affect this connectivity pattern. Thus, neither experience nor orientation of the eye in the head seemed to have influenced axonal targeting. A large body of literature has confirmed and extended these observations, some of which will be detailed below. Another example indicating that axon guidance relies on cues extrinsic to the growing neuron comes from studies in mutant mice. As mentioned above, cortical neurons are significantly displaced in reeler mutants and sometimes the orientation of the cells is inverted. Nevertheless, axonal connections develop virtually normally. Again, these data indicate that the environment of growing axons influences the direction and pathway of axonal outgrowth.

Three major theories have been considered for explaining axonal guidance. Mechanical guidance cues by glial 'tunnels' and the expression of growth-permissive and/or repulsive molecules along future axonal trajectories, diffusable factors originating from target regions or selected guide-posts, and chemical cues presented in a graded fashion on cellular surfaces to allow axonal navigation by

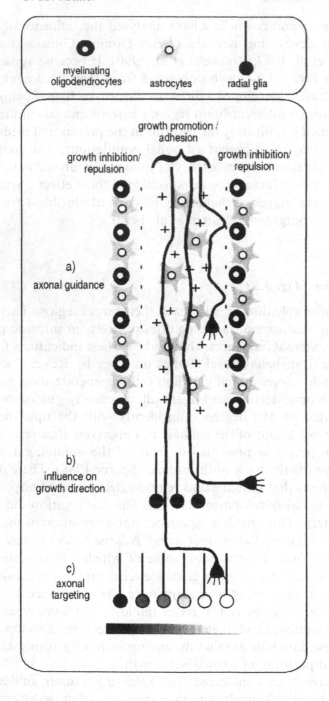

reading such positional information. Experimental evidence for these mechanisms and the inclusion of glial cells in such mechanisms is outlined below.

3.2.2.1 Axonal Guidance by Pre-formed Pathways

Anatomical studies have indicated that axon tracts often follow pathways formed by glial cells which surround enlarged extracellular spaces. In a series of studies, Jerry Silver and collaborators showed such specialisations in a number of different brain regions at time periods when axonal bundles traversed these locations (for review see McKeon and Silver 1995). Two major theories, not necessarily exclusive, have been developed to explain the function of such specialisations. A mechanical model suggests that glial cells delineate an expanded extracellular space essential for axonal growth. This model is supported by the failure of axon elongation in mouse mutations showing a significant reduction of extracellular space size (Silver and Robb 1979). A second model suggests that axons may grow along matrix or surface molecules expressed along the glial trajectories. The presence of the neural cell adhesion molecule (NCAM), and other adhesion molecules like laminin, and N-cadherin at locations of preferential axon growth and the synthesis of such molecules by glial cells is in line with such a mechanism. Additional evidence for the neccessity of glial structures in the development of axonal connections come from studies in the fruit fly *Drosophila*. Mutants which lack major axonal commissures share significant disturbances of glial development. This is true for mutants *spitz*, *Star*, *rhomboid*, *slit*, and *pointed* (Therianos et al. 1995), all of which show gaps in the distribution of glial cells prior to the formation of axon tracts. These and a large body of additional data suggest that axonal outgrowth is significantly guided by growth supporting signals or adhesion molecules expressed by glia. An alternative and possibly supplementatory influence of glial cells on axonal tract formation is linked to molecules repulsive for axonal growth, e.g. those which are expressed by myelinating oligodendrocytes (Caroni and Schwab 1988). Upon formation of the corticospinal tract in mammals, myelinating oligodendrocytes surround the future axon trajectory. Inhibition of the repulsive effect of the myelin associated growth inhibitor by a functional antibody, in vivo, leads to aberrant sprouting of growing axons

Fig. 3.2. Glial influences on axonal growth and targeting. (a) Axonal trajectories are guided by astroglial 'tunnels' containing growth promoting molecules (+) and which are often delineated by growth-inhibiting molecules (−) expressed by myelinating oligodendrocytes or astrocytes. (b) Axonal growth direction can be influenced by molecules expressed on glial surfaces, e.g. midline radial glial cells. (c) Accurate pathfinding of axons within a target region can be accomplished by graded distributions of guidance molecules presented on radial glia.

(Schwab and Schnell 1991). Similar data have also been obtained for other axon tracts being formed late in development (Kapfhammer and Schwab 1992).

Such glial influences on growing axons may not only be important for the development of axon tracts, but may also be implicated in the changing of growth direction of specific sets of axons. One such example is the optic chiasm in mammals with frontal vision where only half of the retinal axons cross to the opposite hemisphere. At the time when retinal axons arrive at the optic chiasm, a pallisade of radial glial cell processes is present at the midline of the brain which are contacted by growing axons (Marcus et al. 1995). At that location, part of the axons turn their growth direction towards the ipsilateral optic tectum, most probably due to inhibitory signals encountered by growth cones (Witzenmann et al. 1993). The recent discovery of an axonal guidance molecule expressed by radial glial cells in the optic tectum (Drescher et al. 1995) may support the notion that glial cells express such guidance signals (see below). However, as neuronal elements are also present close to the midline where 'decision making' by retinal ganglion cell growth cones takes place, it cannot be excluded that these cells are participating in axonal navigation (for review see Guillery, Mason and Taylor 1995).

3.2.2.2 Axonal Guidance by Diffusable Factors

The participation of diffusable factors in axonal navigation has been shown by in vitro studies. Explant cultures of embryonic brain structures allow the co-culturing of source and target structures in artificial, spatial arrangements. Such studies have revealed that both attractive and repulsive diffusable substances secreted from one tissue are capable of influencing axonal growth in remote tissues (Pini 1993; Serafini et al. 1994). To date, there is little evidence that such diffusable guidance molecules are actually derived from glial cells.

3.2.2.3 Axonal Guidance by Graded Distributions of Molecules

Probably the best studied model system for axonal targeting is the retino–tectal projection in vertebrates. The development of simple in vitro systems allowed significant progress in understanding the molecular mechanisms underlying axonal pathfinding over the last decade. The so-called 'stripe-assay', developed by Friedrich Bonhoeffer and collaborators is such an in vitro model system. A strip of retinal tissue which contains nasal and temporal parts of the retina is labelled with a lipophilic fluorescent dye to allow visualisation of outgrowing axons and is transferred to a membrane containing alternating stripes of test-substrates (Bonhoeffer and Huf 1982). When the stripes contain alternating lanes containing membranes from anterior and posterior tectum, then axons from temporal retina grow exclusively on 'anterior' stripes, the in vivo target of these projections. This preference is due to repulsive molecule(s) present in 'posterior' membrane preparations. A similar preference for 'posterior' membranes by nasal axons has also been observed in this system (von Boxberg,

Deiss and Schwarz 1993). A role for glial cells in such effects was suggested by experiments where retinal axons were confronted with astroglial cells derived from different tectal regions and diencephalon (Gooday 1990; Johnston and Gooday 1991). While both nasal and temporal axons extended neurites on diencephalic astrocytes, contacted by both populations during retino–tectal outgrowth, axon outgrowth from temporal retina but not nasal explants was hindered by tectal astrocytes. These data parallel the findings obtained with crude membrane preparations from tectum and suggest that glial cells may be the source of guidance activity. Most recent data support the notion that the molecular basis of axon guidance involves a neuron–glial interaction. Using molecular biological techniques, two genes coding for putative guidance molecules acting during the formation of the retino–tectal pathway have been identified, i.e. RAGS (Drescher et al. 1995) and ELF-1 (Cheng et al. 1995). Both molecules are ligands for Eph receptor tyrosine kinases expressed by retinal ganglion cells. Interestingly, RAGS expression is associated with radial glial cells of the optic tectum. The human homolog of RAGS, AL1, has previously been shown to be expressed by cortical astrocytes and to influence growth of cortical axons (Winslow et al. 1995). The effect of AL1 on cortical axons is strikingly similar to the behaviour of temporal retinal axons when contacting glial cells from posterior tectum. Thus, it appears likely that similar guidance mechanisms to those suggested for the retino–tectal pathway are realised in other brain regions and are also associated with an astroglial cell population. The complementary spatial expression of the receptor (Mek4) for ELF-1 and RAGS in retinal ganglion cells and their ligands in the tectum indicates that the adequate regulation of axonal guidance is based on coordinated neuronal and glial mechanisms.

3.3 Regional Specification/Parcellation

Following the initial formation of long-range axonal connections, target areas undergo significant changes in their overall structure and in both their afferent and intrinsic circuitry. This refinement of axonal and synaptic patterns leads to mature parcellation into functional units. Three examples may illustrate this developmental period and the participation of glial cells in such processes. The primary somatosensory cortex of rodents has a highly compartimentalised appearance, reflecting the pattern of whiskers on the animal's snout. Input carrying information from individual whiskers terminates in restricted circular regions ('barrels') comprising of a ring, formed by neuronal cell bodies in layer IV of the cortex, which extend their dendrites towards the centre of the ring. This highly organised pattern is formed within a few days after ingrowth of thalamo–cortical axons. Prior to the relocation of the initially uniform distribution of neuronal cell bodies to the future barrel walls, astroglial markers already reveal this pattern (Cooper and Steindler 1986; Steindler and Cooper 1987; Steindler et al. 1989). Astroglial cells at the future boundaries of barrels express high amounts of the filament-protein GFAP, as well as the matrix molecules tenascin-C and chondroitin sulfate proteoglycan. The latter share a repulsive effect on neurite growth (Faissner 1993). This led to the hypothesis that astroglial cells may present a 'blueprint' of the future architecture of the barrel cortex. The major argument against this hypothesis is that manipulation of the peripheral sense organs is capable of modifying the transient pattern of glial markers, as well as the mature barrel pattern. In addition, transplantation experiments show that visual cortical tissue is capable of expressing barrels, when transplanted into the target area of somatosensory thalamic afferents (Schlaggar and O'Leary 1991). It is thus conceivable that axonal ingrowth, and most probably neuronal activity, influences the expression of matrix molecules in cortical astrocytes which then influence pattern formation of cortical neurons. A similar series of events has been observed in the developing retino–thalamic projection in the ferret (Müller, Faissner and Altrogge 1995). Due to the partial crossing of retinal axons in the optic chiasm (see above) afferents from both eyes innervate the thalamic dorsal lateral geniculate nucleus (LGNd). While both axon populations initially innervate the entire LGNd, a segregation into eye-specific layers occurs over subsequent development (Sretavan and Shatz 1986). Immunostaining with an antibody directed against the astroglial matrix molecule tenascin-C reveals transient boundaries at the future inter-laminar zones. Similar to the situation in the somatosensory cortex, the confinement of tenascin-C immunoreactivity to the future boundaries occurs after ingrowth of retinal fibres and coincides with the process of pattern formation by retino–thalamic axons, as well as neurons in the LGNd. Further features common to the development of the barrel cortex are the expression of GFAP and proteoglycans by astrocytes situated at the forming boundaries (Hutchins and Casagrande 1990; Robson and Geisert 1994). Studies on the moth *Manduca sexta* by Leslie Tolbert and coworkers indicate that the mechanisms described above are already present in the insect central nervous system and underscore the necessity of glial cells for regional pattern formation. After ingrowth of olfactory sensory axons into the antennal lobe, glial cells accumulate in ring-like structures which subsequently delineate olfactory glomeruli. Destruction of glial cells during early development interferes with the development of glomerular structures (Tolbert and Oland 1989). Recent evidence shows that glial cells that surround future glomeruli transiently express a tenascin-like molecule (Krull et al. 1993).

The available data indicate that local parcellation of some central nervous structures involves a cascade of events initiated by axon–glial interaction which is followed by specific changes in the glial population with the potential to influence axonal and dendritic growth, and neuronal relocation. The astroglial molecules tenascin-C and proteoglycans appear to represent a molecular basis for glial–neuronal interactions. It is suggested that axonal signals induce the patterned expression of such growth-restricting molecules by astrocytes which may impose a constraint on, or even guide, neuronal migration, as well as dendritic and axonal growth. The signalling pathways from axons to glial cells remain to be elucidated.

3.4 Adaptive Plasticity

Two reasons have to be considered for the increasing importance of adaptive changes in brain circuitry during evolution. The first reason appears to reside in the increasing complexity of neuronal interconnectivities which calls for developmental paradigms beyond genetic instruction alone. The increasing diversity of individual organisms has also contributed to an important role of self-organisation as a developmental principle, e.g. slight variations in the position of sense organs may call for significant changes in central nervous connectivities to allow for highly elaborate information processing. One such example is stereoscopic vision in higher mammals. Analysis of the third dimension is achieved by comparison of the two-dimensional pictures obtained by either eye. Subtle differences in the pictures allow computation of depth information. These differences are not only influenced by the form or distance of objects but are also significantly influenced by the distance between the eyes. This parameter is not only highly variable between individuals, but can also be influenced by epigenetic factors, e.g. head deformations during birth. Thus it appears essential to allow for adaptive mechanisms during development which may guarantee adequate matching of neuronal connectivities and the individual's phenotype. The second factor which seems to underly the evolution of highly adaptable brain circuitries resides in the necessity for individuals to cope with a variety of different environmental influences. Social interactions, especially, have gained increasing importance in highly evolved animals and it is conceivable that mechanisms of learning and memory are essential for adequate behavioural adaptability (see Chapter 2).

Adaptive plasticity in the brain can be pinned down to two general rules, usually referred to as the Hebbian rules. The first rule has been formulated by Donald Hebb (1949) and says (in modern terms) that connectivities which successfully participate in synaptic transmission are stabilised or even enhanced. This general rule applies to the elaboration of developing projections, as well as to mechanisms of learning. An axon which innervates an appropriate target will often be active in concert with other axons carrying similar information to the same structure. Consequently, this axonal projection will be maintained. Similarily, associative learning can rely on the same mechanism. An extension of Hebb's postulate was introduced by Gunther Stent (1973). Axons which fail to participate in successful synaptic transmission will decrease their efficacy or will be eliminated. The developmental correlate of this axiom is that axons which innervate an inappropriate target will have a low chance of activating postsynaptic neurons, as they lack the 'support' of coherently active neurons carrying similar information. Therefore such axons may be eliminated or become very weak. Such a mechanism may also be related to 'forgetting'.

Hebbian plasticity is generally considered to be exclusively mediated by neurons. However, cumulative evidence suggests that glial cells may influence these phenomena (for review see Müller 1992a). A more direct participation of glial cells in adaptive plasticity can be assumed with respect to morphological changes of synaptic connectivities. Some examples are summarised below and are also the subject of later chapters (Chapters 14, 15).

3.4.1 Glial Cells and Plasticity in Synaptic Efficacy

The efficacy of synaptic transmission is primarily determined by the amount of transmitter released by axons, the sensitivity of neuronal transmitter receptors, and the gating characteristics of ion channels in the neuronal membrane. However, external influences may also have a considerable influence on these events. The intimate association of astroglial processes with synapses and the accumulating evidence for morphological plasticity of glial processes coincident with synaptic changes (for review see Müller 1992a) may support an important role of these cells in the mechanisms leading to synaptic plasticity. Changes in the extracellular potassium concentration have a significant influence on neuronal excitability (see also Chapters 10, 12). Thus, changes in the astroglial mechanisms for potassium homeostasis may have an impact on neuronal excitability. Indeed, the Na^+/K^+ pump in astrocytes has been shown to increase in efficacy upon strong neuronal activation (Onozuka et al. 1987). Similar influences have been considered with respect to the impact of astrocytes on pH regulation (Deitmer 1992a; Ransom 1992; see also Chapter 11). Again, neuronal signals are known to influence the astroglial mechanisms of pH regulation which could feedback on neuronal excitability, especially due to the pH dependence of transmitter receptors. For both mechanisms, however, no clear-cut relation to adaptive plasticity has been established conclusively. A more direct link between an astroglial function and adaptive plasticity has been suggested in the mammalian hippocampus. Tetanic stimulation of axons innervating the hippocampal area CA1 are known to induce a sustained enhancement of synaptic efficacy, called long-term potentiation. The manifestation of this phenomenon includes signalling molecules released from postsynaptic cells. One of these signalling molecules is arachidonic acid (Williams et al. 1989), which acts on astroglial cells and leads to a prolonged reduction in glutamate uptake (Barbour et al. 1989). It is conceivable that the resulting increase in extracellular glutamate contributes to the enhanced neuronal transmission. Recent evidence from our laboratory shows that astroglial intoxification with the gliotoxin fluoroacetate suppresses tetanus induced long-term potentiation (LTP) in rat hippocampus (Kullmann and Müller, in preparation). However, this failure does not block LTP induced by concomitant afferent stimulation and neuronal depolarisation by current injection. Therefore it is unlikely that astrocytes participate in the process of LTP manifestation, but rather may have an impact on the probability of LTP induction. Such a mechanism may be based on glial influences on one transmitter receptor which is crucial for LTP, i.e. the N-methyl-D-aspartate (NMDA) receptor which mediates the calcium-influx in postsynaptic neurons upon activation by glutamate. The NMDA-receptor is modulated by D-serine, which is exclusively synthesized by astroglial cells and which is released by activation of glutamate receptors on these cells (Schell, Molliver and Snyder 1995).

The examples summarised above clearly indicate the potential of glial cells, especially astrocytes, to influence changes in synaptic efficacy. However, to date, there is no clear proof that such mechanisms are crucial and instrumental for synaptic plasticity.

3.4.2 Glial Cells and Structural Plasticity

With respect to structural plasticity associated with adaptive changes of neuronal circuitries evidence for a glial participation is accumulating. Glial influences can be divided into three major effector cascades: (i) promotion of axonal growth, (ii) supression of axonal growth, and (iii) elimination of synaptic contacts. First indications for glial participation in structural plasticity came from correlative studies. In most structures of the mammalian brain, adaptive structural plasticity is confined to a limited time in development, the so-called critical period. These time periods are characterised by the presence of immature glial cells (Stichel, Müller and Zilles 1991; Müller 1992b). Experimental prolongation of the critical period in the mammalian visual cortex is paralleled by a retarded maturation of the astrocytic population (Steward, Bourne and Gabbott 1986; Müller 1990; Hawrylak and Greenough 1995). Interestingly, structures which maintain the capacity for structural plasticity throughout life contain astrocytes with features of immature cells, e.g. in the olfactory bulb (Doucette 1990).

Direct evidence for the participation of glial cells in structural plasticity comes from both in vitro and in vivo experiments. Transplantation of immature astrocytes in the mature visual cortex, i.e. after termination of the critical period, is capable of reinducing the capacity for activity-dependent plasticity (Müller and Best 1989). The exact mechanism of this effect is not yet understood but appears to be related to activity-dependent elimination of synapses rather than the induction of axonal growth. This is indicated by the finding that transplantation of immature astrocytes mainly affects regressive plasticity, like the loss of synaptic function upon unilateral deprivation, but does not induce a reversal of such effects from previous deprivation when vision is restored (Müller, unpublished observation). A causal relation of astroglial cells to synapse elimination has first been deduced from electron microscopic studies in the developing spinal cord. During the time period of refinement of axonal circuitries, astrocytic processes were often identified in synaptic clefts and shown subsequently to phagocytose presynaptic terminals (Ronnevi 1978). Experimental studies have supported the neccessity of astroglial cells for synapse elimination. In cerebellar cultures, synapses are initially formed in exuberance and are reduced in number during subsequent development. Elimination of astrocytes by gliotoxic manipulations prevents the process of synapse elimination (Meshul, Seil and Herndon 1987). When astrocytes are reintroduced in cultures previously deprived of astrocytes, the process of synapse elimination can be reinstalled. Like the observation in the developing spinal cord, in cerebellar cultures also, astrocytes are found to separate synaptic structures. To date, it is unclear how neuron–glial signalling may guide such synapse elimination. This could either be mediated by specific signals that are presented on ineffective synapses and which initiate the elimination, or it can be envisaged that synapse elimination is a continuous process which is actively suppressed by signals from successfully activated synapses. While synapse elimination occurs quite slowly in visual cortex upon full exclusion of sensory experience, rapid changes occur in sensory deprived afferents in the presence of a competing, active afferent (Antonini and Stryker 1993). This indicates that the mechanism of synapse elimination can be activated significantly by neuronal activity. As the separation of synaptic contacts by astroglial processes has to be linked to morphological plasticity in astrocytes, it is of interest that neuronal activity, as well as activation of astroglial transmitter receptors, indeed triggers such events (Cornell-Bell, Thomas and Smith 1990; Wenzel et al. 1991).

Another set of experiments underscoring the role of astrocytes in structural remodelling of synaptic connections has been obtained in studies on the hypothalamic, neurohypophyseal system. These experiments are summarised in Chapter 14 and therefore are not detailed here.

Beside a role in synapse elimination, astrocytes have also been implicated in trophic mechanisms influencing synaptogenesis during activity-dependent plasticity. Several neurotrophic factors are synthesised and released by astrocytes (for review see Labourdette and Sensenbrenner 1995). Studies on the developing cat visual cortex have shown that interference with the astroglial S-100-β protein, a calcium binding protein with neurite-inducing activity on neurons, affects activity-dependent alterations in neuronal specificity (Müller, Akhavan and Bette 1993). Interestingly, S-100 release from astrocytes can be influenced by the neuromodulator serotonin (Whitaker-Azmitia, Murphy and Azmitia 1990), which similarly influences plasticity in kitten visual cortex (Gu and Singer 1995). It is therefore conceivable that neuron–glial signalling may also regulate synapse formation or stabilisation by the release of astroglial-derived growth factors.

3.4.3 Glial Control of Regeneration and Involvement in the Development of Brain Architecture

The capacity of the brain for regenerative processes shows a remarkable change during evolution. Up to the level of amphibia, central nervous axons can readily regenerate upon transection, whereas in reptiles, birds and mammals regeneration fails in most central nervous structures. Amphibia reveal regeneration in rostral, but not caudal brain structures (Lang et al. 1995). The regenerative failure is mainly due to the expression of growth-inhibitory molecules by myelinating oligodendrocytes (Caroni and Schwab 1988; Kapfhammer and Schwab 1994). A possible explanation for the evolution of a mechanism which prevents regeneration may reside in the evolution of a very complex brain architecture and the importance of adaptive plasticity in the brain. Ordered axonal projections which underly the elaborate patterns of functional topographies in highly evolved brains are stabilised by growth-impermissive factors. Due to the immense energy invested during adaptive plasticity in development, such a mechanism may be of considerable importance for the maintenance of brain function. An additional hypothesis may be based on the very close similarity of developmental structural plasticity and adaptive changes in the mature brain, e.g. synaptic efficacy changes. The occurence of growth-inhibitory molecules may confine adaptive plasticity to local changes within the brain architecture without affecting the global organisation. Such a mechanism may allow the maintenance of adaptive changes using the same mechanisms as during development. Thus, glial cells may play a pivotal role in brain evolution by allowing a compromise between energy consuming developmental mechanisms of circuitry refinement and the lifelong capacity for adaptive brain plasticity, being of considerable importance for the complex and highly adaptable behaviour seen in highly evolved organisms (see also Chapter 2).

3.5 Future Perspectives

The data summarised above clearly show the importance of glial cells in the making of a brain during development. Neuronal migration, axonal outgrowth and pathfinding are phenomena clearly linked to glial mechanisms. Further roles of glia can be considered in adaptive plasticity where glial cells may play a modulatory role or could even be implicated in the adaptive process proper. Experiments which may ultimately allow the unravelling of glial mechanisms in brain plasticity will need tools which selectively interfere with glial cells. To date, such tools are rare or lack a clear-cut selectivity. Both biochemical and physiological studies may allow the development of more specific tools. An additional area for promising new findings will reside in the mechanisms of neuron–glial signalling mechanisms. The wealth of information of putative cascades, including transmitter receptors, will hopefully stimulate more research on intact neuron–glial networks. This may set the stage, ultimately, to tackle the longstanding, yet still only vaguely defined, role of glial cells in higher brain functions, including the control of animal behaviour.

Acknowledgement

The author's work presented was funded by BMBF (316902A), DFG (Mue 908/2/3) and by the Max Planck Gesellschaft.

4

The Retina as a Model of Glial Function in the Brain

ANDREAS REICHENBACH,
SERGUEI N. SKATCHKOV and
WINFRIED REICHELT

Summary

The retina, ontogenetically arising from a lateral outgrowth of the neural tube, can be considered as a rather simply layered, easily accessible model of the brain. There are considerable advantages in using the retina to understand glial influences on neuronal activity and thereby behaviour, (i) the function of the retina, as a visual sensory organ, is well understood, and (ii) in most vertebrates (with the exception of mammals with vascularised retinae) there exists only one type of macroglia, the Müller cell. Müller cells express voltage-sensitive ion channels, neurotransmitter receptors and various transporter systems. They are able to recognise a variety of neuronal signals that may be used to adjust the activity of glial functions in response to neuronal requirements. In turn, Müller cells can control the activity of retinal neurons by fuelling the aerobic carbohydrate metabolism of neurons, and by regulating the extracellular concentration of neuroactive substances such as K^+, H^+, γ-aminobutyric acid (GABA) and glutamate. This allows (i) modulation of general neuronal excitability and metabolic state, (ii) modulation of synaptic transmission, and (iii) modulation of and contributions to extrasynaptic transmission. These mechanisms modify the state of retinal information processing in response to changes in the visual environment, and thereby affect behaviour.

4.1 Introduction

4.1.1 Peculiarities of Retinal Information Processing

Although the synaptic circuits of the vertebrate retina are rather complex, and although almost all known brain neurotransmitters have also been demonstrated in the retina, there are a few basic rules of retinal information processing (see Rodieck 1988). The adequate stimulus for the retina is light, which is detected by two types of photoreceptor cells. The cones function during daylight, and their signals are processed by neurons of the so-called photopic system that allows for high spatial and temporal resolution, as well as for colour information. In contrast, the low threshold of the rods enables them to operate in dark environments, and their signals are processed by neurons of the so-called scotopic system that displays strong convergence; this causes a loss of spatial and temporal resolution but allows for high sensitivity.

'Forward' processing from photoreceptors towards the brain involves the following stations of the photopic system, (i) cones, (ii) at least two types of cone-dependent bipolar cells, responding to either light ON or OFF, and (iii) several types of retinal ganglion cells that send their signals via the optic nerve to the brain (see Fig. 4.6). All these cells use glutamate as their neurotransmitter (see Rodieck 1988). 'Forward' processing is more complicated in the scotopic system which is said to be 'piggy-backed' on the photopic circuit (Strettoi, Raviola and Dacheux 1992). Its stations are as follows, (i) rods, (ii) rod bipolar cells, (iii), AII-type amacrine cells, (iv) the two types of cone-dependent bipolar cells, and/or directly (V) the retinal ganglion cells of the photopic pathways (see Fig. 4.6). Again, glutamate is the neurotransmitter in the first synapses involved (for details, see Rodieck 1988; Strettoi, Raviola and Dacheux 1992).

'Lateral' information processing seems mostly to involve lateral inhibition, serving the enhancement of contrast. It is much more pronounced within the photopic system, and is performed essentially by two classes of cells, (i) the horizontal cells acting within the outer plexiform (synaptic) layer, and (ii) the amacrine cells whose processes lie in the inner plexiform layer (see Fig. 4.7, and Rodieck 1988). The dominant neurotransmitter of these 'lateral' pathways is γ-aminobutyric acid (GABA; see Rodieck 1988).

In addition to glutamate (for 'forward' processing") and GABA (for 'lateral' inhibition), another neutrotransmitter, dopamine, is thought to be important for retinal function. Dopamine, being the transmitter of many amacrine cells, seems to play a leading role in the control of the many processes occurring during dark adaptation of the retina (see Djamgoz and Wagner 1992). These events involve, e.g. (i) a transition from photopic to scotopic dominance, (ii) a reduction or loss of lateral inhibition, that may require ultrastructural and structural alterations of horizontal cells, and (iii), in cold-blooded vertebrates, retinomotoric movements of pigment epithelial and photoreceptor cell processes.

To complete this short description of the retina as a 'model brain', it should be mentioned that the extracellular volume fraction of the retina is extremely small (Reichenbach et al. 1988; Karwoski, Frambach and Proenza 1985). This may cause severe problems in extracellular homeostasis, all the more as the retina is a metabolically very active tissue (Ames et al. 1992). Together, this causes a high production of CO_2 (Ames et al. 1992), and, during light stimulation, marked changes in the extracellular concentrations of neuroactive substances, particularly in the plexiform layers. Among these are accumulation of K^+ ions (increased $[K^+]_e$: Karwoski and Proenza 1977; Steinberg, Oakley and Niemeyer 1980), loss of Ca^{2+} ions (decreased $[Ca^{2+}]_e$: Livsey et al. 1990), and alkalinisation (increased pH_e: Borgula, Karwoski and Steinberg 1989). Large accumulations of glutamate and

GABA must also occur. In this context, one interesting finding is that although mammalian horizontal cells are thought to be GABAergic, they fail to show GABA-uptake in adult retinae (Redburn and Madtes 1986). It should also be mentioned that in response to illumination, the $[K^+]_e$ decreases markedly in the subretinal space (Karwoski and Proenza 1977; Steinberg, Oakley and Niemeyer 1980).

4.1.2 Peculiarities of Retinal Glial (Müller) Cells

It is apparent that the above-mentioned changes produced by neuronal activity will mediate a wealth of interactions with retinal glial cells. It was H. Müller (1851) who discovered the radial trunks of macroglia spanning the thickness of the retina. These cells now bear his name and have been found in the retinae of all vertebrates, where they constitute the dominant type of macroglia. The present review will deal exclusively with the interactions between retinal neurons and Müller cells.

Müller cells have a bipolar, ependymoglial morphology (Figs 4.1, 4.2, 4.3; see also Reichenbach and Robinson 1995a). Their vitread (inner) trunk terminates in an expanded conical endfoot adjacent to the vitreous body. In species with vascularised retinae, Müller cells form additional 'en-passant endfeet' onto retinal blood vessels (Wolburg and Berg 1988). At their opposite end, Müller cells extend apical microvilli into the subretinal space which, particularly in avascular retinae, is the source of nutrients and oxygen delivered by the choriocapillary circulation. Thus, Müller cells contact, and even delimit, all non-neuronal compartments surrounding or penetrating the retina. Further, their abundant side branches form elaborate sheaths around neuronal somata (in the nuclear layers), dendrites and synapses (in the two plexiform layers), and fascicles of optic axons (in the nerve fibre layer).

This intimate morphological contact with retinal neurons is supplemented by the physiological features of Müller cells (Newman 1986c, 1996b; Reichenbach and Robinson 1995b). Their membranes display a variety of voltage-gated ion channels including K^+ channels (dominating inward rectifier, delayed rectifier, and A-type: Newman 1985b; Chao et al. 1994a), Na^+ channels (so far only found in some mammalian species: Chao et al. 1994b), and Ca^{2+} channels (Newman 1985b; Puro, Yuan and Sucher 1996). Further, ligand-gated receptors have been observed for glutamate (several types), $GABA_A$ type, and other signal molecules (see Table 4.1). Moreover, the repertoire of membrane transport proteins involves a glutamate uptake system (Ehinger 1977; Brew and Attwell 1987; Schwartz and Tachibana 1990) and a GABA transporter (Ehinger 1977; Biedermann, Eberhardt and Reichelt 1994), a cystine/glutamate exchanger (Kato et al. 1993) as well as a Na^+/HCO_3^- cotransporter (Newman 1991, 1994, 1996a; Newman and Astion 1991) and other acid/base transporters (Newman 1996b). Finally, Müller cells possess enzymes for degradation of neuroactive substances such as glutamine synthetase, as well as carbonic anhydrase, activity involved in pH regulation, and

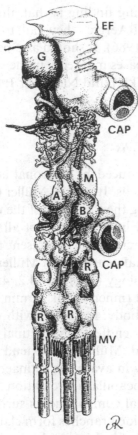

Fig. 4.1. Semi-schematic drawing of the columnar arrangement of neuronal cells along Müller cells. A = amacrine cell, B = bipolar cell, G = ganglion cell, M = Müller cell, R = rod photoreceptor cells; EF = endfoot, MV = microvilli of the Müller cell; CAP = capillaries. All somata and processes of neuronal cells are extensively ensheathed by Müller cell processes. (Modified after Reichenbach et al. 1993, with permission.)

cellular retinoic acid binding protein (CRABP) involved in visual pigment metabolism (for review, see Reichenbach and Robinson 1995b).

In this chapter, we will present recent experimental data and hypotheses to show how Müller cells communicate with neurons within the retina, and thus how they modulate the behaviour of neuronal networks and organisms.

4.2 Müller Cell Functions

4.2.1 Various Preparations Suitable to Study Müller Cell Functions

The structure and location of the retina permits the isolation of the entire living organ, or large functionally intact pieces of it, and to maintain it for many hours

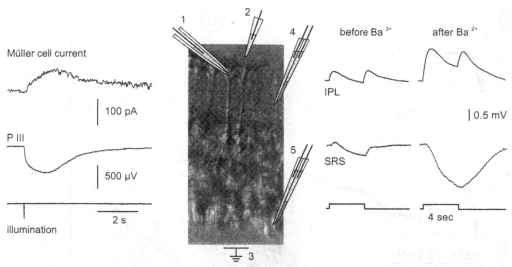

Fig. 4.2. Experimental demonstration of spatial buffering K^+ currents mediated by Müller cells. The centre of the figure shows a lateral view of a living unstained retinal wholemount preparation (vitread side up), containing several Müller cells, and the approximate localisations of the micropipettes used in the different experiments; 1 = voltage-clamp pipette to record currents across the Müller cell membrane, 2,3 = reference electrodes for electroretinogram (ERG) recordings, 4 = ion-sensitive double-barrel microelectrode (ISM) in the inner plexiform layer (IPL), 5 = ISM in the subretinal space (SRS). On the left, the results of a whole-cell voltage-clamp experiment on an isolated light-stimulated wholemount retina is shown. This part of the figure demonstrates outward currents across the Müller cell membrane (upper trace), compared to the slow P III component of the ERG (middle trace) in response to a 60-ms light flash (lower trace) of a retina in which synaptic transmission in the outer plexiform layer (OPL) was blocked; own unpublished results (S. N. Skatchkov and W. Reichelt). On the right of the figure, results of measurements with extracellular ion-sensitive microelectrodes are demonstrated (Frishman et al. 1992). Light-evoked increases of the $[K^+]_e$ in the inner plexiform layer (IPL; upper pair of traces) and decreases of the $[K^+]_e$ in the SRS (lower traces), before (left) and after blockade of the Müller cell K^+ channels by Ba^{2+} (right), during a light stimulus; changes in $[K^+]_e$ are given as voltages at the K^+ sensitive pipette. All light-evoked changes of $[K^+]_e$ are greatly enhanced when spatial buffering by Müller cells is prevented.

as a superfused '*wholemount*' preparation. In cases when the widepread lateral interactions are not of primary interest, retinal *slices* can be cut perpendicularly to the surface, and maintained in a similar way. Both types of preparations allow physiological stimulation by light. Further, as the tissue is transparent and most cell classes display a characteristic morphology and location, it is often possible to identify even unstained cells and penetrate them by microelectrodes (cf. also Fig. 4.2).

It is also possible to obtain preparations of acutely *isolated living cells*, by a combination of enzymatical and mechanical dissociation (Sarthy and Lam 1978;

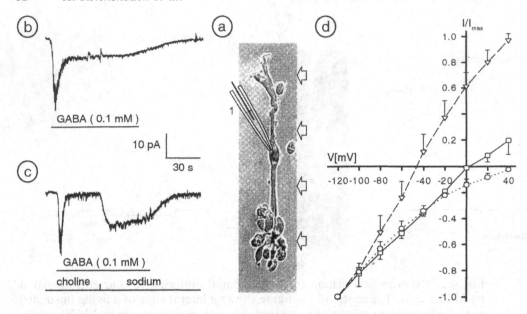

Fig. 4.3. GABA-evoked membrane currents in isolated human Müller cells. (a) A living, unstained isolated Müller cell is shown with the approximate localisation of the voltage-clamping micropipette (1) and the direction of GABA application (arrows). (b, c) current recordings from a human Müller cell exposed to GABA. (b) The first response under control conditions shows two parts, (i) a fast-desensitising transient response caused by activation of the $GABA_A$ receptor, and (ii) a sustained current generated by the GABA uptake carrier. (c) In Na^+-free solution, only the receptor-mediated response can be recorded; if Na^+ is re-supplied, the carrier current develops rapidly. (d) Current/voltage relationships of the receptor-mediated currents, in solutions with symmetrical ($E_{Cl} = -50$ mV; triangles) and asymmetrical $[Cl^-]$ ($E_{Cl} = +5$ mV; squares), respectively; the curve is shifted according to the Cl^- equilibrium potential. Under control conditions, exposure to GABA evokes Cl^- outward fluxes (i.e., positive inward currents by convention). For comparison, the I-V curve of the carrier current is shown (circles); this current shows no reversal potential. The receptor current was recorded in Na^+- and K^+-free solutions; the carrier current was isolated by block of the K^+ conductance by Ba^{2+}, and by block of the $GABA_A$ receptors by bicuculline. Own unpublished data (W. Reichelt and B. Biedermann).

see Figs. 4.3–4.4, Plates 1 and 2). Such Müller cell suspensions may either be purified and used for biochemical or radiochemical experiments, or fixed on glass slides and used for immunocytochemistry, autoradiography, or in-situ hybridisation. Single cells from such suspensions may also be sucked into micropipettes, and used for microbiochemistry (Sarthy and Lam 1978) or single-cell polymerase chain reaction (PCR). Furthermore, such single cells can be penetrated by conventional microelectrodes, or sealed to patch-clamp pipettes for single-channel

Table 4.1. *Evidence for receptor expression by Müller cells*

Signal molecule	Receptor subtype	Animal species	Biological effects/ demonstration	Source of data*
GABA	$GABA_A$	Skate	Depolarisation (Cl^- currents)[1]	aic
"	"	Baboon	Cl^- currents[2]	aic
"	"	Man	Cl^- currents[3]	aic
Glutamate	NMDA	Chick	↑ Cell proliferation[4]	cc
"	"	Man	↑ Cell proliferation[5]	cc
"	"	Chick	↑ AP-1 DNA binding[6]	cc
"	"	Man	↓ K^+ inward currents[7]	cc
"	AMPA/kainate	Chick	↑ AP-1 DNA binding[6]	cc
"	"	Rabbit	↑ $[Ca^{2+}]$[8]	cc
"	" GluR-1, -3, -4	Chick	(Molecular biology)[9]	cc
"	" GluR-4	Rat, goldfish	(Immunocytochemistry)[10]	ir
"	Metabotropic	Salamander	↓ K^+ inward currents[11]	aic
"	"	Man	↓ Cell proliferation[5]	cc
Dopamine	–	Salamander	↑ Membrane resistance[12]	aic
"	–	Salamander	↓ K^+ inward currents[11]	aic
"	D_2	Guinea pig	↓ K^+ inward currents[13]	aic
"	"	"	(Immunocytochemistry)[13]	ir, aic
"	"	Salamander, frog	(Immunocytochemistry)[14]	ir
Noradrenaline	–	Salamander	↑ Membrane resistance[12]	aic
"	β	Rabbit	↑ cAMP, ↑ glycogenolysis[13]	cc
"	α1	Rabbit	↑ Inositol phosphate[15,16]	cc
Carbachol	–	Rabbit	↑ Inositol phosphate[16]	cc
Thrombin	–	Man	↑ $[Ca^{2+}]_i$ ↓ K^+ currents[15]	cc
Substance P	–	Rabbit	↑ Inositol phosphate[18]	cc
VIP	–	Chick	↑ cAMP[19]	cc
Glucagon	–	Chick	↑ cAMP,[19] GS induction[20]	cc

Receptors for growth factors have recently been reviewed by Puro (1995).

*aic = acutely isolated cells, cc = cell culture, ir = intact retina.

[1]Malchow, Qian and Ripps (1989) [11]Schwartz (1993)
[2]Reichelt et al. (1996) [12]Henshel and Miller (1992)
[3]WR and B. Biedermann, unpublished results [13]Biedermann et al. (1995)
[4]Uchihori and Puro (1993) [14]Muresan and Besharse (1993)
[5]Ikeda and Puro (1995) [15]Osborne (1993)
[6]López-Colomé, Murbartián and Ortega (1995) [16]Osborne and Ghazi (1990)
[7]Puro (1995) [17]Puro and Stuenkel (1995)
[8]Wakakura and Yamamoto (1994) [18]Osborne and Ghazi (1989)
[9]López, López-Colomé and Ortega (1994) [19]Koh, Kyritsis and Chader (1984)
[10]Peng et al. (1995) [20]Moscona (1983)

studies or whole-cell voltage-clamp experiments. Finally, isolated Müller cells may be studied by ion- or substance-imaging techniques based on fluorescent dyes.

Another preparation to study properties of Müller cells is *cell culture*. In species with avascular retinae (or retinal regions), the entire glial cell population consists of Müller cells. Small pieces of this type of retinal tissue can be explanted in vitro.

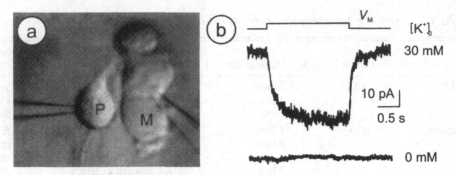

Fig. 4.4. Depolarisation-evoked release of glutamate generated by reversal of the Müller cell glutamate uptake carrier. (a) Release of glutamate from a Müller cell (M) is monitored by recording glutamate-evoked currents from an adjacent Purkinje cell (P). (b) Depolarising a Müller cell from -60 to $+20\,mV$ (top trace) evokes an inward current in the Purkinje cell (middle trace). The Purkinje cell current is generated by activation of its glutamatergic receptors. When extracellular K^+ is omitted (bottom trace), reversed glutamate transport by Müller cells is blocked and no glutamate current is recorded in the Purkinje cell. (Part (a) by courtesy of B. Billups and D. Attwell, (b) modified from Billups and Attwell 1996.).

If no particular effort is spent in supporting the adhesion and/or survival of neuronal cells, virtually all retinal neurons die within several days, and outgrowth from the explants will produce almost pure Müller cell cultures (Reichelt et al. 1989; Scherer and Schnitzer 1989). Under these conditions, the cells lose their characteristic morphology and form monolayers of flat polygonal cells. Certainly, functional changes occur as well. Nevertheless, Müller cell cultures have been successfully used for a variety of studies that required large numbers, or long-term observation, of monotypic cells.

4.2.2 The Role of Voltage-Dependent K^+ Channels for Extracellular K^+ Modulation

As mentioned above, light stimulation of the retina results in neuronal activation-evoked increases of $[K^+]_e$ in the two plexiform layers, and decreases of $[K^+]_e$ in the subretinal space (Karwoski and Proenza 1977; Steinberg, Oakley and Niemeyer 1980). These $[K^+]_e$ changes must be buffered rapidly in order to limit fluctuations in neuronal excitability. Müller cells remove excess K^+ from the extracellular space by uptake mechanisms such as the Na^+/K^+ pump (Reichenbach et al. 1992) as well as by a spatial buffering mechanism (Newman, Frambach and Odette 1984): K^+ currents enter the Müller cells in the two plexiform layers where $[K^+]_e$ is high, whereas K^+ efflux occurs into the vitreous humor (at the endfoot) and into the subretinal space where $[K^+]_e$ is decreased (cf. Fig. 4.9); in vascularised mammalian retinae, further K^+ efflux may occur where the Müller cells contact blood vessels. These spatial buffering currents pass through inwardly rectifying K^+ channels which (i) are the dominating conductivities of Müller cells, open at their physiological membrane potentials of -70 to -90 mV (Brew et al. 1986; Newman 1993; Chao et al. 1994a), (ii) mediate both inward and outward currents (Skatchkov, Vyklický and Orkand 1995), (iii) increase their conductance when $[K^+]_e$ is raised (Newman 1993), and (iv) show a peculiar non-uniform distribution over the Müller cell surface, with high densities at regions which may serve as sinks for spatial buffering currents. In amphibian species, 80–90% of all these K^+ channels are localised to the vitreal endfoot (Newman 1984, 1993; Brew et al. 1986). A similar distribution of K^+ conductivity has been observed in Müller cells from the avascular retina of the rabbit (Reichenbach and Eberhardt 1988), while in mammalian species with vascularised retinae, high K^+ conductance is localised to the vitread endfoot, soma, and, in cat, apical microvilli (Newman 1987).

When compared to extracellular diffusion, this K^+ siphoning (Newman, Frambach and Odette 1984) is estimated to reduce the half-time of K^+ clearance from the plexiform layers by 50–70% (e.g. Newman and Odette 1984; Eberhardt and Reichenbach 1987; Reichenbach et al. 1992). It may also prevent lateral spread of excitation, and, thus, improve visual acuity (Reichenbach et al. 1993).

Experimental studies demonstrate directly that K^+ siphoning is a key mechanism for $[K^+]_e$ homoeostasis. In amphibian species, light-evoked $[K^+]_e$ enhancements in the plexiform layers more than double (Oakley et al. 1992), and in cat, more than triple (Frishman et al. 1992) when K^+ siphoning currents are blocked by Ba^{2+} (Fig. 4.2, upper right). Likewise, the apical K^+ efflux from Müller cells (Fig. 4.2, lower left) plays an important role in buffering the light-evoked $[K^+]_e$ decreases in the subretinal space: when the glial K^+ channels are blocked by Ba^{2+}, the subretinal $[K^+]_e$ decreases are markedly prolonged, and increased in amplitude (Frishman et al. 1992; Oakley et al. 1992; Fig. 4.2, lower right).

In this context, it must be mentioned that the conductance of Müller cell inwardly rectifying K^+ channels can be modulated by physiological retinal neurotransmitters such as glutamate (Schwartz 1993; Puro et al. 1996) and dopamine (Biedermann et al. 1995), as well as by other factors such as thrombin which may be released into the retinal tissue under pathological circumstances (Puro and Stuenkel 1995). Thus, $[K^+]_e$ regulation by Müller cells seems to be under neuronal control. This may play an important role during dark adaptation, or during sleep (Galambos et al. 1994).

4.2.3 The Role of GABA$_A$-Receptor Coupled Cl$^-$ Channels for the Modulation of Extracellular Cl$^-$

In neuronal cells, activation of GABA$_A$ receptors causes an influx of Cl^- ions, and thus a hyperpolarisation of the membrane. In cases of intense inhibitory input, like that probably provided by horizontal cells in the outer plexiform layer, such Cl^- currents may even result in changes of the Cl^- distribution across the membrane, and thus in alterations of neuronal inhibitory mechanisms. It has been proposed that glial $GABA_A$ receptors, together with the outwardly directed driving force for Cl^- in glial cells, may serve a buffering function (Bormann and Kettenmann 1988). $GABA_A$ receptors were not found in Müller cells from many vertebrates studied (Reichelt and coworkers, unpublished results) but are present in cells from skate (Malchow, Qian and Ripps 1989) and from primates (Reichelt et al. 1996), including man (Fig. 4.3). It can be shown that activation of these receptors evokes outward currents which are diminished when the cytoplasmic side of the Müller cell membrane is equilibrated with a low Cl^- solution (Fig. 4.3). Thus, at least in the skate and primate retina, Müller cells are capable of performing extracellular Cl^- homoeostasis.

4.2.4 The Role of the GABA and Glutamate Uptake Carriers for the Regulation of Extracellular Neurotransmitter Concentrations

As shown in Fig. 4.3, Müller cells possess an electrogenic GABA uptake system. It has been found in skate (Qian, Malchow and Ripps 1993) as well as in all mammalian species studied so far (Biedermann, Eberhardt and Reichelt 1994). GABA is thought to be the inhibitory transmitter used by horizontal cells, even in those mammals where adult horizontal cells lack a GABA uptake system. In such mammals, the presence of an active glial GABA uptake carrier would be essential if the accumulation and spread of the transmitter in the extracellular space were to be avoided. GABA uptake by Müller cells has long been known to occur (Ehinger 1977; Sarthy 1982), although the demonstration of internalised GABA is impeded by rapid metabolism; it can be facilitated considerably by inhibition of cell metabolism (Barnett and Osborne 1995) or by inhibition of the enzyme GABA-transaminase (Neal et al. 1972; Cubbells, Walkley and Makman 1988). Of the different known molecular forms of the GABA carrier protein, GAT-3 has been shown to be expressed by Müller cells (Honda, Yamamoto and Saito 1995); the pharmacological properties of this molecule also correspond to the findings in Müller cells (Biedermann, Eberhardt and Reichelt 1994). The transport of GABA is electrogenic, as it involves the inward transport of excess Na^+ ions (Qian, Malchow and Ripps 1993; Biedermann, Eberhardt and Reichelt 1994); the stoichiometry of the cotransport is probably 2 Na^+ plus 1 Cl^- plus 1 GABA (Attwell, Barbour and Szatkovski 1993).

Glutamate uptake occurs by means of a glutamate carrier expressed by Müller cells (Ehinger 1977; Brew and Attwell 1987; Schwartz and Tachibana 1990). There exist several distinct molecular forms of the carrier protein; in Müller cells, the L-glutamate/L-aspartate transporter (GLAST) but not the glutamate transporter (GLT-1) has been demonstrated (Otori et al. 1994; Derouiche and Rauen 1995).

The stoichiometry of the carrier seems to be rather complex and has been a matter of controversy (Schwartz and Tachibana 1990). The group of Attwell devoted a series of studies to this question, and they concluded that an inward transport of 1 glutamate plus 2 Na^+ occurs for 1 K^+ (Barbour, Brew and Attwell 1991) plus 1 OH^- (Bouvier et al. 1992) moved outward. The finding that OH^- anions are outwardly transported demonstrates that the carrier generates extracellular alkalinisation. Because the transporter is electrogenic, glutamate uptake is voltage-dependent and cell depolarisation slows down or even reverses uptake of the excitatory amino acid (Szatkovski, Barbour and Attwell 1990; Fig. 4.4).

4.2.5 The Role of the Na^+/HCO_3^- Cotransporter and of Carbonic Anhydrase in Extracellular pH Modulation

Müller cells contain large stores of carbonic anhydrase, an enzyme that catalyses the hydration of carbon dioxide to carbonic acid (reviewed by Moscona 1983), and seems to be essential for limiting activity-induced extracellular pH changes in the retina (Borgula, Karwoski and Steinberg 1989). Moreover, their cell membrane contains an electrogenic Na^+/HCO_3^- cotransport system, with a stoichiometry of 3 HCO_3^- transported along with 1 Na^+ (Newman 1991). As these cotransporters are concentrated in the basal endfoot membrane of Müller cells, they may be utilising the large volume of the vitreous body as a means of stabilising extracellular pH in the retina. Newman (1994) proposed a mechanism of 'CO2 siphoning' by Müller cells (analogous to K^+ siphoning). Neuron-derived CO_2 diffuses into the Müller cells, where it is rapidly converted by the carbonic anhydrase into H^+ and HCO_3^-; the latter is transported into the vitreous body by the Na^+/HCO_3^- cotransport system of the endfoot membrane (Newman and Astion 1991), and H^+ might be removed by an adjacent Na^+/H^+ exchanger (E.A. Newman, unpublished results; see Fig. 4.6 and Plate 1, and Chapter 11).

4.3 Recognition of Neuronal Signals by Müller Cells

4.3.1 Sensors and Second Messengers

Several different classes of signals are released by activated retinal neurons, including, among others, neurotransmitter molecules, K^+ ions, electrical fields, and metabolic waste products such as CO_2. Neurotransmitter molecules are recognised by ligand-gated ion channels and other receptors of Müller cells. There is now sound evidence for the expression by Müller cells of receptors for glutamate, GABA, catecholamines, and several neuroactive peptides, hormones, and growth factors (Table 4.1). Increases in $[K^+]_e$ are 'detected' by the K^+ channels (immediate depolarisation) and Na^+/K^+ pumps (delayed hyperpolarisation: Reichenbach et al. 1992) of Müller cells. It has also been postulated that their Na^+ channels may act as 'sensors' of the field potentials caused by neuronal action potentials (Chao et al. 1994b).

In many cases, recognition of neuronal signals by membrane receptors of Müller cells is translated into activation of their second messenger systems. One exciting example is ligand-induced elevations of intracellular Ca^{2+}. These are caused by activation of receptors for glutamate (Wakakura and Yamamoto 1994) or adenosine triphosphate (ATP) (Keirstead and Miller, unpublished results). These phenomena have been studied in enzymatically isolated cells, using the calcium indicator Fura-2 and video imaging microscopy techniques. If an influx of extracellular Ca^{2+} ions was allowed, depolarisations evoked an increase in $[Ca^{2+}]_i$ throughout the length of the Müller cell. By contrast, in the absence of extracellular calcium, stimulation of the calcium signalling system triggered a long-latency, wave-like increase in $[Ca^{2+}]_i$ that began in the apical (sclerad) region of the cells and moved toward the endfoot (Keirstead and Miller 1995; Fig. 4.9, Plate 2). This reaction could be stimulated by high KCl-induced depolarisation as well as by agents that evoke release of calcium from intracellular stores, such as caffeine and ryanodine (Fig. 4.9, Plate 2).

In addition to the calcium system, several other second messenger systems are involved in the responses of Müller cells to neuron-derived ligands. These comprise the inositol phosphate system and the adenylate cyclase/cyclic adenosine monophosphate (cAMP) system (examples are shown in Table 4.1). Furthermore, G-proteins are probably involved in the pathway from D_2-dopamine receptor activation to control of K^+ channels.

4.3.2 Long-Term Adaptations to Functional States

Some of the above-mentioned signalling pathways may also serve to induce and/or to maintain cellular features or even fates. From a teleological point of view, it seems to be cogent that the capacity of a given Müller cell function is adjusted so as to meet the needs of its neuronal partners. Indeed, there are some data supporting this view. If cultured Müller cells were maintained in elevated $[K^+]_e$ for 24 h, their Na^+/K^+ pump activity was enhanced under standard conditions (Reichelt et al. 1989). On the other hand, degeneration of retinal neurons was found to cause reduced expression of glutamine synthetase (Härtig et al. 1995) and loss of K^+ inward currents (Pannicke et al. 1995; Skatchkov et al. 1996) in Müller cells (Fig. 4.5). It is presently unknown what signalling pathways may be involved in these regulatory processes.

There are many reports of Müller cell proliferation following retinal damage or detachment (e.g. Rentsch 1979; Erickson et al. 1983; Anderson et al. 1986). The factors that trigger this proliferation are not yet known, but there are likely to be several, because Müller cells in vitro can be stimulated to divide by a variety of

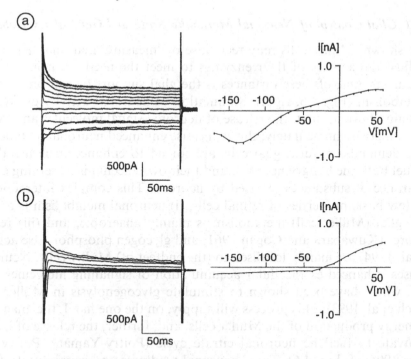

Fig. 4.5. Whole-cell current recordings from dissociated human Müller cells, in response to hyperpolarising and depolarising voltage steps. In cells isolated from control retinae (a), large K^+ dependent inward currents were always recorded; in the vast majority of cells isolated from pathologically altered retinae (b), these inward currents were strongly reduced or even missing. Own unpublished results (W. Reichelt, T. Pannicke and M. Francke).

growth factors, as well as by substances potentially released by dying neurons, such as glutamate and K^+ (for a recent review, see Puro 1995). The converse is also possible, as both the development and the survival of retinal neurons are known to depend on growth factors derived from Müller cells.

4.4 Discussion

In this section, we will discuss the above-mentioned data, as well as additional data from the literature, in the context of glial effects on the functioning of neuronal information processing. These effects will be focussed into three aspects, (i) maintenance of neuronal functional capacity, (ii) modulation of synaptic efficacy, and (iii) contribution to extrasynaptic information processing.

4.4.1 Glial Control of Neuronal Metabolic State and General Excitability

As we have shown, Müller cells may recognise or 'measure' neuronal activity in order to adjust the activity of their enzymes to meet the needs of neighbouring activated neurons. One of these instances is the glial support of neuronal carbohydrate metabolism (Fig. 4.6, right). Stimulation of neuronal activity evokes the following chain of events: first, the release of neuronal signal molecules and 'waste products' will increase immediately; this will cause enhanced neuronal metabolism and fuelling demands; in turn, glial cells are forced to enhance their metabolic activity to fuel both the hungry neurons, and their own mechanisms serving extracellular clearance of substances released by neurons. This complex interaction is based on a few basic properties of retinal cells, (i) neuronal metabolism is mainly aerobic, (ii) glial (Müller cell) metabolism is mainly anaerobic, and (iii) retinal glycogen stores (Kuwabara and Cogan 1961) and glycogen phosphorylase activity (Pfeiffer et al. 1994) are mainly localised to (the endfeet of) Müller cells. Neuronal activity causes enhanced extracellular accumulation of signalling molecules such as K^+ ions, which have been shown to stimulate glycogenolysis in Müller cells (Reichenbach et al. 1993). This process will supply, on the one hand, the anaerobic glycolytic energy production of the Müller cells, and, further, the release of lactate and/or pyruvate to fuel the neuronal citrate cycle (Poitry-Yamate, Poitry and Tsacopoulos 1995; cf. Fig. 4.6). Thus, neuronal readiness and capability to function crucially depend on the ability of Müller cells to recognise neuronal demands, and to adjust their release of metabolic fuel.

Moreover, neurons might suffocate in the CO_2 produced by their own aerobic metabolism if Müller cells did not express carbonic anhydrase, and perform efficient CO_2 export towards the vitreous body (see above, and left of Fig. 4.6). In a wide sense, every homeostatic function of glial cells is necessary to maintain neuronal function. Another example is the expression by Müller cells of CRABP (Bunt-Milam and Saari 1983); this protein is involved in the photopigment recycling of rod photoreceptor neurons (Bunt-Milam and Saari 1983), and, thus, essential for successful dark adaptation. Similar examples will be provided in the next sections. Here we want to emphasise that there is a wide range of glial 'service' functions; any deficiency of such functions will severely impair or even disrupt neuronal information processing. In another view, any qualitative or quantitative alteration of such glial functions may provide a specific and sensitive tool to modulate certain neuronal functions. For instance, even subtle changes in glial K^+ clearance activity may cause $[K^+]_e$ changes large enough to alter neuronal excitability.

4.4.2 Glial Control of Synaptic Transmission in the Neuronal Network

Müller cell processes ensheath all synapses in the two plexiform layers (e.g. Reichenbach et al. 1989), thus facing the synaptic clefts with their membranes

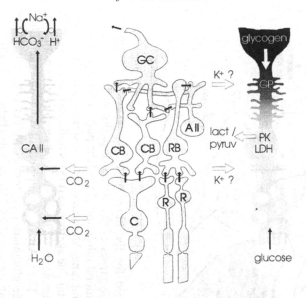

Fig. 4.6. Glial–neuronal interactions in carbohydrate metabolism. At the left and right margin of the figure, a Müller cell is drawn; the centre shows a simplified neuronal assembly containing a retinal ganglion cell (GC), a type II amacrine cell (A II), two different cone bipolar cells (CB), a rod bipolar cell (RB), as well as a cone (C) and two rod (R) photoreceptor cells. Synaptic circuits of the 'forward' information pathways of the neurons are indicated by small black arrows. Release of signals such as K^+ ions by activated neurons will activate the glycogen phosphorylase (GP) of Müller cells (right side), which results in enhanced glycogenolysis (and will induce enhanced glycolysis). By means of the glial-specific enzymes pyruvate kinase (PK) and lactate dehydrogenase (LDH), Müller cells release pyruvate and/or lactate which serves to fuel the Krebs cycle of the neurons (Poitry-Yamate, Poitry and Tsacopoulos 1995). The neuronal Krebs cycle produces CO_2 which, together with water, is taken up by Müller cells, and transformed into HCO_3^- and H^+ by their carbonic anhydrase. These ions are released primarily into the vitreous body by means of the Na^+/HCO_3^- cotransporter (and a Na^+/H^+ exchanger) in the Müller cell endfoot membrane; this process has been called 'CO$_2$ siphoning' (Newman 1991). Original.

(Sarantis and Mobbs 1992). In these membranes, Müller cells possess high affinity uptake sites for most neurotransmitters (see above) and by scavenging transmitters from synaptic clefts, they may control the time during which the transmitters are available to postsynaptic binding sites.

Moreover, the glial uptake of, e.g., glutamate is an important initial step in a process called neurotransmitter recycling (cf. right of Fig. 4.7). Glutamine synthetase, an enzyme which transamidates glutamate to glutamine, has been localised exclusively to Müller cells (reviewed by Moscona 1983). The glutamine synthesised by Müller cells is supplied to retinal neurons, as an essential precursor for their glutamate production; inhibition of the glial enzyme glutamine synthetase causes a

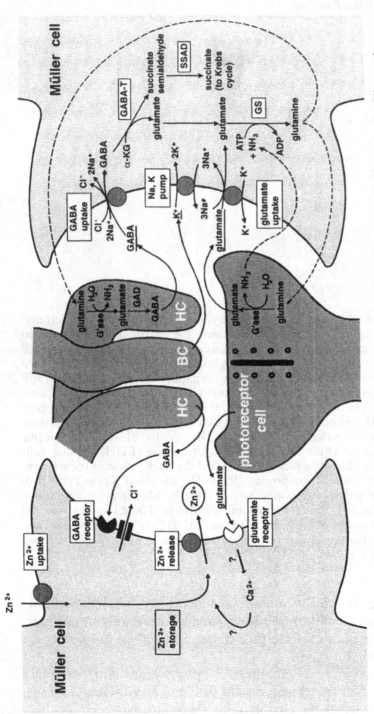

Fig. 4.7. Müller cell modification of synaptic transmission, exemplified for the outer plexiform layer. The excitatory transmitter glutamic acid (glut) is released by the (photoreceptor cell) synapses of the 'forward' pathway. The inhibitory transmitter GABA is used by the (horizontal cell) synapses mediating lateral inhibition. The right part of the figure shows the uptake carriers for both transmitters, localised in the Müller cell membrane. Moreover, the transformation of the active transmitter substances into the inactive substance glutamine by glial glutamine synthetase (GS) is indicated, as a part of the transmitter recycling system (as well as the detoxification pathway for ammonia). The presence of receptors for both types of transmitters in Müller cells is indicated in the left part of the figure. The $GABA_A$ receptor-coupled Cl^- channels allow for Cl^- outfluxes that may buffer Cl^- influxes into neuronal cells. The glutamate receptors of Müller cells may trigger various events. A hypothetical candidate is the release of Zn^{2+} ions that are stored by Müller cells (Behrens, Kadner and Wagner 1996), and may modulate neuronal ion channels. ADP, adenosine diphosphate; ATP, adenosine triphosphate; G'ase, glutaminase; GABA-T, GABA transaminase; GAD, glutamic acid decarboxylase; SSAD, succinic acid semialdehyde dehydrogenase; α-KG, α-ketoglutarate; HC, horizontal cell process; BC, bipolar cell dendrite. Original.

complete loss of neuronal function (Pow and Robinson 1994, and Chapter 5). Similar crucial recycling pathways seem to exist for other transmitter substances (reviewed by Reichenbach and Robinson 1995b).

There are several other ways in which Müller cells modify synaptic transmission. For instance, the function of neuronal GABA$_A$ receptors, as well as of other ligand- and voltage-gated ion channels, is known to depend strongly on Zn^{2+} ions (Harrison and Gibbons 1994). Recently, it has been demonstrated in fish retina that retinal Zn^{2+} stores are essentially restricted to Müller cells (Behrens, Kadner and Wagner 1996; Fig. 4.8). Thus, if there are conditions resulting in (different levels of) Zn^{2+} release by Müller cells, the cells may exert strong control of the efficacy of GABAergic transmission, and, thus, of lateral inhibition. It has already been mentioned that Cl^- release by Müller cells after stimulation of their own GABA$_A$ receptors may be necessary to maintain Cl^- concentration gradients, sufficient to support neuronal inhibition.

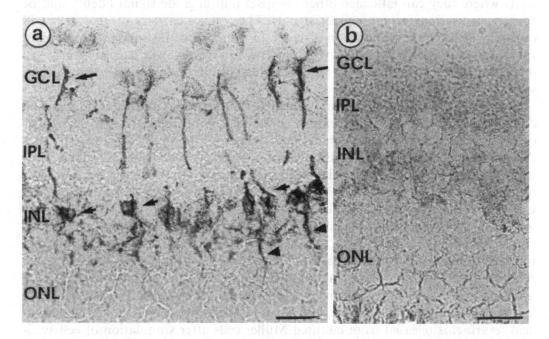

Fig. 4.8. (a) Histochemical demonstration of Zn^{2+} stores (modified Neo-Timm method) in Müller cells of the fish retina (courtesy of U. D. Behrens). Dark adapted goldfish retinae were incubated in Na$_2$S in phosphate buffered saline; cryosections were used for physical development. (b) The specificity of Zn^{2+}-staining was established in control sections after acid treatment which abolished the reaction product. Short arrows point to Zn^{2+}-positive Müller cell bodies in the inner nuclear layer (INL); long arrows show the endfeet, arrowheads the distal processes of Zn^{2+}-positive Müller cells. Calibration bars: 20 mm.

In this context, it should be recalled that the conductivity of glial inward rectifier K^+ channels, mediating spatial buffering of extracellular K^+ ions, is under control of neurotransmitters such as glutamate (Schwartz 1993) and dopamine (Biedermann, Eberhardt and Reichelt 1994). This means that synaptic release of, e.g. glutamate, may stimulate glial receptors, inhibit the spatial buffering K^+ currents, and finally cause elevated $[K^+]_e$ which, in turn, will depolarise the neuronal cell membranes and enhance the glutamate-induced excitation.

4.4.3 Glial Control of and Contribution to Extrasynaptic Signal Transmission

It has been shown in the preceding sections that Müller cells are not only able to recognise neuronal signals, but also to control the propagation of such signals through the extracellular space. The high density of synapses in both plexiform layers creates a high probability of diffusion of neurotransmitters out of synaptic clefts where they can influence other synapses and degrade signal fidelity and/or cause sensitisation for subsequent signals. The uptake carriers of glial cells will normally restrict the volume or distance in which the transmitter can spread. Inhibition of the activity of these transporters, however, may be caused by changes in membrane potential or pH, that will then result in enhanced extrasynaptic spread of the neurotransmitter.

Further, there is accumulating evidence of signalling pathways originating directly from Müller cells. Release of preloaded, labelled GABA from Müller cells has been observed after stimulation by high $[K^+]_e$, veratridine, or ethylenediamine (Sarthy 1983). The GABA release induced by both high $[K^+]_e$ and veratridine appears to be caused by depolarisation (in the latter case, via activation of tetradotoxin (TTX)-sensitive Na^+ channels), and to involve entry of extracellular Ca^{2+} by voltage-sensitive Ca^{2+} channels. By the same kind of mechanism, preloaded, labelled glycine is also released by Müller cells (Sarthy 1983). In contrast, ethylenediamine-induced GABA release is Ca^{2+}-independent, and seems to be due to a carrier-mediated homoexchange (Sarthy 1983). Similarly, glutamate may be released from Müller cells by a non-vesicular process involving the glutamate uptake carrier; such outward currents were evoked by high $[K^+]_e$- induced depolarisations (Szatkovski, Barbour and Attwell 1990). Another neuroactive amino acid, taurine, is released from cultured Müller cells after stimulation of cell swelling by high $[K^+]_e$ or hypo-osmotic solutions, as well as by application of ammonia, in a swelling-independent manner (0.25–5 mM; Faff-Michalak et al. 1994). Finally, it appears to be possible that a particular neuroactive signalling molecule, nitric oxide, can be released by activated Müller cells. Müller cells have been shown to express nitric oxide synthase at least in some species, or under particular conditions (Liepe et al. 1994; Dighiero et al. 1994; Huxlin 1995), albeit NO release by Müller cells has not yet been demonstrated, and nothing is known about mechanisms that might stimulate such a release. The release of GABA, glycine, or taurine by Müller cells may exert an inhibitory effect on the surrounding neurons, whereas glial release of glutamate or K^+ will evoke their excitation. Thus, these (and other) substances may act as 'gliotransmitters' involved in processes of plasticity of neuronal pathways, such as adaptation to various levels of background illumination.

Beyond this, it should also be noted that Müller cells possess several potential mechanisms for information propagation that might act in parallel to the neuronal 'forward' signalling chain directed from outer retina (where the photoreceptor cells recognise the light stimuli) to the inner retina (where the information is encoded by retinal ganglion cells, before it is sent to the brain). These are (i) the currents mediating K^+ siphoning, (ii) the Ca^{2+} waves, and perhaps (iii) the transport of HCO_3^- ions involved in CO_2 siphoning. If compared with synaptic transmission, particularly along the multisynaptic rod pathway, spatial buffering K^+ currents arrive certainly faster in the inner retina (left of Fig. 4.9). For the amphibian optic tectum where similar radial glial cells occur, it has been speculated that such a redistribution of K^+ ions may (slightly) depolarise the neurons at the end of the synaptic pathway before the 'regular' signal arrives; this mechanism might

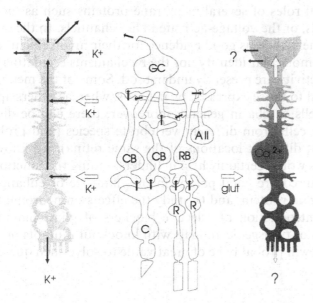

Fig. 4.9. Hypothetical long-range signalling by Müller cells. Abbreviations as in Fig. 4.6. The left part of the figure shows spatial buffering K^+ currents, with K^+ influxes in the plexiform layers, and outfluxes of K^+ into both the vitreous body and the subretinal space. The right part of the figure symbolises the Ca^{2+} waves which arise in the sclerad part of Müller cells and travel towards the endfoot. These waves may trigger the release of, as yet unknown, signalling molecules. Original.

generate some sensitisation or facilitation of signal transmission (Laming 1989a, 1992). By contrast, the Ca^{2+} waves (right of Fig. 4.9) are much slower than synaptic transmission. Further, their occurrence probably requires a certain threshold level of retinal stimulation. Thus, we may imagine these Ca^{2+} waves as rather rare, slow events which might be involved in some long-term regulation of neuronal signalling (see, e.g. Leibowitz 1992; Smith 1992).

Müller cells are also involved in 'lateral' intercellular signalling networks; amphibian (frog and toad) Müller cells are interconnected by gap junctions (Uga and Smelser 1973) that permit extensive electrical coupling (Attwell, Brew and Mobbs 1986). Mammalian Müller cells display gap-junctional coupling to astrocytes (Robinson et al. 1993). Presently, any functional interpretation of these findings must remain highly speculative.

4.5 Future Perspectives

The data presented in this chapter suggest that on different time scales, glial–neuronal signalling may be intimately involved in development, function, and pathology of the retina. Nevertheless, there remain many open questions with respect to properties and functions of Müller cells. For instance, nothing is known about the functional rôles of several membrane proteins such as the out-ward-rectifying K^+ channels, or the voltage-activated Na^+ channels. In the case of inward-rectifying K^+ channels, there is good evidence for their involvement in K^+ clearance, but neither their molecular identity nor the mechanisms regulating their expression and their conductivity are presently understood. Some of the membrane proteins seem to be identical to those expressed by neurons, whereas others appear to be specific for Müller cells or glia in general; moreover, there can be distinct differences between Müller cells from different vertebrate species (and probably also between Müller cells at different locations of the same retina). To know the reasons for these differences would certainly help in understanding the functions of Müller cells. What are required are good paradigms to eliminate or enhance the activity of a given specific glial protein, and to study the effects on neuronal function and behaviour. The introduction of selective blockers of glial channels or carriers, and the generation of transgenic animals with knockout mutants or over-expression of certain genes, will probably be of great value to solve such questions.

Acknowledgements

The authors wish to thank E. A. Newman (Minneapolis) and P. Laming (Belfast) for critical comments, D. Attwell and B. Billups (London), U. Behrens and H.-J. Wagner (Tübingen), and B. Biedermann and M. Francke (Leipzig) for their per-mission to use unpublished data, and J. Grosche (Leipzig) for his advice in com-puter graphics.

5

Metabolic Trafficking Between Neurons and Glia

STEPHEN R. ROBINSON, ARNE SCHOUSBOE,
RALF DRINGEN, PIERRE MAGISTRETTI,
JONATHAN COLES and LEIF HERTZ

Summary

In order to understand potential involvement of glia in behaviour, it is necessary to know about metabolism in neurons and glial cells and about the transfer of metabolites between the two cell types (metabolic trafficking). The present chapter provides such information. Only limited information can be obtained from experiments using intact brain tissue, necessitating the use of several different model systems, which are described in some detail. The reliability of the individual model systems is greatly supported by the fact that widely different models have provided analogous, although not always identical results.

The best studied metabolic interactions between neurons and glia are those involved in the metabolism of glutamate and γ-aminobutyric acid (GABA), and in the supply of precursors for these amino acid transmitters. Glial cells, and especially astrocytes, are indispensable for de novo formation of glutamate and GABA precursors from glucose and for the clearance and metabolism of these transmitters after their release from neurons. Metabolic trafficking seems also to occur during the degradation of glucose for the generation of energy.

When neurons are dependent on glia for metabolites or precursors of amino acid transmitters, they are vulnerable to changes in glial metabolism. This fact has been elegantly demonstrated in studies that have shown that inhibition of specific metabolic steps occurring only in glia has pronounced behavioural consequences. These effects can be reversed when the inhibited reaction is bypassed by administration of its endproduct. Such studies provide a firm biochemical basis for understanding the ways in which glia contribute to behaviour.

5.1 Introduction

A thorough knowledge of metabolic pathways in neurons and glia makes it possible to interfere with neuronal–glial interactions via drugs which act at very specific metabolic steps. Subsequently, these drugs can be tested in behavioural paradigms. Some of the drugs that act exclusively on glia have been found to exert profound behavioural effects, thereby allowing the unequivocal conclusion that metabolic reactions occurring in glia are essential for certain behaviours.

The neuronal–glial interactions which will be described in this chapter are associated with the metabolism of glucose. Glucose is the only nutrient which both is present in the systemic circulation at high concentrations and readily crosses the blood–brain barrier into the central nervous system. Some reactions in the metabolism of glucose do not take place in both cell types. Such metabolic compartmentation necessitates the transport of metabolites from one cell type, to another where they are utilised as substrates. Such interactions have been called 'metabolic trafficking' (Tildon 1993).

Glucose is not only needed for generation of energy [in the form of adenosine triphosphate (ATP)], but also for the production of a diverse range of metabolites, including the neurotransmitters glutamate and GABA. Glutamate is the major excitatory transmitter in the mammalian central nervous system, while GABA is the major inhibitory transmitter. Strong evidence is found for the involvement of glutamate in learning, whereas much less work has been done with GABA (Chapter 15). Neurons have a considerable demand for new precursors of glutamate and GABA because only a proportion of glutamate released from glutamatergic neurons is re-accumulated by these neurons (possibly with considerable differences between subpopulations of glutamatergic neurons). The majority of glutamate released by neurons is taken up into adjacent glia. Part of the glutamate accumulated into astrocytes is converted to glutamine, which is subsequently released from astrocytes into the extracellular fluid (glutamine has no transmitter activity), where some is taken up by neurons, to be used as a precursor for glutamate synthesis (Hertz et al. 1992, 1996; Schousboe, Drejer and Hertz 1988; Schousboe et al. 1993).

5.2 Methods and Models Used for Investigating Metabolic Trafficking Between Neurons and Glia

5.2.1 Principles

Detailed information about neuronal and astrocytic metabolism in general, and metabolic interactions in particular, cannot be obtained from studies of intact brain tissue in vivo, as these studies do not allow measurements in single cells. Moreover, a large proportion of the volume of all grey matter is composed of 'neuropil' (Fig. 5.1), which consists of densely intermingled neuronal and glial processes (Peters, Palay and Webster 1991). Glial cells, mainly astrocytes, account for close to one half of the volume in the neuropil. Exchange of metabolites between different cell types in the neuropil is facilitated by the large surface area of the cell processes, and the neuropil is the site of increased energy metabolism during neuronal activity (Kadekaro, Crane and Sokoloff 1985).

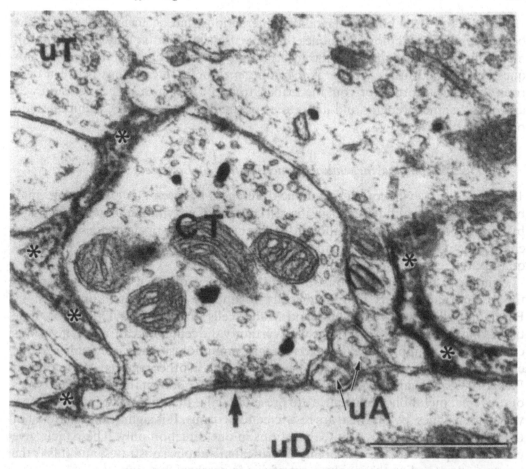

Fig. 5.1. Electron micrograph showing the ultrastructural organisation of a small section of the neuropil. The tissue has been labelled (gold particles) for tyrosine hydroxylase, a key enzyme in the production of the neurotransmitter noradrenaline, as well as being immunolabelled with a ligand that binds to β-adrenergic receptors. At the top left-hand corner there is an unlabelled terminal (uT). In the centre, there is a noradrenergic presynaptic terminal (CT) with prominent mitochondria and cytosolic staining for tyrosine hydroxylase (black grains). This terminal apposes a weakly labelled neuronal cell body in the upper right of the micrograph, an unlabelled dendrite (uD) at the bottom of the micrograph, and two unlabelled axons (uA; small arrows). The large arrow indicates a synapse between the noradrenergic terminal and the unlabelled dendrite. Throughout the remainder of its circumference, the terminal apposes astrocytic processes (indicated by asterisks), that are strongly labelled for the β-adrenergic ligand. This micrograph shows that even in a tiny portion of the neuropil, there are numerous potential routes for metabolic trafficking between neurons and glia. In addition, it demonstrates that glia are targets of noradrenergic terminals. Bar = 0.5 μm. (From Aoki and Pickel 1992a.)

In order to learn about the metabolic interactions that occur in the brain, it has been necessary to employ techniques that give us insights into many facets of brain metabolism. When combined, the information garnered by these diverse techniques has allowed firm conclusions regarding metabolic interactions between neurons and glia. In order for you, the reader, to appreciate how this conclusion was arrived at, some strengths and limitations of the different research techniques are briefly discussed below.

5.2.2 *Immunocytochemical Demonstration of Enzymes*

The most direct evidence for metabolic differences between glia and neurons may be demonstration of differences in the cell content of enzymes in intact brain tissue by immunocytochemistry. Although content of enzyme protein does not equal enzyme activity, such measurements provide qualitative information and semi-quantitative estimates of enzyme activities.

Immunocytochemical demonstration of enzymes is often performed on parts of the brain that possess morphologically distinctive glial populations, such as Bergmann glia in the cerebellum, and Müller cells in the retina. The use of these tissues makes it easier to determine with certainty the cellular localisation of various enzymes and amino acids. However, elegant immunohistochemical studies at the electron-microscopic level have also been carried out in other regions (Aoki, Joh and Pickel 1987; Aoki and Pickel 1992a). Such studies have shown that several enzymes of universal metabolic importance are present in glia, but are absent from neurons; very few enzymes, by contrast, are restricted to neurons. It is significant that most of the glial-specific enzymes catalyse reactions in one direction only. These facts give glia a monopoly over the availability of critical metabolic substrates, and this is the key to understanding the involvement of glia in cerebral function.

5.2.3 *Autoradiographic Determination of Rates of Glucose Utilisation*

The 2-[^{14}C]deoxyglucose method allows the calculation of metabolic rates by determining the rate at which radioactive 2-deoxyglucose is accumulated and trapped intracellularly as 2-deoxyglucose-phosphate, which for all practical purposes is not metabolised further (Sokoloff et al. 1977; Dienel and Cruz 1993). This method has been able to distinguish between energy metabolism in neuronal somata and in the neuropil (Kadekaro, Crane and Sokoloff 1985), but its resolution of about 100 μm is generally not high enough to provide information about events in individual cells.

5.2.4 *Metabolism in Model Systems*

On account of the shortcomings of the in vivo methods, model systems made up of one specific cell type are commonly used. Primary cultures (i.e. cultures of cells obtained directly from an animal) consisting of glia (commonly astrocytes) or neurons (commonly glutamatergic or GABAergic) have provided detailed and consistent information about metabolism in these cells. Studies using highly homogenous cultures of one cell type (monotypic cultures) have been of great importance in delineating how each of the different cell types react metabolically, how they may interact (which in some cases has also been studied in neuronal–astrocytic co-cultures), how these interactions can be disturbed pharmacologically, and how such pharmacological impairments may be reversed.

It is important to characterise the model systems in order to ascertain how closely they resemble their in vivo counterparts. However, even if the cells appear to be perfectly normal and the cultures are highly homogenous, there are still differences between the situation in culture and in vivo. For example, about 15% of the neuropil in the brain is composed of extracellular space, whereas in vitro the volume of the incubation medium is orders of magnitude larger than the volume of the cultured cells, and it may serve as a sink for released metabolites. This difference may influence the uptake and release of many compounds of interest, as has been described for non-cultured tissue (Larrabee 1995). It should also be kept in mind that a consequence of establishing monotypic cultures is that the cells can only form synapses with their own kind. Thus, a glutamatergic culture is not only a preparation in which all the neurons release glutamate as their transmitter, but it is also a culture in which the cells receive only glutamatergic innervation.

Astrocyte cultures can be prepared with no neuronal contamination, provided well established techniques are used (Juurlink and Hertz 1985, 1992); however, most, if not all, cultures of neurons from the mammalian central nervous system do contain a small proportion (approximately 5% by volume) of glia. For some types of experiments, this glial contamination may be an important source of error. On the other hand, an absence of neuronal–glial contact may impair neuronal differentiation. It also drastically changes the morphology of the region where most neuronal–glial interactions occur: the neuropil. The cultures still contain a large amount of a neuropil-like structure (Peng, Juurlink and Hertz 1991), but instead of glial processes which are so prominent in the neuropil in vivo, the neuronal processes in the 'neuropil' in vitro are separated by large extracellular spaces. Thus, the paucity of glial elements in pure neuronal cultures is both their strength and weakness, and it is always necessary to relate observations made in vitro to the in vivo situation.

Although some differences are found between cultured astrocytes from different brain regions (Juurlink and Hertz 1993), these are often minor. Neuronal cultures, in contrast, vary widely metabolically from one preparation to another (e.g. glutamatergic cerebellar granule cell neurons versus GABAergic cerebral cortical interneurons [Peng, Zhang and Hertz 1994]). This may be a reflection of corresponding differences between the same neurons in situ. If so, the differences may reflect regional variability, differences between glutamatergic and GABAergic neurons, or differences between neurons expressing different kinds of receptors. On the other hand, the observed differences might be a tissue culture artifact, especially since the characteristics of cerebellar granule cells depend upon the precise culturing conditions (Peng and Hertz 1993). Therefore, it is not possible to draw any firm conclusions about metabolism in 'neurons' without specifying the type of neurons studied.

In spite of these shortcomings, primary cultures of neurons and astrocytes have provided a very powerful and efficient means of obtaining information about metabolism at the cellular level. For example, all conclusions about neuronal–glial interactions in glutamate metabolism drawn on the basis of results obtained with cultured cells (Schousboe, Drejer and Hertz 1988; Hertz et al. 1992) have held when tested in intact brain.

5.2.5 *Immunocytochemical Staining for Amino Acids*

One way of analysing metabolic fluxes at the cellular level in intact preparations is to inhibit a specific enzyme or uptake site. Immunocytochemistry can then be used to examine changes that occur in the amino acid contents of various cell types (Pow and Robinson 1994). Such studies have provided unequivocal indications of metabolic trafficking between neurons and glia in the intact nervous system. Due to their methodological complexity, these studies have up till now only been carried out in selected cases and their design has benefited greatly from information obtained from simpler systems, such as primary cultures. In contrast to tissue culture experiments, these experiments can be related to behaviour, for example by investigating if an altered supply of a metabolite to neurons is reflected by changes in signal transduction.

5.2.6 *Energy Metabolism in Retinal Cells*

The retina is part of the central nervous system, which can be used as an experimental model of the central nervous system (Ames and Nesbett 1981; Chapter 4). The honeybee retina has provided impressively clear-cut information in a series of pioneering investigations of neuron–glial interactions (Coles and Tsacopoulos 1981; Tsacopoulos 1995; Tsacopoulos and Poitry 1995). Thus, this is the only preparation in which it has been demonstrated that glucose is exclusively taken up into glial cells and not into neurons (Tsacopoulos et al. 1988). In bee retina, the increased metabolism in the photoreceptor neurons at the onset of stimulation causes pH changes in the extracellular space and in glial cells within 10 s. These changes in pH may be a reflection of processes involved in transferring a glucose metabolite to photoreceptors (Coles et al. 1996a). This illustrates the possibility of rapid and tight coupling between the metabolic pathways of the two cell types. However, being an invertebrate, the honeybee's retina is anatomically and physiologically different to that in vertebrates. For example, it has an inside-out organisation, and it receives its oxygen from the air, rather than from the systemic circulation, which has very little oxygen-carrying capacity (Osorio 1991).

Photoreceptor cells and Müller cells (a type of radial glia) have been dissociated from vertebrate retinae by enzymatic digestion, and both cell types seem to survive intact. It has also been possible to obtain Müller cells with adjacent photoreceptor cells still enclosed within Müller cell processes (Nilius and Reichenbach 1988). These preparations appear to have a great deal of potential for investigations into metabolic trafficking between neurons and glia, although the possibility of regional differences must be kept in mind.

5.2.7. Conclusion

The conclusion to be drawn from this brief survey of methodology is that it is not a simple task even to demonstrate that metabolic trafficking does occur between neurons and astrocytes in the normal, mammalian central nervous system. However, by combining evidence obtained using a multitude of different techniques it has, indeed, been possible to derive not only qualitative information but also semiquantitative data and to utilise this information in studies in vivo, including learning experiments.

5.3 Glucose Metabolism

5.3.1 Glycolysis

Glucose is a substrate containing six carbon atoms, which during glycolysis is broken down in the cytosol to two molecules of pyruvate (three carbon atoms) (Fig. 5.2). Only some of the intermediates between glucose and pyruvate are shown in the figure, but they are all phosphorylated and therefore do not easily leave the cell. Although the formation of pyruvate from glucose (glycolysis) yields only a small amount of energy (ATP), it appears that some important processes in the central nervous sytem are partly dependent upon glycolytically derived energy, not only in culture (Kauppinen et al. 1988) but also in the brain in vivo (Rosenthal and Sick 1992).

5.3.2 Glycogenolysis

Glucose can be stored as glycogen in a process which is regulated by certain transmitters, for example noradrenaline and vasoactive intestinal peptide (VIP) (Magistretti, Sorg and Martin 1993). Breakdown of glycogen (glycogenolysis) leads to the production of more ATP than glycolysis because the formation of glucose phosphate from glucose, but not from glycogen, requires energy. In the

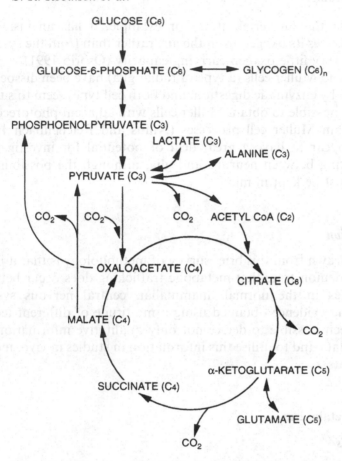

Fig. 5.2. Glucose metabolism: glucose, containing six carbon atoms, is completely degraded to CO_2 through glycolysis to pyruvate (three carbon atoms) and oxidative metabolism in the TCA cycle. Pyruvate is condensed with oxaloacetate (four carbon atoms) to form citrate (six carbon atoms); two CO_2 are released, and oxaloacetate is regenerated in one turn of the cycle; there is no net synthesis of any TCA cycle constituent. Pyruvate can also be condensed with CO_2 to provide net synthesis of oxaloacetate and it is interchangeable with lactate and alanine. Malate can leave the TCA cycle to form pyruvate, and phosphoenolpyruvate can be formed from oxaloacetate. α-Ketoglutarate can be used for synthesis of glutamate. The latter three reactions lead to leakage of TCA cycle constituents from the cycle, requiring synthesis of new TCA cycle intermediates.

mature central nervous system, glycogen is virtually restricted to astrocytes (Peters, Palay and Webster 1991; Hamprecht and Dringen 1994). Astrocytic glycogen can be subsequently broken down (glycogenolysis) by the astrocyte-specific enzyme, glycogen phosphorylase.

Central nervous system activity is correlated with an increased turnover of glycogen (Swanson et al. 1992). This includes at least some cases of learning

(O'Dowd et al. 1994a,b; Chapter 15). Since glycogen is virtually restricted to astrocytes, utilisation of glycogen indicates astrocytic participation in the ongoing activity. It might be argued that the astrocytic involvement amounts to no more than a supply of a metabolic substrate to neighbouring neurons. However, astrocytic glycogen is not converted to glucose, which is then released; instead it is converted in the astrocytes to glucose phosphate, and then via pyruvate to lactate which can be released (Dringen et al. 1993a). Energy production during the glycolytic phase is for the benefit of the astrocytes, whereas lactate after metabolic trafficking can be used as an energy substrate also by adjacent neurons.

The importance of glycogenolysis as an energy source must be in the short-term, since glycogen stores in the brain are depleted within minutes if glycogen serves as the only metabolic substrate. However, the breakdown of glycogen occurs so rapidly (twice as fast as glycolysis from glucose in mouse astrocytes exposed to elevated K^+ (Subbarao, Stolzenburg and Hertz 1995) that glycogen is an ideal substrate for the provision of large amounts of energy within a short time.

Glycogen can be synthesised not only from glucose but also from pyruvate, lactate, alanine or tricarboxylic acid (TCA) cycle constituents, like glutamate, in a gluconeogenic process (Dringen et al. 1993b; Huang, Shuaib and Hertz 1994; Schmoll et al. 1995a). Gluconeogenesis proceeds through the same intermediates as glycolysis (Fig. 5.2), but different enzymes are involved. One of these is fructose-1,6-biphosphatase, an enzyme that is restricted to glia (Schmoll et al. 1995b).

5.3.3 *Oxidative Metabolism*

Pyruvate can be readily and reversibly reduced to lactate in a reaction that is catalysed by lactate dehydrogenase. This process enables glycolysis to continue in the absence of oxygen, with the build-up of a high concentration of lactate, but it occurs even under oxygenated conditions, when cyclic metabolic processes, such as the malate–aspartate shuttle, are capable of transferring reducing equivalents from the cytosol to the mitochondria. Pyruvate can also be transaminated to alanine, by alanine aminotransferase. The reaction velocities for these conversions are sufficiently high, compared to the rates of generation and subsequent breakdown of pyruvate, that in most instances alanine, lactate and pyruvate can be regarded as interchangeable. It should, however, be kept in mind that the formation of alanine involves introduction of an amino group, as will be discussed in more detail later. Subsequent metabolism of lactate or alanine requires that these compounds are initially reconverted to pyruvate. The ratio between pyruvate and lactate reflects the cytosolic redox potential, and the lactate concentration is generally about 10-fold higher than the pyruvate concentration. In the central nervous system the extracellular concentration of lactate, measured by microdialysis, is approximately 1 mM, but it increases as a result of neuronal activity (Korf et al. 1993). The concentration of alanine in cerebrospinal fluid is 30–50 µM (Ferraro and Hare 1985; Roettger and Goldfinger 1991), but it might be higher in the extracellular fluid in brain (Fabricius, Jensen and Lauritzen 1993).

Pyruvate generated by glycolysis can be oxidised to carbon dioxide and water in the mitochondrial TCA cycle, producing a substantial amount of ATP. Initially, pyruvate is converted to acetyl coenzyme A (acetyl CoA), and the acetyl moiety (two carbon atoms) is condensed with the TCA cycle intermediate, oxaloacetate (four carbon atoms), to form citrate (six carbon atoms) (Fig. 5.2). Through a series of reactions, leading to the removal of two carbon atoms, oxaloacetate is eventually regenerated from citrate, while the two carbon atoms are completely oxidised and large amounts of ATP are produced by oxidative phosphorylation. In each turn of the cycle, two new carbon atoms are introduced and two carbon atoms are oxidatively degraded to CO_2. One molecule of oxaloacetate is consumed and one molecule of oxaloacetate is generated. Thus, there is no net production of TCA cycle intermediates. This cycling could continue indefinitely (as long as glucose is available and energy is required), except for the fact that the cycle is leaky: TCA cycle intermediates are used for the synthesis of other compounds.

In the central nervous system, the most important diversions of TCA cycle constituents are for the synthesis of glutamate and GABA, which can be formed from α-ketoglutarate (Fig. 5.3). Glutamate and the TCA cycle constituent α-ketoglutarate are rapidly interconverted in two different reactions: oxidative deamination/reductive deamination, and transamination. The former process is catalysed by glutamate dehydrogenase and ammonia is either added (for formation of glutamate) or removed (for conversion of glutamate to α-ketoglutarate). Other amino acids cannot be formed in a direct reaction between the corresponding ketoacid and ammonia. The most common transamination process is that between glutamate and oxaloacetate, yielding α-ketoglutarate and aspartate (or in the opposite direction glutamate and oxaloacetate). This transamination is catalysed by aspartate aminotransferase.

Glutamate can be transaminated with pyruvate, forming α-ketoglutarate and alanine, or alanine can be transaminated with α-ketoglutarate, forming glutamate and pyruvate. The former of these reactions is involved in the formation of alanine during glycolysis, the latter in the re-conversion of alanine to pyruvate for further oxidative metabolism. The latter reaction may also be important in synthesis of transmitter glutamate, where alanine may provide the amino group (but not the carbon skeleton) of glutamate.

Glutamate can be amidated to glutamine by the addition of ammonia (Fig. 5.3). This process requires energy (conversion of ATP to adenosine diphosphate (ADP)), and is catalysed by glutamine synthetase, which is present in glia (both astrocytes and oligodendrocytes) (Norenberg and Martinez-Hernandez 1979; D'Amelio, Eng and Gibbs 1990; Tansey, Farooq and Cammer 1991) but absent from neurons. Hydrolysis of glutamine to glutamate requires no energy and is catalysed by a different enzyme, phosphate-activated glutaminase (PAG). The

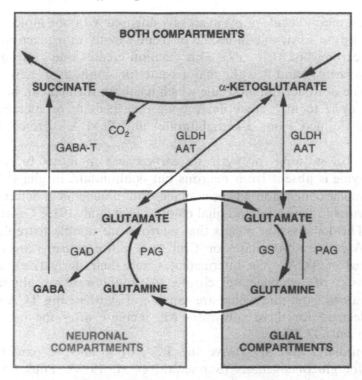

Fig. 5.3. Synthesis, release and metabolism of glutamate and GABA. The section of the TCA cycle from α-ketoglutarate to succinate is identical to Fig. 5.2. Glutamate can be formed from α-ketoglutarate in a reversible reaction catalysed by either GLDH (glutamate dehydrogenase) or AAT (aspartate aminotransferase). Glutamate can be formed from glutamate in an irreversible reaction, catalysed by GS (glutamine synthetase) and re-converted to glutamate in a likewise irreversible reaction, catalysed by PAG (glutaminase). GABA can be formed from glutamate in an irreversible reaction catalysed by GAD (glutamate decarboxylase) and metabolised to succinate in a likewise irreversible reaction, catalysed by GABA transaminase (GABA-T).

presence of this enzyme in both neurons and astrocytes was shown in primary cultures (Kvamme et al. 1982; Hogstad et al. 1988) and confirmed histochemically in intact tissue (Aoki et al. 1991; Würdig and Kugler 1991). Therefore, neurons cannot generate glutamine from glutamate, whereas both neurons and glia can form glutamate from glutamine (Fig. 5.3). GABA is produced by decarboxylation of glutamate, catalysed by glutamate decarboxylase, which only occurs in GABAergic neurons (Fig. 5.3). Glutamate is also used for synthesis of other compounds such as glutathione.

Due to the leakiness of the TCA cycle it is extremely important that pyruvate (or lactate or alanine) can be used for net production of new TCA cycle constituents. In this process, one molecule of pyruvate is condensed with one molecule of CO_2 (pyruvate fixation) to form one molecule of oxaloacetate, in a reaction catalysed by pyruvate carboxylase (Fig. 5.2). This reaction creates one molecule of oxaloacetate (but no energy) and it is the major route for synthesis of new TCA cycle constituents. The oxaloacetate molecule which has been formed can be converted in the TCA cycle to any other TCA cycle intermediate or metabolite, including glutamate (formed from α-ketoglutarate) and GABA (formed from glutamate) (Fig. 5.3).

Immunohistochemical staining for pyruvate carboxylase in intact brain has shown that this enzyme is absent from neurons but is abundant in glia (Shank et al. 1985), and a similar conclusion has been made from biochemical determination of enzyme activities in neuronal and glial cultures (Yu et al. 1983; Cesar and Hamprecht 1995). This localisation means that neurons are unable to replenish their supply of TCA cycle intermediates on their own. Since neurons are being continuously depleted of TCA cycle intermediates and their derivatives, there needs to be a transfer of oxaloacetate, citrate, α-ketoglutarate or glutamine (Figs 5.2, 5.3) to neurons from glia which are capable of synthesising TCA cycle constituents. The demand for these substrates will increase after the neuronal release of glutamate and GABA.

TCA cycle intermediates can also leave the TCA cycle and be oxidatively degraded or used for gluconeogenesis (Sonnewald et al. 1993). Thus, malate can exit the mitochondrial membrane and be converted to pyruvate in the cytosol (Fig. 5.2). This reaction is catalysed by cytosolic malic enzyme, which is restricted to glia (Kurz, Weisinger and Hamprecht 1993; McKenna et al. 1993). Studies using radioactively labelled acetate and glucose have shown that in the mouse brain, the formation of pyruvate from TCA cycle intermediates takes place predominantly in glia (Hassel and Sonnewald 1995). Pyruvate can be reintroduced into the TCA cycle via acetyl coenzyme A for complete degradation to CO_2 and water.

5.4 Neuron-Glia Interactions in Turnover of Glutamate and Glutamine

5.4.1 Metabolic Compartmentalisation in Vivo

Early papers showed that glucose metabolism in brain is not straightforward (e.g. Vrba 1962), and abnormal precursor–product relations for specific radioactivities in whole-brain tissue gave rise to the concept of a GABA–glutamate–glutamine cycle (for review of the older literature on metabolic compartmentalisation, see Hertz 1979), in which GABA is accumulated into astrocytes, converted to glutamine, and then returned to neurons as a precursor of GABA (Fig. 5.3). The concept of a GABA–glutamate–glutamine cycle received support from the finding that glutamine synthetase is a glial-specific enzyme.

5.4.2 Model Systems

Cell culture experiments have supported the existence of a glutamate–glutamine cycle by consistently showing: (1) uptake kinetics in neurons and astrocytes that favour astrocytic uptake of glutamate; (2) intense conversion of glutamate to glutamine in astrocytes; (3) release of glutamine from astrocytes; (4) uptake of glutamine into neurons; and (5) utilisation of glutamine as a precursor for neuronally released glutamate or GABA (Hertz et al. 1992; Peng et al. 1993; Schousboe et al. 1993). Cultured astrocytes also take up GABA, but since the release rates of GABA from GABAergic neurons and the uptake rates of GABA into astrocytes are several-fold lower than the corresponding rates for glutamate, the neuronal requirements for GABA precursors are probably much lower than for glutamate precursors.

The formation of glutamine from glutamate after its accumulation into astrocytes only requires glutamine synthetase activity. The formation of glutamine from GABA is more complex: first GABA is transaminated by GABA-transaminase (an enzyme concentrated in, but not confined to glia) to succinic semialdehyde. This in turn is converted to succinate, a TCA cycle constituent, which is then metabolised in the TCA cycle to α-ketoglutarate. The latter is further converted to glutamate and then amidated to glutamine (Figs 5.2, 5.3).

In order for glutamine supply to neurons by glia to match the amount of neuronally released glutamate and GABA taken up into astrocytes, all astrocytic glutamate and GABA should be converted to glutamine, none completely degraded to CO_2 and water (and thus removed from the system); no glutamine should be metabolised to glutamate (or CO_2) in astrocytes; all extracellular glutamine should be accumulated in neurons, none in astrocytes; and all glutamine accumulated into neurons should be converted to glutamate or GABA, and none oxidatively degraded. Cell culture experiments have shown that none of these prerequisites are met (Hertz et al. 1992; Peng et al. 1993; Schousboe et al. 1993; Sonnewald et al. 1993; Huang et al. 1994a,b): (1) glutamate leaves the TCA cycle as indicated by a pronounced formation of labelled lactate from labelled glutamate and is very actively metabolised to CO_2 and water in astrocytes, and in brain slices; (2) glutamine is converted to glutamate in astrocytes and is further metabolised to CO_2 and water, not only in astrocytes but also in neurons; (3) glutamine is not preferentially accumulated by neurons, and (4) glutaminase activity is not substantially higher in neurons than in astrocytes.

Given these diversions of neuronally released glutamate, the situation must be more complex than a simple glutamate–glutamine cycle. Specifically, new TCA constituents need to be generated so that they can serve as precursors for the synthesis of additional glutamate. Given that the synthesis of new TCA constituents is entirely dependent on the activity of the glial enzyme, pyruvate carboxylase (Yu et al. 1983; Shank et al. 1985; Kaufman and Driscoll 1992; Cesar and Hamprecht 1995), de novo synthesis of neuronal glutamate must be ultimately dependent on metabolic processes occurring in glia. There are several potential steps where new TCA intermediates can be released by glia for uptake by neurons. Citrate for example, is released in large amounts by cultured astrocytes. It is unclear, however, whether citrate is a viable precursor of neuronal glutamate, since it cannot be used for this purpose by cultured cerebellar granule cells (Westergaard et al. 1994). α-Ketoglutarate is also released from primary cultures of astrocytes (Westergaard, Sonnewald and Schousboe 1994). It is accumulated by highly regulated transport systems into synaptosomes (Lehmann, Kapkov and Shank 1993), and exogenous α-ketoglutarate is able to increase the glutamate release from brain slices. α-Ketoglutarate can also sustain transmitter release of glutamate in cultured glutamatergic cerebellar granule cells, if administered together with alanine (which in vivo may be supplied by astrocytes) to provide the amino group (Peng, Schousboe and Hertz 1991). Thus, exogenous α-ketoglutarate is a suitable glutamate precursor in experiments with a cultured glutamatergic neuron, but this does not necessarily mean that it is the only glutamate precursor travelling from astrocytes to neurons in the functioning brain.

5.4.3 Studies in Retina

The strongest evidence for the operation of a glutamate–glutamine cycle in the intact central nervous system comes from exposure of the isolated rabbit retina to methionine sulphoximine, a relatively selective inhibitor of the glial enzyme, glutamine synthetase. This drug completely depletes some retinal neurons (bipolar cells and ganglion cells) of glutamate, even when the incubation medium contains large amounts of glutamate and glutamine (Pow and Robinson 1994). This finding unequivocally shows that these neurons depend upon glutamine synthesis in their glial Müller cell neighbours for their entire supply of glutamate, and that they have no access to extracellular glutamate or glutamine, probably because the neurons are completely invested by glial processes (Reichenbach and Robinson 1995b). These findings have been confirmed in organotypic cultures of hippocampal slices (Laake et al. 1995), with the exception that extracellular glutamine could be utilised directly by the neurons, perhaps because the glial ensheathment is less extensive in hippocampal slices. It is in support of this concept that iontophoretically administered glutamine to brain tissue causes excitation of neurons expressing glutamatergic receptors.

In photoreceptor cells, methionine sulphoximine causes a substantial reduction, but not always a total depletion of intracellular glutamate (Pow and Robinson 1994). This difference from ganglion and bipolar cells probably reflects the fact that the photoreceptor cells protrude into the subretinal space, from which they may receive some of their glutamate by direct uptake from the extracellular fluid (Fig. 5.4). This interpretation is consistent with electrophysiological evidence that

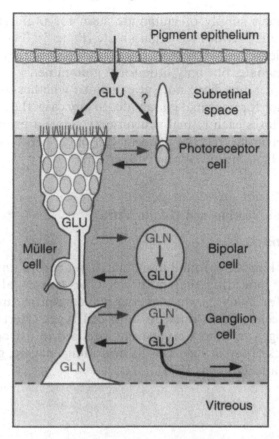

Fig. 5.4. Cartoon of glutamatergic pathways in the vertebrate retina. The Müller glial cells span the width of the retina, with processes extending into the subretinal space. Two glutamatergic neurons, bipolar cells and ganglion cells, receive all their glutamate by breakdown of glutamine supplied from Müller cells, and some of their released glutamate is accumulated into Müller cells. The photoreceptor cells receive some of their glutamate via Müller cell glutamine, but they may also accumulate some glutamate directly from the subretinal space. The ganglion cells send their output to the diencephalon.

the function of photoreceptors is inhibited by interfering with their uptake of glutamate (Yang, personal communication).

In an even more convincing experiment, rabbit retinae were incubated in medium containing only the non-physiological D-isomer of glutamate, which was absent from the tissue prior to incubation (Pow and Crook 1996). This isomer is transported by a glutamate uptake carrier and converted to D-glutamine by glutamine synthetase, which is not stereospecific. However, the subsequent hydrolysis of glutamine to glutamate by glutaminase can only take place with L-glutamine, not D-glutamine, as the substrate. Therefore, the neurons which depend upon astrocytic glutamine for their supply of glutamate stain for D-glutamine, supplied from adjacent Müller cells, but not for D-glutamate (Plate 3). The adjacent Müller cells must rapidly release the synthesised D-glutamine, since they stain intensely for accumulated D-glutamate, but only little for D-glutamine.

Immunocytochemical studies of retina have not yet examined whether α-ketoglutarate is an additional precursor for neuronal glutamate. In any case, the sheath of Müller cell processes that encloses each retinal neuron may act as a barrier to exogenous substrates, thereby ensuring that the neurons can only access α-ketoglutarate that has been released from neighbouring Müller cells.

5.5 Energy Metabolism of Neurons and Glia in Vitro

5.5.1 Enzymes and Substrates

Mitochondrial forms of creatine kinase are found in mammalian neurons and glia (Hemmer and Walliman 1993), indicating that both cell types are capable of oxidative metabolism. Staining for many enzymes in energy metabolism, and for glucose transporters has also been demonstrated in both cell types (Hertz and Peng 1992a). By contrast, glycogen is almost exclusively localised in astrocytes. It is abundant in primary cultures of astrocytes, as is its degrading enzyme, glycogen phosphorylase (Hamprecht and Dringen 1994).

5.5.2 Glycolysis

Neurons and astrocytes in primary cultures are both able to carry out glycolysis. Mouse astrocytes in primary cultures have even under non-stimulated conditions a glycolytic activity which is at least as high as the rate of glucose utilisation of the cerebral cortex in vivo (Cummins, Glover and Sellinger 1979; Pellerin and Magistretti 1994; Peng, Zhang and Hertz 1994), and twice as high as the mean rate of glucose utilisation in cerebellar granule cells. Some important energy-requiring processes in rodent astrocytes, like uptake of potassium ions (K^+) and glutamate, depend upon glycolytically derived ATP rather than on oxidatively generated ATP, not only in culture (Kaupinnen et al. 1988; Huang et al. 1994a), but also in vivo (Rosenthal and Sick 1992). Production of labelled CO_2 from glucose requires initial glycolysis, producing enough labelled pyruvate for further oxidative metabolism (Fig. 5.2). Cultured astrocytes release a substantial amount of lactate into the medium, leading to an accumulation of lactate in the millimolar range within a couple of hours (Hertz, Drejer and Schousboe 1988; Walz and Mukerji 1988). The production of pyruvate must proceed very quickly, since production of labelled CO_2 from [U-^{14}C] glucose increases rectilinearly from the time astrocyte cultures are exposed to the radioisotope (L. Peng and L. Hertz, unpublished experiments).

Table 5.1. *Changes in rates of glycolysis, glycogenolysis and oxidative metabolism in neurons and astrocytes in response to glutamate, potassium and noradrenaline. Large arrow: pronounced stimulation; small arrow: less pronounced stimulation; small arrow in parenthesis: possible small stimulation; dash: no effect. For references, see text*

	ASTROCYTES			NEURONES		
	Glycolysis	Glycogen breakdown	Oxidative metabolism	Glycolysis	Glycogen breakdown	Oxidative metabolism
Elevated K⁺	↑	⬆	No change	↑	No change	⬆
Elevated glutamate	⬆	No change	No change	(↑)	No change	⬆
Elevated noradrenaline	↑	⬆	⬆	No change	No change	No change

As indicated in Table 5.1, glucose utilisation in cultured astrocytes is stimulated to a modest degree by an elevation of the K^+ concentration (Cummins, Glover and Sellinger 1979; Peng, Zhang and Hertz 1994) and by noradrenaline (Subbarao and Hertz 1990a; Hertz 1992; Yu et al. 1993). It can be greatly increased by extracellular glutamate (Pellerin and Magistretti 1994; Takahashi et al. 1995). The increase in glucose utilisation by either glutamate or elevated K^+ is mirrored by an enhanced release of lactate (Walz and Mukerji 1988; Pellerin and Magistretti 1994). It is not a result of stimulation of glutamate receptors, but reflects the increased energy demand for active uptake of glutamate.

The increase of glycolysis in astrocytes by glutamate and excess K^+ is secondary to stimulation of Na^+/K^+-ATPase activity, and in both cases it is blocked by the Na^+/K^+-ATPase inhibitor, ouabain (Pellerin and Magistretti 1994; Peng, Juurlink and Hertz 1996). Elevated K^+ might directly stimulate the extracellular potassium-sensitive site of this enzyme (Hajek, Subbarao and Hertz 1996). The stimulation by glutamate is exerted at the intracellular, sodium-sensitive site of the Na^+/K^+-ATPase and is secondary to active glutamate uptake coupled to sodium entry (Pellerin and Magistretti 1994).

Glucose utilisation in glutamatergic granule cells (but not in all types of neurons) can be increased by an elevation of extracellular K^+, but not appreciably by glutamate or noradrenaline (Peng, Zhang and Hertz 1994; L. Peng and L. Hertz, unpublished experiments). The extracellular concentrations of K^+ and glutamate are elevated during activation of a given cortical area, for example by sensory stimulation, and during seizures (see Walz and Hertz 1983; Magistretti, Pellerin and Martin 1995). The stimulation of glycolysis by glutamate and elevated K^+ couples neuronal activity directly with glucose utilisation. Since the increase in glucose utilisation occurs mainly in glia, these cells are likely to be the predominant source of the 2-deoxyglucose signal detected in autoradiographic or positron emission topography (PET) studies during activation (Magistretti, Pellerin and Martin 1995). This may also apply to the increase in 2-deoxyglucose uptake that occurs during a certain stage of the Gibbs–Ng one-trial aversive learning task (Sedman et al. 1992; Chapter 15).

5.5.3 Glycogenolysis

Since little, if any, glycogen is present in neurons, no stimulated glycogenolysis occurs in these cells. In astrocytes, glycogenolysis is stimulated by K^+-induced depolarisation. This response has been observed in a variety of preparations including retinal Müller cells (Reichenbach et al. 1993), brain slices (Hof, Pascale and Magistretti 1988) and cultured astrocytes that have been treated with dibutyryl cyclic adenosine monophosphate (cAMP) (Subbarao, Stolzenburg and Hertz 1995). In the latter preparation potassium-stimulated glycogenolysis proceeds twice as fast as glycolysis. At least in cultured astrocytes, the glycosyl units of glycogen are released as lactate (formed from pyruvate), not as glucose (Dringen, Gebhardt and Hamprecht 1993a). This means that energy derived from glycolysis must be utilised by the astrocytes themselves. Energy produced during subsequent oxidative metabolism could be available not only for astrocytes but also for neurons, provided there is metabolic trafficking of lactate from astrocytes to neurons.

Certain neurotransmitters, including noradrenaline, VIP, adenosine and serotonin bind to astrocytic receptors (Fig. 5.1) and potently evoke glycogenolysis in cultured astrocytes (Subbarao and Hertz 1990b; Sorg and Magistretti 1991; Chen et al. 1995). Many of the same transmitters also stimulate formation of glycogen; this a long-term effect, and it is dependent on protein synthesis (Sorg and Magistretti 1992; Magistretti, Pellerin and Martin 1995).

5.5.4 Oxidative Metabolism

CO_2 production from glucose in astrocytes is not stimulated by extracellular glutamate or by elevated extracellular K^+, although there may be a brief stimulation of oxygen consumption followed by a drop below the resting level (Peng, Zhang and Hertz 1994; L. Peng and L. Hertz, unpublished experiments).

Noradrenaline stimulates virtually all steps of oxidative metabolism of glucose in astrocytes (Subbarao and Hertz 1991; Huang et al. 1994b), but glutamate does not. Pyruvate carboxylation, which occurs only in astrocytes, increases during exposure to an elevated K^+ concentration (Kaufman and Driscoll 1992). The extent of this increase is almost as large as the K^+-induced increase in glycolysis, but is far smaller than the stimulation of glycogenolysis by elevated K^+. Neither noradrenaline (Chen 1995) nor glutamate (Kaufman and Driscoll 1992) has an effect on pyruvate carboxylation.

Neuronal function, including electrophysiological activity in brain slices is readily maintained with either glucose or pyruvate/lactate as the substrate (Larrabee and Horowicz 1956; Schurr, West and Rigor 1988; Izumi et al. 1994). Cultured cerebellar granule cells have a rate of oxidative metabolism which is comparable to that of astrocytes. Their rate of glycolysis is somewhat higher than their rate of oxidative metabolism, but lower than the rate of glycolysis in astrocytes (Peng, Zhang and Hertz 1994). Cultured granule cells resemble astrocytes in the fact that they release pyruvate/lactate into the incubation medium, but they do so at about half of the rate. Furthermore, during exposure to radioactive glucose there is no release of labelled CO_2 from cultured granule cells during the first 15 min (Peng, Zhang and Hertz 1994). This delayed appearance of labelled CO_2 has been confirmed by Takahashi et al. (1995), and is in contrast to the immediate appearance of labelled CO_2 from cultured astrocytes (see above).

Elevated K^+ concentrations stimulate CO_2 production from glucose, lactate and pyruvate in glutamatergic granule cells to an even greater extent than they stimulate glycolysis (Peng, Zhang and Hertz 1994). The glutamate receptor agonist, kainate, causes a huge increase in the rate of oxidative metabolism in primary cultures of cortical neurons (Frandsen, Quistorff and Schousboe 1990). By contrast, no stimulatory effect of noradrenaline on oxidative metabolism has been demonstrated in neurons (Subbarao and Hertz 1990b).

5.6 Metabolic Trafficking Between Neurons and Glia

5.6.1 Studies in Retina

A unique feature of the honeybee retina is that it has been clearly demonstrated that metabolite transfer from glial cells to neurons is obligatory for the maintenance of neuronal function (Coles and Tsacopoulos 1981; Tsacopoulos, Coles and Van de Werve 1987; Tsacopoulos et al. 1988). The link between glycolysis and oxidative metabolism in the photoreceptors is a transfer of the pyruvate metabolite, alanine (Tsacopoulos et al. 1994; Tsacopoulos and Poitry 1995), which is present in the extracellular space in extremely high concentrations (Cardinaud et al. 1994). Formation of alanine from pyruvate probably occurs in a transamination with glutamate, which in the transamination process is converted to α-ketoglutarate. Glutamate is, in turn, regenerated from α-ketoglutarate by reductive amination with NH_3, accumulated from the extracellular space (Tsacopoulos 1995; Coles et al. 1996a).

The situation is different in the mammalian retina, since isolated guinea-pig photoreceptors in vitro can utilise either glucose (which they in vivo may receive from the systemic circulation), or lactate (Poitry-Yamate, Poitry and Tsacopoulos 1995). It is highly likely that lactate is normally transferred from Müller cells to photoreceptors because the release of lactate into the incubation medium is substantially lower when photoreceptors remain attached to the Müller cells than when the two cell types are dissociated. Since mammalian photoreceptors, unlike those in the honeybee retina, are able to utilise glucose, these experiments show that metabolic trafficking between neurons and glial cells is not obligatory in vertebrates. A second major difference is that lactate, rather than alanine, is the major metabolite transferred. This probably reflects the facts that NH_3 is highly toxic to the mammalian central nervous system, including the retina (Reichenbach et al. 1995), and that it almost exclusively reacts with glutamate to form glutamine (Cooper and Plum 1987). This does not mean that alanine cannot be formed by mammalian glial cells, since the oxidative metabolism of glutamate yields ammonia or an amino group which may then combine with pyruvate to form alanine. A supply of alanine (or another amino acid) is essential if neurons are to use α-ketoglutarate as a precursor of glutamate (Peng, Schousboe and Hertz 1991).

5.6.2 *Other Regions of the Nervous System*

Larrabee (1992) examined the conversion of glucose to lactate and alanine and the further fate of these metabolites in an intact chain of sympathetic ganglia from chick embryos, incubated in a bath. This was a complex undertaking because lactate (or pyruvate or alanine) is released as an end product of glycolysis, and is also re-accumulated for further metabolism in the TCA cycle (Fig. 5.2). These experiments have shown that about half of the glucose which is metabolised appears in the bath as lactate or alanine in the extracellular space prior to oxidation. Although the tissue can metabolise both glucose and lactate, lactate is the preferred substrate in this tissue at this developmental stage, since more CO_2 is generated from lactate than from glucose when both substrates are present at the same concentration. These experiments clearly show that there is extensive trafficking of lactate and alanine into and out of cells in an intact preparation. They are unable to distinguish, however, whether these metabolites travel back and forth between cells of the same kind or whether there is metabolic trafficking between different types of cells.

During the onset of intense central nervous system activity, such as seizures, the rates of glycolysis and of subsequent oxidation are uncoupled from each other. The rates of glycolysis and vascular perfusion increase several-fold, whereas oxidative metabolism (in spite of adequate oxygen supply) is almost unaltered; this situation leads to an accumulation of lactate which is so massive that it may result in a release of lactate into the systemic circulation (Bolwig and Quistorff 1973; Brodersen et al. 1973; Fox and Raichle 1986; Ting and Degani 1993). Such an elevation in extracellular lactate would favour neuronal lactate uptake over uptake of glucose, particularly if some cell types are primarily dependent on glycolytic activity (perhaps glia), while others depend mainly on oxidative metabolism (perhaps neurons).

5.6.3 Cultured Cells

Uptake and release of pyruvate, lactate and/or alanine across astrocytic and neuronal membranes can proceed fast enough to supply metabolic demands, so trafficking of these metabolites is a real possibility (Tildon et al. 1993; Westergaard et al. 1993; Hamprecht and Dringen 1994; Dringen et al. 1995; L. Hertz, unpublished experiments). Nonetheless, studies of kinetics for uptake and release of these metabolites have failed to find a preferential uptake of either pyruvate or lactate into cultured neurons. The kinetics for alanine, on the other hand, suggest that it may be released by astrocytes and taken up by neurons when the extracellular concentration of alanine is 50 mM (Westergaard et al. 1993). This concentration is comparable to the 30–50 mM of alanine reported for human and cat cerebrospinal fluid in vivo (Ferraro and Hare 1985; Roettger and Goldfinger 1991).

5.6.4 Synopsis

In the preceding pages, we have seen that glycolytic flux is greater in astrocytes than in neurons; that at least one half of glucose carbon is converted to lactate or alanine before complete degradation of glucose; and that neuronal function (in contrast to glial function) is readily maintained with lactate as the substrate. Given these facts, some astrocytically produced pyruvate/lactate or alanine is almost certainly accumulated into neurons and utilised as a metabolic substrate also in the mammalian retina and central nervous system. This may especially be the case when neuronal activity is suddenly increased.

An increase in extracellular glutamate massively stimulates glycolysis in astrocytes, but has no effect on their glycogenolysis or oxidative metabolism, while an increase in extracellular K^+ massively stimulates glycogenolysis, and mildly stimulates astrocytic glycolysis, but also has no effect on their oxidative metabolism. In other words, elevated extracellular K^+ or glutamate can double or triple pyruvate production by astrocytes, but this is not accompanied by a comparable increase in their utilisation of pyruvate (only pyruvate carboxylation is elevated). In at least some types of neurons, by contrast, an increase in extracellular glutamate has little effect on glycolysis but it dramatically increases their oxidative metabolism. An increase in extracellular K^+ concentration also increases glycolysis in some neurons, but the effect on oxidative metabolism is much more pronounced. Taken together, these differences indicate that when neuronal activity is increased, there must be a net loss of pyruvate, lactate and/or alanine from astrocytes. Under extreme conditions, this loss may be large enough that some lactate is released from the brain to the systemic circulation; under less extreme conditions, it is likely to be consumed by the increased oxidative metabolism in some neurons.

In principle, pyruvate, lactate or alanine could be trafficked from neurons to glia. If all cells in the central nervous system release a substantial fraction of their glucose carbon as pyruvate or a pyruvate metabolite during glucose degradation, it would be surprising if some pyruvate molecules that had been generated in neurons were not oxidatively degraded by glia. However, with the distinctly higher glycolytic rates in astrocytes, and with glycogenolysis being an exclusively glial process, it is doubtful that there will be situations in which there is a net transfer of pyruvate or its metabolites from neurons to glia.

Noradrenaline must act in a different way, since it stimulates both glycogenolysis and oxidative metabolism in astrocytes, yet leaves neuronal metabolism unchanged (Table 5.1). This is consistent with conclusions from immunohistochemical studies (Fig. 5.1) and lesion experiments that many monoaminergic transmitter systems, especially noradrenaline, have glia as a major target (Stone and Ariano 1989; Aoki and Pickel 1992a; Stone et al. 1992a,b). Therefore, when noradrenaline stimulates glycogenolysis, excess pyruvate, lactate and/or alanine must be oxidised by astrocytes instead of by neurons.

5.7 Implications of Metabolic Trafficking for Behaviour

The potential importance of metabolic trafficking for behaviour has been demonstrated by the application of toxins that target specific metabolic steps in glia. For example, methionine sulphoximine selectively blocks glutamine synthetase. When injected into the eye, this drug has no observable effect on the retinal distribution of GABA, glycine or taurine (Pow and Robinson 1994), it does not cause neuronal or glial loss, and the photoreceptor hyperpolarisation in response to light (a-wave of the electroretinogram) remains absolutely normal (Barnett et al. 1996). Nonetheless, such injections in rats eliminate the b-wave of the electroretinogram (due to bipolar cells) within 30 min or less (Barnett et al. 1996), and in cats they shift ocular dominance in visual cortical areas V1 and V2 towards the saline-injected control eye within 4 h or less (Robinson et al. 1994). In both instances, the loss of a response to light is accompanied by a loss of immunocytochemically detectable glutamate in retinal neurons. Although these experiments do not directly show that glia normally modulate neuronal excitability, they do provide a powerful demonstration that by reducing the activity of glutamine synthetase or the provision of glutamine to neurons, glia possess the potential to modulate glutamatergic transmission. Glutamine production in astrocytes also appears to be essential for consolidation of one-trial aversive learning in newly hatched chicks (Gibbs et al. 1996). This topic is discussed in depth in Chapter 15 in the present volume.

Fluoroacetate inhibits metabolism of citrate in the TCA cycle. While neurons and glia both metabolise citrate, only glia are able to take up fluoroacetate at an appreciable rate: hence this toxin is specific for astrocytes. Unless high concentrations are used (which also reduces the cell specificity), fluoroacetate has little effect on ATP production in astrocytes (Hassel et al. 1994; Swanson and Graham 1994), probably because astrocytes rely mainly on glycolytically derived energy. However, it impairs de novo synthesis of glutamate from glucose because oxaloacetate cannot be converted to α-ketoglutarate (Fig. 5.2). This may explain the observation by Keyser and Pelmar (1994) that glutamatergic transmission is significantly impaired when fluoroacetate is applied to hippocampal slices and the finding by Gibbs et al. (1996) that intracranial injection of fluoroacetate abolishes learning in a similar manner to methionine sulphoximine (see Chapter 15). Administration of fluoroacetate to rats has recently also been found to abolish certain somatic reactions to stress (L.R. Watkins, personal communication), suggesting that glutamatergic transmission is involved in the establishment of these reactions.

Glycogen is broken down at a certain stage of memory consolidation in day-old chicks (O'Dowd et al. 1994a). As discussed in more detail in Chapter 15 in this volume, it is likely that glycogenolysis is secondary to the release of noradrenaline, since it is prevented by the β-adrenergic antagonist, propranolol. Propranolol also inhibits learning in day-old chicks, and noradrenaline stimulates glycogenolysis in chick astrocyte cultures at a developmental stage similar to that in the newly hatched chick (O'Dowd et al. 1995). Very similar events may be involved in learned attraction of rat pups to the odour of their mother (Coopersmith and Leon 1995; M. Leon, personal communication). It is unknown why inhibition of glycogenolysis in astrocytes impairs learning. Is it on account of reduction of ATP production during glycolysis in astrocytes when demand for energy increases, on account of deficient ATP production in neurons when less pyruvate is available for metabolic trafficking, or on account of both neuronal and astrocytic metabolic energy deficiency?

5.8 Concluding Remarks

This chapter has summarised information about metabolic trafficking, and potential metabolic trafficking in the central nervous system. Compelling evidence has been presented from the honeybee retina to show that energy production in some neurons is entirely dependent upon metabolic trafficking from glia. In the mammalian central nervous system differences from the honeybee retina appear to exist both in terms of the metabolites transferred (lactate versus alanine) and in the ability of the neurons to metabolise glucose directly, although it may not be the preferred substrate. Nonetheless, glycolysis has a special functional importance for mammalian glia, and under certain conditions the rate of glycolysis in glia may increase dramatically without any corresponding increase in their oxidative metabolism. Under the same conditions, oxidative metabolism is substantially increased in neurons. Neuronal production of pyruvate to sustain this increase may be delayed, as suggested by the long delay between exposure to [^{14}C]glucose and production of labelled CO_2. It is highly likely that in such circumstances pyruvate, or a pyruvate metabolite, is released from astrocytes and taken up and metabolised by neurons. In any case, there is no doubt that in the vertebrate central nervous system the neuronal supplies of TCA cycle constituents and their derivatives (including glutamate and GABA) are absolutely dependent upon metabolic trafficking from astrocytes.

6

Transmitter Receptor and Uptake Systems in Astrocytes and Their Relation to Behaviour

HAROLD K. KIMELBERG, TUULA O. JALONEN, CHIYE AOKI and KEN McCARTHY

Summary

Studies during the past decade have shown that glial fibrillary acidic protein (GFAP)-containing astrocytes in primary cultures prepared from neonatal rodent brains can exhibit receptors and uptake transporters for a wide variety of neurotransmitters. However, the expression of receptors and transporters in cultured astrocytes is quite plastic, and current work using systems that are more likely to represent the in vivo state, such as brain slices, immunocytochemistry at the electron microscope level and freshly isolated cells, have shown that GFAP(+) cells in these systems show a more limited repertoire of receptors and transporters. This chapter compares and contrasts receptor and transporter expression in astrocytes in primary cultures with the more in vivo-like systems. So far, β-adrenergic receptors, several glutamate receptors and two glial-specific glutamate transporters have been shown to be present in the non-cultured systems, while several transmitter receptor systems known to be present on cultured astrocytes have been shown to be absent. Clearly, further work is needed to determine how receptors and transporters vary with region and development stages and whether there is marked localisation so that some receptors and transport systems are present on very few astrocytes. Since the actions of transmitters are so critical to behaviour, understanding of the patterns of expression on astrocytes in vivo and their function is of critical importance for a true understanding of the cellular and molecular bases of behaviour.

6.1 Introduction

Behavioural changes ranging from sensory–motor through mood and cognitive behaviour depend on and are affected by changes in transmitter–receptor interactions. These interactions are generally thought to be purely attributable to interactions of transmitter with receptors located on neurons, particularly at synapses. The neurons are then proposed to connect synaptically to form circuits, still undefined as far as behaviour is concerned. However, elementary purposeful behaviour can be modelled in artificial neural networks, using properties known to be associated with neurons and synapses, so it is thought that such network paradigms are essentially correct (Crick 1994; Chalmers 1995). With the identification of receptors and uptake systems for transmitters on astrocytes in primary cultures, it became self-evident that behaviourally related transmitter effects could also involve astrocytes via transmitter–astrocyte receptor interactions (Hertz and Richardson 1984). However, supporting such a general proposal would require the conceptual and technical effort already expended on understanding behaviour based on purely neuronal interactions (Crick 1994). One hopeful development might be that when neuronal-based hypotheses start to identify clear patterns, then this work may have immediate implications for the degree of involvement of astrocytes.

Transmitter uptake systems also play a critical role in the control of neural activity by terminating transmitter activity. These systems were also earlier considered to be restricted to neuronal presynaptic sites, but work on cultures and in situ has shown transporters, especially for excitatory amino acids and γ-aminobutyric acid (GABA), on astrocytes. It is well established that astrocytes are linked by gap junctions to form a syncytium (McCarthy, Enkvist and Shao 1995), and since it was found that waves of intracellular Ca^{2+} increases can be propagated through this syncytium (Cornell-Bell et al. 1990), this led to speculation that these may resemble neural networks (Finkbeiner 1992). However, there is no evidence to date to support such an intriguing hypothesis, but it could be incorporated into a general theory of behaviour and consciousness once such a general theory begins to be achieved.

At a more prosaic level, it should be borne in mind that the documentation of transmitter interactions with astrocytes has been mainly done on primary astrocyte cultures consisting of 95% or more, of flat GFAP(+) type 1 astrocytes. Although these have provided simple experimental systems in which the neuron–centric view of transmitter-related activities could be challenged, there is a clear need for confirming the data obtained from astrocyte cultures in systems that can be more reliably viewed as representing astrocyte properties in situ. Clearly, once an astrocyte property has been established in situ or in vivo, astrocyte cultures expressing this property can serve as good models, as is done for neurons for example. There are currently several approaches used in determining the transmitter receptor and uptake properties of astrocytes in situ or in vivo:

1 Microscopy, especially at the electron microscopic (EM) level or by co-localisation with GFAP at the light microscopic level, using antibody labelling to determine the cellular localisation of receptors in situ. As discussed later, adrenergic β receptors have clearly been shown to be on astrocytes using this approach. Transmitter uptake can be similarly localised by receptor antibody, and also by autoradiographic studies of uptake of radiolabelled transmitters.

2 Using lesioning studies selectively to eliminate or increase the astrocyte component using selective astrocytic toxins (e.g. fluoroacetate) or neuronal elimination leading to astrogliosis (either by tract sectioning, neuronal toxins such as kainate or transgenic knockouts). These approaches are important as they can also address function, but it is difficult to establish direct versus secondary effects (Sontheimer 1995).

3 Studying functional effects of transmitters on GFAP(+) astrocytes in slices by patch-clamp electrophysiology or Ca^{2+} imaging using Ca^{2+}-specific dyes and microscopy (Steinhäuser et al. 1994; Porter and McCarthy 1995b). These methods can also be used to measure transmitter uptake when it is electrogenic.

4 Using cells within a few hours of isolation from the brain and studying electrophysiological or Ca^{2+} responses to transmitters in single GFAP(+) astrocytes. The $GABA_A$ receptor (Fraser et al. 1995) and glutamate, serotonin and adenosine triphosphate (ATP) receptor-mediated Ca^{2+} responses (see section 2 and Kimelberg et al. 1995a, 1997), have recently been studied in such cells. Such preparations can also be used for studying transmitter uptake (Dave and Kimelberg 1994).

In this chapter, we will emphasise the different systems used in relation to the findings discussed. Also, we have selected a few receptors and uptake systems that have been clearly located to astrocytes, namely glutamate and adrenergic receptors and excitatory amino acid uptake systems, rather than attempt an encyclopaedic review, since there are already sufficient reviews to give an overview of our present state of knowledge (Schousboe 1980; Hertz 1982; Kimelberg 1983, 1988, 1995; Federoff and Vernadakis 1986; Walz 1989; Hertz, McFarlin and Waksman 1990; Malhotra, Shnitka and Elbrink 1990; Sontheimer 1992; Kimelberg, Jalonen and Walz 1993; Aschner and LoPachin, Jr 1993b; Montgomery 1994; McCarthy, Enkvist and Shao 1995). A section on receptor-activated ion channels in astrocytes is also included as changes in the membrane conductances of astrocytes can affect extracellular K^+ clearance and electrical circuits in the brain.

We cannot, as yet, ascribe any particular animal behaviour to any of these astrocytic systems, but such studies as described in this chapter will lay the necessary data bases upon which astrocytic involvement in specific behaviours can be ruled in or out. Identification of the chemical bases of behaviour is a subject fraught with difficulties even for the much better-studied neuronal systems, so it is perhaps not surprising that the relation of transmitter-related properties of astrocytes has not yet been clearly correlated with any behavioural changes. Other chapters in this volume document those cases in which other changes in astrocytes and other glial cells have shown some general correlation with behavioural changes.

6.2 Receptors in Cultured Versus Acutely Isolated Astrocytes

Receptors for transmitters on glial cells were first shown in predominantly non-neuronal primary cultures prepared from neonatal rats (Gilman and Schrier 1972; Narumi, Kimelberg and Bourke 1978; McCarthy and De Vellis 1978; van Calker,

Muller and Hamprecht 1979). When the astrocyte-specific marker glial fibrillary acidic protein (GFAP) (Eng et al. 1971) became available and widely used, it was found that these same cultures were 95% or more astrocytic as determined by immunocytochemical staining for GFAP (Bock 1978). It was subsequently shown that these astrocyte cultures could also exhibit a number of other 'neuron-like' properties, such as voltage-gated Na^+, K^+, and Ca^{2+} channels, as well as receptors and high-affinity uptake systems for neurotransmitters (Federoff and Vernadakis 1986; Duffy and MacVicar 1993; Steinhäuser 1993; Kimelberg and Aschner 1994; Sontheimer, Black and Waxman 1996). The receptors found on cultured and other astrocytes have been summarised in several reviews (van Calker and Hamprecht 1980; Federoff and Vernadakis 1986; Murphy and Pearce 1987; Kimelberg 1988, 1995; Murphy 1993; Kimelberg and Aschner 1994). Therefore the details of receptor expression and action seen in primary astrocyte cultures will not be recapitulated here. Suffice to say that around ten adrenergic and related aminergic receptors, including their subtypes, nine amino acid and two purinergic, and at least eight peptide receptors have so far been found and studied in cultured astrocytes. All this was quite surprising to many neuroscientists (Somjen 1988; Kimelberg and Norenberg 1989; Sontheimer 1992; Tower 1992; Dierig 1994). The ease of obtaining $\geq 95\%$ pure proliferating astrocyte cultures from neonatal rodents, which can then be readily studied by a variety of biochemical, molecular and physiological techniques, has undoubtedly contributed to the continued popularity of these cultures. At the time of writing, such cultures continue to be the primary experimental model for studying astrocyte functions at the cellular and molecular levels, but the emphasis is beginning to shift. However, it should be emphasised that primary astrocyte cultures were very important in sensitising the neuroscience community to the complexity of astrocyte properties and their potential involvement in many aspects of central nervous system (CNS) function. It was also recognised that the fidelity of such cultures in reflecting the properties of astrocytes in vivo, could not be assumed a priori, and they might best be viewed as providing hypotheses that could be more definitively answered by subsequent studies in situ or in vivo (Kimelberg 1983). But alternative experimental systems were not obvious, and work on the primary astrocyte cultures yielded many fascinating results at a rapid rate.

Nonetheless a number of the properties shown by the cultures have been shown to be a property of astrocytes in situ, such as glutamate uptake (Ottersen 1989; Torp et al. 1991; Lehre et al. 1995), and β-adrenergic receptor expression (Aoki 1992 and see following section). However, examples of differences between in vitro and in vivo have emerged as more in situ studies have been done. For example, in the case of receptors it has been recently reported that the 5-hydroxytryptamine (serotonin, 5-HT_{2A}) receptor, routinely found in primary astrocyte cultures (Nilsson, Hansson and Rönnbäck 1991; Deecher et al. 1993), is rarely found on GFAP(+) astrocytes in rat brain sections when probed with cyclic deoxyribose nucleic acids (cDNAs) for the receptor (Hirst et al. 1994), although it has been reported in rat brain sections using an antibody (Whitaker-Azmitia, Clarke and Azmitia 1993) and messenger ribose nucleic acid (mRNA) for 5-HT receptor has been detected in corpus callosum (Matute and Miledi 1993). Glial cells, either oligodendrocytes or astrocytes, identified electrophysiologically in spinal cord slices from P3–P18 rats, were found to have glycine receptors, whereas primary cultures of these cells had not been found to have such receptors (Kirchhoff et al. 1996).

The use of freshly isolated cells, the fourth approach mentioned in the introduction, has been used by some of the authors of this chapter to study the Ca^{2+} responses of acutely isolated GFAP(+) astrocytes, studied less than 6 h after isolation, to glutamate, ATP, adenosine and 5-HT (Kimelberg et al. 1995a, 1997). These cells frequently showed increases in intracellular Ca^{2+} in response to 50 µM L-glutamate (60 % of cells studied; Fig. 6.1). Responses to 10 µM ATP or 10 µM 5-HT were much less frequently observed. Culturing such cells in medium containing 10% horse serum did not alter the response to glutamate but greatly increased the response to ATP and 5-HT to 70 and 50%, respectively (Fig. 6.1, middle group). In primary cultures prepared from 1-day-old rats and grown for 4 weeks in serum-containing medium the responses to glutamate were only around

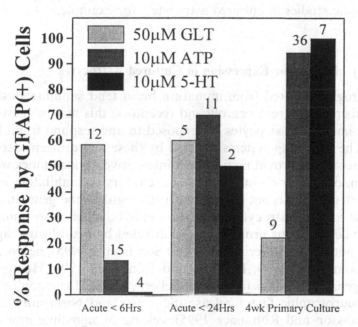

Fig. 6.1. Percentage response of GFAP(+) cells to ATP, 5-HT or glutamate, as indicated, for cells acutely isolated from the cortices of postnatal 5–8 day rats (left-hand set of bars), the same cells cultured for 24 h in serum containing medium (middle set of bars), or 4 week primary astrocyte cultures (right-hand set of bars). Numbers above individual bars are total number of cells tested for each condition.

20%. In contrast, 90 and 100 % of the cells responded to ATP and 5-HT, respectively (Fig. 6.1, right hand group). Studies by others have frequently shown that almost all cells in primary cultures respond to ATP and 5-HT (Kastritsis, Salm and McCarthy 1992; Neary et al. 1996).

The same acutely isolated cell that failed to respond to ATP or 5-HT often responded to glutamate. Thus the lack of response to ATP and 5-HT would either be due to actual differences in receptor expression or their coupled second messenger systems, or selective damage to these receptors during isolation. However, selective damage seems less likely, as we found that culturing in serum-free medium, in contrast to serum-containing medium, did not up-regulate the response. Also, GFAP-negative cells in the same acutely isolated preparation sometimes showed responses to ATP (data not shown). Thus, some of the receptor responses seen in primary astrocyte cultures may reflect up-regulation in response to culture conditions. This appears to apply to ATP and serotonin but not to glutamate, and interestingly AMPA and mGluR, but not ATP, responses on astrocytes have been seen in situ (Porter and McCarthy 1995a). The implications are that we need to seriously study appropriate in situ and in vivo preparations to be able to determine which astrocyte properties actually exist on astrocytes in vivo. The results of these studies will then also allow rational assessment of which receptors are appropriate for detailed mechanistic studies in cultured astrocytes, for example.

6.3 Plasticity of Receptor Expression in Cultured Astrocytes

Since individual astroglia cultured from immature brain tend simultaneously to express a large number of different neuroligand receptors, this may suggest that during development immature astrocytes are exposed to and respond to multiple neurotransmitters. The signalling systems affected by these neurotransmitters are often diverse and interactive, providing potential integrative opportunities within astrocytes reminiscent of a neuron's integration of excitatory and inhibitory input. Whereas neuronal integration seems, in large part, to regulate the generation of action potentials, the roles of astrocytic integration may be much more complex, or less clear. Astrocytic functions proposed to be affected by neuroligand signalling systems include potassium buffering (Roy and Sontheimer 1995), neurotransmitter uptake (Barbour et al. 1989; Hansson and Rönnbäck 1992; Huang and Hertz 1994), glycogenolysis (Magistretti and Pellerin 1996; Tsacopoulos and Magistretti 1996), neurotrophic factor release (Schwartz and Nishiyama 1994), volume changes (Hansson and Rönnbäck 1995), release of signalling molecules and changes in morphology (Narumi, Kimelberg and Bourke 1978; Shain et al. 1987; Canady and Rubel 1992). Complicating the situation further, it seems likely that the fine processes of a given astrocyte which radiate outward to ensheathe distant neuronal elements may function autonomously from one another. Indeed, the neurotransmitter environment and functions affected by neurotransmitters may vary among the processes of an individual astrocyte in vivo. However, certain signals such as increases in intracellular calcium may be propagated to the astrocytic cell body and beyond into distant processes and through gap junctions into adjacent astrocytes to coordinate these responses (Dani and Smith 1995). These more encompassing astrocytic responses would, presumably, be required to regulate the transcription/translation of gene products involved in maintaining and adjusting astrocytic functional responses. Signals propagated into adjacent astrocytes may be involved in activating a syncytium of astrocytes to affect a larger volume of the cellular milieu. In large part, these are issues of compartmentalisation, geometry and localised receptor stimulation. As a result, it will be difficult to investigate these issues using cultured astrocytes which fail to exhibit the complex morphological features characteristic of these cells in vivo and cannot, of course, mimic the complex interactions seen in vivo. For these reasons, a number of investigators have recently turned to the study of astrocytes in slices, as discussed in other sections of this chapter.

Early in the study of astroglial receptors, the question was often raised of whether the expression of receptors by these cells was the result of their in vitro environment (Kimelberg 1983). The importance of this question was underscored by the fact that no one had been able to demonstrate that astrocytes in situ expressed neurotransmitter receptors (given technical advances, this is no longer the case, see below). One experimental approach taken by a number of investigators to address this question was to determine if astroglia in vitro were heterogeneous with respect to their expression of neuroligand receptors. The presumption is that if astroglia grown under identical conditions were heterogeneous, culture conditions were not the predominant factor in the expression of astroglial receptors. Two basic approaches were used in these studies. First, experiments were designed to determine if astroglia cultured from different brain regions exhibited different properties, both qualitatively and quantitatively (see Fig. 6.2 for an example of these type of studies for glutamate uptake). Second, experiments were carried out to see if there was heterogeneity among individual astroglia cultured from a single brain region. Both approaches provided evidence that cultured astroglia were heterogeneous with respect to their ability to respond to an array of neuroligands. For example, Wilkin and coworkers reported that β-adrenergic agonists and vasoactive intestinal peptide (VIP) differentially stimulate cAMP levels in cortical and cerebellar astroglia (Wilkin, Marriott and Cholewinski 1990). Similarly, when a panel of ligands known to increase intracellular calcium levels through different receptors were applied to cortical astroglia, video-based imaging demonstrated that individual astroglia varied in their ability to respond to different neuroligands (McCarthy and Salm 1991). Hence, astroglia prepared from a single brain region also varied markedly in their neuroligand responsiveness. Overall, these studies clearly demonstrate that an astroglial cell's in vitro milieu alone does not control the nature of the receptors expressed.

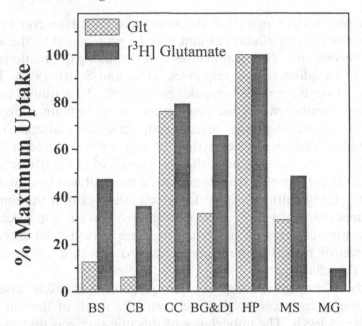

Fig. 6.2. Relative percentage uptake of [³H]-L-glutamate in cultures prepared from different brain regions (modified from Amundson, Goderie and Kimelberg 1992) and the relative distribution of the astrocyte specific glutamate transporter (Glt) in the same regions in situ quantitated by immunoblots (Lehre et al 1995b). The highest value, which for both cases was the hippocampus (HP), was set at 100%, and each other region expressed as a percentage of that. CC, cerebral cortex; BG and DI, basal ganglia and diencephalon; MS, mesencephalon; BS, brainstem; CB, cerebellum; MG, meninges.

It is generally accepted that astroglia isolated from neonatal rodents are immature when placed in culture, but whether or not astroglia differentiate in culture is intensely debated. It is likely that neuronal growth and synapse formation continue during the early postnatal period of rodent development and the neurotransmitters being released change. Together, these observations suggest that if astrocyte receptors are to match their milieu in vivo, they must exhibit some degree of plasticity. Calcium-sensitive indicator dyes and video-based imaging have been used to investigate the possibility that individual astroglia qualitatively change their sensitivity to neuroligands over time in vitro (Shao and McCarthy 1993). In these experiments, the calcium responsiveness of the same astroglial cells was examined over the course of days in vitro. Examples where the progeny of a single cell division yielded daughter cells which were qualitatively distinct with respect to their ability to respond to neuroligands were observed, as well as astroglia which actually diversified in the absence of cell division (Shao and McCarthy 1993). Two conclusions arise from these studies. First, astroglia within a given clone vary with respect to their sensitivity to neuroligands. Second, the responsiveness of a given astroglial cell changes qualitatively with time in culture. Given that these changes occur in the absence of neurons and in the same chemical milieu, they appear to be programmed in astroglia by the time they are removed from the animal. While these findings seem predictable given the biology of developing brain, they are surprising given that qualitative changes in receptor expression are rare, whereas quantitative changes, such as occur with receptor desensitisation, are common. Whether mature astrocytes in vivo retain the ability to qualitatively shift their neuroligand responsiveness, however, remains unknown.

6.4 Studies on Astrocytes in Non-Cultured Systems

As noted above, primary cultures of astroglia have been extremely valuable for establishing the potential of these cells to contribute to brain function. However, it seems naive to think that astroglia, isolated from developing brain, grown in a plastic dish and in a foreign chemical and cellular milieu would differentiate into normal mature astrocytes. With this in mind, a number of laboratories have revisited the study of astrocytes in situ, with better techniques and, we think it is fair to say, more understanding of potential astrocyte properties and function based on the culture work. As noted, approaches used to study astrocytes in situ include electrophysiology, confocal imaging of ion-sensitive indicator dyes and immunocytochemistry. Each of these avenues has yielded results suggesting that astrocytes in vivo recognise and respond to neurotransmitters but which specific ones and what are the functional consequences of these interactions largely remains for future work.

6.4.1 Ultrastructural Localisation of β-adrenergic Receptors in Astrocytes in Situ

Receptor autoradiography has contributed much to our understanding of the laminar organisation and chemically specific synaptic transmission within the cerebral cortex, for it was with this method that the distinct tangential bands of receptor-rich zones were first visualised (reviewed by Herkenham 1987). In the rat visual cortex, for example, both β-adrenergic receptors and N-methyl-D-aspartate (NMDA)-type glutamate receptors are enriched in supragranular layers 1 through 3 but are relatively scarce in layer 4 (Monaghan and Cotman 1985; Aoki, Kaufman and Rainbow 1986; Maragos, Penny and Young 1988). In contrast nicotinic acetylcholine receptors are prominently concentrated in layers 4 and 6 (Clarke et al. 1985). However, while providing valuable information about subtypes of receptors and their laminar distribution, receptor autoradiography at the light microscope level is limited in resolution to a macroscopic level. Thus, details about the pre- versus postsynaptic localisation or of the individual cell types that express the receptors (e.g. interneurons versus pyramidal neurons versus glia) are difficult to discern by receptor autoradiography. Some attempts have been made to overcome this limitation. One example is to determine whether nicotinic receptors in layer 4 are localised to thalamic afferents by combining lesion of thalamo–cortical afferents with receptor autoradiography (Liu et al. 1993). Results from such an approach has suggested that they may be. More recent results, however, indicate that the loss of nicotinic receptors following deafferentation might be due to loss of thalamic regulation of the receptor's expression within cortical neurons (Broide, Robertson and Leslie 1996). These results point to the difficulty of interpreting receptor autoradiography results beyond the macroscopic level, because the most parsimonious explanation does not necessarily reflect reality. Recently, another approach, namely immunocytochemistry, that uses antibodies directed against receptor molecules, has begun to provide new information that both complements and extends the data obtained by receptor autoradiography. Not only can immunocytochemistry yield cellular and subcellular localisations of receptors but it can potentially provide information about conformation changes of receptors if antibodies are directed against post-translationally modified domains of the molecule. On the other hand, antibodies may recognise conformational states of the molecule that are not ligand-binding. Thus, care must be taken in interpreting data obtained from immunocytochemistry in ways that differ from interpreting receptor autoradiography. Summarised below is the current state of knowledge gained regarding the cellular and subcellular distribution of β-adrenergic receptor by immuno-electron microscopy, and especially its location on astrocytes.

Successful cloning of the gene for the mammalian β-adrenergic receptor (Dixon et al. 1986) led immediately to elucidation of the receptor molecule's functional domains, including understanding of its topography in relation to the plasma membrane and identification of sites that are phosphorylated or involved in determining ligand-binding specificity, desensitisation and sequestration (Strader et al. 1983; Dixon et al. 1986; Bouvier et al. 1988; Zemcik and Strader 1988). Another consequence of the successful cloning was the generation of antibodies directed specifically to the N-terminus, C-terminus and the third intracellular loop portion of the receptor molecule (Strader et al. 1987). As will be described, these antibodies have provided data that complement those gained previously by using antisera directed against whole receptor molecules (Strader et al. 1983; Aoki, Joh and Pickel 1987). With the use of these antibodies it became possible to localise receptors within intact tissue of various brain regions at varying developmental stages. Moreover, by combining the immunocytochemical localisation of β-adrenergic receptors with the immunocytochemical localisation of catecholaminergic terminals, it is possible to determine whether the two elements are likely to form synaptic and/or non-synaptic relationships. The immunoperoxidase label that can be applied following receptor–antibody binding provides greater sensitivity than the previous ultrastructural method of using a ferritin-labelled receptor ligand (Muntz et al. 1988).

As expected, the antibody directed against the third intracellular loop portion of β_2-adrenergic receptors recognises neurons. Within neurons, perikaryal organelles involved in protein synthesis, i.e. the Golgi apparatus and endoplasmic reticulum, as well as plasma membranes, are immunoreactive (Aoki et al. 1989; Aoki and Pickel 1992a). Dendritic shafts and spines also are immunoreactive. What was surprising, however, was the frequent recognition of plasma membranes that are apparently not part of or continuous with pre- or postsynaptic regions. This observation supported the proposal that norepinephrine may operate as a neurotransmitter via 'volume transmission' in addition to conventional point-to-point synaptic transmission. This was an idea put forth first by investigators noting that noradrenergic terminals rarely form morphologically identifiable synaptic junctions (Descarries, Seguela and Watkins 1991). This view is compatible with the notion that the locus coeruleus–norepinephrine system is involved in setting the behavioural states of vigilance and orientation toward sensory stimuli, while the GABAergic and glutamatergic systems mediate fast point-to-point transmission, such as sensory perception via circuits to and within the visual cortex (reviewed by Sillito 1984; Tsumoto 1990).

More surprising are the results obtained when using the C-terminus antiserum to the β-receptor. It was observed that the predominant sites of immunoreactivity were the fine processes of astrocytes (Aoki 1992 and Fig. 6.3). For example, within layer 1 of adult rat visual cortices, greater than 90% of the immunoreactive profiles encountered are astrocytic (Aoki, manuscript in preparation). It is apparent that, in spite of the fact that these astrocytic sites cannot be directly involved in synaptic transmission, they are in the immediate proximity of or within a few micrometers of catecholaminergic (presumably noradrenergic) axons, and can therefore presumably be receptive to neuronally released norepinephrine. The remaining 10% of the immunoreactive profiles are mostly dendritic, although axonal labelling also is evident. These immunoreactive neuronal profiles are not necessarily adjacent to immunoreactive astrocytic processes. Instead, the immunoreactive astrocytic profiles typically are adjacent to asymmetric (presumably excitatory (Gray 1959)) axo-spinous junctions (Fig. 6.3). Based on these observations, Aoki (1992) hypothesised that β-adrenergic receptors on astrocytes may be involved in boosting neural processing of sensory information by stimulating glycogenolysis (reviewed by Stone and Ariano 1989; Magistretti and Pellerin 1996; Chapter 5). Stimulation of β-adrenergic receptors has also been reported to reduce the uptake of L-glutamate in primary astrocyte cultures which, if it occurs in vivo, would also lead to increasing glutamatergic activity prior to desensitisation (Hansson and Rönnbäck 1991).

The above distribution pattern is compatible with earlier results that used an antiserum directed against the whole purified receptor molecule from frog erythrocytes (Aoki, Joh and Pickel 1987). Using this polyclonal antiserum which, presumably, consisted of a collection of IgGs immunoreactive to the C-terminus, N-terminus, intracellular loop and extracellular loop domains, it was noted that the

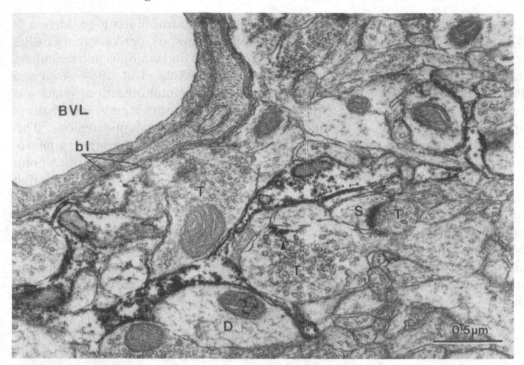

Fig. 6.3. Electron micrograph showing astrocytic profiles near a blood vessel immunopositive for β-adrenergic receptors. Asterisks are placed within the cytoplasm of immunoreactive astrocytic processes. Note the immunoreactivity along a gap junction formed by an astrocytic profile (three double-sided arrows). Frequently, astrocytic processes containing β-adrenergic receptor-immunoreactivity are so fine that their diameters are merely the thickness of two plasma membranes (large open arrow within a dendritic profile, D). T = terminal; S = dendritic spine; bl = basal laminae; BVL = blood vessel lumen (see text for further details).

antigenic sites included perikarya of neurons, dendritic shafts, dendritic spines, presynaptic terminals and also fine astrocytic processes. This finding also is compatible with another laboratory's report using another β-adrenergic receptor antibody (Liu et al. 1993). The reason for the rather selective immunolabelling of astrocytic processes by the C-terminus antiserum remains unknown. One possibility is that there is prevalence of one conformational state of the receptor within astrocytes, relating to the degree of phosphorylation of the C-terminus by β-adrenergic receptor kinase and of the agonist-promoted desensitisation (Bouvier et al. 1988).

Other receptors have been localised to glia in situ using the approach described above. Use of antibodies to dopamine D_2 receptors (Sesack, Aoki and Pickel 1994), NR1 subunits of the NMDA-type glutamate receptors (Aoki et al. 1994) on astrocyte plasma membranes, and more recently NR2A/B also have been found, predominantly on the membranes of the processes of cortical astrocytes

(Conti et al. 1996). Alpha amino, 3-hydroxyl, 5-methyl, 4-isoxazole proprionic acid (AMPA) subunits of glutamate receptors (Conti, Minelli and Brecha 1994; Farb, Aoki and LeDoux 1995) and α_2-adrenergic receptors (Aoki et al. 1994; Rosin et al. 1996) also have shown antigenic sites on astrocytic plasma membranes.

6.4.2 Transmitter-Induced Currents in Astrocytes in Slice Preparations

The hippocampus has long been recognised as an excellent model for examining synaptic interactions between specific neuronal groups, largely due to its laminar organisation, which permits the preparation of brain slices where the major neuronal pathways remain intact. Within the hippocampus CA3 pyramidal neurons send glutamatergic input to CA1 pyramidal neurons via the Schaeffer collateral pathway, forming excitatory synapses in several regions of the CA1 including the stratum radiatum. When hippocampal slices from young animals ranging in age from 7 to 16 days are loaded with calcium-sensitive indicator dyes, astrocytes are the principal cells that take up and trap the dye (Porter and McCarthy 1995a,b). Confocal microscopy, which has the ability to collect light from optically-thin sections tens of microns deep into tissue slices was used to study the neuroligand Ca^{2+} responsiveness of astrocytes in situ using calcium-sensitive indicator dyes. All cells studied were subsequently identified as astrocytes by their staining for GFAP.

In the first series of experiments, the effect of perfusion with glutamatergic ligands on astrocytic calcium levels was examined (Porter and McCarthy 1995b). The results of these experiments indicate that astrocytes within hippocampal slices respond to glutamate, kainate, AMPA, *trans*-1-amino, cyclopentane-1,3-dicarboxylic acid (t-ACPD) and NMDA with increases in $[Ca^{2+}]_i$. Preincubation with tetradotoxin (TTX) to block Na^+-dependent neuronal action potentials failed to block calcium increases mediated by either glutamate, kainate, AMPA or t-ACPD, but did block approximately half the responses to NMDA. Preincubation with receptor antagonists or removal of extracellular calcium suggested that hippocampal astrocytes exhibit both ionotropic and metabotropic glutamatergic receptors. The finding that approximately half of the NMDA responses were blocked by TTX suggests that, in these cases at least, NMDA was indirectly affecting astrocytes via the stimulation of neurons. The observation that astrocytes responded to NMDA in the presence of TTX suggests that either certain astrocytes exhibit this receptor subtype or that NMDA was causing TTX-insensitive neuronal release of transmitters (possibly through an effect on presynaptic nerve terminals). Additional experiments will be required to distinguish between these possibilities.

In another series of experiments, the effect of purinergic ligands on hippocampal astrocytes was examined (Porter and McCarthy 1995b). Both ATP (P2-receptor agonist) and adenosine (P1-receptor agonists) are known to be important neurotransmitters in the CNS. In vitro, astroglia exhibit calcium responses primarily to ATP and not adenosine (Kastritsis et al. 1992). When hippocampal slices were perfused with these ligands, the majority of astrocytes responded to both adenosine and ATP; however, most of the responses to ATP (but not all) were blocked by the adenosine receptor antagonist, theophylline. Furthermore, a selective P2-receptor antagonist that is less susceptible to breakdown than ATP failed to increase $[Ca^{2+}]$ in all but a few astrocytes. This behaviour corresponds well with recent findings on GFAP(+) astrocytes acutely isolated from rat cerebral cortex (see section 3 and Kimelberg et al. 1995a, 1997). Duffy and MacVicar (1995) have shown an α_1-mediated $[Ca^{2+}]_i$ increase in astrocytes, identified electrophysiologically and by dye-coupling, in the CA1-3 region of hippocampal slices from P21–42 rats to perfusion with specific agonists.

The above findings suggest that the release of glutamate or adenosine/ATP (converted in vivo to adenosine via ecto-ATPases) from neurons leads to calcium increases in astrocytes in vivo. To demonstrate this more directly, the Schaeffer collateral pathway, which provides excitatory glutamatergic input to CA1 pyramidal neurons, was stimulated electrically while recording astrocytic calcium responses in the dendritic field of CA1 pyramidal neurons (Porter and McCarthy 1996). Stimulation of the Schaffer collaterals [50 Hz, 2 s; a level of stimulation commonly used to study long-term potentiation (LTP)] rapidly increased astrocytic intracellular $[Ca^{2+}]$, which then declined over tens of seconds after stimulation. Astrocytic responses were blocked by TTX, omega-conotoxin MVIIC (a voltage-dependent calcium channel blocker reported to inhibit neurotransmitter release in the hippocampus) and MCPG (a selective metabotropic glutamate receptor antagonist). These findings seem best explained by neuronal action potentials causing the release of glutamate which then stimulate metabotropic glutamatergic receptors on astrocytes leading to calcium mobilisation from internal stores. When these experiments were carried out in the presence of 4-aminopyridine (4-AP; a K^+ channel antagonist) to increase neuronal activity following stimulation, both metabotropic and ionotropic glutamatergic receptor antagonists were required to block astrocytic responses. These findings suggest that while astrocytes exhibit both metabotropic and ionotropic glutamatergic receptors in situ, they are differentially activated depending on the level of neuronal activity.

6.5 Transmitter-Induced Electrical Changes in Astrocytes

6.5.1 Effects of Transmitters on Astrocyte Membrane Potentials

The first studies aimed at finding out exactly what functions glia might have were electrophysiological and were done in isolated tissues and preceded the work on cultures. These studies were of glia in the amphibian optic nerve; a resilient tissue that could be kept viable in a dish and which had accessible glial cell bodies and only a few neuronal cell bodies (Kuffler, Nicholls and Orkand 1966). Measurements of membrane potentials were made using sharp microelectrodes. In contrast to the dogma of that day, which was unscientifically based on indirect inferences, these direct measurements recorded large, negative membrane potentials which corresponded to the Nernst potential for K^+, indicating a high intracellular $[K^+]$ and dominant K^+ channels in the glial cell membrane. The selective K^+ conductance of the amphibian glial cells led Kuffler and his colleagues (Kuffler, Nicholls and Orkand 1966) to propose the K^+ 'spatial buffering hypothesis', by which K^+ released from active neurons could be removed from the extracellular space through the K^+ channels in the plasma membrane (Kuffler and Nicholls 1976). Later work in the mammalian brain in vivo showed that glial cells, most probably astrocytes, also had very negative membrane potentials (Grossman 1972; Somjen 1975; Takato and Goldring 1979; Greenwood, Takato and Goldring 1981). The cells were identified as glial cells, based on the lack of change of their membrane potentials when stimulating the tissue; they were therefore also termed 'idle' cells.

Early experiments impaling 'glia' (= astrocytes?) in olfactory cortical slices from guinea pigs showed that perfusion with glutamate resulted in a prompt depolarisation of their membrane potentials. However, since it was considered at that time (see preceding paragraph) that glial cells did not have receptors but did have a highly K^+-sensitive membrane potential, the depolarisation was thought to be due to raised extracellular K^+ released from glutamate-activated neurons (Constanti and Galvan 1978). These studies also routinely failed to detect a conductance change to injected current during addition of glutamate or GABA; evidence that the membrane potential depolarisations were not due to changes in membrane conductances but were Nernstian responses to a changing transmembrane K^+ gradient (Krnjevic and Schwartz 1967; Constanti and Galvan 1978). In view of later work in cultures, and more importantly in slices (discussed later) the failure to see a conductance change was likely due to methodological limitations.

Work by Bowman and Kimelberg (1984) and Kettenmann et al. (1984) in primary astrocyte cultures showed marked depolarisations to applied glutamate and kainate. Since these effects could not be due to accumulation of extracellular K^+ in these neuron-free, perfused astrocyte monolayers, the depolarisations were attributed to glutamate receptors or electrogenic glutamate uptake. Later work showed that in these cortical astrocyte cultures, the depolarisation was via a kainic acid (KA)/AMPA type receptor (Sontheimer et al. 1988). However, electrogenic glutamate uptake was found to be the basis of the glutamate-induced depolarisation in acutely isolated astrocytic Müller cells from the amphibian retina (Brew and Attwell 1987; Barbour, Brew and Attwell 1991), and primary cultures of cerebellar astrocytes (Wyllie et al. 1991). Later, in situ hybridisation studies detected transcripts for the AMPA receptor in Bergmann glial cells in tissue sections. It was found that this receptor lacked the GluR2 subunit, making it Ca^{2+} permeable (Burnashev et al. 1992; Müller et al. 1992; Seeburg 1993). This type of receptor was also expressed by primary cultures of the Bergmann glia (Jonas 1993), and is thus an example of how primary cultures can reproduce the in vivo state. In contrast, acutely isolated glial cells from P9–12 (P = post-partum) hippocampus showed a high level of GluR2 by single-cell reverse transcriptase polymerase chain reaction (RT-PCR) (Steinhäuser and Gallo 1996). It is also beginning to appear that NMDA receptors, absent from cultured astrocytes, are present in some glial cells in situ (Steinhäuser and Gallo 1996).

Walz and Schlue (1982) were the first to show that serotonin (5-HT) hyperpolarised glial cells. As did Kuffler and Nicholls (1964) they used a simple, in this case, invertebrate model; the neuropil glial cells of the leech CNS, which could also be conveniently impaled with sharp microelectrodes. They showed that the hyperpolarisation was likely due to activation of a K^+ conductance. Recently, these studies in the neuropil glial cells have been extended by Munsch and Deitmer (1992), measuring $[Ca^{2+}]_i$ with fura-2 in the exposed cell. They found that 5-HT increased $[Ca^{2+}]_i$, and that this was largely dependent on external Ca^{2+}. Using current injection with two electrodes, they also found a decrease in membrane resistance which was ascribed to an increased Ca^{2+}-dependent K^+ conductance.

6.5.2 Transmitter-Induced Currents in Astrocytes in Slice Preparations

Electrophysiological studies on astrocytes in situ in mammalian brain slices or tissue are being currently done using patch-clamp methodology (MacVicar et al. 1989; Burnard, Crichton and MacVicar 1990; Clark and Mobbs 1992; Steinhäuser, Jabs and Kettenmann 1994), and have shown conductance changes in voltage-clamped astrocytes or presumed glial cell bodies in hippocampal slices when glutamate and GABA are perfused. In the whole-cell patch-clamp recordings, the possibility of the astrocyte responses being secondary to neuronal activation and release of K^+, on which Constantini and Galvan had earlier based their interpretation of indirect effects (see above), were considered to be avoided in the voltage-clamped, whole-cell mode, since changes in the slope of current–voltage relationships for specific ion currents would more reliably indicate a conductance change directly induced by applied transmitters.

In a recent study using whole-cell voltage clamping, Steinhäuser, Jabs and Kettenmann (1994) perfused GABA and glutamate onto P9–12 mouse hippocampal slices. Besides $GABA_A$ receptor-mediated currents, it was found that in electrophysiologically 'passive' GFAP(+) astrocytes, glutamate decreased the resting K^+ conductance and that most glutamate-mediated responses were through the kainate receptor. A small group of these cells also had NMDA-activated currents. High concentrations of glutamate of 1 mM were presumably needed because of glutamate uptake. However, in a study on P21–42 rat hippocampal slices, Duffy and MacVicar (1995) failed to show any astrocytic responses to glutamate or the metabotropic glutamate receptor agonist t-ACPD, and kainate caused brief Ca^{2+}

changes in only 25 % of the cells. In contrast, norepinephrine and the alpha-1-agonist phenylephrine evoked complex $[Ca^{2+}]_i$ signals in 100% of the astrocytes tested. The differences in the glutamate responses in these two studies could be because of species differences, age-difference, or because too low glutamate concentrations were used in the second set of studies. However, clear indication of age-dependency of the glutamate-mediated events has been shown in a study on rat hippocampal slices, where metabotropic glutamate receptors mediated the phosphorylation of GFAP in immature but not in adult rats (Wofchuk and Rodnight 1994). GABA- and glycine-induced chloride currents and block of K^+ conductance mediated by $GABA_A$ receptor activation have also been shown in astrocytes in rat spinal cord slices (Pastor et al. 1995).

Various complexities and difficulties do arise in the interpretation of whole-cell recordings from slice preparations. A decrease in detected net current could indicate either an inhibition of one type of K^+ current or increase in another K^+ current in the opposite direction; e.g. decrease in delayed rectifier K^+ outward current or increase in an inward rectifying K^+ current with the outward current being unaffected (see Barres, Chun and Corey 1990). This increased inward current could, besides being a direct result of transmitter exposure, also result from elevated $[K]_e$ due to K^+ release from contiguous, glutamate-activated neurons in the tissue preparation. Therefore the net current detected with the whole-cell configuration does not specify the underlying conductance changes. Another complication arises from the uncertainty that, although the soma from which the recordings are made are voltage-clamped, the processes may not be. Further complications in slices are that the added transmitter only diffuses relatively slowly to the cell under study, is taken up by other cells or can affect release of transmitters within the slice by actions on presynaptic receptors.

6.5.3 *Ionotropic Transmitter Receptor Channels in Astrocytes*

Ionotropic glutamate receptor channels activated by L-glutamate or its specific analogues NMDA, AMPA or kainate and variably permeable to K^+, Na^+ and Ca^{2+}, are some of the most intensively studied receptor ion channels. The ionotropic glutamate receptor channels, especially the NMDA receptor channel, have been suggested to play important roles in brain maturation (Facchinetti et al. 1996), some pathological conditions and in behavioural disorders such as schizophrenia (Goldstein et al. 1994). The NMDA receptor has only rarely been found in cultured astrocytes, but is seen in astrocytes in situ (Steinhäuser, Jabs and Kettenmann 1994; Puro, Yuan and Sucher 1996). The AMPA or kainate-activated receptors are found in most astrocyte preparations (Pearce and Murphy 1993; Kimelberg, Jalonen and Walz 1993; Jensen and Chiu 1993). In cultured trout astrocytes glutamate, kainate and quisqualate-induced inward currents are carried mainly by Na^+ (Clasen, Jeserich and Krüppel 1995). Comparison of the neuronal (granule cells) and astrocytic (type-2 astrocytes) receptor channels in cerebellar cultures showed striking similarities in the whole-cell currents, single-channel function and pharmacology of their AMPA/kainate receptor channels (Wyllie and Cull-Candy 1994). In cultured cortical type-1 astrocytes, glutamate activated inward currents are mainly carried by the electrogenic glutamate uptake system and kainate-activated Na^+-dependent currents (Stephens, Djamgoz and Wilkin 1993). In type-2 cortical astrocytes, kainate seems to activate currents carried by both Na^+ and Ca^{2+} (Stephens, Djamgoz and Wilkin 1993; Meucci et al. 1996).

Other ionotropic receptor channels found in astrocytes are the $GABA_A$ receptor chloride channels, which have been found in rat optic nerve and acutely isolated hippocampal astrocytes (Butt and Jennings 1994a; Fraser et al. 1995). In astrocytes cultured from spinal cord, two different types of $GABA_A$ receptors have been characterised; in both fibrous and protoplasmic astrocytes the local anaesthetic pentobarbitone, as well as the benzodiazepine diazepam, increased GABA-induced currents, but the inverse benzodiazepine agonist DMCM reduced GABA-induced currents in 'fibrous' astrocytes and increased them in 'protoplasmic' astrocytes (Rosewater and Sontheimer 1994). Similar results have been obtained from acutely isolated rat hippocampal astrocytes (Fraser et al. 1995). Ion channel activities related to adrenergic receptor activation have surprisingly, in view of the evidence that these receptors exist on astrocytes in situ (see section 6.4.1), not been much studied in astrocytes (adrenergic receptor activation in astrocytes reviewed by Stone and Ariano (1989) and Shao, Enkvist and McCarthy (1993)). However, Bowman and Kimelberg (1988) showed conductance changes in type 1 astrocytes in primary culture which were mediated by α_1 receptors and seemed to involve a change in Cl^- conductance.

Serotonin is known to directly modulate both K^+ and Cl^- ion channels in neurons via G protein-linked metabotropic receptors and also to activate an ionotropic receptor channel ($5-HT_3$). Activation of channels via the metabotropic $5HT_{2A}$ receptor have recently been reported by one of the authors in primary astrocyte cultures (see section 6.5.4). Another very important receptor channel in the brain, the nicotinic acetylcholine (ACh) receptor, has so far not been reported in astrocytes, though the metabotropic muscarinic ACh receptor has been found (Van der Zee et al. 1993; Guizzetti et al. 1996). It thus seems that astrocytes lack some of the very important ionotropic transmitter receptor ion channels found to be essential in many neuronal functions. In contrast, astrocytes have an abundance of metabotropic receptors, especially using Ca^{2+} signalling pathways.

6.5.4 Metabotropic Receptors and Calcium-Mediated Events in Astrocytes

Astrocytes are known to show great plasticity in their receptor expression and function depending on their developmental stage, region or experimental conditions. For example the metabotropic glutamate receptor agonist t-ACPD induces phosphoinositol hydrolysis over 10 times more in astrocytes cultured in serum-free compared to serum-containing culture media. This difference was shown to be specific for glutamate receptors as no such difference was detected for carbachol or noradrenaline (Miller, Bridges and Cotman 1993). Metabotropic (mGluR$_5$) receptor expression was found to be enhanced when astrocytes were cultured in chemically defined media, and it was suggested that this resembles reactive gliosis in vivo (Miller et al. 1995). The amount of mGluR$_5$ present in astrocytes has been found to decrease drastically in brain with development (Van den Pol, Romano and Ghosh 1995). Metabotropic RNAs encoding glutamate, acetylcholine and serotonin receptors have been found in corpus callosum tissue, and in situ hybridisation studies detected the message in astrocytes in situ (Matute and Miledi 1993).

One consequence of the activation of metabotropic receptors is a rise in intracellular Ca^{2+}. This usually involves a first, fast peak of calcium release from intracellular stores via the IP$_3$ pathway, and often a second long-lasting elevation and/or oscillation of Ca^{2+} mediated by Ca^{2+} influx, at least partially through Ca^{2+} channels, such as the voltage-sensitive L-type Ca^{2+} channel (Charles et al. 1991; Van den Pol, Finkbeiner and Cornell-Bell 1992; Duffy and MacVicar 1993; Kim, Rioult and Cornell-Bell 1994). Among a plethora of possible effects, the increased $[Ca^{2+}]_i$ can lead to increased and transient activation of Ca^{2+}-sensitive K^+, Cl^- and Ca^{2+} channels, which may then cause alteration of the astrocyte membrane potential, followed by further voltage-dependent channel activation. An example of small-conductance K^+ and Ca^{2+} channels opening following 5HT$_{2A}$ receptor activation in a cultured astrocyte is shown in Fig. 6.4. However, astrocytes respond to serotonin by release of Ca^{2+} from intracellular stores, concomitant with inward K^+ and Ca^{2+}-channel activation only when cultured for over 24 h in media containing horse serum, and no such responses have so far been seen in acutely isolated cortical astrocytes (Margraf et al. 1995). Other metabotropic receptors linked to increases in $[Ca^{2+}]_i$ in primary astrocyte cultures are bradykinin B$_2$ receptors inducing $[Ca^{2+}]_i$ elevation together with mainly inward currents (Gimpl et al. 1992; Stephens, Djamgoz and Wilkin 1993). Many of the metabotropic receptors also activate cyclic adenosine monophosphate (cAMP)-mediated intracellular pathways, which in contrast may lead to decreased Ca^{2+} currents, but increased K^+ currents (see review by Morga and Heuschling 1996).

In conditions where long-lasting excessive transmitter release from neurons, or reduced uptake by astrocytes, occurs, $[Ca^{2+}]_i$ may stay permanently elevated, which will lead to overactivation of Ca^{2+}-sensitive ion channels, triggering Ca^{2+}-mediated cell metabolism, and, if prolonged, eventually to cell death. If more than one transmitter is released at any time close to the astrocyte receptors (which certainly is expected to occur in vivo), multiple synergistic interactions, as well as antagonistic effects may follow. These complex transmitter/ion channel and ion channel/ion channel interactions in astrocytes could form a net of

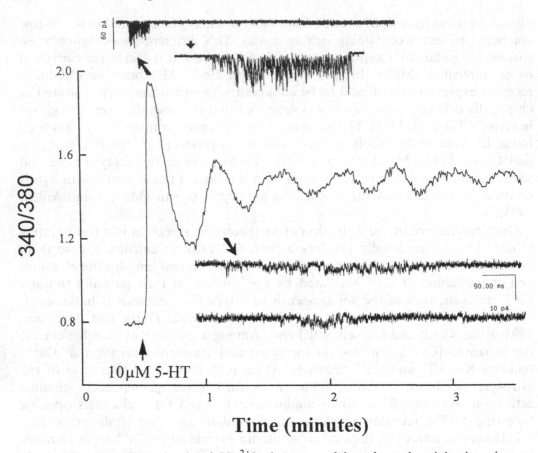

Fig. 6.4. 5-HT-stimulated $[Ca^{2+}]_i$ changes and ion channel activity in primary cultured astrocytes. For the $[Ca^{2+}]_i$ changes (main tracing) the recording was from a cell in a 21-day primary culture which had been grown in 10% horse serum. For the ion channel activities (times at which the channel activities appeared shown by the bold arrows pointing from the Ca^{2+} tracing) the cell was from the same type of culture, except it was grown for 8 days. The burst-type opening of multiple small-conductance K_{Ca} channels (calcium-dependent potassium channels, upper channel traces) starts typically 15–30 s after 5-HT addition and inactivates within 10–30 s. The more sustained Ca^{2+} channel activity (lower channel traces) starts after the peak sK_{Ca} is over and continues some minutes after 5-HT is removed (Jalonen et al., unpublished data).

signalling systems, which via the astrocytes' ability to regulate the neuronal environment will modulate neuronal firing and therefore ultimately affect behaviour. Far more speculatively, these could form astroglial networks contributing to information storage and processing and behavioural manifestations of consciousness.

6.6 Transmitter Transporter Systems in Astrocytes

Uptake systems are very important in determining the concentrations of transmitters remaining in the synaptic cleft and therefore the magnitude and duration of transmitter effects. Astrocytes in vivo have long been known to contain a very active uptake system for the excitatory amino acids (EAA) glutamate and aspartate, as determined by immunocytochemistry (Rothstein et al. 1994; Lehre et al. 1995), measuring uptake of radiolabelled EAAs by autoradiography (Hertz 1979) and immuno-labelling for EAAs (Laake et al. 1995). Astrocytes in primary culture duplicate these active uptake systems in density of transporters, their kinetics and pharmacology. Glutamate uptake studies on astrocyte cultures from different brain regions show the same relative rank order as the recent localisation of the dominant astrocyte-specific glutamate transporter (GLT) form of the excitatory amino-acid transporters (Fig. 6.2). Three separate cyclic deoxyribose nucleic acids (cDNAs) encoding three different transporters have now been described. In rat brain two of these localise to astrocytes [GLT-1 and L-glutamate/L-aspartate transporter (GLAST)] while a third (EAAC1) is found in neurons (Rothstein et al. 1994; Kanai et al. 1995).

Altering the activities of the astrocytic EAA transporters has been shown to alter neuronal function. Keyser and Pellmar (1994) lesioned astrocytes in guinea pig hippocampal slices with fluoroacetate. This resulted in inhibition of post-synaptic potentials, which could have been due to loss of a variety of metabolic or other support functions of astrocytes. It was also found that the response to added glutamate was prolonged. More recently, Rothstein et al. (1996) specifically reduced the levels and activities of the three EAA transporters individually by chronic intraventricular administration of the specific antisense mRNAs in mice. They found that only reduction of the astrocytic GLT-1 or GLAST increased steady state [glu]$_e$ levels while similar reductions in the neuronal EAAC1 had no effect. Thus such lesion studies can address the question of functional relevance. We and others have recently shown that raising medium [K$^+$], as seen in cerebral ischaemia, leads to reversal of the glial transporter in cultured astrocytes and this may be one source of the raised [EAAs]$_e$ seen in these conditions which are considered to lead to neuronal toxicity (excitoxicity) (Szatkowski and Attwell 1994; Kimelberg et al. 1995). All these data suggest that alterations in the functioning of the astrocyte EAA transporter will have profound effects on extracellular glutamate levels, thereby affecting normal as well as pathological brain function.

The presence of other transporters on astrocytes have only been clearly established in primary cultures and at much lower activities than the EAA transmitters. These include the Na$^+$-dependent and fluoxetine-sensitive high affinity uptake system for 5-HT. In cultures, the 5-HT system is dependent on serum, whereas the glutamate uptake system is unaffected by growth in serum-free medium (Kimelberg et al. 1992). High affinity uptake has also been shown by autoradio-

!graphy in astrocytes freshly isolated from rat cerebral cortex (Dave and Kimelberg 1994). It may be that many transporters are present in very localised regions, so !that they would only be infrequently seen in isolated cells or in situ. Inhibition of 'uptake systems for transmitters such as serotonin have profound effects on mood, appetite and other affective and non-affective behaviours (Cowley et al. 1990; Fuller, Wong and Robertson 1991).

6.7 Functional and Behavioural Implications of Transmitter Receptors and Uptake Systems on Astrocytes

What are the implications of these transmitter interactions on the many proposed functions of astrocytes? The potential roles of astrocytes in neuronal development and migration, extracellular ion homeostasis and blood flow regulation have been extensively reviewed (Kimelberg 1983; Federoff and Vernadakis 1986; Somjen 1988; Malhotra, Shnitka and Elbrink 1990; Tower 1992; Aschner and LoPachin 1993b; Murphy 1993; Kimelberg and Aschner 1994; Montgomery 1994; Kimelberg 1995). The experimental bases for many of these suggestions remain frustratingly indirect, but there is sufficient general physiological and morphological data from a variety of systems to indicate that it would be surprising if astrocytes were not involved in a large number of CNS functions, but each hypothesis has to be supported by careful experimentation. To go beyond the general, we first need precise information as to what degree the marked regional localisation seen for receptors and transporters in the brain refer to astrocytes and to neurons. Of course, the major localisations of receptors and transporters, such as dopamine in the striatum and glutamate in the hippocampus, clearly are referable to neurons. The primary astrocyte cultures have been of great value in showing the many and varied properties that astrocytes can have. However, as pointed out many times in this chapter continuing studies have shown differences in receptor expression between the cultures and astrocytes in situ. Thus primary astrocyte cultures cannot be automatically trusted to give data of sufficient reliability to indicate what receptors and transporters astrocytes have in vivo.

A large number of hypotheses have been put forward concerning the role of astrocytes in brain function, as noted and referenced throughout this chapter. Astrocytes in vitro exhibit properties that support each of these hypotheses. Essentially, however, these hypotheses remain untested in vivo. Establishing the role of astrocytes in brain and behaviour is even more difficult and faces many of the same difficulties encountered in determining the precise roles of neurons in the brain. Thus, we know that neurons carry information and that disruption of specific pathways elicit changes in behaviour, but we have little idea of the actual processes underlying behaviour. At a minimum, it seems likely that astrocytes may play a central role in modulating neuronal activity. This could occur in a large number of ways related to the hypotheses noted above. For example, small changes in $[K^+]_e$, determined by astrocytic uptake or release, could markedly affect neuronal excitability in a given region. Subtle astrocytic shape changes could alter the strength of neuronal synaptic connections and ephaptic transmission, and hence information flow. The really hard question is whether astrocytes play roles in behaviour independent of their effects on neurons. Even the most chauvinistic glial supporters would be unlikely to say that there is currently any evidence for such roles; but who knows? Furthermore, it will probably be difficult, and quite possibly artificial, to consider the contributions of neurons and astrocytes to behaviour as independent entities.

Acknowledgements

Original work of the authors quoted in this chapter was supported by NIH grants NS 19492 (HKK), NS 20212 (KDM), NS 30944 and EY 08055 (CA). Also RCD 92-53750 from NSF and RG-16/96 from HFSP to Ca^{2+}. We thank Erin Grasek for help in preparing the manuscript.

7

Glial Regulation of the Neuronal Microenvironment

EVA SYKOVÁ, ELISABETH HANSSON,
LARS RÖNNBÄCK and CHARLES NICHOLSON

Summary

The astrocytes in the brain form gap-junction coupled networks which constitute the link between blood and the neurons. All communication between astroglia and neurons occurs through the very narrow extracellular space (ECS), and the astroglia have a high capacity to maintain ionic, amino acid, neurotransmitter and water homeostasis in this space. Extracellular glutamate is taken up into the astroglial syncytium by high-affinity, high-capacity uptake carriers. Glutamate induces rapid astroglial swelling. The activation of both ionotropic and metabotropic glutamate receptors, glutamate uptake carriers and redistribution of Na^+ and K^+ ions are important components in the glutamate-induced rapid astroglial swelling. Furthermore, the Na^+-K^+-$2Cl^-$-co-transporter and a Na^+/K^+-ATPase seem to be activated during the glutamate-induced astroglial swelling process.

Changes in ECS composition and geometry are a consequence of neuronal activity and the role of glia in K^+, pH and amino acid homeostasis and cellular swelling. They result from repetitive neuronal activity, seizures, anoxia, injury and many other pathological states in the central nervous system (CNS) and may significantly affect signal transmission in the CNS. Cellular swelling is compensated for by ECS volume shrinkage and by a decrease in the apparent diffusion coefficients of neuroactive substances diffusing in the ECS, and the movement of substances in the intercellular channels is hindered. The molecules of the ECS matrix and the varying size of the fine glial processes may form diffusional barriers and/or channel the diffusion of substances in the CNS. This can either increase efficacy of synaptic as well as non-synaptic transmission, by greater accumulation of substances, or induce damage to the nerve cells if these substances reach toxic concentrations. The dynamic changes in the composition and structure of the neuronal microenvironment can affect the efficacy of signal transmission and therefore result in behavioural and plastic changes. Thus the extracellular communication channel may be regarded as predominantly under the control of the glial cells.

7.1 Introduction

Behavioural changes, plastic changes and the establishment of memory are believed to involve a persistent change in the strength of communication between neighbouring neurons, i.e. a persistent change in synaptic efficacy (Squire 1987). Only recently, it has been shown that the efficacy of signal transmission in the brain is critically dependent on neuron–glia interaction, on glial cell function and on changes in the cellular microenvironment (Nicholson 1980; Syková 1992b, 1997). In this chapter, we would like to show how persistent changes in glia, in neuron–glia communication and in the neuronal microenvironment can affect the efficacy of signal transmission and therefore result in behavioural and plastic changes.

It is now widely accepted that the ECS is a communication and modulation channel (Nicholson 1980; Syková 1983, 1992; Fuxe and Agnati 1991; Bach-y-Rita 1993), whose ionic and chemical composition, size and geometry depend on neuronal activity and glial cell function. Experiments employing ion-selective microelectrodes (ISMs) (Syková, Hník and Vyklický 1981; Syková 1992a), have revealed that transmembrane ionic fluxes during neuronal activity and pathological states result in transient changes in the ionic composition of the CNS extracellular space. Ionic homeostasis in the CNS is ensured by a variety of mechanisms in both neurons and glial cells (Syková 1983, 1992b; Walz 1989; Chesler 1990; Deitmer and Rose 1996). It has been shown that the impairment of ionic homeostasis due to insufficient glial cell function can lead to the impairment of signal transmission. This is particularly due to activity-related extracellular K^+ increase and acid shift in extracellular pH.

CNS local architecture is composed of neurons, neural connections, glial cells and molecules of the extracellular matrix (Fig. 7.1). By local architecture, we mean the size of the pores between the cells (size of the intercellular channels) and the geometry of the ECS. The local architecture is altered during glial swelling, astrogliosis, demyelination, and changes in the components of the extracellular matrix (e.g. proteoglycans, laminin, fibronectin, tanescin, adhesion molecules etc.), i.e. during changes which affect the size of the intercellular channels, extracellular macromolecules and ECS geometry. In this sense, local CNS architectures differ during development and ageing, and persisting changes exist during ongoing neuronal activity, 'soft' pathologies, in response to trauma and after cell death during severe pathological states. We can therefore also assume that changes in the local CNS architecture occur during learning, memory formation and behavioural changes.

ECS size and geometry affect the movement (diffusion) of various neuroactive substances in the CNS. Although synaptic transmission is the major means of communication between nerve cells, it is not the only one. Substances can be released non-synaptically, diffuse through ECS and bind to extrasynaptic, high-affinity binding sites. This type of non-synaptic transmission by diffusion was

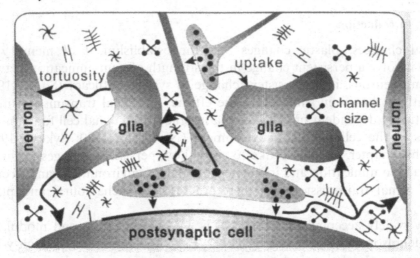

Fig. 7.1. Schematic of CNS architecture. The CNS architecture is composed of neurons, axons, glial cells, cellular processes, molecules of the extracellular matrix and intercellular channels. The architecture affects movement (diffusion) of substances in the brain, which is critically dependent on channel size, extracellular space tortuosity (λ), and cellular uptake. (Modified from Syková 1997.)

recently termed 'diffusion transmission' (Bach-y-Rita 1993) or 'volume transmission' (Fuxe and Agnati 1991). The neuroactive substances may diffuse through the ECS to target neurons, glia or capillaries without requiring synapses. This mode of communication can function between neurons as well as between neurons and glial cells, and may be a basis for the mechanism of information processing in functions involving large masses of cells such as vigilance, sleep, chronic pain, hunger, depression, plastic changes etc. On the other hand, impairment of the ionic homeostasis and glial swelling during pathological states lead to compensatory shrinkage of the ECS, i.e. to dramatic changes in ECS architecture (volume and geometry) which can contribute to the impairment of CNS function and neuronal damage.

7.2 Role of Glia in Ionic Homeostasis

Measurements of dynamic changes in the extracellular concentration of biologically important ions in vivo as well as in vitro became possible with the introduction of ion-selective microelectrodes (ISMs) (for review see Syková 1983, 1992a; Nicholson 1993). An ISM that consists of a liquid membrane (liquid ion-exchanger, ion-carrier) placed in the tip of a glass microelectrode is a miniaturised potentiometric sensor. When introduced into tissue or solution where the activity of the respective ion is to be measured, a Nernst potential develops across the ion-exchanger membrane, i.e. one measures a potential that changes logarithmically with the activity of the ion for which the ion-exchanger is selective. To eliminate distortion by any electrical activity including membrane, synaptic and action potentials, double-barrelled microelectrodes are used, which have an ion-exchanger in one channel, while the other channel serves as the reference electrode. Since the reference electrode also records electrical activity in the tissue, the signal from it can be used to cancel out the undesired component (Fig. 7.2).

7.2.1 Activity-Related Transient Changes in Extracellular K^+, pH and Ca^{2+}

Dynamic changes in $[K^+]_e$ have been recorded in the immediate vicinity of individual neurons. In one example, recordings were made in the mesencephalic reticular formation (MRF) of the rat which is recognised as a structure with a high spontaneous activity level. During a burst of spontaneous action potentials, $[K^+]_e$ steadily increases by as much as 0.2 mM (Syková, Rothenberg and Krekule 1974). The neurons start to fire again at the same time the K^+ elevation returns to the 'resting' K^+ baseline (Fig. 7.2), suggesting that accumulation of K^+ in the ECS blocks spontaneous activity.

Adequate stimulation, such as innocuous stimuli, acute nociceptive stimuli, or peripheral tissue injury of a hind paw, results in activity-related transient K^+ and pH_e changes in the spinal dorsal horn (Svoboda et al 1988; Syková and Svoboda 1990). In the visual cortex of the cat (Singer and Lux 1975) and in the ectostriatum of chicks (Syková et al. 1990), a rise in $[K^+]_e$ and pH shifts accompany neuronal activity during visual stimulation of the receptive field. Pure-tone acoustic stimulation over a frequency range of 500 Hz to 0.25 kHz produced changes of about 1 mM K^+ in the organ of Corti, with the maximal change between supporting cell and inner hair cell (Johnston et al. 1989). The K^+ and pH changes evoked by adequate stimulation are generally of smaller amplitude than those evoked by electrical stimulation, with an increase in $[K^+]_e$ of about 1–3 mM and an acid shift of up to about 0.05–0.1 pH units, but they can last longer. For example, after peripheral injury the $[K^+]_e$ increase and pH_e decrease in the spinal dorsal horn begin 2–10 min after injury, reach their maximum in 15–40 min and then persist for more than 2 h.

An activity-related increase in extracellular K^+ concentration ($[K^+]_e$), alkaline and acid shifts in extracellular pH (pH_e) and a decrease in extracellular Ca^{2+} concentration ($[Ca^{2+}]_e$) have been found to accompany neuronal activity in a variety of animals and brain regions, in vivo as well as in vitro (for reviews see Syková 1983; Chesler 1990; Syková 1992b). It has been recognised that their origin and mechanisms are similar, but the amplitude and sequence vary with brain region. Most frequently, neuronal activity results in an increase in $[K^+]_e$, a decrease in $[Ca^{2+}]_e$ and a fast extracellular alkaline shift, followed by a slower but longer-lasting acid shift (Fig. 7.2; Syková, Rothenberg and Krekule 1974;

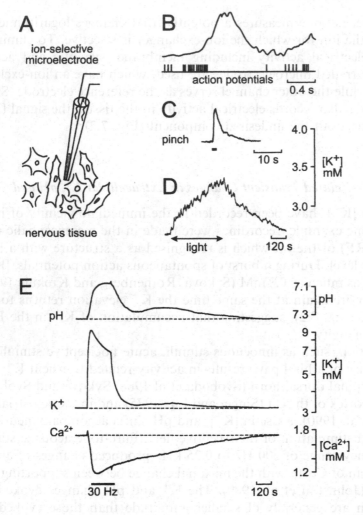

Fig. 7.2. (A) Diagram of experimental set-up for recording with a double-barrelled ion-selective microelectrode. Activity-related elevations of $[K^+]_e$ recorded with K^+-selective microelectrode. (B) Elevation in unstimulated reticular formation of the rat is associated with spontanous bursts of cell firing recorded by the reference barrel. (C) Transient increase in the L4 spinal segment of the rat in response to a pinch of the toes of the hind paw. (D) Increase in the ectostriatum of 2-day-old chick evoked by light stimulation of the contralateral eye. (E) Simultaneous recordings of transient pH_e, $[K^+]_e$ and $[Ca^{2+}]_e$ changes in spinal dorsal horn of the frog evoked by tetanic stimulation at 30 Hz. (Part (B) adapted from Syková et al. 1974; (C) from Svoboda et al. 1988; (D) from Syková et al. 1990 and (E) from Chvátal et al. 1988.)

Syková and Svoboda 1990; Jendelová and Syková 1991). After sustained adequate stimulation of the afferent input or after repetitive electrical stimulation, the ionic transients reach a certain steady state, the so-called 'ceiling' level, which in the mammalian cortex is about 7 mM K^+ (Heinemann and Lux 1977) and in the mammalian spinal cord 6–8 mM K^+ (Kříž, Syková and Vyklický 1975; Syková and Svoboda 1990). The alkaline shifts in mammalian cortex, cerebellum or spinal cord do not exceed 0.02 pH units, while the acid shifts are about 0.2 pH units. For example, after the tetanic stimulation of the sciatic nerve (30–100 Hz) the $[K^+]_e$ 'ceiling' level in the adult rat or cat spinal cord is attained in 5–8 s, while the 'ceiling' level of the acid shift is reached in 10–20 s. When stimulation is continued beyond this, a gradual decrease of both transients, $[K^+]_e$ and pH_e, occur after the ceiling levels are reached (Fig. 7.2) due to homeostatic mechanisms in neurons and glia (see Chapters 10, 11).

7.2.2 Ionic Changes During Postnatal Development and Gliogenesis

Stimulation-evoked transient changes in $[K^+]_e$ and pH_e in the rat spinal cord are different during early postnatal development, presumably because of incomplete glial cell function. Glial cells play an important role in buffering changes in the concentration of ions and small molecules in the tortuous extracellular space. The extensive area of glial cell membranes across which ions and small molecules can move provides an efficient transport system to minimise the drastic changes in the extracellular space which impair neuronal function. Besides their role in K^+ and amino acid homeostasis, glial cells play an important role in buffering changes in extracellular pH.

Studies on K^+ and pH_e in the spinal cord during maturation underscore the role of glial cells in the maintenance of extracellular ionic homeostasis. Both $[K^+]_e$ and pH_e activity-related changes were studied in spinal cords during early postnatal days, since glial cell proliferation, maturation and myelination occur postnatally, and more slowly than maturation of neurons. In the neonatal rat spinal cord, stimulation-evoked changes in $[K^+]_e$ are much larger than in the adult animal. In the ECS, alkaline shifts dominate, while in adult animals acid shifts dominate (Fig. 7.3; Jendelová and Syková 1991; Syková et al. 1992). For example, at P3–P6 (P = postnatal day), the $[K^+]_e$ changes evoked in the dorsal horn by a single electrical stimulus were as large as 1.5–2.5 mM. Such changes in $[K^+]_e$ can be evoked in the adult rat spinal cord only with stimulation at a frequency about 30 Hz (Svoboda et al. 1988). At P3–P6 single, as well as repetitive electrical stimulation, evoked a dominant alkaline shift which was followed by a smaller post-stimulation acid shift when the stimulation was discontinued. At P10–P14, when gliogenesis in rat spinal cord gray matter peaks, the K^+ ceiling level decreases and the stimulation evokes acid shifts of about 0.1–0.2 pH unit, which are preceded by scarcely discernible alkaline shifts, as is also the case in adult rats. In other series of

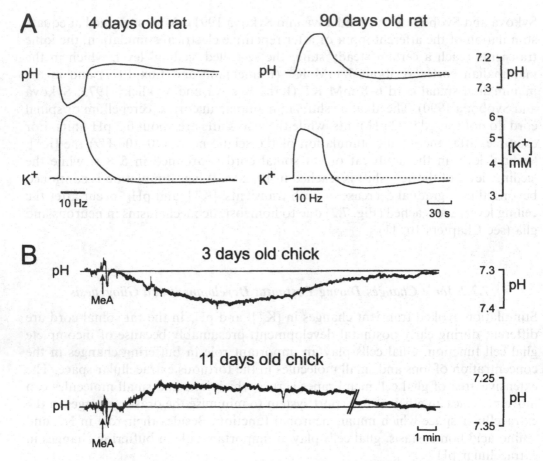

Fig. 7.3. (A) Stimulation-evoked pH_e and $[K^+]_e$ changes in the spinal dorsal horn of 4-day-old rats and adults. The stimulation of the dorsal root at a frequency of 10 Hz evoked a typical alkaline shift in a 4-day-old pup, which was accompanied by an increase in $[K^+]_e$. In adult rats, a stimulation of even 100 Hz evoked a smaller increase in $[K^+]_e$. The change in pH_e was biphasic; first an acid shift occurred, and then a poststimulation alkaline shift. Note the poststimulation undershoots in $[K^+]_e$. (B) Age-related pH responses to taste aversive substance (methylantranilate, MeA) stimulation in a 3-day-old and an 11-day-old chick. (Part (A) from Jendelová and Syková 1991; (B) from Ng et al. 1991.)

studies, we have shown that neither light nor taste aversive substance (methyl-anthranilate) stimulation of anaesthetised chicks yielded reliable evidence of acid shifts in neostriatum until after 10 days posthatching (Fig. 7.3; Ng et al. 1991). It is possible that at least with respect to pH responses, glia are functionally immature in 1- to 3-day-old chicks.

Activity-related $[K^+]_e$ and pH_e changes in spinal cords were also studied after 'early' postnatal X-irradiation (PI), a procedure which blocks gliogenesis but leaves the neurons intact (Syková et al. 1992). In X-irradiated animals, the stimulation-evoked $[K^+]_e$ increase is larger than in control animals, and stimulation evokes a dominant alkaline shift. These results show that postnatal X-irradiation which blocks gliogenesis impairs the normal development of K^+ and pH_e homeostasis.

7.2.3 Extracellular K^+ Homeostasis

K^+ and pH homeostasis in the CNS is ensured by a variety of mechanisms in both neurons and glial cells (for reviews see Syková 1983, 1992b; Chesler 1990; Deitmer and Rose 1996). After returning to the prestimulation $[K^+]_e$ values, a transient decrease in $[K^+]_e$ occurs below the original K^+ baseline, the so-called poststimulation K^+-undershoot (Heineman and Lux 1975; Kříž, Syková and Vyklický 1975). This K^+-undershoot is blocked by ouabain or during hypoxia. These findings suggest that the recovery of the activity-related $[K^+]_e$ change is dependent at least partly on Na^+/K^+ pump activity in neurons and presumably also in glial cells. Besides the Na^+/K^+ pump, the ECS K^+ homeostasis is maintained by three other mechanisms ensured by glia: (1) K^+ spatial buffering, (2) KCl uptake and (3) Ca^{2+}-activated K^+ channels.

7.2.4 Spatial Buffering of Potassium

Many experiments have shown a transient increase in extracellular potassium, $[K^+]_e$, (e. g. Syková 1983) from about 3 mM in the vertebrate brain to somewhere below 12 mM and lasting typically for a few seconds. The 6–8 mM level appeared to be a 'ceiling' in adult spinal cord (Kříž, Syková and Vyklický 1975) and 12 mM level in the adult brain (Heinemann and Lux 1977) under normal conditions, although it was exceeded dramatically during spreading depression and ischaemia (Vyskočil, Kříž and Bureš 1972; Nicholson and Kraig 1981). There are obviously mechanisms that effectively control $[K^+]_e$.

One of the prime candidates for $[K^+]_e$ regulation is the so-called spatial buffering (SB) mechanism. First described qualitatively by Orkand, Nicholls and Kuffler (1966) in the leech, the concept was based on the property of glial cells to behave as almost perfect K^+ electrodes. The idea is that if one end of an elongated glial cell is bathed in elevated $[K^+]_e$ (Fig. 7.4), then that part of the cell will become depolarised and will set up a current circuit through the cell. But since glial cells are predominantly permeable to K^+, the transmembrane currents must be borne by K^+, and so K^+ will enter the glial cell at site of high $[K^+]_e$ and leave elsewhere, thus dissipating the difference in extracellular K^+.

Gardner-Medwin, Coles and Tsacopoulos (1981) published evidence for SB by glial cells in the retina of the bee followed by a series of extensive experimental and theoretical papers (Gardner-Medwin 1983a,b, 1986; Gardner-Medwin and

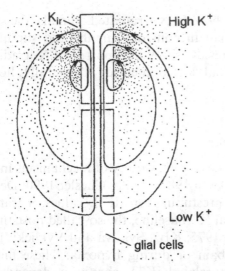

Fig. 7.4. A rise in $[K^+]_e$ localised to one end of a glial cell or ensemble of coupled glial cells leads to localised depolarisation and inward current flow carried exclusively by K^+ through inward rectifier channels (K_{ir}). Current leaves at remote sites through similar channels again mediated by K^+. By this means the initial rise in $[K^+]_e$ is rapidly dissipated. (Modified from Nicholson 1983.)

Nicholson 1983). The essence of these papers is two-fold. First Gardner-Medwin devised an ingenious experimental approach: if the SB mechanism exists, then passing a current across the brain should induce a change in $[K^+]_e$. This was completely verified in a series of experiments in the cerebellum of the rat (Gardner-Medwin and Nicholson 1983). In the latter studies, it was confirmed that current-induced $[K^+]_e$ changes occurred even after metabolic poisoning of the tissue showing they were a basic membrane property and not due to active transport. The current-passing method was also applied successfully in the retina by Karwoski et al. (1989).

The second major contribution of Gardner-Medwin was to develop a complete theoretical framework for the description of spatial buffering (SB) (Gardner-Medwin 1983b, 1986). The theory is quite complex, but in its essentials it combines together the theory of ionic diffusion in the presence of electric fields, using the classic Nernst–Planck equation, and then couples that to a cable-theory description of the glial cells. This theory accurately predicted the results of the current passing experiments and also led to a description of conditions under which SB would be important.

In most of his papers, Gardner-Medwin was careful not to identify unequivocally the cells responsible for SB as glial cells. The most compelling evidence that they are indeed glial cells has probably come from the extensive work of Newman. By developing a technique for isolating and removing single Müller cells from the vertebrate retina, Newman was able to show regional specialisation and K^+ 'siphoning' to the endfeet (Newman 1984, 1985a, 1986a) and to generalise his findings into a quantitative model for the CNS (Odette and Newman 1988). Other investigators added more information on SB in the retina (Immel and Steinberg 1986; Reichenbach 1991; Oakley et al. 1992).

Thus SB has been established under experimental conditions and justified theoretically. What has never been truly addressed is the relative importance of SB compared to other mechanisms for controlling $[K^+]_e$ in the short term. The original work of Kříž, Syková and Vyklický (1975) and Heinemann and Lux (1975) attributed the control of $[K^+]_e$ to the Na^+/K^+ pump (based in part on the undershoot in $[K^+]$ after prolonged stimulation of neuronal populations – such an undershoot cannot be generated by SB mechanisms). Later work on the bee retina (Coles and Orkand 1983) established that both SB and active transport were involved and recent studies have strengthened this view (Newman 1996b).

7.2.5 Extra- and Intracellular pH Homeostasis

Extra- and intracellular pH (pH_i) homeostasis is ensured by a variety of mechanisms in neurons and glia, as described in Chapter 10. The membrane transport processes which lead to the changes in pH_i and pH_e are either non-specific (both in neurons and glia) or specific for neurons or glia. In summary, we can divide them into acid loaders and acid extruders. From a number of studies it is evident that in neurons, acid loaders dominate (making the pH_e alkaline), while in glia acid extruders dominate (making the pH_e acid). There is a considerable evidence for the neuronal origin of the alkaline shifts and the glial origin of the activity-related acid shifts. For example, stimulation-evoked alkaline shifts are abolished by the blockage of synaptic transmission by Mn^{2+} or Mg^{2+}, while the acid shifts are unaffected (Jendelová and Syková 1991). To examine to what extent activity-related $[K^+]_e$ changes in spinal cord result in acid shifts in pH_e, isolated spinal cords of frogs and rats were superfused with Ringer's solutions containing elevated K^+ (Chvátal et al. 1988; Jendelová and Syková 1991). Increases in $[K^+]_e$ to 10 mM resulted in concomitant acid shifts of about 0.2 pH units. The application of K^+ evoked similar changes at P4 and P11; however, the rise in K^+ and the decrease in pH_e were slower at P10–P14, presumably due to the dramatic decrease in the extracellular space volume which slowed down diffusion of K^+ into the spinal cord (Syková and Chvátal 1993; Lehmenkühler et al. 1993b). It is therefore evident that a rise in $[K^+]_e$ results in an acid shift in pH_e.

Stimulation-evoked alkaline shifts in the isolated rat spinal cord are substantially blocked by the γ-aminobutyric acid (GABA) antagonist picrotoxin and by glutamate receptor antagonists and channel blockers such as MK801 (non-competitive NMDA receptor antagonist and channel blocker) and CNQX (competitive AMPA/kainate receptor antagonist) (Syková et al. 1992; Jendelová et al.

1994). Activity-related extracellular acid shifts are therefore a consequence of neuronal acidosis, extracellular K^+ increase, glial depolarisation and alkaline shift in glial pH_i, all leading to stimulation of classic acid extrusion systems in glial cells (for more details see Chapter 10).

7.3 Role of Glia in ECS Volume and Geometry

7.3.1 The Diffusion Parameters of the Brain Extracellular Space

Diffusion analysis provides information about how different types of molecules distribute and transfer information in the brain extracellular space. There are now extensive data ranging from a description of the behaviour of small ions less than 100 M_r to macromolecules up to 70,000 M_r. A second benefit of diffusion analysis comes from allowing diffusing molecules to probe the structure of the extracellular space and reveal its geometry. This approach has led to the description and measurement of volume fraction (α) and tortuosity (λ) (Fig. 7.1 and Fig. 7.5; see below). Finally, diffusion analysis can also reveal information about functional processes such as the kinetics of uptake of molecules by neurons and glia.

7.3.2 The Conceptual Basis of Diffusion in the CNS

The various things that can affect the substance as it distributes in the medium are encapsulated in the fundamental diffusion equation:

$$\frac{\partial C}{\partial t} = \frac{D}{\lambda^2}\nabla^2 C + \frac{Q}{\alpha} - \frac{f(C)}{\alpha} \tag{7.1}$$

where concentration (mM) is $C \equiv C(\mathbf{x}, t)$, distance (cm) is denoted by the vector $\mathbf{x}$ (which is (x, y, z) and is frequently reduced to r in a spherically symmetric system) and time (s) is denoted by t.

The structure of the tissue is introduced through the two non-dimensional factors, λ the tortuosity and α, the volume fraction. Tortuosity is a measure of how diffusing molecules are hindered by cellular obstructions and volume fraction of the extracellular space is the ratio of the extracellular space to total tissue volume in a given region.

The term on the left of the equals sign in Eq. (7.1) represents the way that the concentration changes with time at any location. The first term on the right of the equal sign in Eq. (7.1) describes the contribution of diffusion itself. The free diffusion coefficient is D ($cm^2\,s^{-1}$) while ∇^2 represents the second spatial derivative in the appropriate coordinate system. The second term is the source-term, $Q \equiv Q(\mathbf{x}, t)$ ($mM\,s^{-1}$) which can describe local iontophoretic, pressure pulse or even the distributed release of a substance from blood vessels or cells. The third term, $f(C)$) (mM s^{-1}), represents uptake of material from the extracellular space, typically into cells, or degradation of the migrating substance by enzymatic attack or other means. It is often taken as zero or a linear function of C (Nicholson 1992) but it may also embody more complex uptake, such as Michaelis–Menten kinetics (Nicholson 1995).

The basic experimental paradigm for measuring brain diffusion properties consists of the defined release of a substance from a source that is sufficiently small to be approximated by a point (Fig. 7.5), and the measurement of the concentration of that substance in the volume surrounding the source at various times and distances. This paradigm can be modelled with precision and experimental measurements have verified its correctness.

For the basic paradigm, the solution of Eq. (7.1) may be expressed as (a restatement of equations in Nicholson and Phillips 1981; Nicholson 1992):

$$C(r, t) = \frac{Q}{8\pi D^* \alpha r} [h(r, t, \theta) - h(r, t, -\theta)] \text{ and } h(r, t, \theta)$$
$$= [g(r, t, \theta) - g(r, t - d, \theta)] \exp(r, \theta) \tag{7.2}$$

where $D^* = D/\lambda^2$, $\theta = \sqrt{k'/D^*}$, $g(r, t, \theta) = H(t)\text{erfc}(r/2\sqrt{D^* t} + \theta\sqrt{D^* t})$.

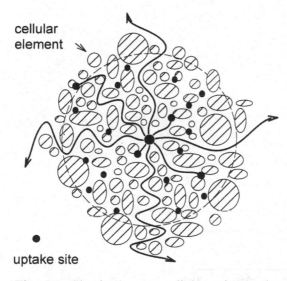

cellular element

uptake site

Fig. 7.5. The brain extracellular microenvironment consists of spaces between cellular elements, depicted here by the hatched ellipses. A microelectrode (central black circle) releases a substance by iontophoresis or infusion. The substance is constrained both by the reduced volume fraction (α) of the extracellular space and the tortuosity (λ). Tortuosity is represented by the wiggling lines emanating from the source. Diffusing molecules may be taken up or degraded at sites indicated by filled circles. In addition there may be a convective flow imposed on the diffusion process. (Modified from Nicholson 1995.)

In this solution an apparent diffusion coefficient (ADC) has been defined as $D^* = D/\lambda^2$. $H()$ is the Heaviside step function and erfc( ) is the complementary error function.

The source term Q is the rate of release of substance by a point source electrode. For iontophoresis $Q = In/F$, where I is the current (amps), n is the transport number for the substance and electrode, and F is Faraday's Electrochemical Equivalent. The duration of the source is d (s). Uptake of the diffusing substance from the extracellular space is represented in Eq. (7.2) by a linear process defined by k' (s^{-1}) so that

$$f(C) = \alpha k' C$$

Equation (7.2) is the basis of the tetramethylammonium (TMA$^+$) method (Nicholson and Phillips 1981; Nicholson 1992, 1993) and is better appreciated as a graph (Fig. 7.6). Note the dramatic effects of the geometrical parameters α and λ in amplifying the concentration (compare agar and brain) and the equally significant influence of uptake, $k' = 0.05 \, \text{s}^{-1}$.

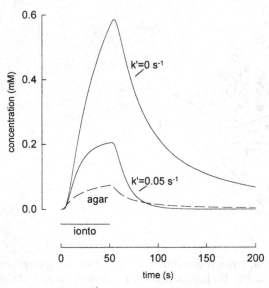

Fig. 7.6. TMA$^+$ iontophoresis curves computed from average parameters. Lowest curve shows diffusion in a dilute agar gel (free medium) with $\alpha = 1$, $\lambda = 1$. The two upper curves show concentrations produced by the same source, in a brain with $\alpha = 0.21$, $\lambda = 1.54$ with linear uptake ($k' = 0.05 \, \text{s}^{-1}$) and no uptake ($k' = 0$). For all curves: $r = 100 \, \mu\text{m}$; iontophoretic current, 100 nA for 50 s; $n = 0.4$; $D = 1.3 \times 10^{-5} \, \text{cm}^2 \, \text{s}^{-1}$ (TMA$^+$ at 37°C). (After Rice and Nicholson 1995.)

7.3.3 Structure of the Extracellular Space

Recent studies suggest that dextrans above 40 kDa (Nicholson and Tao 1993) and albumins above 14.5 kDa (Tao and Nicholson 1996) are significantly more hindered than the much smaller molecule TMA$^+$ ($M_r = 74$). One explanation for this is that the extracellular space is not homogeneous but rather the pore space varies in size so that small molecules can access all the spaces but larger ones are restricted. This would increase the measured tortuosity when larger molecules were used. The idea gains some support from the older morphological literature where spaces of variable size, including 'lakes', were described (Van Harreveld, Crowell and Malhotra 1965; Bondareff and Pysh 1968; Pysh 1969), but these morphological studies were the subject of controversy about the effects of histological fixation.

The actual width of the spaces can be gauged by noting that the Stokes radius (hydrodynamic radius) of 70 kDa dextran is approximately 8 nm (see Nicholson and Tao 1993), although the shape is not well-defined. The dimensions of 66 kDa bovine serum albumin (BSA) are about 14×4 nm, i.e. it is an ellipsoid (see Tao and Nicholson 1996). Since both the 70 kDa dextran and 66 kDa albumin appear appreciably hindered in slices bathed in normal solution, the smallest spaces should be less than the diameters of these molecules. Conventional figures for the width of extracellular space are about 13–14 nm (Villegas and Fernández 1966).

Another possibility is that the extracellular matrix, consisting of long-chain glycosaminoglycans such as hyaluronate, is sufficiently dense to form an obstructive polymer. If enough hyaluronate were present it could significantly affect the diffusion of molecules, especially large ones (Ogston and Sherman 1961; Laurent et al. 1975) and might even lead to macromolecular crowding, which has been invoked recently to explain a variety of intracellular phenomena (Zimmerman and Minton 1993), including volume regulation (Minton, Colclasure and Parker 1992; Garner and Burg 1994). There has long been an issue of whether or not the extracellular space contains glycosaminoglycans and related molecules (e.g. Schmitt and Samson 1969; Margolis et al. 1986). Recent work with appropriate antibodies and other techniques has revealed hyaluronate in most regions of the brain and spinal cord (Bignami et al. 1992, Bignami, Hosley and Dahl 1993; Fuxe et al. 1994). These studies also indicated that the distribution of hyaluronate was probably not uniform but often associated with perikarya or around axons.

7.4 Methods of Measuring Extracellular Space Diffusion Parameters

7.4.1 TMA$^+$ Method to Determine Extracellular Volume Fraction (α) and Tortuosity (λ)

The TMA$^+$ method is the primary method for determining diffusion parameters in brain tissue today (Nicholson and Phillips 1981; Nicholson 1992, 1993) and has been used in several laboratories (McBain, Traynelis and Dingledine 1990; Svoboda and Syková 1991, Lundbaek and Hansen 1992; Lehmenkühler et al. 1993b; Lo et al. 1993; Syková et al. 1994, Syková, Mazel and Roitbak 1996). A micropipette releases TMA^+ by iontophoresis into either the brain slice or a control gel. An ISM located about $100\text{-}150\,\mu m$ from the release electrode measures the concentration of the probe ion as a function of time and the diffusion parameters are determined by fitting Eq. (7.2) using $Q = In/F$. TMA^+ is sensed with an ISM containing p-chloro-tetraphenylborate dissolved in 3-nitro-o-xylene (originally marketed as Corning 477317). The shank of either the ISM or the source electrode is heated and bent through about $30°$, prior to filling with electrolytes, so that both electrode shafts can be glued parallel to each other.

The baseline concentration of TMA^+ must be determined during the experiment in order to calculate α. To do this, the physiological saline that bathes the preparation or covers the surface of the brain, contains $0.5\text{-}1.0$ mM of TMA^+ and the ISM is calibrated periodically in it (Nicholson and Phillips 1981). To maintain a constant transport number (n), a continuous forward bias current of $20\text{-}50$ nA is applied to the iontophoresis electrode, then the current is stepped to $100\text{-}200$ nA for $20\text{-}100$ s to determine the diffusion characteristics of the tissue. The iontophoresis micropipette is filled with either 0.1 M or 1 M TMA-chloride.

The ISM is connected to an impedance-buffer amplifier followed by a D/A converter which transfers the signal to a PC. Appropriate calibration and curve fitting procedures are performed to fit Eq. (7.2) with the program VOLTORO. Control diffusion measurements are made in a 0.3% agarose (NuSieve; FMC BioProducts) or agar (Nobel; Difco) made up in 50 mM NaCl and $0.5\text{-}1.0$ mM TMA^+ and n and D obtained (for dilute gel: $\alpha = 1$, $\lambda = 1$, and $k' = 0$). In the brain, α, λ, and k' are extracted.

7.4.2 Integrated Optical Imaging to Determine Apparent Diffusion Coefficient and λ for Fluorescent Macromolecules

Nicholson and Tao (1993) developed an integrative optical imaging (IOI) method and applied it to the analysis of fluorescent dextran molecules in agarose gel and the brain extracellular microenvironment. Later the method was applied to albumin molecules (Tao and Nicholson 1996). The method uses a precisely defined source of fluorescent molecules pressure ejected from a micropipette, and is based on a detailed theory of the intensity contributions from out-of-focus molecules in a three-dimensional medium to a two-dimensional image (Tao and Nicholson 1995). The fluorescing molecules are imaged with a cooled CCD (charge-coupled device) camera and the output of the camera is transferred directly to a PC for quantitative analysis.

Dextrans have M_r values of of 3, 40, and 70 kDa, while albumins have M_r values of 14.4 kDa (lactalbumin), 45 kDa (ovalbumin) and 66 kDa (bovine serum albumin). All molecules are tagged with Texas Red and are obtained from Molecular Probes, Eugene, OR. Macromolecules are ejected from the source electrode using pressure rather than iontophoresis. Indeed, this is usually essential for uncharged species. In this method the substance, or substances in the micropipette are released by a brief pulse of nitrogen delivered by an electronically controlled valve. If the pulse is very brief compared to the subsequent diffusion measurement time course, then the concentration can be described by (Nicholson 1985, 1992):

$$C = (UC_f\lambda^3/8\alpha(D\pi t)^{1.5})\exp[-(r^2\lambda^2/4Dt) - k't] \tag{7.3}$$

where a volume U (cm^3) at concentration C_f (mM) is ejected and the other parameters are as in Eq. 7.2. If the volume is larger, then a more elaborate equation is needed (see Nicholson 1992 for details). The pressure pulse has the advantage that more than one substance can be delivered at a known concentration and the substance need not be charged. The disadvantage is that it is hard to calibrate the exact volume delivered, so that measurements of α are less accurate and therefore only λ can be measured.

The theory of how the image of the diffusing cloud of molecules maps onto the plane of the CCD camera is quite complex (Nicholson and Tao 1993; Tao and Nicholson 1995) but it can be reduced to the basic equation:

$$I(r', \gamma) = E(\gamma)e^{-(r'/M\gamma)^2} \text{ and } \gamma^2 = 4D^*t \tag{7.4}$$

where I is the intensity of the fluorescence, E is an amplitude term embodying the point spread function of the objective (but it does not depend on distance), r' is distance in the slice, M is the magnification of the optical system. By fitting the exponential term to the spatial distribution at a sequence of times, D^* can be determined (see Nicholson and Tao 1993).

7.5 Diffusion Parameters Obtained in Brain and Spinal Cord in Vivo with TMA$^+$ Method

7.5.1 Homogeneity

The ECS diffusion parameters in CNS differ, i.e. they are not homogeneous in all brain regions. For example it has been recognised that the TMA$^+$ diffusion parameters in the sensorimotor cortex of young adult rats in vivo are heterogeneous (Lehmenkühler et al. 1993b). The mean volume fraction gradually increases from $\alpha = 0.19$ in cortical layer II to $\alpha = 0.23$ in cortical layer VI. In subcortical white matter (corpus callosum), the volume fraction is always lower than in layer VI, often between 0.19 and 0.20. These typical differences are apparent in each individual animal. The mean tortuosity values are typically in the range of 1.51–1.65, and k' values vary between 3.3 and 6.3×10^{-3} s^{-1}. Significantly lower α values than in the cortex and corpus callosum have been found in the rat hippocampus in vivo (Mazel et al. 1996) and in vitro (see later). Exceptionally low values of α were found in area CA1 (about 0.12 in stratum pyramidale and 0.16 in stratum radiatum), while in CA3 and dentate gyrus α values were considerably higher, about 0.16–0.19. One explanation for this may be that the pores of the ECS are not homogeneous, i.e. that sizes vary in diameter. An issue raised by these data is whether the pores of the ECS in certain anatomical regions are different but homogeneous or whether the average pore size is smaller or larger. There is also a certain heterogeneity in the spinal cord, the mean values of the volume fraction being highest in the ventral horn ($\alpha = 0.23$) and lowest in the white matter ($\alpha = 0.18$) (Šimonová et al. 1996). Significant differences in various brain regions have also been found in tortuosity, showing that the local architecture is significantly different.

7.5.2 Anisotropic Diffusion

Is there some degree of anisotropy in brain tissue? Isotropy is defined as a state of constant λ in any direction from a point source, while anisotropy indicates a difference in λ in different axes. To test for anisotropy, the ECS diffusion parameters are measured in three orthogonal axes x, y and z. Anisotropic diffusion can channel the migration of substances in the ECS (preferred diffusion in one direction, e.g. along the axons) and may, therefore, account for a certain degree of specificity of the diffusion transmission. The structure of cells and axons can channel the migration of substances in the ECS and this could be a mechanism for a specificity of diffusion transmission of signals. Indeed, anisotropic diffusion was described using the 'TMA$^+$-method' in molecular layer of the cerebellum (Rice, Okada and Nicholson 1993). Since the molecular and granular layers of the cerebellum have distinct diffusion characteristics, the extracellular molecular traffic will be different in the two regions. The anisotropy of the white matter and molecular layer of the cerebellum could enable different modes of diffusion transmission in these regions.

Diffusion parameters are substantially different in the myelinated and unmyelinated white matter of the rat during postnatal development (Prokopová, Voříšek and Syková 1996). Isotropic diffusion was found in corpus callosum and spinal cord white matter of rats with incomplete myelination. In myelinated spinal cord and corpus callosum, the tortuosity is higher (the apparent diffusion coefficient is lower) when TMA$^+$ diffuses across the axons than when it diffuses along the axons. In white matter of the rat spinal cord at postnatal day 12–14 (P12–14) mean λ along the axon fibres was 1.36, while λ across the axons was 1.82. In the corpus callosum anisotropic diffusion was found at P20–22 (mean λ along the axon fibres was 1.44, while λ across the axons was 1.69). Preferential diffusion pathways were also found along myelinated axon bundles in the living brain using

Texas Red-labelled dextran injected into neostriatum of adult rats (Bjelke et al. 1995). These results confirm the hypothesis that there are preferential diffusion pathways of chemical signals along the myelinated axons in white matter tracts.

7.5.3 Activity-Related Volume Changes in the ECS

Transmembrane ionic fluxes are accompanied by the movement of water and cellular, presumably particularly glial, swelling. Changes in ECS diffusion parameters (ECS volume decrease, tortuosity increase and ADC decrease) are the consequences of activity-related transmembrane ionic shifts and cellular swelling. In the spinal cord of the rat or frog, repetitive electrical stimulation results in an ECS volume decrease from about 0.24 to 0.12–0.17, i.e. the ECS volume decreases by as much as 30–50% (Svoboda and Syková 1991). The changes in ECS diffusion parameters persist for many minutes or even hours after the stimulation has ceased, suggesting long-term changes in neuronal excitability and neuron–glia communication (Fig. 7.7).

7.5.4 ECS Diffusion Parameters During Development and Ageing

Compared to healthy adults the ECS diffusion parameters significantly differ during postnatal development (Lehmenkühler et al. 1993b). The ECS volume in the cortex and subcortical white matter (corpus callosum) is about twice as large ($\alpha = 0.36$–0.46) in the newborn rat as in the adult rat ($\alpha = 0.19$–0.23), while the variations in tortuosity are not statistically significant at any age (Fig. 7.7). A reduction in ECS volume fraction correlates well with growth of blood vessels. The constancy of the tortuosity shows that diffusion of small molecules is no more hindered in the developing brain than in that of the adult. The large ECS pores may allow migration of larger substances during development (e.g. growth factors) and better conditions for cell migration. On the other hand, the large ECS in neonatal brain could significantly dilute ions, metabolites and neuroactive substances released from cells, relative to release in adults, and may be a factor in prevention of anoxia, seizure and spreading depression in young individuals. The diffusion parameters could also play an important role in the developmental process itself.

Morphological changes during ageing, including cellular loss, loss of dendritic processes, astrogliosis, demyelination and swollen astrocyte processes, are accompanied by changes in ECS diffusion parameters (Mazel et al. 1996; Syková et al. 1996). The α in the cortex, corpus callosum and hippocampus of senescent rats (aged 26–32 months) is significantly lower than in young adults, e.g. in the cortical layer V about 0.18 instead of 0.21, in the white matter about 0.15 instead of 0.19, in the gyrus dentatus of the CA3 region of the hippocampus about 0.16 instead of 0.21. Moreover, in hippocampus the tortuosity λ was significantly higher in CA3

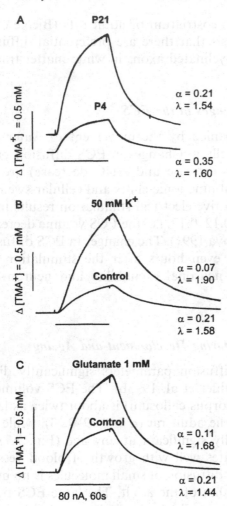

Fig. 7.7. Tetramethylammonium ion (TMA$^+$) diffusion curves and ECS diffusion parameters in brain and spinal cord of the rat during physiological and pathological conditions. Volume fraction (α) and tortuosity (λ) and non-specific uptake (k', not shown) were determined from extracellular concentration–time profiles of TMA$^+$ by real-time iontophoretic method. Representative records of the TMA$^+$ diffusion curves, with α and λ shown with each curve: (A) diffusion curve from layer VI in the cortex of a 4-day-old (P4) and a 21-day-old (P21) rat; (B) and (C) diffusion curves in isolated rat spinal cords at P10 and curves from the same spinal cords after a 20-min application of 50 mM K$^+$ or 1 mM glutamate in iso-osmotic superfusing solution.

stratum radiatum, 1.49 instead of 1.41. It is reasonable to assume that there is a significant decrease in ADCs of many neuroactive substances in ageing brain which accompanies the morphological changes, and can contribute to impaired signal transmission, greater susceptibility to anoxia, changes in behaviour and memory impairment.

7.5.5 ECS During Pathological States

Pathological states, e.g. anoxia/ischaemia, are accompanied by a lack of energy, seizure activity, excessive release of transmitters and neuroactive substances, neuronal death, glial cell loss or proliferation, glial swelling, production of metabolites and loss of ionic homeostasis. Others are characterised by inflammation, oedema or demyelination. It is therefore evident that they will be accompanied not only by substantial changes in ECS ionic composition (see Syková 1983, 1992b) but also by various changes in ECS diffusion parameters according to the different functional and anatomical changes.

7.5.5.1 Anoxia/Ischaemia

Dramatic K^+ and pH_e changes occur in the brain and spinal cord during anoxia and/or ischaemia (Syková and Svoboda 1990; Syková 1992b; Syková, Šimonová and Svoboda 1994; Xie et al 1995). Within 2 min after respiratory arrest in adult rats, blood pressure begins to increase and pH_e begins to decrease (by about 0.1 pH unit), while $[K^+]_e$ is still unchanged. With the subsequent blood pressure decrease, the pH_e decreases by 0.6–0.8 pH units to pH 6.4–6.6. This pH_e decrease is accompanied by a steep rise in $[K^+]_e$ to about 50–70 mM; decreases in $[Na^+]_e$ to 48–59 mM, $[Cl^-]_e$ to 70–75 mM, $[Ca^{2+}]_e$ to 0.06–0.08 mM, and pH_e to 6.1–6.8; accumulation of excitatory amino acids; negative DC slow potential shift; and a decrease in ECS volume fraction to 0.04–0.07. The ECS volume starts to decrease when the blood pressure drops below 80 mm Hg and $[K^+]_e$ rises above 6 mM (Syková et al. 1994a).

During hypoxia and terminal anoxia, the ECS volume fraction in rat cortex or spinal cord decreases from about 0.20 to about 0.04, while tortuosity increases from 1.5 to about 2.2 (Lundbaek and Hansen 1992; Syková et al. 1994a). The same ultimate changes were found in both neonatal and adult rats, in grey and white matter, in the cortex, corpus callosum and spinal cord. However, the time course in white matter was significantly slower than in grey matter; and the time course in neonatal rats was about 10 times slower than in adults (Voříšek and Syková 1997). This corresponds to the well-known resistance of immature CNS to anoxia. Linear regression analysis revealed a positive correlation between the normoxic size of the ECS volume and the time course of the changes. The slower changes in extracellular space volume fraction and tortuosity in the nervous tissue during development can contribute to slower impairment of signal transmission, e.g. due to lower accumulation of ions and neuroactive substances released from cells and their better diffusion from the hypoxic area in uncompacted ECS.

In recent studies using diffusion-weighted ^{1}H magnetic resonance scanning/ imaging (MRS/MRI), the apparent diffusion coefficient of water (ADC_W) was measured during terminal anoxia in rats. Anoxia evokes similar decreases in the apparent diffusion coefficient of ADC_W (measured by the NMR method) and ADC_{TMA} (measured by the iontophoretic method and ISMs). Comparison of ADC_W and ADC_{TMA} in rats 8–9 days of age revealed the same time course, both corresponding to the decrease in ECS volume fraction (Van der Toorn et al. 1996). Although water moves freely across the cellular membranes, TMA^+ stays predominantly in ECS. Since the total amount of tissue water is not believed to increase (Krizaj et al. 1996), this study (Van der Toorn et al. 1996) shows that changes in ADC of brain tissue water measured by diffusion-weighted in vivo magnetic resonance (MR) techniques, predominantly report on extra- and intracellular volume changes resulting from water shift from the extra- to intracellular compartment.

Full recovery to 'normoxic' diffusion parameters is achieved after successful recovery from severe ischaemia (Syková et al. 1994b). Beginning 5–10 min after this recovery, the ECS volume fraction significantly increases above the 'normoxic' values to an α about 0.30; λ and k' were not significantly different from the values found under normoxic conditions.

The observed substantial changes in the diffusion parameters during and after progressive ischaemia and anoxia in vivo could, therefore, affect the diffusion in ECS and aggravate the accumulation of ions, neurotransmitters, and metabolic substances during ischaemia and thus contribute to ischaemic brain damage. On the other hand, changes in the diffusion parameters may persist long after the ischaemic event and affect non-synaptic transmission in CNS. It should be noted that the changes in the diffusion parameters may also affect the access of drugs used to treat nervous diseases to cellular elements.

7.5.6 ECS Volume and Geometry During Inflammation and Demyelinating Diseases

The expansion of the ECS during inflammatory and demyelinating diseases alters diffusion parameters, and may affect the accumulation and movement of ions, neurotransmitters, neuromodulators and metabolites in CNS. Changes in ECS diffusion parameters can be expected during inflammation during which brain oedema may develop. In an experimental model, inflammation was evoked by intracerebral inoculation with a weakly pathogenic strain of *Staphylococcus aureus* (Lo et al. 1993). There was a lack of changes in water content of the inoculated region, indicating that there was no significant development of brain oedema. Acute inflammation and increase in blood–brain barrier (BBB) permeability in the abscess region resulted in rather mild changes in ECS diffusion parameters, i.e. volume fraction tended to be somewhat larger and the tortuosity somewhat smaller.

Dramatic changes in the ECS diffusion parameters were found in the spinal cord of rats during experimental autoimmune encephalomyelitis (EAE), an experimental model of multiple sclerosis (Šimonová et al., 1996). EAE, which was induced by the injection of guinea-pig myelin basic protein (MBP), resulted in typical morphological changes in the CNS tissue, namely demyelination, inflammatory reaction, astrogliosis, BBB damage and in paraparesis at 14–17 days post-injection of MBP. Paraparesis was accompanied by increases in α in the dorsal horn, in the intermediate region and in the ventral horn, as well as in white matter, from about 0.18 to about 0.30. There were significant decreases in λ in the dorsal horn and in the intermediate region and decreases in k' in the intermediate region and in the ventral horn (Šimonová et al. 1996). Although the inflammatory reaction and the astrogliosis preceded and greatly outlasted the neurological signs, the BBB damage had a similar time course. Moreover, there was a close correlation between the changes in ECS diffusion parameters and the manifestation of neurological signs. The observed changes in ECS diffusion parameters may affect synaptic as well as non-synaptic transmission and intercellular communication, and therefore recovery from acute EAE, and manifestation of neurological signs in EAE rats.

7.6 Diffusion Results Obtained in Brain Slices and Isolated Tissue with TMA$^+$, Dextrans and Albumins

The first diffusion measurements on slices were made by Hounsgaard and Nicholson (1983) on the molecular layer in cerebellar slices of the guinea pig using the TMA$^+$ method. The values of the α were 0.28 and λ were 1.84 and uptake was not measured. Later studies on the isolated turtle cerebellum revealed that it was anisotropic (Rice, Okada and Nicholson 1993) and this was not taken into account in the guinea pig study. In fact, anisotropy was not seen in the orginal studies on intact cerebellum (Nicholson and Phillips 1981), probably because the limited computing facilities available then did not allow uptake to be incorporated into the diffusion equation, so reducing the resolution of the method. Some theoretical issues relevant to slices were discussed by Nicholson and Hounsgaard (1983). The following sections will be confined to some of the recent studies.

7.6.1 Anisotropy

The study by Rice, Okada and Nicholson (1993) measured anisotropy of λ in three orthogonal axes of the molecular and granular layers of the isolated turtle cerebellum using the TMA$^+$-method. There was a different tortuosity factor, λ_i, associated with each axis of that layer. The x- and y-axes lay in the plane parallel to the pial surface of this lissencephalic cerebellum with the x-axis in the direction of the parallel fibres. The z-axis was perpendicular to this plane. The tortuosity values were $\lambda_x = 1.44$, $\lambda_y = 1.95$, and $\lambda_z = 1.58$. By contrast, the granular layer was isotropic with a single tortuosity value, $\lambda_{Gr} = 1.77$. Heterogeneity between the molecular and granular layer was revealed by a striking difference in α, for each layer. In the molecular layer $\alpha = 0.31$ while in the granular layer $\alpha = 0.22$.

These results are significant in the context of volume transmission and this was demonstrated by measuring local changes in $[K^+]_e$ and $[Ca^{2+}]_e$ following micro-iontophoresis of a cerebellar transmitter, glutamate. The ratios of ion shifts in the x- and y-axes in the granular layer were close to unity, with a ratio of 1.04 ± 0.08 for the rise in $[K^+]_e$ and 1.03 for the decrease in $[Ca^{2+}]_e$. In contrast, ion shifts in the molecular layer had an $x{:}y$ ratio of 1.44 for the rise in $[K^+]_e$ and 2.10 for the decrease in $[Ca^{2+}]_e$. The preferred diffusion direction of glutamate along the parallel fibres could help constrain an incoming excitatory stimulus to stay 'on-beam'.

7.6.2 Macromolecules

Using the IOI method, it became possible to explore how macromolecules behaved in the extracellular space. Dextrans, tagged with either tetramethylrhodamine or Texas Red, were injected with a pressure-pulse into agarose gel or rat cortical slices and imaged and either D (agarose) or D^* (brain tissue) determined (Nicholson and Tao 1993) enabled λ to be calculated. Values of λ for the 3 and 10 kDa dextrans were 1.77 and 1.86, respectively (these values are based on additional data obtained after the original study, see Tao and Nicholson (1996) and differ slightly from the original values). Tortuosities for the 40 and 70 kDa dextrans had significantly larger values of 2.16 and 2.25, respectively. This study suggests that the extracellular space may have local constrictions that hinder the diffusion of molecules above a critical size that lies in the range of many neurotrophic compounds.

An obvious question raised by the success of the optical method of measuring tortuosity is how the results obtained with the smallest fluorescent molecule (3 kDa dextran) compare to data obtained with the TMA$^+$-method in rat cortical slices. We examined this question recently (Tao et al. 1995). We found that the value of λ measured with 3 kDa dextran was in the range 1.6–1.9, while that obtained from TMA$^+$ measurements was in the range 1.4–1.7. We are still analysing these data, but the small differences between the two methods are probably due to the size, or other characteristics such as charge, of the molecules used. The most recent study (Tao and Nicholson 1996) with the IOI method has extended it to look at the diffusion of lactalbumin, ovalbumin and bovine serum albumin in rat cortical slices. These naturally occurring globular proteins are good models for other diffusible factors in the brain and, in contrast to the dextrans, are negatively charged. The proteins selected had comparable molecular weights to those of the previously studied dextrans, they were: lactalbumin ($M_r = 14.5$ kDa), ovalbumin (45 kDa) and bovine serum albumin (BSA; 66 kDa) and each was labelled with Texas Red fluorescent dye. These measurements produced λs of 2.24 for lactalbumin, 2.50 for ovalbumin and 2.26 for BSA. Comparison with previous studies on dextrans and TMA^+ shows that the λs for the albumins are similar to those obtained with 40 kDa and 70 kDa dextran and averaged about 2.25. These studies confirm that proteins the size of albumin can diffuse through the brain extracellular space but are all hindered to a similar extent as 70 kDa dextran.

7.6.3 Studies in Isolated Tissues in Modified Conditions

The isolated tissues discussed here include conventional mammalian brain slices with a thickness of 300–400 μm and the isolated turtle cerebellum. Both of these preparations permit precise control of the tissue environment.

7.6.3.1 Ischaemia

The TMA^+ method can address the changes in diffusion properties of the extracellular space when oxygen and glucose are withdrawn by studying extracellular potassium, volume fraction and tortuosity in rat hippocampal CA1, CA3 and cortical slices during ischaemia (Pérez-Pinzon, Tao and Nicholson 1995). The ischaemia model consisted of a slice submerged in artificial cerebrospinal fluid containing 5 mM potassium, from which oxygen and glucose were removed until anoxic depolarisation occurred. In vitro ischaemia caused $[K^+]_e$ to rise to 45, 12 and 32 mM in CA1, CA3 and cortex, respectively. During normoxia values of α were 0.13, 0.20 and 0.20 and values of λ were 1.50, 1.54 and 1.64 in the three regions. These data confirm the small volume fraction of CA1 in comparison with the two other regions, as originally demonstrated by McBain, Traynelis and Dingledine (1990). During ischaemia α decreased to 0.05, 0.12 and 0.11 in the three regions. Only in CA3 did λ change significantly (to 1.78).

7.6.3.2 Osmotic Stress

The issue of how water distributes in brain tissue under different conditions has assumed increased importance recently in trying to understand the origins of diffusion-weighted MRI and light scattering from tissue. This was addressed in a recent study that looked at water compartmentalisation and extracellular tortuosity after osmotic changes in cerebellum of the turtle (Krizaj et al. 1996). The water distributions were quantified by combining extracellular diffusion analysis using the TMA^+ method with wet-weight and dry-weight measurements. Changes in the tortuosity of the extracellular space were also measured. Isolated cerebellae were immersed in normal, oxygenated, physiological saline (302 mosmol kg^{-1}), hypotonic saline (238 mosmol kg^{-1}) and a series of hypertonic salines (up to 668 mosmol kg^{-1}) and the osmolarity was varied by altering the NaCl content. The volume fraction was 0.22 in normal saline, 0.12 in hypotonic medium and 0.60 in the most hypertonic medium. Tortuosity was 1.70 in the normal saline, 1.79 in the hypotonic and 1.50 in the most hypertonic saline. The water content, defined as ((wet-weight)−(dry-weight))/wet-weight, of a typical isolated cerebellum was 82.9%. It increased to 85.2% in hypotonic saline and decreased to 80.1% in the most hypertonic saline. One of the most remarkable observations was the 60% volume fraction in the most hypertonic medium.

7.7 Regulation of ECS Volume and Geometry by Glial Cells

It is generally accepted that the ECS volume decrease is primarily due to astrocytic swelling, although swelling of neurons, particularly of dendrites and axons, also occurs. Activity-related or CNS damage-related ionic changes and release of amino acids result in pulsatile or long-term glial swelling, which leads to a compensatory decrease in the ECS volume and increased tortuosity (i.e. decrease in ADC). In turn, an ECS volume decrease is predicted to result in a greater accumulation of neuroactive substances which can ultimately induce damage to the nerve cells by reaching toxic concentrations. A number of different mechanisms have been proposed to lead to astrocytic swelling, namely: osmotic imbalance, uptake of extracellular K^+, acid–base changes, glutamate uptake and excitatory amino acid-induced swelling, blockage of Na^+/K^+ pump activity and accumulation of fatty acids and free radicals (Kempski et al. 1991; Walz, Klimazsevski and Paterson 1993). For the most part, these mechanisms of swelling have been confirmed only in tissue culture and they were only recently compared with changes in the ECS volume and geometry.

The mechanisms of changes in ECS volume and geometry were studied using the TMA$^+$ method in the cerebral cortex of the in vivo rat (Cserr et al. 1991), isolated rat spinal cord (Vargová and Syková 1995), brain slices (Chebabo et al. 1995) and isolated turtle cerebellum (Krizaj et al. 1996). The observed mechanisms might be similar to those of cellular swelling, although there are some differences in the effects of cellular swelling on ECS volume and tortuosity. In the in vivo rat studies, acute hypernatraemia caused a reduction in ECS volume fraction from 0.18 to 0.10–0.15 and the increase in tortuosity from 1.57 to 1.65, with little change in intracellular volume, demonstrating cellular volume regulation in the intact animal (Cserr et al. 1991). The application of hypotonic solution, of physiological saline with elevated $[K^+]_e$, or of glutamate resulted in a dramatic ECS volume decrease and an ECS tortuosity increase (Fig. 7.7; Vargová and Syková 1995; Krizaj et al. 1996). Measurements of ECS volume fraction and water content showed that hypotonic solutions caused water to move from the extracellular to intracellular compartment, while hypertonic solutions caused water to move from the intracellular to the extracellular compartment, with relatively small changes in total water in both cases.

The superfusion of isolated rat spinal cords with solutions containing 10 mM K^+ or low doses of glutamate or glutamate receptor agonists [*N*-methyl-D-aspartate (NMDA) or α-amino, 3-hydroxy, 5-methyl, 4-isoxazole proprionic acid (AMPA), at 10^{-5} M], was used as a model of changes in ECS diffusion parameters during neuronal activity and stimulation. This resulted in the shrinkage of the ECS by as much as 20–25% and an increase in λ from about 1.5 to about 1.8. Specific antagonists blocked the effects of NMDA and AMPA. Superfusion with 50 mM K^+ or higher concentrations of glutamate (at 1–10 mM) or the glutamate receptors agonists NMDA or AMPA (at 10^{-4} M) represented changes during pathological events such as anoxia, ischaemia or injury. Solutions containing 50 mM K^+ induced a decrease in α to as low as 0.04–0.05 and an increase in λ to as high as 2.1–2.2 (Fig. 7.7). Application of NMDA or AMPA resulted in a drop in α to 0.04–0.07 and in large increases in λ to as high as 1.85–2.10. Glutamate in relatively high concentration (1–10 mM) was less effective. Further measurements in the isolated rat spinal cord also revealed that changes of 0.2–0.4 pH units and greater of the superfusing solution lead to changes in ECS volume: namely, an alkaline shift in pH causes an ECS volume increase and an acid shift causes an ECS volume decrease (Vargová and Syková 1995). The ECS volume changes evoked by all these swelling-inducing substances were reversible upon superfusion of spinal cord with physiological solution. In many cases, the ECS volume changes started to recover towards control values already during application of swelling-inducing substances, apparently because the cells started to regulate their volume (a phenomenon called regulatory volume decrease, RVD) (Hoffman and Simonsen 1989).

It is reasonable to assume that ions as well as neurotransmitters released into the ECS during neuronal activity or pathological states interact not only with the postsynaptic and presynaptic membranes, but also with extrasynaptic receptors, including those on glial cells. Stimulation of glial cells may lead to activation of ion channels, second messengers and intracellular metabolic pathways, and to changes in their volume which is accompanied by dynamic variations in the ECS volume, particularly swelling and re-arrangement of their processes. In addition to their role in maintenance of extracellular ionic homeostasis, glial cells may thus, by regulating their volume, influence extracellular pathways for neuroactive substances.

7.7.1 Volume Regulation by Astroglia

Astrocytes are involved in the regulation of electrolyte concentrations and water volume in the ECS of the CNS (Kimelberg 1991). The function of the glial cells as a potassium buffering system suggests that excess potassium in the ECS during neuronal activity is carried away from the neurons into the glial cells. Increased excess external K^+ would depolarise the astrocytes and open Cl^- channels. KCl would passively enter the cells driven by Donnan forces and water would follow the osmotic gradient and lead to cell swelling. The swelling of most cells leads to transport changes that seem designed to effect a shrinkage of the cells back to control levels, RVD, which involves both a decrease in cell osmolyte content and a decrease in cell volume. These transport changes may be related to stretch-activated ion channels (SACs) (Christensen 1987). Calcium is believed to play a fundamental role in cellular volume regulation. The majority of cells shown to have a Ca^{2+}-dependent RVD process are cells in which osmolyte efflux occurs predominantly via K^+ and Cl^- conductances. It is not clear, however, how Ca^{2+} performs its function to modulate RVD. It has been suggested that calcium must enter the cell to initiate cellular volume regulation. The biological actions of Ca^{2+} can be mediated through several biochemical pathways such as production of secondary intracellular messengers, the exocytic insertion into the plasma membrane of vesicles containing ion channels, and phosphorylation or dephosphorylation of existent transporters (McCarthy and O'Neil 1992). Changes in $[Ca^{2+}]_i$ produced by glutamate also appear to produce subsequent changes in the concentrations of several other potentially important second messengers such as phospholipase C and protein kinase C.

Astrocytes also show marked depolarisation of their membrane potentials after swelling, suggestive of ion channels being activated (Kimelberg and O'Connor 1988). Long-term osmolyte accumulation may also be mediated by amino acids which may have a protective function against acute changes in the osmotic environment while playing their role in osmotic homeostasis. It seems that an intimate relationship exists between cell volume control, ion fluxes and intracellular pH (Kempski, Gross and Baethmann 1982). An important mechanism leading to swelling could be transmitter-stimulated carbonic anhydrase activities, such that H^+ and HCO_3^- are created by the hydration of CO_2 and transported out of the cells via the Na^+/H^+ and Cl^-/HCO_3^- carriers. This would lead to an accumulation of NaCl and therefore to a net increase in osmolarity, drawing water into the cell. It has also been suggested that extracellular acidification leads to a stimulation of both carriers and NaCl and water accumulation. Decrease in astrocytic cell–cell coupling due to astrocytic swelling could have marked effects on astrocytic function, such as reducing spatial buffering of K^+ and diffusion of substances taken up by astrocytes through the syncytium, with possible final removal from the CNS at the astrocytic end-feet surrounding brain capillaries. Thus this effect would constitute a major compromise of astrocyte function and implies that swollen astrocytes, encountered in a number of pathological states may be deleterious. If this is true in the living brain, there is the possibility of creating dynamic ways of extraneuronal information processing within the nervous system.

7.7.2 A New Method for the Registration of Relative Changes in Cell Volume at the Single Cell Level

A method was developed for the measurement of relative volume variations in individual cells using a microspectrofluorimetric system. The cells were loaded with a highly fluorescent, intracellular probe (fura-2/AM). The isosbestic point of the probe was used consistently, where the probe is ion-insensitive and the fluorescent signals emitted are related only to the intracellular dye concentration (Eriksson et al. 1992). For volume measurements of the glutamate-induced swelling of astrocytes, the fura-2 Ca^{2+} probe was used and, by varying the excitation wavelengths, changes in intracellular Ca^{2+} transients were recorded simultaneously with the relative volume variations of the individual cells. Using this method relative changes in cell volume were followed with high time-lapse resolution.

7.7.3 Glutamate Induced Astroglial Rapid Swelling – Mechanisms and Probable Physiological Implications

Astroglia have been shown to express ionotropic glutamate receptors of the kainate (KA) and AMPA types (Pearce 1993). These receptors constitute integrated parts of ion channels and their activation leads to depolarisation of the plasma membrane. Some groups have also reported on the expression of NMDA receptors on astroglial cells. Astroglia also express different metabotropic glutamate receptors (mGluRs). These constitute a heterogeneous family of receptors coupled to multiple second messenger systems that include increases in phosphoinositide hydrolysis (Schoepp, Bockaert and Sladeczek 1990), activation of phospholipase D (Boss and Conn 1992), decreases in cyclic adenosine monophosphate (cAMP) formation (Schoepp, Johnson and Monn 1992), increases in cAMP formation (Winder and Conn 1992), and modulation of the ion channels (Lester and Jahr 1990). Using the selective mGluR agonist, 1-aminocyclopentane-1,3-dicarboxylic acid (1S, 3R-ACPD), considerable progress has been made towards understanding the role of the mGluRs in the CNS. This progress has involved the measurement of phosphoinositide hydrolysis (Schoepp, Bockaert and Sladeczek 1990; Conn and Desai 1991) or intracellular Ca^{2+} mobilisation (Mayer and Miller 1990). Ca^{2+} has been considered important in initiating cell volume regulation, since intracellular, rather than extracellular, Ca^{2+} activates the ion fluxes that underlie volume regulation (Davis and Finn 1985). Recent electrophysiological experiments have suggested another mGluR agonist, L-AP4, to have affinity for a G-protein-linked glutamate receptor which decreases cAMP formation in a pertussis-toxin-sensitive manner (Tanabe et al. 1992; Thomsen et al. 1992; Trombley and Westbrook 1992).

The mGluR agonist 1S,3R-ACPD which activates inositol phosphate (IP)-metabolism, and L-AP4, which inhibits cyclic AMP formation, all cause a volume

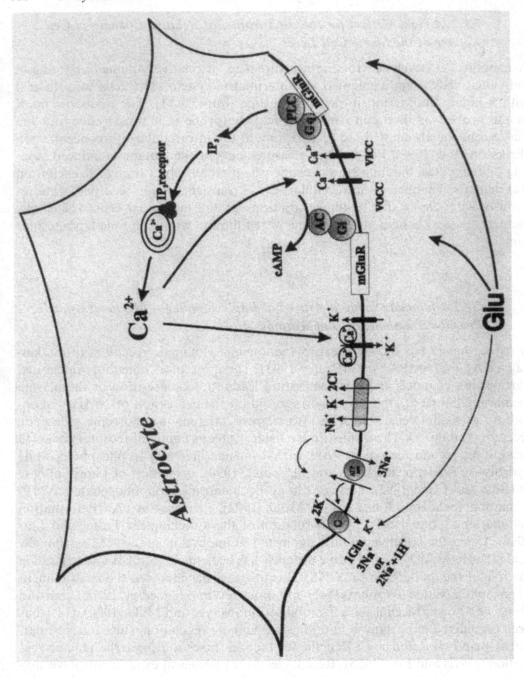

increase within some few minutes (Fig. 7.8; Hansson, 1994). These agonists interact with receptors coupled to IP_3 synthesis, intracellular Ca^{2+} increases followed by an influx of calcium via Ca^{2+} channels in the cell membrane and opening of an outward K^+ rectifier, as well as to a G_i-protein and the opening of an inward K^+ rectifier. At least one Na^+-K^+-$2Cl^-$-co-transporter and a Na^+/K^+-ATPase are affected, and an electrogenic Na^+-dependent glutamate carrier, through which glutamate is taken up into the astrocytes. The astroglial swelling induced by glutamate is not only the result of these processes, but requires another, until now unidentified mechanism, probably some ketamine sensitive, ion-channel complex for K^+ outflow and probably Na^+ influx. The ionotropic glutamate receptors, which could be blocked with CNQX, DNQX and NBQX (selective non-NMDA receptor antagonists), did not stimulate a volume increase in isolated astrocytes. The excitatory amino acid receptors are also coupled to Na^+ channels (Sontheimer et al. 1988). An influx of Na^+ through glutamate receptor-coupled ion channels, together with the resultant Ca^{2+} influx and elevated cytosolic Cl^-, may be of importance in astrocytic swelling (McCarthy and O'Neil 1992; O'Connor and Kimelberg 1993). It has long been known that astrocytes actively take up glutamate via a Na^+-dependent mechanism (Hertz 1979). This glutamate transporter or carrier system also leads to a volume increase (Schneider, Baethmann and Kempski 1992), which could only be partially blocked by the glutamate uptake inhibitors, dihydrokainic acid, L-3-hydroxyaspartic acid or L-pyrrolidine-2,4-dicarboxylic acid (L-2,4,PDC) (Hansson 1994). The glutamate taken up is converted to glutamine through the action of the astrocyte specific enzyme, glutamine synthetase, and this glutamate–glutamine pathway constitutes the locus of the small glutamate pool in brain tissue. Release from this pool could occur as a result of the swelling of astrocytes, since the swelling of isolated cells and in many vertebrate and invertebrate tissues is known to lead to the release of taurine, glutamate, aspartate, and other amino acids as part of the process of RVD, by which swollen cells regain their normal volume (Kimelberg 1991).

Fig. 7.8. Schematic drawing of an astroglial cell summarising possible interactions between Glu and receptors, ion channels and transport carriers of importance for understanding the molecular mechanisms behind Glu-induced swelling. Glu interacts with metabotropic Glu receptors activating PLC and IP_3 and leading to a mobilisation of intracellular Ca^{2+} $[Ca^{2+}]_i$. This, in turn, induces opening of Ca^{2+} channels and opening of an outward rectifying Ca^{2+} dependent K^+ channels. Glu can also interact with mGluRs which inhibit adenylate cyclase and lead to a decrease in cAMP production. This inhibition of cAMP formation could lead to the opening of L-Ca^{2+} channels and, furthermore, through activation of a G protein (G_{ia}), to opening of an inward rectifying K^+ channel. There is also an activation of the Na^+-K^+-$2Cl^-$ co-transporter. Na^+/K^+-ATPase is activated as is also the Na^+-dependent Glu carrier. Glu is taken up into the cell.

NMDA receptor-mediated ischaemic swelling and glutamate-induced swelling, and the subsequent cell death, have both been demonstrated in neurons. Ketamine and MK 801, well known noncompetitive antagonists of the NMDA receptor, completely abolished the glutamate-induced swelling in cultured astrocytes. MK 801 has been identified as a potent anticonvulsant as well as a protective agent for ischaemia-induced neuronal degeneration (Gill, Foster and Woodruff 1987). One explanation of these effects is that MK 801, like ketamine, blocks the ion channels independent of the NMDA receptor (Chan and Chu 1989).

7.7.4 Glial and Neuronal Glutamate Uptake Carriers

Glutamate transporters help to terminate the postsynaptic action of the neurotransmitter glutamate (Nicholls and Attwell 1990) and keep the extracellular glutamate concentration at low levels (1–3 mM). This is important, as low glutamate levels in the synaptic cleft amplifiy the signal-to-noise ratio upon release of this amino acid from presynaptic terminals. Furthermore, excessive stimulation of particularly NMDA receptor bearing neurons can lead to neuronal injury and/ or death ('excitotoxicity'). The transport of glutamate across the plasma membranes of neurons and glial cells proceeds via high- and low-affinity transport systems (Schousboe 1981; Hansson, Erikssonn and Nilssan 1985; Kanai and Hediger 1992). Both astroglial cells and neurons possess similar, although not identical, glutamate uptake carriers on their plasma membranes (Kanner and Schuldiner 1987). However, the capacity of neurons to take up glutamate seems to be less than that of glia, even though the anatomy of the synaptic cleft might favour a neuronal removal of glutamate after its release from the presynaptic region. The uptake capacity of glutamate by astroglia, however, is considered to be sufficient to account for all glutamate released by neurons. Although the precise contribution of either neuronal re-uptake and astroglial glutamate uptake is uncertain, it is likely that astroglia which have a greater driving force for uptake than neurons, must figure prominently in the overall process and especially in the protection of neurons from glutamate excess (Schousboe 1981). Furthermore, the astroglial carriers could be important in maintaining defined levels of the extracellular glutamate. In addition, glial glutamate uptake plays an integral role in the glutamine cycle, which has been proposed to generate terminal glutamate via glial glutamine synthetase and diffusion of the glutamine so formed to the terminals for hydrolysis to glutamate. It is interesting, in that context, that the expression of astroglial glutamate carriers is most prominent in those brain regions with the most extensive glutamate transmission. Three different glutamate transport systems have been described in astrocytes (Flott and Seifert 1991): the Na^+-dependent uptake (Hansson, Erikssonn and Nilssan 1985; Kanai and Hediger 1992), the Cl^--dependent transport mechanism, and the Ca^{2+}-dependent transport system. The Na^+-dependent glutamate transporter has recently been cloned and is different from neuronal subtype(s) (Kanai and Hediger 1992; Pines et al. 1992; Levy et al. 1993).

7.8 Discussion and Future Perspectives

The experiments and data reviewed in this chapter show that we can now study the behaviour of the extracellular space in unprecedented detail. We are able to reveal both local structure and dynamic behaviour. Several new ideas are emerging from these ongoing investigations. We now discuss some of these.

A non-specific feedback suppressing neuronal activity may exist in the CNS: (1) Neuronal activity results in the accumulation in $[K^+]_e$; (2) K^+ depolarises glial cells, and this depolarisation induces an alkaline shift in glial pH_i; (3) The glial cells therefore extrude acid; and (4) the acid shifts in pH result in a decrease in the neuronal excitability (Fig. 7.9; Ransom, 1992, Syková 1992b, 1997). The cellular swelling is compensated for by ECS volume shrinkage and is accompanied by increased tortuosity, presumably by the crowding of molecules of the ECS matrix and by the swelling of fine glial processes. These long-term changes in CNS architecture may affect (1) synaptic transmission (width of synaptic clefts, permeability of ionic channels, concentration of transmitters, dendritic length constant, etc.), (2) non-synaptic transmission by diffusion (diffusion of diffusible factors such as

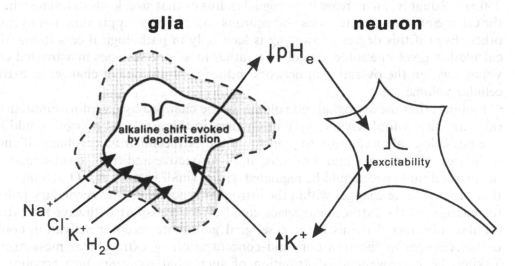

Fig. 7.9. Schematic of the mechanism of nonspecific feedback suppressing neuronal excitability. Active neurons release K^+ which accumulates in the ECS and depolarises glial cells. This causes an alkaline shift in glial pH_i and an acid shift in pH_e. Extracellular acidosis further suppresses neuronal activity. Transmembrane ionic movements and transmitter release result in glial swelling, ECS volume decreases and therefore in the greater accumulation of ions and neuroactive substances in the ECS.

ions, transmitters, neuropeptides, neurohormones, growth factors and metabolites), (3) neuron–glia communication, (4) ECS homeostasis. The long-term changes in local architecture would therefore affect the efficacy of signal transmission, and may be the basis of plastic behavioural changes.

Glial swelling is a consequence of the role of glia in ionic (particularly K^+, pH) and amino acid (glutamate) homeostasis, and it generally accompanies the phenomena of repetitive neuronal activity, seizures, anoxia, injury and many other pathological states in the CNS. Activity-related or CNS damage-related ionic changes and release of amino acids result in pulsatile or long-term glial swelling, which leads to a compensatory decrease in the ECS volume and increased tortuosity (i.e. decreases in ADC). In turn, an ECS volume decrease would result in a greater accumulation of neuroactive substances. This can either increase synaptic or non-synaptic efficacy or induce damage to the nerve cells by reaching toxic concentrations. Chemical and physical properties of the ECS as described by ECS diffusion parameters therefore significantly affect signal transmission in the CNS.

What are the possible physiological consequences of astroglial swelling? Estimations have shown that the extracellular space of the brain represents 10–20% of its total volume. Furthermore, the total astroglial volume has been estimated to be approximately 30% of the brain cell volume. If we assume that the astrocyte is a sphere with processes and with a diameter of 15–20 µm, then a 10% increase in cell volume corresponds to an increase in the radius of approximately 250 nm. Roughly, an increase in astroglial radius of that size, leads to a state where the cell membranes of astrocytes and neurons come in close approximation to each other. Even if this degree of swelling is seen only in pathological conditions, the calculation gives one some idea of how rather moderate changes in astroglial cell volume within the overall glial network induce very prominent changes in extracellular volume.

Findings that the astroglial cell volume can be changed by receptor stimulation, raise the question of whether volume changes in the astroglial network could be one physiological mechanism for control of the extracellular fluid volume. If such is the case, the concentrations of ions, and neuroactive and trophic substances in the extracellular space could be regulated within small brain areas. Or, could it be that rapid volume changes within the astroglial syncytium, with secondary pulsatile changes of the extracellular space could direct transport pathways for extracellular substances? If this is the case, glial glutamate receptor activation could induce changes in the transport and concentration of extracellular messengers. Taking the heterogeneous distribution of such glial receptors into account, a foundation is beginning to emerge for extensive and dynamic signalling pathways. Another possibility is that astroglial swelling leads to a narrowing of the astroglial cell processes in the synaptic regions, providing a morphologically closer interaction between neurons and glia, and an economy of the signalling substances (cf Smith 1992). In addition, this mechanism could quite simply protect synaptic regions from substances in the extracellular space. It is difficult to make calculations to evaluate the reliability of these possibilities and, therefore, they must be considered only as hypotheses for the present.

With the above discussion in mind, the glutamate-induced rapid astroglial swelling might also have physiological consequences, and furthermore might have consequences for behaviour in the sense that glutamate is the most well known excitatory transmitter in brain and that it has been implicated in mental processes such as learning and memory. From this point of view, it is therefore interesting that glutamate-induced atroglial swelling can have effects on the concentrations and transport capacities of the neuroactive substances in the extracellular space with on one hand local effects on glutamate transmission, probably involved in neuronal events such as LTP, and on the other hand, also have implications for neuronal excitability in larger brain areas.

In summary, we can tentatively say that for classical synaptic transmission of information, the neuron is the dominant player but in the realm of volume or extracellular transmission, the regulating element is the glial cell. Glia accomplish their role by modulating both the geometry of the extracellular space and the chemical composition. Thus, as we increasingly see the extracellular milieu as being the critical communication channel in long-term behavioural processes, we will increasingly identify a pivotal role for the glial cell in brain function.

8

Role of Periaxonal Glia in Nerve Conduction

N. JOAN ABBOTT

Summary

In vertebrates, both the glial cells of the central nervous system (oligodendrocytes and astrocytes) and of the peripheral nervous system (Schwann cells) form close associations with nerve axons. Some of these ensure the insulation of the axon by the myelin sheath, but other more dynamic interactions also occur. Although invertebrate glia do not form true myelin, they also form close associations with axons. Axon-associated glia express a variety of K^+ channels, and in some cases Na^+ and Ca^{2+} channels have been observed. Communication from axon to glial cells has been demonstrated in both invertebrate and vertebrate nervous systems, mediated by K^+ and by neurotransmitters. There is also some evidence for chemical signalling from glial cells to axon. Glial cells appear to induce or stabilise the pattern and clustering of ion channels in the axon membrane, and in some cases there is a close correspondence between the channel subtypes present in the neighbouring glial and axonal membranes. The glial K^+ channels and transporters may contribute to clearance of periaxonal K^+ during high frequency stimulation. In some invertebrate preparations, there is well documented transfer of macromolecules from glial cells to axon. Some of these processes offer mechanisms by which glial cells could modulate axonal function and hence behaviour.

8.1 Introduction: Glial Cells Associated with Synapses and Axons

Dynamic interactions between the neurons of the nervous system and their associated glial cells play important roles in the development of the nervous system, and in shaping behaviour in the adult. In synaptic zones, glial cells can influence neural activity both pre- and postsynaptically, and can therefore contribute to the modulation of neural integration and hence behaviour. By contrast, most axons are designed as 'executive links', relaying information in a relatively stereotyped way, to preserve the detail and accuracy of the information transmitted. Thus 'spiking' axons carrying all-or-none action potentials use a frequency code to convey information without distortion over long distances. It might then be expected that the glial cells associated with axons would have relatively fixed functions in maintaining the structure and integrity of the conducting axons, for example, by providing the insulating sheath that determines the conduction properties of myelinated vertebrate axons. However, recent work on the glial cells associated with axons in vertebrates and invertebrates shows that the axon–glial unit is engaged in a series of dynamic interactions. Some of these do indeed help to maintain the reliability of axonal signalling in a variety of physiological and pathological conditions, but some of the mechanisms present also offer means for modulating axonal activity. This review will present key features of axon–glial cell anatomy and glial membrane properties, then discuss the role of axon-associated glia in axonal organisation, action potential conduction, ion regulation and trophic support, and conditions in which glial activity could modulate axonal firing and hence influence behaviour.

8.2 Anatomy of Axon–Glial Relations

There are several different patterns of axon–glial anatomy. In vertebrates, axons within the central nervous system (CNS) are typically ensheathed by oligodendrocytes, either as a loose wrapping enveloping a group of unmyelinated axons or as a multilamellar organisation forming the myelin sheath (Fig. 8.1) (Szuchet 1995). Individual oligodendrocytes may ensheath from less than five to more than 30 axons. Each segment of myelin is separated from the neighbouring segment by a node of Ranvier, a short gap in which the axon membrane is exposed. The overlapping oligodendrocyte lamellae form expanded lips around and projecting into the node. Astrocytic processes have been observed preferentially associated with the nodes of Ranvier (Fig. 8.1) (Waxman and Black 1995), and in certain sites, astrocytes provide a lattice-like framework that together with the oligodendrocytes shapes the geometry of the parallel bundles of axons (Maggs and Scholes 1990; Suzuki and Raisman 1992). In vertebrate peripheral nervous system (PNS), Schwann cells of neural crest origin act in the same capacity as oligodendrocytes, ensheathing axons and forming (peripheral) myelin. Differences between central and peripheral ensheathing glia contribute to the differential capacity for neural regeneration in CNS and PNS (Schwab 1995; Stuermer 1995), and to the selective pattern of damage in demyelinating diseases (Campagnoni 1995).

In invertebrates, true myelin is absent, and the pattern of axon–glial association is more varied, from axon bundles with few intercalated glial cells as in some bivalve interganglionic connectives, to the multilamellated glial sheets with 'pseudo-nodes' surrounding axons in certain crustacea and annelids (Roots 1995). Division into classes of glia is less clear cut than in vertebrates, and glia are generally described by their shape and location (e.g. ensheathing, perineurial, neuropilar, connective), although axon-associated glia of the PNS are still termed 'Schwann cells' (Abbott 1995). The axons of the squid stellar nerve show many

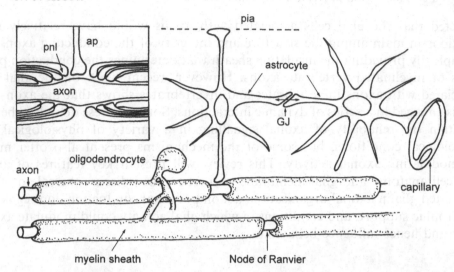

Fig. 8.1. Diagram showing two main types of axon-associated glia in vertebrate CNS: oligodendrocytes forming the myelin sheath around the axons, and astrocytes which may send fine processes to the nodal region, in addition to other processes to capillaries or the pial surface. Gap junction (GJ) coupling is shown between two astrocytes. Inset shows nodal region in longitudinal section, with multiple wrappings of myelin sheath; pnl, paranodal loop; ap, astrocytic process. Not to scale. (See sections on anatomy in Kettenmann and Ransom 1995).

variants of glial ensheathment, from the epithelial-like layer of elongated Schwann cells surrounding single giant axons, to arrangements where single Schwann cells ensheath several smaller axons (Fig. 8.2) (Brown et al 1991; Brown and Abbott 1993; Abbott et al 1995).

Certain anatomical specialisations are present that may offer clues to physiological function. Thus in vertebrate myelinated axons, the 'paranodal apparatus' is the term given to the complex of Schwann cell microvilli packed with mitochondria, and the extracellular material that fills the nodal gap, a structure suggesting an active role in translocation mechanisms or ion regulation in the node (Rosenbluth 1995). In the paranodal region, adjacent paranodal loops of Schwann cells are joined by tight junctions, limiting access to the reduced extracellular spaces within the myelin. The periaxonal space in the paranodal region narrows to a uniform 2–4 nm width, apparently stabilised by 'transverse bands' spanning the space and corresponding to diagonal arrays of intramembranous particles (IMPs) seen in freeze-fracture replicas of the Schwann cell membranes. IMPs are also associated with other membrane proteins, including ion channels and 'recognition molecules'; the density of IMPs has been used to follow the expression of these molecules (Waxman and Black 1995).

Gap junctions and dye- and electrical-coupling have been observed between glial cells both in vivo and in vitro, strongly between astrocytes, weakly between

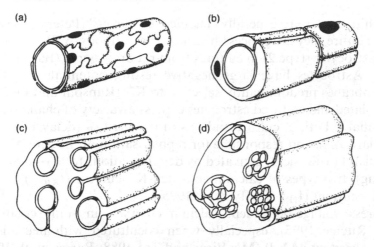

Fig. 8.2. Diagram illustrating four types of ensheathment of axons by Schwann cells in the squid stellar nerve: (a) giant axon surrounded by an epithelial like monolayer of several Schwann cells; (b) ensheathment of a medium-sized axon (1.5–10 μm diameter) by a single Schwann cell; (c) several small (0.5–1.0 μm diameter) axons ensheathed by a single Schwann cell; (d) bundles of the smallest axons (< 0.5 μm diameter) ensheathed by single Schwann cell. (From Abbott et al. 1995, with permission.)

oligodendrocytes, and between oligodendrocytes and astrocytes, including those associated with nodes of Ranvier (Ransom 1995). Dye-coupling occurs between non-myelinating but not between myelinating Schwann cells of vertebrate nerve (Konishi 1990a), and those of the squid giant axon are weakly coupled (Brown et al 1991; Brown and Kukita 1996). In addition, the squid Schwann cells show a system of transcellular tubules (the 'tubular lattice') greatly expanding the area of Schwann cell membrane accessible to the periaxonal space (Brown and Abbott 1993). Cell:cell coupling and glial membrane expansion become relevant in consideration of the role of glia in ion regulation and trophic support (see below).

8.3 Glial Cell Ion Channels

Early studies with microelectrodes found no evidence for voltage-dependent ion currents in glial cells (Somjen 1995), but with the improvements in technique that now permit patch clamp studies of cells both in culture and in situ, it is clear that axon-associated glia are between them capable of expressing almost all the ion channel types described for axons. However, differences between species and between cultures under different conditions suggest that not all channels are functionally expressed in the adult in situ, and moreover that there may be anatomical segregation of channels between different parts of the cell.

Astrocytes in white matter are generally classified as 'fibrous' (Peters, Palay and Webster 1976); in culture they are process-bearing. The antibody A2B5 recognises a class of fibrous astrocytes (type 2) in cultures from rat optic nerve (Barres, Chun and Corey 1990). Astrocytes have large negative resting potentials (~ -80 to -90mV), and membranes predominantly selective to K^+ (Ransom and Goldring 1973b). Freshly isolated and cultured astrocytes express a variety of channel types. K^+ currents identifiable both in culture and in situ include I_{DR} (delayed rectifier, activated by depolarisation and responsible for repolarisation of the action potential in excitable cells), I_A (transient, activated by depolarisations to ~ -40 mV and rapidly inactivating), two types of calcium-activated K^+ current ($I_{K(Ca)}$), and an inward rectifier K^+ current (I_{IR}) (Duffy et al. 1995).

Astrocytes express voltage-dependent calcium channels in some conditions (Sontheimer and Ritchie 1995), especially when cocultured with neurons, or exposed to agents elevating cAMP (MacVicar and Tse 1988; Barres et al. 1990a; Corvalen et al. 1990). A proportion (typically $\sim30\%$) of cultured astrocytes, and astrocytes in situ or freshly isolated by the 'tissue print' method, also express Na^+ channels (Clark and Mobbs 1994; Sontheimer and Ritchie 1995). Again, neural influence can be detected. Thus Na^+ channels were virtually absent in astrocytes cultured from optic nerve of enucleated animals in which axons had degenerated (Minturn et al. 1992), but could be partially restored by coculture with neurons (Barres et al. 1990a). By contrast, Na^+ channels in spinal cord astrocytes were downregulated by cocultured neurons, or by exposure to neuron-conditioned medium, implicating a soluble factor (Thio et al. 1993). Shorter-term modulation may also occur: Marrero et al. (1989) showed that Na^+ currents in the glial layer at the surface of the frog optic nerve were transiently increased by nerve impulses, seconds after stimulation. However, in all cases, the astrocytic Na^+ channels are present at very low density and would be inactivated at the normal resting potential, so they are unlikely to be able to generate action potentials (Somjen 1995; Sontheimer and Ritchie 1995).

Oligodendrocyte membranes are also predominantly permeable to K^+, behaving like K^+-selective electrodes (Kettenmann 1987; Butt and Tutton 1992). A sodium current channel (I_{na}) could be demonstrated in immature cells, but not later (Sontheimer et al. 1989b; Barres et al. 1990a,b). Although at least four types of K^+ current have been detected in culture, the adult in situ phenotype appears simpler, with I_{DR} and I_{IR} the predominant channel types (Barres, Chun and Corey 1990). I_{DR} and I_A would be most active during very large depolarisations, only likely in cells with either Na^+ channels or neurotransmitter receptors (Vartanian et al. 1988; Butt and Tutton 1992; Clark and Mobbs 1992). K_{IR} would be most active at the resting potential.

Cultured Schwann cells of some species express Na^+ channels (Sontheimer and Ritchie 1995), and Ca^{2+} currents have been reported in one study (Amedee et al. 1991), but generally K^+ currents predominate, including I_{DR}, I_A and I_{IR} (Chiu 1991, 1995; Duffy, Fraser and MacVicar 1995). A high conductance anion channel is also reported (Quastoff, Strupp and Grafe 1992). A change in channel expression appears to accompany maturation, with a progressive downregulation of I_{IR} and reduction in negative resting potential with days in culture (Konishi 1990a,b; Wilson and Chiu 1990a,b). Myelinating and non-myelinating Schwann cells show a different pattern of ionic currents in whole cell clamp, but this may reflect location of ion channels in the fine myelinating lamellae, beyond the detection of the patch electrode (Chiu 1995; Sontheimer and Ritchie 1995). Contact with neurites has been reported to modify expression of functional potassium channels in cultured mouse Schwann cells (Fig. 8.3) (Despeyroux, Amedee and Coles 1994).

   The ion channels of axon-associated glia in invertebrates have been less well studied, but follow a similar pattern. Squid Schwann cells, like those of vertebrates, have a low resting potential (~ -40mV), but a predominantly K^+-selective membrane (Lieberman, Abbott and Hassan 1989; Abbott et al. 1995; Villegas 1995). Impalements with microelectrodes show spontaneous hyperpolarisations in a proportion of the cells, compatible with the presence of calcium-dependent K^+ channels, activated by calcium entry on electrode penetration (Abbott et al. 1995). Patch clamp studies of Schwann cells freshly isolated from axons demonstrate a calcium current, and both I_{IR} and $I_{K(Ca)}$ (Brown, Inoue and Tsutsui 1996). Taken together, these studies show that in both vertebrates and invertebrates, K^+ channels are likely to be the most important in axon-associated glial function, but that other channels may influence electrical properties in certain locations and developmental stages.

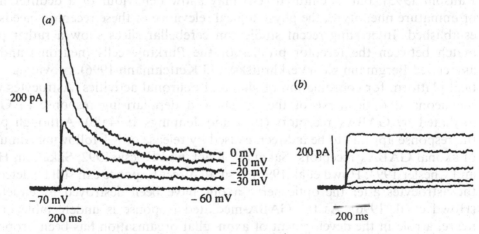

Fig. 8.3. Neurons influence Schwann cell K^+ currents. (a) On an isolated Schwann cell, depolarising voltage steps from a holding potential of -70 mV evoked a K^+ current with two components, a fast transient current followed by a delayed sustained current. (b) The same voltage protocol applied to a typical Schwann cell attached to a neurite evoked only a delayed sustained K^+ current. (From Despeyroux, Amedee and Coles 1994, with permission.)

8.4 Axon–Glial Communication

Given the close anatomical association of axons and their adjacent glia, communication between the cells is possible, both by surface contact, and via soluble signals. Surface adhesion and recognition molecules are important in determining the anatomical relations of axons and their associated glia, during initial development (McKeon and Silver 1995), during differentiation, in maintaining the normal adult anatomy, and in response to injury (Faissner and Schachner 1995). Glia associated with axons both produce and respond to growth factors under certain conditions, including nerve growth factor (NGF) and brain-derived neurotrophic factor (BDNF) (Sendtner 1995). In addition to these long-term interactions mediated by surface molecules and growth factors, there are now several examples of axon–glial cell communication by short-term signalling.

Axons release K^+ during the action potential, and as the glial membranes are sensitive to K^+, much of the early literature concentrated on K^+ as a putative axon–glial signal (Pentreath 1982). Indeed, changes in the metabolism and glucose uptake of optic nerve glia do occur in the presence of raised $[K^+]$ (Orkand, Bracho and Orkand 1973; Salem et al. 1975). However, nerve impulses cause changes in a number of other substances in the glial microenvironment, including calcium and protons, which could also influence glial activity (Orkand 1995). Recently, interest has focused on the possibility that axon–glial signalling may involve neurotransmitters.

Cultured astrocytes have been found to express receptors for virtually all the chemical transmitter molecules liberated by neurons (see Kettenmann and Ransom 1995), but as cultured cells may show behaviour of a dedifferentiated or immature phenotype, the physiological relevance of these receptors needs to be established. Interesting recent studies on cerebellar slices show a rather precise match between the receptor profiles of the Purkinje cells (neurons) and their associated Bergmann glia (Verkhratsky and Kettenmann 1996), providing a practical platform for coordination of glial and neuronal activities. Astrocytes within the neonatal optic nerve of the rat show a depolarising response to GABA, mediated by $GABA_A$ receptors (Butt and Jennings 1994a,b). Although part of the response appears to be indirect, caused by release of K^+ following stimulation of axonal $GABA_A$ receptors (Sakatani, Black and Kocsis 1992; Sakatani, Hassan and Chesler 1994; Howd et al. 1995), a small direct response can still be detected in the astrocytes after the optic nerve axons have been destroyed by enucleation (Howd et al. 1996). As the GABA-mediated response is undetectable in adult nerve, a role in the development of axon–glial organisation has been proposed.

Oligodendrocytes and Schwann cells in culture respond to a smaller range of neurotransmitters than do astrocytes (Lyons, Morrell and McCarthy 1994; Yoder, Tamir and Ellissman 1996), but it has proved difficult to determine whether these axon-associated glia express receptors in situ. Perisynaptic Schwann cells of the frog neuromuscular junction (Jahromi, Robitaille and Charlton 1992) respond to axonal stimulation with a rise in $[Ca^{2+}]_i$; acetylcholine (ACh) or ATP may be responsible, as the effects can be mimicked by bath application of these agents (Jahromi, Robitaille and Charlton 1992; Reist and Smith 1992). Freshly-isolated Schwann cells responded to ATP and bradykinin with a rise in $[Ca^{2+}]_i$, but showed no response to histamine or glutamate (Lyons, Morrell and McCarthy 1994). Maintenance of the response to ATP in culture was dependent on contact with neurons (Lyons et al. 1995). Stimulation of optic nerve axons caused a rise in $[Ca^{2+}]_i$ in the nearby glial cells (Fig. 8.4), a response mimicked by application of glutamate (Kriegler and Chiu 1993).

Among invertebrates, the giant axon of the squid provides extensive evidence not only for Schwann cell receptors in situ, but also for their involvement in axon–glial signalling. In a series of studies beginning in the 1970s, J. Villegas and co-workers have demonstrated a complex array of receptors on the giant axon Schwann cell, which are linked physiologically (Villegas 1995). Axon stimulation releases a signal or signals, probably including glutamate, since it can be mimicked by application of glutamate agonists, and inhibited by glutamate receptor antagonists (Lieberman, Abbott and Hassan 1989; Evans et al. 1995). Glutamate acts on Schwann cell receptors of predominantly non-NMDA metabotropic type (Evans et al. 1992), triggering a further cascade of actions in which the Schwann cell releases acetylcholine (ACh), that acts back on Schwann cell autoreceptors, causing elevation of cAMP and membrane hyperpolarisation. In this state the membrane is more K^+ selective (Coles and Abbott 1996), compatible with the opening of K^+ channels, activated by a rise in intracellular calcium (Abbott et al. 1995). Octopamine, a squid stress hormone, potentiates the action of the ACh-dependent system, and a Schwann cell derived vasoactive intestinal (VIP)-like peptide may also be involved (Fig. 8.5) (Evans, Reale and Villegas 1986; Villegas 1995).

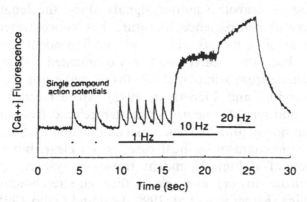

Fig. 8.4. Axon–glial signalling. Calcium fluorescence from glial cells associated with axons in neonatal rat optic nerves in response to axonal stimulation to generate single action potentials or bursts of activity at 1–20 Hz. (From Kriegler and Chiu 1993, with permission.)

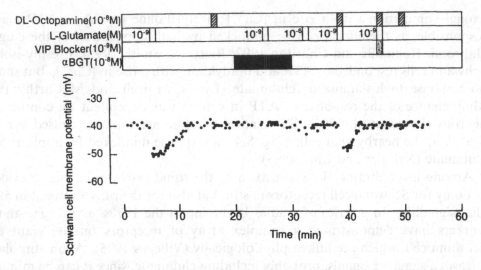

Fig. 8.5. Axon–Schwann cell signalling in squid giant axon. Release of a VIP-like peptide in response to a 1-min pulse of 10^{-9} M L-glutamate in the presence of 10^{-8} M DL-octopamine, after the cholinergic component of the response has been blocked by exposure to 10^{-8} M α-bungarotoxin (αBGT). The response to the release of the endogenous peptide is blocked in the presence of 10^{-9} M of the VIP blocking agent (pCl⁻ D-Phe⁶,Leu¹⁷)VIP. Each point represents the potential difference recorded in a different Schwann cell. (From Evans et al. 1995, with permission.)

Activation of opiate receptors blocks parts of the pathway (Evans, Reale and Villegas 1986). Although not studied in such detail, a similar system involving glial cell cholinergic receptors may be present in the ensheathing glial cells of crustacean giant axons (Grossfeld, Hargittai and Lieberman 1995).

How widespread is release of neurotransmitter signals along the length of conducting axons? The classical neuroscience literature has concentrated on neurotransmitter release at axon terminals via a calcium-dependent process involving synaptic vesicles, but some early studies documented release of amino acids, especially glutamate from stimulated lengths of nerve not containing terminals (Grossfeld, Hargittai and Lieberman 1995). More recently, evidence has accumulated for non-synaptic neurotransmitter release from axons and dendrites as well as from non-neural cells such as endothelium and smooth muscle (Vizi et al. 1983). The mechanism in most cases is not clear, but possibilities include reverse action of sodium-dependent transport systems during depolarisation (e.g. the glutamate carrier), and release through stretch-activated channels opened by cell swelling (Kimelberg et al. 1990; Levi and Gallo 1995). In the case of the axon, a signal released as a by-product of axon membrane depolarisation thus becomes a suitable candidate for communication between the axon and its associated glial cells.

In summary, in addition to axon–glial signalling using K^+, axon tracts in both the central and peripheral nervous systems of both vertebrates and invertebrates have available a series of putative signalling molecules that can be released from axons by bursts of action potentials, and that are capable of eliciting specific responses from the associated glial cells via action on membrane receptors. These signals enable the glial cells to match their activities to those of active axons. The need for such signalling will become clearer following discussion of the role of glial cells in axonal functions.

8.5 Signals Produced by Glial Cells

The examples of axon–glial interaction discussed so far involve glial cells responding to an axonally-released signal. Of equal interest to axon–glial interaction is whether axons can respond to glial-released signals. During development, glial cells synthesise and release a number of growth factors, including NGF and BDNF that influence neurite outgrowth and axonal development (Labourdette and Sensenbrenner 1995). Schwann cells do not normally express NGF/BDNF, but do so after nerve lesion, whereas ciliary neurotrophic factor (CNTF) is expressed when Schwann cells stop dividing and start myelinating (Sendtner 1995).

In normal adult physiology, glia-to-axon signalling is less well established. Glial cells in culture can be shown to release a variety of substances including ATP and amino acids (GABA, taurine; Levi and Gallo 1995), and as noted above, the squid Schwann cell produces ACh and possibly a (co-released?) VIP-like peptide (Fig. 8.5) (Evans et al. 1995; Villegas 1995). These squid Schwann cell signals act back on autoreceptors on the Schwann cell, and are therefore likely to be part of an amplification cascade, but it is not known if they also exert effects on the axon. However bath-applied carbachol raises the cyclic guanosine monophosphate (cGMP) level within squid giant axons, consistent with the possibility of a response to Schwann cell-produced ACh in vivo (Allen and Rouot 1995). Evidence for axonal receptors to a variety of glial-released agents is available for non-myelinated vertebrate axons, including the rabbit vagus (Armett and Ritchie 1961) and neonatal rat optic nerve (Sakatani, Black and Kocsis 1992; Sakatani, Hassan and Chesler 1994). Neurotransmitter receptors are now recognised to occur on many areas of the neuron surface outside synaptic zones (Ramcharan and Matthews 1996).

8.6 Role of Glia in Axonal Excitability and Conduction

A major function of the glial cells of myelinated nerves is to produce myelin to insulate the surface of the axon, reducing the effective membrane capacitance, and increasing membrane resistance. As a result, action potential conduction velocity is increased (Waxman and Black 1995) and the metabolic cost of conduction reduced (Chiu 1991). The axon appears to produce recognition molecules that initiate myelination. The thickness of the myelin sheath and the length of the internodes correlate with the diameter of the axon, as required for optimal conduction velocity, suggesting that signalling from axon to Schwann cell regulates the extent and geometry of the myelin sheath. Among invertebrates, glial enwrapment of axons appears to bring similar benefits, with conduction velocities up to 220 m/s achieved in the shrimp *Penaeus japonicus* (Roots 1995).

The ion channels of the vertebrate myelinated axon are not uniformly distributed; voltage dependent Na^+ channels are clustered predominantly at the node (up to $1000/\mu m^2$), and fast K^+ channels in the paranode. This has been proposed as a way of avoiding K^+ accumulation in the node, where it could influence the membrane potential and hence activation of Na^+ channels (Chiu 1995). Astrocytic processes are clearly associated with Na^+ channel-rich parts of the axon membrane, in the node of Ranvier, in 'hot spots' of channel clustering not located at nodes (as in non-myelinated portions of retinal ganglion cell axons (Hildebrand and Waxman 1983), and in artificially demyelinated axons at sites where nodes will later form (Sims et al. 1985b). It is not yet clear whether the ion channel cluster attracts the astrocytic process and encourages its adhesion, or whether the astrocytic process specifies the site of channel clustering. However, it appears that the nodal clustering is stabilised by the paranodal junctional contacts between oligodendrocyte/Schwann cell loops and the axon membrane. In rare examples of 'ectopic' oligodendrocyte processes contacting nodes of Ranvier, the axonal membrane shows a marked reduction in density of intramembranous particles (IMPs), consistent with reduction in Na^+ channel insertion (Black, Waxman and Hildebrand 1985; Waxman and Black 1995). There is thus circumstantial evidence for the regulation of Na^+ channel location by glial cell processes.

An equivalent pattern appears to determine ion channel distribution in the internodal axon membrane, where Na^+ channel expression is low ($\sim25/\mu m^2$); this appears to be due to active suppression by the adjacent glial cell, since in animals depleted of glia by X-irradiation, there is a significantly higher density of IMPs than in controls (Black et al., 1985, Black Waxman and Hildebrand 1985). The mechanism controlling suppression of Na^+ channel expression is not known.

The role of perinodal astrocytes in regulating axonal Na^+ channel density is intriguing. Mammalian astrocytes in vitro can express Na^+ channels with biophysical properties similar to those of neuronal Na^+ channels. Black et al. (1994a,b) described the expression of mRNA for Na^+ channel subtypes II and III, as well as the putative glial specific Na^+ channel Na-G, in cultured astrocytes, and in both membrane and cytoplasm of perinodal astrocytes. There is thus an interesting association between Na^+ channel-rich sites in the adjacent astrocytic process and axon membrane. Similar observations concerning Schwann cell Na^+ channel expression led to the suggestion that the associated glia (perinodal astrocytes in the CNS, Schwann cells in the PNS) may act as local factories for axonal Na^+ channels (Gray and Ritchie 1985). There is as yet no direct evidence for this hypothesis.

If present, this may not be the only function of glial Na^+ channels, since some glial Na^+ channels appear to have no neuronal counterpart. Schwann cells isolated from squid giant axons have a small Ca^{2+} current, but appear not to express the Na^+ channels present in the giant axon (Brown, Inoue and Kukita 1996), making it unlikely that axonal Na^+ channels are synthesised by these Schwann cells. Alternative or additional functions for glial Na^+ and Ca^{2+} channels could include amplification of axon–glial signalling by potentiating the local depolarising effects of transmitter-mediated activation (Chiu 1995).

The glial–axonal interactions at sites of Na^+ channel clustering in developing and mature vertebrate axons can also be observed in partially demyelinated axons, where Na^+ channels appear to be clustered at remaining contacts with Schwann cells (PNS) or astrocytes (CNS) (Black and Waxman 1995). These 'hot spots' or 'phi-nodes' may be sufficient to sustain excitability in these axons.

In addition to influencing ion channel distribution, axon-associated glia may exert dynamic effects on axonal excitability. Thus axonal conduction can be modulated by several agents reported to be released by glial cells, including ACh in rabbit vagus nerve (Armett and Ritchie 1963) and GABA in neonatal rat optic nerve (Sakatani, Black and Kocsis 1992; Sakatani, Hassan and Chesler 1994). It remains to be shown that such signalling occurs in situ.

8.7 Role of Axon-Associated Glial Cells in Ion Regulation

Nodal Na^+ channels and paranodal fast K^+ channels are the major channel types involved in axonal excitability, but internodal ion channels are now recognised to play a role in axonal function. While the paranodal junctions restrict diffusion in the periaxonal space of the internode for molecules the size of horseradish peroxidase, small ions can enter, as shown by penetration of lanthanum tracer (Mackenzie, Ghabriel and Allt 1984). Electrophysiological studies with microelectrodes have demonstrated that part of the action current during an action potential flows along the periaxonal space (Barrett and Barrett 1982). Slow K^+ channels are concentrated in the node, but are also present in the internode. Direct microelectrode recording from the periaxonal space provides evidence that internodal K^+ channels are activated during saltatory nerve conduction (David, Barrett and Barrett 1992); they also appear to be important in setting the axonal resting potential. Calculations show that K^+ accumulation in the 20 nm wide internodal periaxonal space during a single propagated action potential could exceed 10 mM for stimulation frequencies > 100 Hz, if clearance occurred only by extracellular diffusion (Chiu 1991). Studies with voltage-sensitive dyes do indeed suggest K^+ accumulation in a restricted paranodal periaxonal space during repetitive stimulation (Lev-Ram and Grinvald 1986). Such observations have led to interest in the possibility that the axon-associated glial cells may be involved in K^+ regulation in order to ensure that K^+ accumulation does not compromise nerve conduction.

If extracellular Na^+ depletion and K^+ accumulation occur during nerve conduction, both with disadvantageous physiological consequences, to what extent can they be counteracted by axon-associated glial cells? As we have seen, all types of glial cells have a variety of K^+ channels, and perinodal astrocytic processes show a clustering of Na^+ channels. Both oligodendrocytes and Schwann cells express the inwardly rectifying channel K_{IR} maximally activated at the resting potential, and assuming these are present in the paranodal membrane, they could siphon K^+ in the paranodal region into Schwann cells (Konishi 1990a,b; Wilson and Chiu 1990a,b). K_{IR} channels have recently been detected in the nodal microvilli of Schwann cells (Mi et al. 1996). As the Schwann cells also contain delayed rectifier K^+ channels in regions away from the node (Mi et al. 1995), their activation at a distal site could provide an exit path for K^+, as required for K^+ clearance by 'spatial buffering' (Fig. 8.6). The greatly expanded Schwann cell membrane in the paranodal region ($\sim \times 10$ the area of the local axon membrane; Berthold and Rydmark 1983) would favour this kind of K^+ siphoning.

Cell swelling and vacuolation of Schwann cells in the paranodal region during repetitive stimulation suggest entry of K^+ and water (Wurtz and Ellisman 1986).

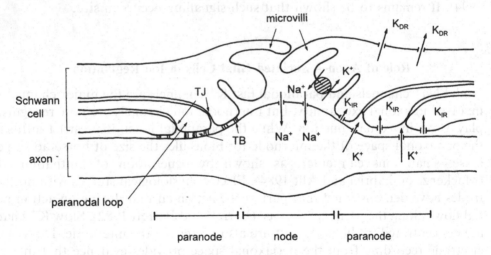

Fig. 8.6. Diagram to show role of Schwann cell ion channels and transporters in ion regulation around the node and paranodal regions of the myelinated axon. Tight junctions (TJ) restrict access to the extracellular spaces within the myelin sheath, and 'transverse bands' (TB) maintain a narrow periaxonal space in the paranodal region. Axonal voltage-activated Na^+ channels are clustered in the nodal region, whereas K^+ channels are mainly in the paranodal membrane. Within the Schwann cell membranes, the inward rectifier K^+ channels (K_{IR}) adjacent to the axon, and the delayed rectifier channels (K_{DR}) away from the axon surface, would facilitate K^+ siphoning during periods of axonal activity. The Schwann cell Na/K-ATPase transporters (hatched circle) would enable the Schwann cell to act as a sink for K^+ and source for Na^+. (Based on information in Chiu 1995; Mi et al. 1996.)

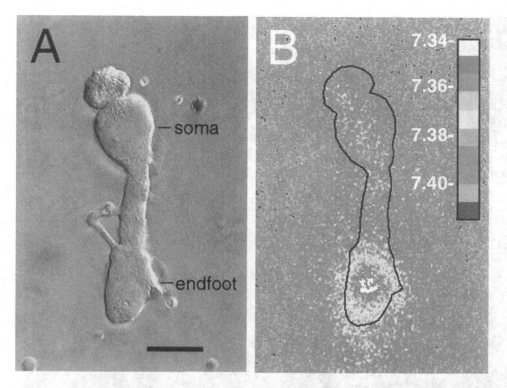

Plate 1. Depolarization-evoked acid efflux generated by the Müller cell $Na^+/$ HCO_3-co-transport system. (A) Micrograph of a dissociated salamander Müller cell. Scale bar, 20 mm. (B) Image of extracellular pH for the cell shown in (A), measured by imaging the pH-indicator dye BCECF fixed to a coverslip. The cell Na^+/HCO_3-co-transporter is activated by depolarization ($[K^+]_e$ raised from 2.5 to 50 mM). The resulting acid efflux is largest at the cell endfoot, indicating that co-transporters are preferentially localised to this cell region. The pseudo-colour image is calibrated in pH units (bar at right). (From Newman 1996a.)

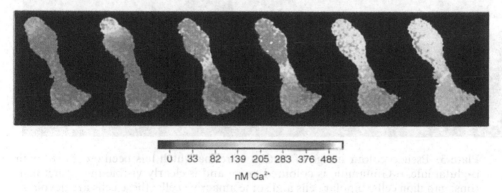

Plate 2. Calcium wave in a dissociated salamander Müller cell. The Ca^{2+} wave, evoked by addition of 100 nM ryanodine in the absence of extracellular Ca^{2+}, begins at the apical end of the cell and travels towards the cell endfoot. Intracellular Ca^{2+} concentration is imaged using the Ca^{2+}-indicator dye Fura-2. Images were obtained at 7-s intervals. (From Keirstead and Miller 1995.)

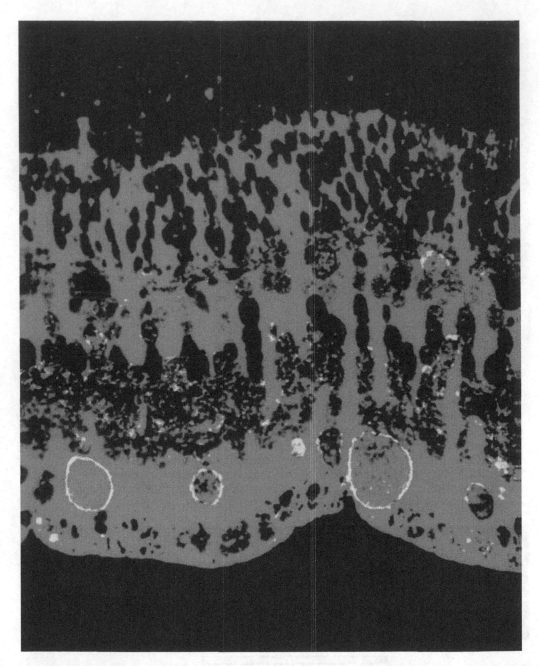

Plate 3. Pseudo-colour image of section of retina which has been incubated with D-glutamate. D-Glutamine is coloured green and is clearly visible in distinct neurons: ganglion cells, bipolar cells and some amacrine cells; these cells are devoid of glutamate (coloured red). The remaining cells, including Müller cells, stain intensely for glutamate. (From Pow and Crook 1996.)

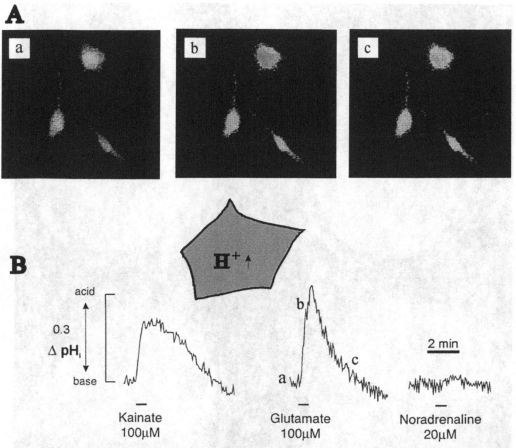

Plate 4. Intracellular acidosis of cultured rate cerebellar astrocytes induced by glutamate (A, B) and kainate, but not by noradrenaline (B). (A) Video imaging of BCECF-AM loaded cells before (a), during (b) and after (c) bath application of 100 μM glutamate. (B) BCECF ratio signal at 440 nm/495 nm excitation wavelengths. (A from T. Brune and J. W. Deitmer, unpublished; B modified from Brune and Deitmer 1995.)

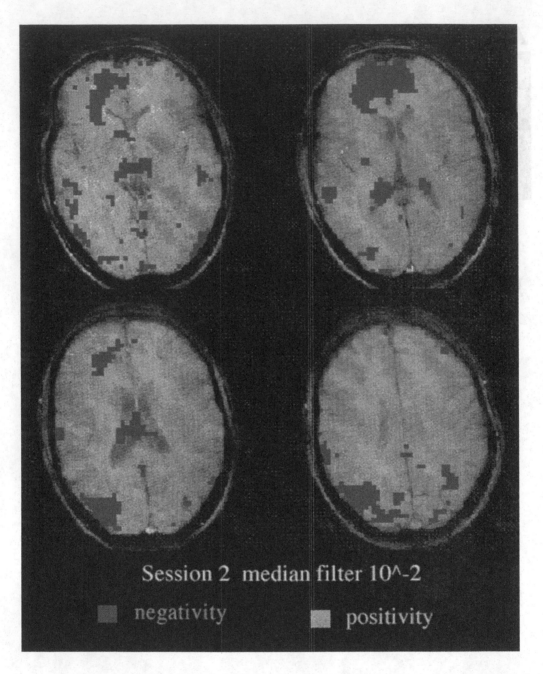

Plate 5. Functional magnetic resonance imaging (fMRI) of regional blood flow of a highly trained subject producing SPS-negativity at C_z (blue) and SPS-positivity at C_z (orange). Coloured shading indicates significant differences in blood flow changes between achieved SPS-negativity and positivity. Four successive slices of the brain are shown (see text for description). (From Birbaumer et al. 1998.)

As the swelling persists in Cl^--free conditions (Konishi 1991), it appears not to be necessarily accompanied by entry of Cl^-, confirming that K^+ siphoning rather than KCl entry is involved. The mechanisms may be particularly important in immature and remyelinating axons, where the myelin sheath is relatively loose, and the location of K_{IR} channels to the innermost turn of the Schwann cell adjacent to the axon could siphon K^+ accumulated along the length of the internodal periaxonal space (Chiu 1995). Bath application of Cs^+, a blocker of K_{IR}, did not affect conduction of high frequency bursts of action potentials, but did alter the threshold for excitation (Baker et al. 1987). Hoppe et al. (1991) were unable to demonstrate any change in K^+ accumulation or removal with the K^+ channel blocker Ba^{2+}, but these experiments are complicated by the effects of Ba^{2+} on the axonal K^+ channels. In sucrose gap recording from the rabbit vagus nerve, changes in Schwann cell membrane potential contribute to the recorded potential (Robert and Jirounek 1994). Ba^{2+} caused a reduction in resting $[K^+]_e$ and an increase in stimulated $[K^+]_e$ (Fig. 8.7), interpreted as showing that Schwann cell K^+ channels contribute to removal of axon-liberated K^+ ions.

K_{IR} channels are also found on perinodal astrocytes and as these are electrically coupled to oligodendrocytes, they may share in the K^+ siphoning process. The advantage of the astrocytes is that because of their strongly coupled syncytial arrangement, and end-feet away from the axon on blood vessels and the pial surface (Fig. 8.1), K^+ siphoning through astrocytes can occur over a greater distance (Newman 1995).

In the case of the squid giant axon, the electrical coupling between Schwann cells of the ensheathing monolayer acts within the same plane as the propagation

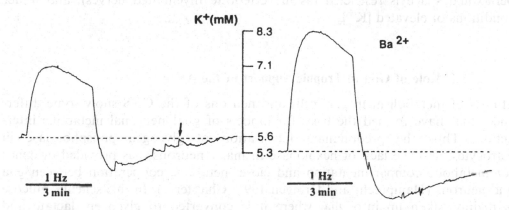

Fig. 8.7. Role of Schwann cells in K^+ regulation in the rabbit vagus nerve. Application of 1 mM barium (Ba^{2+}) reduced the resting level of extracellular K^+, but increased both the maximal level of K^+ accumulation during 1 Hz axonal stimulation and the post-stimulation undershoot. By comparing changes in potential and $[K^+]$, it was concluded that Schwann cell K^+ channels contributed to K^+ clearance in this preparation. (From Robert and Jirounek 1994, with permission.)

of the axonal action potential, and is hence unlikely to contribute to K^+ spatial buffering. Electrical coupling between squid Schwann cells may therefore play other roles in the coordination of function (Abbott et al. 1995; Pichon et al. 1995; Brown and Kukita 1996). Brunet and Jirounek (1994) have demonstrated a slowly propagating depolarisation in the syncytial Schwann cells of the stimulated vagus nerve, which may have counterparts in other systems.

In addition to passive mechanisms for K^+ removal, axon-associated glial cells have a number of carrier-mediated transport mechanisms that can contribute to K^+ regulation, including the ouabain-sensitive Na/K-ATPase, and the bumetanide-sensitive Na-K-2Cl cotransporter (Ballanyi 1995; Newman 1995). In studies on the giant axon of the squid *Alloteuthis*, K^+ clearance from the axon surface during repetitive stimulation depends on the presence of healthy Schwann cells (Abbott et al. 1988; Astion et al. 1988; Brown 1993). The undershoot of the action potential recorded with sharp microelectrodes has been used to monitor periaxonal $[K^+]$. The decline of undershoots over 5–10 s stimulation increased in the presence of ouabain or bumetanide, suggesting the presence of a carrier-mediated contribution to periaxonal K^+ clearance under conditions of elevated extracellular K^+ (Pichon et al. 1995). This is likely to be predominantly on Schwann cells, given the much greater membrane area they present to the periaxonal space (Brown and Abbott 1993). In studies on axons of the squid *Sepioteuthis* examined with voltage clamp and axial microelectrode recording, under conditions where little K^+ accumulation occurred, extracellular diffusion could account for K^+ clearance, and neither blocking Schwann cell K^+ channels nor adding ouabain caused a change in clearance (Inoue, Tsutsui and Brown 1997). Taken together, these studies suggest that Schwann cells contribute to K^+ clearance at sites where diffusion from the periaxonal space is restricted (as in vertebrate myelinated nerves), and under conditions of elevated $[K^+]_e$.

8.8 Role of Glia in Trophic Support of the Axon

Studies of metabolism in glial cells and neurons of the CNS show some differences that have formed the basis for models of glial–neuronal metabolic interaction. Thus the predominant localisation of glycogen phosphorylase in astrocytes, and the lack of hexokinase in many neurons, has provided evidence for metabolic compartmentation and close metabolic cooperation between glia and neurons (Hamprecht and Dringen 1995; Chapter 5). In this scheme, glucose is mainly taken up into glia, where it is converted to glycogen, lactate and pyruvate. Lactate and pyruvate can then form energy substrates for neurons, particularly in periods of increased activity (Magistretti et al. 1993). It is not yet known whether similar metabolic compartmentation occurs in axon tracts. In vertebrate nerve, metabolic reliance of axons on glial cells is unlikely to be universal, as the degree of ensheathment of axons by glia is very variable, with little or no glial ensheathment in some non-myelinated axon bundles, such as olfactory and vagus nerves. The high metabolic requirements of small axons, which need to sustain ion gradients by active transport, yet have a disadvantageous surface area:volume ratio, mean that small axons may need to manage their metabolism themselves.

Better documented is the transfer of large molecules from glial cell to axon, demonstrated in some invertebrate preparations. There is evidence for transfer of polypeptides and proteins (10–200 kDa) from the ensheathing glia to the axoplasm of giant axons in the squid and the crayfish (Sheller and Bittner 1992; Sheller et al. 1995), permitting survival of the axon when supply of substances from the cell body is restricted. The mechanism for transfer is unclear, but may involve vesicle formation from glial cell processes penetrating the axon (Buchheit and Tytell 1992). However, as most demonstrations of transfer have involved axonal dissection or damage (Fishman, Tewari and Stein 1990), it is not clear to what extent such molecular trafficking occurs in normal physiology, and whether it can be modulated by axonal activity. The same is true of occasional observations of protein transfer to axons after injection into axon-associated glia in vertebrates (Duncan et al. 1996).

8.9 Can Glial Cells Modulate Axonal Activity in Normal Behaviour?

From the above discussion, it is clear that glial cells are able to respond to axonal activity in a variety of ways that appear to be important in the support and homeostatic functions of the axons. Glial cells are thus regulating behaviour in the sense that in the absence of their activity, axonal function and hence behaviour would be unreliable or disturbed. In the case of the passive redistribution of K^+ by glial cells, this simply aids homeostasis, but when active transport is involved, as with the Na/K-ATPase, stimulation of the transport system in activated glia could have more subtle effects, including reducing the basal level of extracellular $[K^+]$ after a period of activity (Ballanyi, Grafe and Ten Bruggencate 1987; Ballanyi 1995). Modulation of extracellular $[K^+]$ ($[K^+]_e$) would have several effects on axonal function, including changing the threshold for excitability, and influencing the pattern of activity during bursts of action potentials (Leng, Shibuki and Way 1988). Reductions in basal $[K^+]_e$ have indeed been observed in vertebrate spinal cord and optic nerve following stimulation (Kříž, Syková and Vyklický 1975; Sakatani, Hassan and Chesler 1994). Moreover, as sodium pump activity can be modulated by neurotransmitters and hormones (Sweadner 1995), this is an example of a situation in which glial cell activity can feed back to modify axonal activity and hence behaviour. As methods for simultaneously recording glial and axonal activity are applied to both CNS and PNS axon tracts, further examples of such modulation are likely to emerge.

8.10 Conclusions

This review has discussed the dynamic axon–glial interactions involved in development, in normal physiology, and in recovery from neural damage. The interactions help establish the proper anatomy underlying coordinated behaviour, improve reliability of axonal conduction, and offer opportunities for glial modulation of axonal function. Studies are now required to follow up the promising observations from cultured cells, using advantageous intact or semi-intact preparations, to establish their roles in vivo.

Acknowledgements

Our work on squid axon–glial interaction has been supported by the Wellcome Trust and the BBSRC, UK.

9

Transplantation of Myelin-Forming Glial Cells into the Spinal Cord: Restoration of Normal Conduction in Previously Demyelinated Axons

JEFFERY D. KOCSIS and STEPHEN G. WAXMAN

Summary

It is well established that myelination is associated with an increase in conduction velocity, a reduction in relative refractory period, and enhanced ability to conduct high-frequency sequences of action potentials in normal axons. In demyelinated and dysmyelinated axons, there is a decrease in conduction velocity, an increase in relative refractory period, and impaired ability to transmit high-frequency action potential trains. Under some circumstances, remyelination by endogenous glial cells is associated with reversal of these functional abnormalities and restoration of nearly normal axonal conduction. This opens up the questions of (i) whether it is possible to repair the de- or dysmyelinated nervous system by transplantation of exogenous myelin-forming glial cells; and (ii) whether myelin formation by transplanted glia can favourably alter axonal conduction in the de- or dysmyelinated central nervous system. This chapter summarises recent studies in our laboratory which have shown that it is possible to enhance conduction in demyelinated and dysmyelinated axons by transplantation of myelin-forming glial cells. Conduction velocity, relative refractory period, and ability to conduct high-frequency impulse trains returned to levels close to normal as a result of myelination by transplanted oligodendrocytes or Schwann cells. These results provide a striking example of the modulation of axonal conduction properties by glial cells and, importantly, suggest that it may be possible to restore normal, or nearly-normal, function to de- and dysmyelinated axons via cell transplantation.

9.1 Introduction

Axons are the conductile elements that connect the receptive part of the neuron, i.e. the cell body and dendrites, with other neurons, and their function is to conduct action potentials. Within the mammalian nervous system, many axons are myelinated, and this constitutes an important adaptation which shapes their conduction properties. In myelinated axons, the myelin forms a high resistance, low capacitance shield and conduction velocity is linearly related to fibre diameter; in contrast, in non-myelinated fibres, conduction velocity is proportional to (diameter)$^{1/2}$. As a result of this, above a critical diameter of 0.2 µm, myelinated axons conduct more rapidly than their nonmyelinated counterparts of the same diameter (Waxman and Bennett 1972). The energetics of conduction are also more favourable in myelinated axons, allowing the conduction of sequences of action potentials at higher frequencies than in non-myelinated axons.

Disorders involving the myelin sheath provide an important opportunity to examine the roles of myelin in determining the conduction properties of axons. Axons that have sustained damage to their myelin [i.e. *demyelinated* axons which are characteristic of multiple sclerosis and are also observed in contusive spinal cord injury and spinal cord compression (Gledhill, Harrison and McDonald 1973; Blight 1985; Byrne and Waxman 1990)], and axons that have not acquired normal myelin sheaths (i.e. *dysmyelinated* axons, which are observed in disorders such as the leukodystrophies) display conduction velocities that are substantially lower than those of normally myelinated fibres of the same diameter. In addition, it is well established that the refractory period for transmission is increased in demyelinated axons (Smith, Blakemore and McDonald 1983) and that abnormally myelinated axons are unable to conduct impulses at frequencies as high as those in normal axons (Honmou et al. 1996).

Studies on the production of new myelin sheaths, in models of dys- and demyelinating diseases, have provided an additional route for determining the roles of glial cells in modulating the conduction properties in axons; these studies are aimed at the clinically important possibility of restoring normal, or nearly-normal, conduction to de- or dysmyelinated axons via approaches that promote myelin repair. Microelectrode studies have demonstrated relatively normal action potential conduction following myelin formation by *endogenous* oligodendrocytes or following invasion of peripheral Schwann cells in some experimental models of central nervous system (CNS) demyelination (Smith, Blakemore and McDonald 1981, 1983; Blight 1989; Felts and Smith 1992). A number of studies have demonstrated that transplanted glial cells can also form compact myelin with relatively normal morphological characteristics within the demyelinated CNS (Waxman and Brill 1978; Blakemore and Crang 1985; Duncan, Hammang and Gilmore 1988; Rosenbluth et al. 1990; Gout and Dubois-Dalcq 1993; Lachapelle et al. 1994). However, the presence of compact myelin per se does not necessarily ensure reliable conduction of action potentials. Secure conduction requires the formation of internodal myelin segments of the appropriate length (Huxley and Stämpfli 1949; Waxman and Brill 1978) and the clustering of sodium channels at the newly formed nodes of Ranvier (Waxman 1977; Ritchie and Rogart 1977; Moore et al. 1978; Hines and Shrager 1991).

Despite the need for physiological studies, most research to date, on the transplantation of cells to systems that lack myelin, has focused on morphological aspects of myelin formation and has not examined the effects of myelination, by exogenous transplanted glial cells, on axonal conduction. In this chapter, we summarise research in which we have used electrophysiological methods (Kocsis and Waxman 1980, 1983) to study the conduction of action potentials along dysmyelinated or previously demyelinated axons in several experimental models, following myelination by transplanted glial cells. Our results demonstrate that myelination by exogenous, transplanted glial cells can in fact enhance the conduction properties, including conduction velocity, refractory period, and ability to transmit high-frequency impulse trains of dysmyelinated and demyelinated axons so that they conduct action potentials in a nearly normal manner.

9.2 Transplantation of Myelin-Forming Glial Cells into the Dysmyelinated Spinal Cord

We carried out our first electrophysiological studies on transplant-induced myelination on dorsal column axons in the myelin-deficient (*md*) rat (Utzschneider et al. 1994). This experimental model was chosen because this mutant lacks CNS myelin, as a result of a point mutation in proteolipid protein gene (Boison and Stoffel 1989; Zeller, Dubois-Dalcq and Lazzarini 1989; Hudson et al. 1989; Simons and Riordan 1990). The absence of myelin within the CNS of this mutant permits definitive confirmation that physiological changes are due to myelination by exogenous, transplanted glial cells, and are not due to background myelination by endogenous cells (Duncan et al. 1988; Duncan, Hammang and Gilmore 1988). Previous electrophysiological studies in the *md* rat CNS demonstrated that action potentials can propagate along dysmyelinated *md* axons with slow conduction velocities similar to those of premyelinated axons (Waxman et al. 1990), and showed that, although the dysmyelinated fibres of the *md* dorsal columns display decreased conduction velocities, they are capable of secure action potential conduction at relatively normal frequencies (Utzschneider, Black and Kocsis 1992).

For our studies in the *md* model (Utzschneider et al. 1994), glial cell suspensions were prepared from the spinal cords of female littermates of the animals to be transplanted, at 4–5 days postnatal. Cells were cultured overnight, and were then concentrated at 50 000 per μl. For transplantation, recipient rats were anaesthetised with halothane and a dorsal laminectomy was performed at the thoracolumbar junction. Injections of 1.0 μl of cell suspension were made via a glass micropipette, into two or three sites along the dorsal columns of the spinal cord and the transplant sites were marked for subsequent identification. Conduction in the transplanted spinal cords was studied on postnatal days 20, 21, or 22, corresponding to 15–17 days following cell transplantation. For these studies, following deep pentobarbitone anaesthesia, animals were perfused with chilled, oxygenated high sucrose solution (containing 124 mM sucrose, 26 mM $NaHCO_3$, 3 mM KCl, 1.3 mM NaH_2PO_4, 2 mM $MgCl_2$ and 10 mM dextrose) and the spinal cord was then carefully removed and allowed to equilibrate to room temperature over

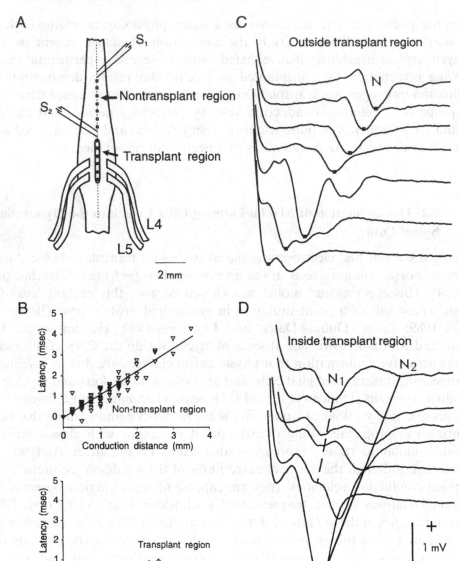

30–45 min prior to positioning in a recording chamber. Field potential and single cell recordings were obtained as described by Utzschneider et al. (1994).

The transplanted spinal cords studied in this series ($n = 10$) each displayed an opaque white patch, which corresponded to a zone of myelination, extending for several millimetres along the longitudinal axis of the dorsal surface of the spinal cord. Histological examination revealed that there were numerous oligodendrocytes within these patches, and most axons had become myelinated. Rostral and caudal to these areas of myelination, the histology was similar to that of non-transplanted *md* spinal cords and there were few or no myelinated axons within the dorsal columns.

Figure 9.1 shows recordings obtained along the course of dorsal column axons, both outside of the transplant zone and within the transplant region where they had become myelinated. These field potential recordings provide a measure of the pooled behaviour of dorsal column fibres. Conduction velocity is 0.9 ± 0.03 m/s (mean $\pm$ SEM) outside of the transplant region. Within the transplant region, two negativities are apparent in the field potentials, probably representing conduction in two populations of axons (those that have become myelinated and those that have not become myelinated). The increment in latency with increasing conduction distance is consistently smaller for the first negativity (N_1) than for the N_2 negativity; the change in latency, per increment of conduction distance, for the N_2 response is similar to that seen in the adjacent, non-transplanted dorsal column, and represents the conduction velocity in axons that have not been myelinated. By contrast, the latency per increment of conduction distance for the N_1 response,

Fig. 9.1. Increased conduction velocity in dorsal column axons of myelin-deficient (*md*) rat 16 days following transplantation of myelin-forming cells. Field potentials from transplant region (~3 mm in length) and non-transplant region are shown. (A) Two stimulation sites (S_1 and S_2) provide recording tracks within the transplant region and more rostrally outside the transplant region. The recording interval is 0.5 mm for both tracks. (B) Aggregate conduction latencies in non-transplant (upper graph) and transplant regions (lower graph) in the *md* dorsal columns. The upper graph shows the latency of the main N negativity (from 100 recording sites from 17 recording tracks) outside the transplant region. The slope of the linear regression indicates an average conduction velocity of 0.9 ± 0.03 m/s. The lower graph shows a significantly smaller increase in latency with increasing conduction distance within the transplant region, with an average conduction velocity of 3.2 ± 0.23 m/s. (C) Field potentials outside the transplant region usually show a single main negativity with occasional early or late components. (D) Field potentials from transplant region of the same animal show separate negativities (N_1 and N_2) with increasingly distinct latencies as the recording electrode is moved further away from the stimulus site. Conduction velocity for the N_1 component is increased. The stimulus site is outside the transplant region, indicating propagation of the impulse across the dysmyelinated–myelinated junction. (Modified from Utzschneider et al. 1994.)

representing conduction in axons that have acquired myelin following transplantation, is reduced. Our field potential analysis indicates, in fact, that conduction velocity of the most rapidly conducting fibres within the transplant region increased 3 to 4-fold to (3.2 ± 0.2 m/s), compared to the conduction velocity outside the transplant region (0.9 ± 0.03 m/s). Moreover, in experiments where the conduction track encompassed both myelinated and non-myelinated regions, conduction velocity increased by a factor of approximately 2-fold as the action potential propagated into the myelinated region.

Notably, field potentials could be observed to propagate either into, or out of, the transplant area in all six of the spinal cords in which this was studied. Thus impedence mismatch, which can block conduction at sites where the pattern of myelination changes abruptly (Waxman and Brill 1978), did not block conduction at this crucial interface following transplantation. Within the transplant region, dorsal column fibres displayed frequency-following properties that were virtually identical to those of fibres outside of the transplant region (Fig. 9.2). The ability of fibres within the transplant region to carry high-frequency inpulse trains, following stimulation at frequencies as high as 100 Hz, was similar inside and outside of the transplant region.

Intracellular recordings, obtained from dorsal root ganglion (DRG) neurons while the axons of these cells were antidromically stimulated within the dorsal columns, were used to assess the functional consequences of myelination by transplanted cells at the single-cell level (Fig. 9.3). Stimulating electrodes were placed at the dorsal root entry zone and within the dorsal columns at the rostral edge of the transplant region. Recordings from 67 axons which conducted through the transplant region demonstrated that mean conduction velocity was approximately 3-

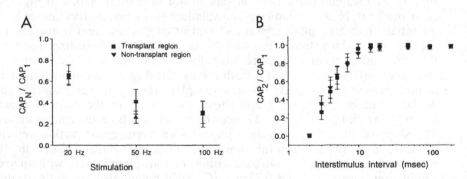

Fig. 9.2. (A) The ability of *md* axons to follow tetanic stimuli is similar inside and outside the transplant region. The graph shows the ratio of the amplitudes of the first (CAP_1) and last (CAP_N) compound action potentials (CAPs) for repetitive stimuli at 20 Hz (10 s), 50 Hz (10 s), and 100 Hz (2 s). (B) Double-shock experiments showing the ratio of test CAP (CAP_2) to control CAP (CAP_1) for interstimulus intervals of 2–200 ms. The time-course recovery for impulse conduction is similar inside and outside the transplant region.

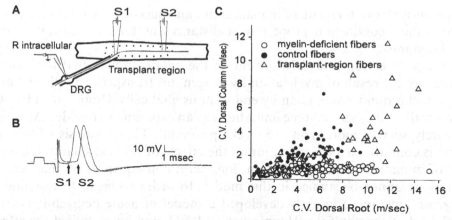

Fig. 9.3. (A) Single-cell recording of action potential conduction through the transplant region. The schematic shows the placement of two stimulating electrodes in the transplant zone and an intracellular recording electrode in a dorsal root ganglion cell. (B) Action potentials recorded from dorsal root ganglion cell following stimulation at two sites (S_1, S_2) in the transplant region. Propagation of the action potential from stimulating electrode S_2 to the dorsal root ganglion cell demonstrates that conduction occurred through the zone of potential impedance mismatch, from the transplant zone to non-transplanted parts of the host nervous system. From the latency shift and interstimulus distance, a conduction velocity of 2.6 m/s within the transplant zone can be calculated for this axon. (C) Aggregate data on conduction velocity for axons within *md* transplant regions, *md* non-transplant region, and control spinal cord.

fold faster for axons in the transplant region, than for non-transplanted *md* dorsal column axons. Conduction velocity in transplanted axons was comparable with that in age-matched controls in which myelination had occurred normally (transplanted rats, 2.3 ± 0.3 m/s; $n = 67$; *md* rats, 0.76 ± 0.02 m/s; $n = 258$; age-matched controls 1.9 ± 0.13 m/s; $n = 95$). Dorsal column conduction velocities are plotted in Fig. 9.3C as a function of dorsal root conduction velocity for axons from each of the three experimental groups. Axons in the transplant region display conduction velocities that are significantly greater than axons with comparable dorsal root conduction velocities from non-transplanted *md* rats. As seen in Fig. 9.3B, propagation of action potentials from the transplant region, into non-transplanted zones, was also demonstrated at the single axon level in these experiments, providing additional evidence that conduction proceeded securely through the region of potential impedance mismatch at the junction between myelinated and non-myelinated axon segments.

These observations in the *md* rat spinal cord provide a clear demonstration of enhanced axonal conduction in the spinal cord following myelination by transplanted glial cells. Enhancement of conduction was not confined to the immediate site of cell injection; notably, our results show that transplanted glial cells can migrate away from their site of implantation, and successfully myelinate axons to improve their conduction properties at distances as far as 5–10 mm along the dorsal columns.

The lack of endogenous CNS myelin in the *md* rat implies that the functional changes are the result of myelination by exogenous, transplanted cells and are not due to background myelination by endogenous glial cells. Despite its advantages, however, the *md* CNS has some limitations as an experimental model. Affected *md* rats rarely survive more than 3–5 weeks postnatal. Thus, analysis of this model system is confined to an examination of the effects of cell transplantation into the CNS of immature hosts. In addition, long-term consequences of glial cell transplantation cannot be studied in this model. In order to begin to examine these issues, we have more recently developed a model of acute demyelination in the spinal cord of the adult rat (Honmou et al. 1996), and have studied the effects of glial cell transplantation in this model.

9.3 Demyelination of Dorsal Columns in the Adult Rat

To determine whether it is possible to reconstruct demyelinated white matter within the adult central nervous system via transplantation of exogenous glial cells, we have transplanted suspensions of cultured Schwann cells, in some cases transfected with a *Lac Z* reporter gene, together with astrocytes derived from immature rats, into demyelinated dorsal columns of the spinal cord in adult rats (Honmou et al. 1996). In these studies, an acute demyelinating lesion, with minimal endogenous remyelination, was produced by X-irradiation and injection of ethidium bromide using a modification of the method of Blakemore and Patterson (1978). The ethidium bromide–X-radiation model provides a lesion which remains glial cell-free for more than 5–6 weeks in contrast to most other models, in which endogenous remyelination can commence within days of demyelination. In this model, X-irradiation (40 Grays surface dose) is delivered to the T-10 level of the spinal cord; at 3 days post-irradiation, demyelination is induced within the dorsal column via injection of ethidium bromide which chelates nucleic acids so as to induce oligodendrocyte death and demyelination. Histological and ultrastructural examination (Fig. 9.4A, B) confirmed that axons within the lesion were totally demyelinated and the lesion site was essentially free of glial cells (Honmou et al. 1996). Demyelinated lesions encompassed 70–80% of the transverse extent of the dorsal columns and, using this demyelination protocol, measured 7–8 mm along the rostro–caudal axis of the spinal cord. At intervals ranging from 1 to 6 weeks following induction of the lesion, there was no evidence of axonal ensheathment or remyelination by endogenous oligodendrocytes or Schwann cells.

For these studies, Schwann cells cultured from neonatal (P1–P3) (P = postpartum) rat sciatic nerve were prepared for transplantation by the method of Brockes, Fields and Raff (1979). Primary astrocyte cultures from neo-

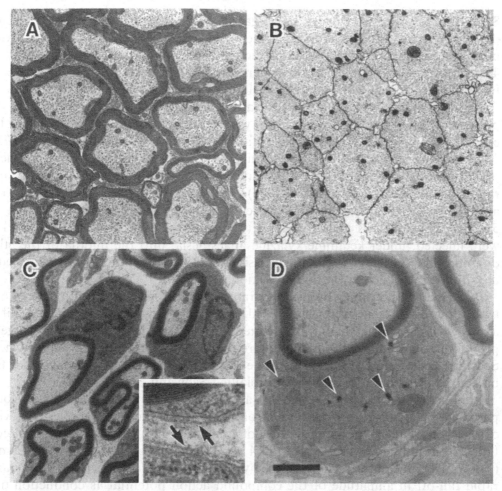

Fig. 9.4. Electron micrographs showing normal (A) and demyelinated (B) axons in the dorsal columns. All demyelinated spinal cords that received cell injections showed clear evidence of remyelination (C) of the demyelinated axons. Examination at higher magnification (inset in C) showed the presence of a basal lamina (arrows) as well as extracellular collagen fibrils surrounding the individual fibres. (D) Schwann cells carrying the β-gal gene (reaction product indicated by arrow heads) could be detected in the lesion by treating the tissue with the substrate X-Gal. Scale bar, 4 μm for (A), (B) and (C); 2 μm for (D); 0.6 μm for inset in C. (Modified from Honmou et al 1996.)

natal rat optic nerve were established using the method of McCarthy and de Vellis (1980). Histological identification of transplanted Schwann cells was accomplished using a replication-defective BAG retroviral vector (Price, Turner and Cepko 1987) containing the j2 packaging line (Mann, Mulligan and Baltimore 1983) for transfection of the bacterial β-gal gene, which we used as a reporter, into

Schwann cell primary cultures. The β-gal gene was cloned into the pDOL vector derived from the Maloney murine leukaemia virus (Mo-Mu LV), which provides a promoter for the β-gal gene, for construction of the BAG vector. The simian virus 40 early promoter and the Tn5 neomycin-resistant gene were inserted downstream from the β-gal gene to facilitate selection of transfected colonies. Supernatants from packaging cells were utilised for transfection of Schwann cells cultured in the presence of polybrene (8 μg/ml), which were rapidly proliferating under the influence of forskolin and glial growth factor (Brockes, Fields and Raff 1979). Contamination by fibroblasts was eliminated prior to transfection by treatment of cultures with cytosine arabinoside and cell lysis with anti-Thy 1.1 antibody and rabbit complement (Porter et al. 1986). Following incubation in the neomycin analog G-418, transfected Schwann cells were selected, and suspensions of 5×10^4 Schwann cells and astrocytes (in a ratio of approximately 3:2) in 1 μl were injected, under ketamine/xylazine anaesthesia, into the middle of the ethidium bromide–X-irradiation induced lesion. Cell transplantation was performed 3 days following ethidium bromide injection.

By 3 weeks following Schwann cell transplantation, essentially all of the axons within the lesion zone were myelinated, with the exception of the finest calibre axons which are normally non-myelinated (Fig. 9.4C). The presence of β-gal gene product in Schwann cells surrounding remyelinated axons, in experiments where Schwann cells were transfected with the *Lac Z* reporter gene, confirmed that the new myelin had been formed by transplanted Schwann cells (Fig. 9.4D).

Conduction in the demyelinated dorsal columns was severely impaired, as compared with controls (Fig. 9.5). In control rats in which there were no lesions, with conduction of the compound action potential for 5 mm through the dorsal columns, its amplitude was reduced to $13.4 \pm 4.4\%$ ($n = 5$) of the amplitude at 2 mm (Fig. 9.5B1). In contrast, within the demyelinated dorsal columns there was a more rapid fall-off in amplitude of the compound action potential as conduction distance increased (Fig. 9.5B2), and at a conduction distance of 5 mm, the amplitude of the compound action potential had decreased so precipitously that a response could not be detected, demonstrating conduction block in the demyelinated axons. These changes were reversed as a result of cell transplantation. Following myelination by transplanted cells, a relatively normal pattern of conduction was restored and there was a smaller amplitude decrement with distance, which was indistinguishable from controls (Fig. 9.5B3), demonstrating that propagation of action potentials had penetrated substantially farther within the lesion without block. Conduction velocities were also restored to near-normal following transplantation. Conduction velocity was decreased substantially compared to its control values (10.2 ± 0.9 m/s) in the demyelinated dorsal column (0.90 ± 0.1 m/s) at 36°C. Essentially normal conduction of velocities were restored (11.4 ± 0.7 m/s) in lesions that had been remyelinated by transplanted Schwann cells.

To study conduction in single axons that traverse the lesion site, we used intra-axonal recording methods with arrays of stimulating electrodes that were posi-

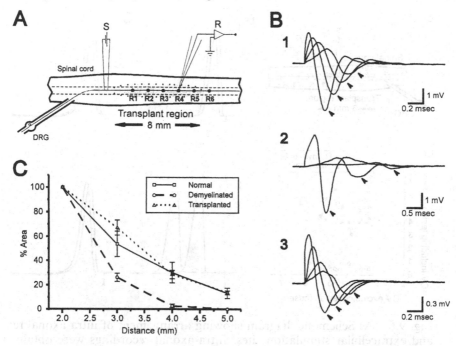

Fig. 9.5. (A) Schematic diagram showing the dorsal surface of spinal cord with the positions of the stimulating (S) and recording (R) electrodes. Shaded region indicates the area of demyelination or remyelination. (B) Compound action potentials recorded at 1 mm increments along the dorsal columns in control (1), ethidium bromide–X-irradiation demyelinated (2) and transplant-induced remyelinated (3) axons. (C) Compound action potential area (% Area) plotted versus conduction distance for normal, demyelinated, and transplant-induced remyelinated dorsal columns (*n* = 5). (Modified from Honmou et al. 1996.)

tioned on the dorsal surface of the spinal cord within the lesion and on the demyelinated dorsal column at distances up to several millimetres rostral and caudal to the lesion. Axons were impaled at a site between the two arrays of stimulating electrodes within the non-demyelinated region, so that conduction along axon segments running through, and excluding, the lesion could be studied (Fig. 9.6A). In demyelinated spinal cords that had not received a transplant, conduction velocity was abruptly decreased within the region of demyelination (Fig. 9.6B). In axons that had been myelinated following transplantation of Schwann cells, conduction velocities were essentially restored to normal so that they were the same within the lesion (where axons had been remyelinated by transplanted Schwann cells) and outside of the lesion (where demyelination had not occurred) (Fig. 9.6C, D). Action potentials, evoked by stimulation within the transplant region, propagated into the non-demyelinated portion of the spinal cord (Fig. 9.6A, C), demonstrating that conduction had successfully traversed the zone of potential

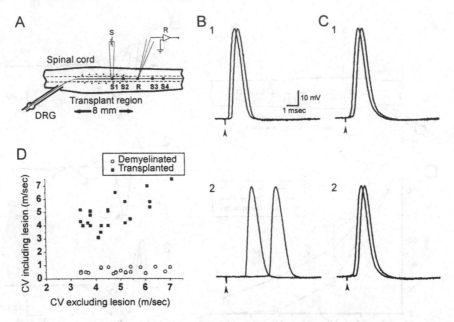

Fig. 9.6. (A) Schematic diagram showing arrangement of intra-axonal recording and extracellular stimulation sites. Intra-axonal recordings were obtained from dorsal column axons outside of the lesion, where the axons were normally mye-linated (R). Stimulating electrodes were positioned within and outside (S1–S4) of the lesion zone to assess conduction velocity over both the demyelinated or remyelinated parts of the axons, and from a normally myelinated segment of the same axon. (B) Pairs of action potentials recorded at comparable conduction distances from a spinal cord that did not receive a transplant for a conduction path that either included the demyelinated lesion (2) or excluded (1) the lesion. Note the increased conduction latency due to slowed conduction through the demyelinated region. (C) Similar stimulation-recording protocol as (B) but for transplant-induced remyelinated axons. The conduction latencies through the remyelinated part of the axon trajectory are similar to those of the axon segment outside of the lesion zone. (D) Plot of conduction velocities of axon segments within the lesion versus conduction velocities of the axon segment outside of the lesion, for demyelinated and transplant-induced remyelinated groups. Note the increase in conduction velocity in axons remyelinated by transplanted cells. (Modified from Honmou et al. 1996.)

impendence mismatch at the junction between remyelinated and normal parts of the host nervous system.

Refractory period was prolonged, and ability to conduct action potential impulse trains of high frequency were impaired as a result of demyelination, but both of these abnormalities were reversed by remyelination. To study refractory periods for transmission, we used paired pulse stimulation protocols. In axons remyelinated following transplantation, the relative refractory period was reduced so that it approached, or was even less than, control values. As shown in

Fig. 9.7A, the onset of recovery occurred sooner, and the slope of recovery was greater in axons following remyelination. The ability of dorsal column axons to carry high-frequency trains was impaired following demyelination, and the amplitude of the field potential of the demyelinated axons was reduced compared to controls at frequencies of 50 Hz and higher. Following transplantation of Schwann cells, this abnormality was reversed and remyelinated axons were able to follow high frequency stimulation as well as controls, with amplitude decrements at high stimulus frequencies that were smaller than in control dorsal columns (Fig. 9.7B).

9.4 Implications for Functional Repair of the CNS

These studies show that, as a result of myelination by transplanted glial cells in both the immature and adult rat spinal cord, there are significant changes in the conduction properties of spinal cord axons. Conduction velocity, refractory

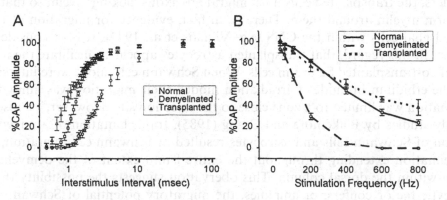

Fig. 9.7. (A) Paired pulse stimuli using varying interstimulus intervals were applied to study the refractory period for transmission in normal, demyelinated, and transplant-induced remyelinated axons. Compound action potentials resulting from the second of two paired stimuli were plotted at increasing interstimulus intervals for normal, demyelinated, and transplanted spinal cord axons. Amplitude recovery was reduced in the demyelinated axons as compared to normal axons, but transplant-induced remyelinated axons exhibited faster recovery properties than control axons. (B) To study high frequency following capability, the compound action potential amplitudes of the last response of a train (0.5 s, 36°C) over the first response was plotted at various frequencies for normal, demyelinated and transplant-induced remyelinated axons. The demyelinated axons showed reduced frequency–response properties. Transplantation-induced remyelinated axons showed recovery in their frequency–response properties as compared to those of the demyelinated axons; at higher frequencies, the remyelinated axons showed less amplitude decrement than controls. (Modified from Honmou et al. 1996.)

period, and ability to conduct at high frequencies are restored to values close to those seen with normal myelination.

The possibility of grafting myelin-forming glial cells, or their precursors, into the CNS as a therapeutic strategy for dysmyelinating and demyelinating disorders has been under active investigation by a number of laboratories, but only a small number of studies have examined the effects of introduction of exogenous cells on conduction in CNS axons. Myelination within the CNS can be mediated by both cultured oligodendrocytes and Schwann cells (Blakemore and Crang 1985; Duncan et al. 1988; Groves et al. 1993). Schwann cells provide a potential advantage because they can be derived from peripheral tissues and, in principle, could be derived from the host by biopsy of a nerve such as the sural, thus permitting transplantation of autologous cells and obviating the necessity for immunosuppression. Moreoever, since the immune attack in inflammatory disorders such as multiple sclerosis is directed against CNS but not peripheral nervous system (PNS) myelin (Waxman 1993), Schwann cell remyelination might have the additional advantage of being resistant to further immunological damage.

In order for transplantation strategies to be successful in dys- and demyelinating disorders, the transplanted cells must migrate to axons lacking myelin so that they can form myelin around them. There is, in fact, evidence for migration of transplanted glial cells within the CNS (e.g. Vignais et al. 1993). It is of considerable interest, in this regard, that transplanted astrocytes appear to facilitate the migration of co-transplanted Schwann cells. When Schwann cells alone were introduced into the ethidium bromide–X irradiation model, their migration was limited and myelination was limited to a zone close to the injection site. However, as observed in early studies by Blakemore and Crang (1985), transplantation of a mixed suspension of Schwann cells and astrocytes resulted in Schwann cell migration, with remyelination extending throughout the entire 8 mm extent of the demyelinated region within the dorsal column. This obervation suggests the possibility that an astrocytic factor confers, or amplifies, the migratory potential of Schwann cells. Characterisation of astrocyte factors that influence Schwann cell migration might ultimately contribute to the development of transplantation procedures that optimise the migratory potential of Schwann cells, thus facilitating their role in remyelination following transplantation.

Numerous resident astocytes are present although there is no endogenous myelin within the CNS of the *md* rat. In the *md* spinal cord, introduction of Schwann cells and combinations of Schwann cells and astrocytes results in myelination of the *md* axons, but Schwann cell migration is less robust than in the astrocyte-free environment that exists in the ethidium bromide–X-irradiation lesion (Duncan et al. 1988). One explanation for these results is that resident astrocytes may impede Schwann cell migration. Consistent with this hypothesis, the layer of resident astrocytes at the glial limitans, which delineates the junction between the spinal cord and CNS, constitutes a barrier to Schwann cell migration (Sims et al. 1985a).

The enhanced conduction that we observed in transplanted spinal cords suggests that, as a result of axon–glial interactions, there is reorganisation of dorsal
column axons. In normal myelinated fibres, the axon membrane is spatially non-
uniform and contains a heterogeneous distribution of Na^+ channels which are
aggregated at nodes of Ranvier at a density of about $1000/\mu m^2$, with a much lower
density (less than $25/\mu m^2$) in the internodal part of the axon membrane under the
myelin (Waxman 1977; Ritchie and Rogart 1977; Shrager 1989). During normal
PNS development, aggregation of Na^+ channels is dependent on axonal interactions with glial cells prior to myelination (Waxman and Foster 1980; Wiley-
Livingston and Ellisman 1980). Although prior morphological studies demonstrated the formation of compact myelin following transplantation of myelin-
forming precursor cells into the ethidium bromide–X-irradiation lesion within
the adult spinal cord, it could not be predicted, a priori, whether axon–glial cell
interactions in the pathological environment of the lesion would permit the formation of the high nodal Na^+ channel densities required for secure conduction
along newly myelinated fibres. In addition, morphological studies have demonstrated that internode distances, myelin sheath thickness, and axon diameter in the
spinal cord are altered following endogenous remyelination compared to normal
(Harrison and McDonald 1977). Since these changes can interfere with conduction
(Waxman and Brill 1978), it was not possible to predict whether myelination by
exogenous cells would reverse conduction abnormalities in previously demyelinated axons. In our experiments, conduction proceeded for much longer distances
in the transplant zones as compared to non-transplanted demyelinated regions,
indicating that conduction block had been reversed; these results are consistent
with the ideas that (i) clustering of Na^+ channels at nodes of Ranvier had occurred
in axons remyelinated by transplanted cells; and (ii) impedence mismatch did not
block conduction along axons myelinated by transplanted glial cells.

The studies reviewed here demonstrate that conduction velocities, in spinal cord
axons that were myelinated by transplanted glial cells, return to levels close to
those in controls. Remyelinated CNS axons often display reduced internodal
spacing (Harrison and McDonald 1977). These observations can be reconciled if
it is recalled that there is a hyperbolic function, with a broad maximum, that
relates internode distance and axonal conduction velocity (Huxley and Stämpfli
1949); reductions of 3-fold or less in internode distance have been predicted to
result in conduction velocities that are close to normal along remyelinated axons
(Brill et al. 1977).

In our studies on the ethidium bromide X-irradiation model, we observed that
Schwann cell remyelination is associated with a relative refractory period shorter
than in controls, and with enhanced frequency-following capability. Whether these
alterations might foster clinical recovery or, on the other hand, interfere with
normal axonal coding so as to interfere with normal function, is not known.
The reduced refractory period and enhanced high-frequency conduction capability
of transplanted axons may reflect differences in organisation of the nodes along

Schwann cell-remyelinated, as compared to oligodendrocyte-remyelinated axons (Peters 1966); (Berthold and Rydmark 1995), or could be due to altered ionic regulation at nodes of Ranvier along Schwann cell-remyelinated axons within the spinal cord following cell transplantation, since it is clear that extracellular ion concentrations, which are regulated by glial cells, can effect axonal conduction within the CNS (Kocsis, Malenka and Waxman 1983).

Important questions, including the nature of the cell types that are optimal for transplantation, the long-term effects of glial cell transplantation, and the functional consequences of shorter-than-normal refractory period and higher-than-normal frequency-following capabilities, remain to be explored. Nevertheless, the results described above indicate that repair of demyelinated white matter, via transplantation of exogenous myelin-forming cells, can restore relatively secure impulse conduction with near-normal conduction velocity within the host CNS. Moreover, this functional restitution of demyelinated spinal cord white matter can be accomplished by Schwann cells which, under appropriate circumstances, can migrate for millimetres within the lesion so as to myelinate extensive lengths of the demyelinated axons. Although much work remains to be done, these results suggest that it may become possible to induce functional recovery, in some dysmyelinating and demyelinating disorders, via strategies that include cell transplantation in the CNS.

Acknowledgements

Research in the authors' laboratories has been supported in part by the Medical Research Service, Veterans Administration, and by grants from the National Institutes of Health, National Multiple Sclerosis Society, The Myelin Project and the Nancy Davis Foundation for Multiple Sclerosis.

10

Contributions of Potassium Currents and Glia to Slow Potential Shifts (SPSs)

UWE HEINEMANN and WOLFGANG WALZ

Summary

This paper reviews evidence that glial cells contribute to the generation of slow shifts in local field potential recordings and in the electroencephalogram (EEG). Glial cells are often spatially extended and electrically coupled. They sense rises in $[K^+]_e$. Changes in $[K^+]_e$ are associated with most conditions where slow potential shifts are recorded. Local accumulation of K^+ leads to depolarisation of glial cells, which spreads along the glial syncytium. As a result, the local depolarisation in glial membrane potential is smaller than expected from the change in $[K^+]_e$ and a driving force for K^+ uptake develops while at remote sites K^+ is released from glia. The potassium inward currents into glia are associated with generation of slow negative field potentials, while at remote sites the K^+ outflux leads to generation of positive field potentials. Evidence for this hypothesis from different parts of the central nervous system is reviewed in this chapter.

10.1 Introduction

Many physiological and pathophysiological conditions are associated with the generation of slow field potential and EEG changes. These include slow shifts in the steady potential during sleep (Caspers, Speckmann and Lehmenkühler 1980), the generation of slow negative shifts during the preparation of a voluntary movement (Kornhuber and Deecke 1964), the period between a conditioning and imperative stimulus (Walter et al. 1964), during spindling activity in the EEG, stimulation of peripheral nerve fibres or receptors (Heinemann, Lux and Gutnick 1977) and of afferent or efferent pathways in the brain (Lux and Neher 1973), seizure activity (Ayala et al 1973) and different patterns of abnormal activity such as spreading depressions, hypoxia, ischaemia and hypoglycaemia (Caspers and Speckmann 1969; Somjen 1975; Nicholson et al. 1977; Lehmenkühler et al. 1988). In addition, many pharmacological manipulations such as application of excitatory amino acids will cause local negative field potential shifts (Heinemann and Pumain 1979).

Except for slow potentials in sleep and in preparation of a task where technically difficult measurements of ionic changes with the very high ohmic and movement-sensitive ion-selective microelectrodes in freely moving animals would be required, all these conditions have been shown to be associated with rises in extracellular potassium concentration ($[K^+]_e$). Conversely manipulations which lead to reductions of extracellular potassium concentration can be associated with positive field potential shifts (Heinemann and Lux 1975). Thus, it was shown that antidromic activation of the pyramidal tract causes profound inhibition in deep cortical layers with an associated decrease in $[K^+]_e$ and generation of a positive field potential. Likewise, following rises in $[K^+]_e$ induced by repetitive stimulation, seizures, spreading depression and transient hypoxia, the $[K^+]_e$ undershoots baseline and this undershoot is associated with a positive shift of the steady potential. Since glial cells are very sensitive to changes in $[K^+]_e$, this has led to the hypothesis that glial cells could contribute to generation of such slow potentials. This hypothesis was supported by findings where local iontophoretic application of potassium induced slow potential shifts both in intact preparations but also in a gliotic scar devoid of neurons (Heinemann and Dietzel 1984).

However, persistent depolarisations are also observed during most of these manipulations in neurons (Caspers and Speckmann 1969; Speckmann et al. 1972; Lehmenkühler et al. 1988, 1993a). Moreover, focal application of glutamate and its various agonists can also induce slow potential shifts associated with strong neuronal and glial membrane depolarisations as well as rises in $[K^+]_e$ (Lambert and Heinemann 1986). The generation of slow potentials by glutamate is not observed when glutamate is injected into gliotic tissue devoid of neurons (Alici et al. 1996). Therefore it is likely that neurons also contribute to the generation of slow potentials and some authors have taken the position that the generation of slow potentials in the EEG is purely a function of steady neuronal depolarisation. Three questions have therefore to be addressed:

- Can glial cells contribute to generation of slow potentials?
- Do glial cells contribute to generation of slow potentials?
- To what extent do glial cells contribute to generation of slow potentials?

This review will address these questions by discussing relevant studies in the mammalian central nervous system.

10.2 Glial Properties in Situ Compatible with a Contribution to Generation of Slow Potential Shifts

In order for glial cells to supply the current for the slow potential shifts, the following four criteria must be met:

- When neuronal elements are active, neighbouring glial cells must always be depolarised.

- A large enough population of glial cells has to undergo that depolarisation at the same time.
- There has to be electrotonic continuity of spatially extended glial cells and/or the glial syncytium from the active to the inactive region.
- The length constant of the glial syncytium has to be compatible with the spread of current.

In this context, it is important to investigate these criteria in astrocytes in vivo or in situ (brain slices or isolated preparations) where these cells are part of a functional module consisting of neurons and astrocytes with their natural connections, extensions and specialisations intact. Cultured or transformed astrocytes in isolation are not a good model in this context. Therefore, in this review only astrocytic properties from in vivo or in situ preparations are considered.

10.2.1 Membrane Potential Responses of Astrocytes

In general, astrocytes have about a 20 mV more negative membrane resting potential than neighbouring neurons (Somjen 1995). This is mainly due to the relatively reduced Na^+ permeability of astrocytes compared to neurons. This is also the reason why astrocytes are more sensitive to increases in extracellular K^+ than neurons. They react with larger depolarisation amplitudes to these extracellular K^+ increases. However, at least two in situ studies find that the membrane potential of astrocytes is not an exclusive potassium equilibrium potential. Ballanyi et al. (1987) found evidence for a non-negligible Cl^- conductance in glial cells of the olfactory cortex. The same was found for astrocytes from hippocampal slices with induced gliosis (Walz, Paterson and Wuttke 1996). The Cl^- equilibrium potential of astrocytes in these two preparations is close to the membrane resting potential, thus assuming high resting potentials. Still, the K^+ equilibrium potential is the most negative ion equilibrium potential of these astrocytes. Since many of the voltage-sensitive ion channels found in cultured astrocytes seem to exist in a subset of adult astrocytes in situ (Kressin et al. 1995; Jabs, Paterson and Walz 1996), this situation means that once their threshold is reached their activation should contribute to depolarisations of the astrocytic membrane. It is not clear what role these voltage-sensitive channels play during normal activity in the adult brain. If they are activated during neuronal activity their effect on the astrocytic membrane potential would be a depolarisation rather than a hyperpolarisation. A membrane mechanism that could lead to a hyperpolarisation is the electrogenic Na^+/K^+ pump. If this pump is stimulated by extracellular K^+, the electrogenic current created by its operation would result in a hyperpolarisation, as it does in cultured rat but not mouse astrocytes (Walz and Kimelberg 1985). However, the electrogenic current will contribute only if the specific membrane resistance is high enough to cause a voltage drop. One would assume that the relatively low specific membrane resistance of astrocytes would render such a hyperpolarisation non-significant. Transient polarisation of astrocytes in brain slices perfused with 10 mM K^+-containing salt solution for a short period did not lead to any transient hyperpolarisation (Walz, Paterson and Wuttke 1996). If, however, in slices from guinea-pig olfactory cortex the lateral olfactory tract was stimulated, glial cells underwent a depolarisation from -80 to -60 mV and at the end of the longer-lasting stimulation periods (>30 s) when the membrane slowly repolarised, there was an after-hyperpolarisation of approximately 5 mV. This after-hyperpolarisation was ouabain-sensitive, indicating that it was created by the electrogenic current of the Na^+/K^+ pump. Alternatively, it could reflect the undershoot which follows stimulus-induced elevations in $[K^+]_e$ and which is generated by the activity of the Na^+/K^+ pump in neurons activated by sodium load. These hyperpolarisations were only apparent to strong, longer lasting stimuli and it is questionable if they could be observed during normal physiological activity. The same was noted during repetitive stimulation of cat cortex. In any event, the presence of after-hyperpolarisations did not prevent the large amplitude depolarisations (>20 mV) created by the extracellular accumulation of K^+ released from active neurons.

Substances other than K^+ released from active neurons, could also contribute to glial membrane potential changes. In situ, all of these substances, kainate (glutamate), GABA and dopamine cause a depolarisation in the glial cells (Walz and MacVicar 1988; MacVicar et al. 1989; Mudrick-Donnan et al. 1993; Jabs, Paterson and Walz 1996). The depolarisation response is mediated by three contributing factors: changes in the extracellular microenvironment, modulation of ion channel conductances and electrogenic uptake. In some cases, transmitter induced glial depolarisations were clearly dependent on simultanous increases in $[K^+]_e$. An example are the Müller cells in the retina which in situ show a clear depolarisation when exposed to kainate, but no such depolarisation when studied after acute isolation (Pannicke and Reichelt, in preparation). GABA can also induce rises in $[K^+]_e$ but the GABA-dependent depolarisation may have a component mediated by Cl^- influx into neurons, as is the case in spinal cord where glycine receptors have been identified in astroglia. As pointed out above, the membrane resting potential of glial cells is very close to the K^+ equilibrium potential, the most negative ion equilibrium potential. Thus even signals like glycine or GABA that increase a Cl^- conductance in astrocytes will lead to a depolarisation. The best studied uptake systems in astrocytes are those for amino acids, and all of these cause depolarisations (Sarantis and Attwell 1990; Schwartz and Tachibana 1990; Biedermann, Eberhardt and Reichelt 1994; Pannicke et al. 1994). The contribution of such an electrogenic uptake under physiological conditions should be much less than the K^+-induced depolarisation. Other modulating factors exist; the most prominent is probably the activity-induced acidification of the ECS. This acidification, however, will again result in depolarisation of the membrane (Walz and Wuttke 1989 and Chapter 11).

10.2.2 Extracellular Potassium During Neuronal Activity and Glial Membrane Depolarisation

Astrocytes in situ sense increases in the extracellular K^+ concentration (Somjen 1995). The relationship is in most conditions somewhat sub-Nernstian in mammalian tissue. This can be explained by the simultaneous K^+ uptake leading to an increased intracellular K^+ concentration rather than a stationary one and by the modulatory effects described above. Orthodromic stimulation in a variety of preparations leads to a depolarisation of glial cells that persists longer than the stimulation or the activity of neurons, including synaptic potentials (Somjen 1995). Lothman and Somjen (1975) studied the relationship of stimulation-induced K^+ increases and glial membrane potentials in the spinal cord of the cat. They found K^+ increases up to 8 mM with corresponding glial depolarisations of 25 mV. An amplitude of 25–30 mV seems to be the maximal depolarisation achievable by neuronal pathways in vivo and in brain slices (Ballanyi, Grafe and Ten Bruggencate 1987). If more physiological stimuli are used, like light flashes, glial cell depolarisation is much smaller (8 mV) as are the simultaneous rises in $[K^+]_e$, but there is never any hyperpolarisation phase (Kelly and Van Essen 1974; Karwoski and Proenza 1977). During seizure-like events, the glial depolarisations are up to 35 mV, which corresponds to the 10–12 mM ceiling level (Heinemann and Lux 1977). This ceiling level is only increased during spreading depression waves and hypoxia or ischaemia. Under these conditions glia can depolarise very strongly to levels a few mV below zero potential.

In some conditions super-Nernstian depolarisations in glial cells have also been described (i.e. beyond that predicted by the Nernst equation for the distribution of K^+). One such condition is the penicillin focus in cat neocortex. Local application of penicillin induces rises in $[K^+]_e$ which are maximal in layer IV/V. These local field potentials are associated with large rises in $[K^+]_e$ and glial cells become depolarised with a sub-Nernstian slope (Futamachi and Pedley 1976). In more superficial layers, rises in $[K^+]_e$ are much smaller while glial cells are still almost maximally depolarised. When plotting the relationship between glial cell membrane potential and rises in $[K^+]_e$ in such layers, it was found that glial cells depolarised more than expected from local $[K^+]_e$ accumulation.

Studies using membrane potential-sensitive dyes in glial cells are lacking; thus, it is not possible to estimate the extent of the direct depolarisation of glial cells by extracellular K^+. Presumably, the extent of this direct depolarisation is limited to the region of the ECS that contains raised K^+ levels. There is, however, a spread of the depolarisation to areas not experiencing raised external K^+ by currents through gap junctions (see below).

10.2.3 Electrical Coupling of Glial Cells

As shown in Fig. 10.1, if glial cells constitute a syncytium that is electrotonically coupled, and one part of this syncytium is depolarised by a positive shift of the K$^+$ equilibrium potential, these currents *could* spread to other parts of the syncytium and depolarise those parts that do not experience any neuronal activity and in turn lead to a negative extracellular potential with the same time course. Two conditions are absolutely necessary for this to happen:

(i) astrocytes have to be coupled by gap junctions or they must be spatially oriented through different layers and

(ii) the length constant in the resulting syncytium has to be compatible with the expected spread of the depolarisation.

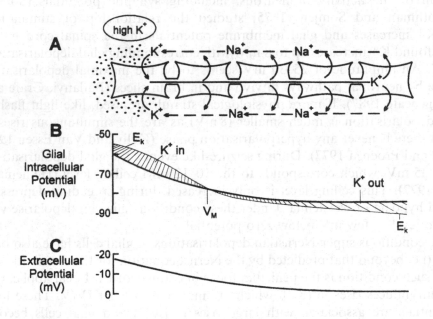

Fig. 10.1. Schematic illustration of the spatial buffer concept. (A) A glial syncytium is shown with the left-hand cell exposed to high extracellular K$^+$. The K$^+$ currents into this cell are shown, as well as the intracellular spread of the K$^+$ currents across gap junctions into areas of the syncytium which are not exposed to elevated K$^+$. Depending on the length constant, K$^+$ currents are leaving the cell. The extracellular return current is mainly carried by Na$^+$ and by Cl$^-$ (not shown for simplicity). (B) Spread of depolarisation along the syncytium in (A). Shown is the membrane potential and potassium equilibrium potential. At the site of high K$^+$, the equilibrium potential is more positive than the membrane potential, causing a K$^+$ driving force inward. At the more distant parts, the equilibrium potential is more negative causing an outward driving force for K$^+$. (C) Estimated contribution of such an intracellular glial potential spread to the extracellularly measured potential.

There can be no doubt that astrocytes in situ are dye-coupled. Virtually all astrocytes, when injected with a dye small enough to pass gap junctions, will lose some of the dye to neighbouring astrocytes. Most mammalian astrocytes show widespread dye-coupling with each other (Ransom 1995); the dye can appear in as many as 100 other cells when injected into one astrocyte. The spread of the dye seems to be spherically outward from the injected cell. There seems to be every reason to assume that astrocytes that are dye coupled are also coupled electrically, as is evident from cell culture studies. In cell culture, adjacent astrocytes are strongly coupled to one another with an average junctional conductance of 13 mS, which represents approximately 235 gap junctions (Dermietzel et al. 1991). Enkvist and McCarthy (1994) reported an increase in dye-coupling of astrocytes by glutamate and high K^+. This can possibly be mediated by intracellular alkalinisation, which is caused in astrocytes by high K^+ and which increases gap junctional conductance. In summary, the coupling of astrocytes seems to be sufficient to allow the required spread of current to non-depolarised regions of the syncytium.

In addition, it must be noted that astrocytes can also be spatially oriented. Such an example is the area CA1 in the hippocampus, where astrocytes in the stratum radiatum orient their processes parallel to the main axis of pyramidal cell dendrites. Their processes reach from the stratum pyramidale towards the stratum moleculare (Nixdorf-Bergweiler, Albrecht and Heinemann 1994). Similar long-ranging glial cells are Müller cells in the retina and Bergmann glia in the cerebellum.

10.2.4 The Length Constant of the Syncytium

The length constant is the distance along a process to the site where a voltage amplitude has decayed to 37% of its value due to leakage of current across the cell membrane. It is obvious that a low specific membrane resistance will decrease the length constant and therefore the length a significant amount of a current can travel in the processes of the glial syncytium. Since astrocytes have a relatively low membrane resistance, this issue of a restricted length constant is seen as the largest problem in dealing with a glial contribution to slow extracellular potentials (Somjen 1973). This problem is compounded by the inaccessibility of the glial syncytium in situ to measurements of the length constant and by the fact that the ionic channels of astrocytes in situ seem to be unequally distributed. Barres et al. (1990b) measured the length constant of an acutely isolated astrocyte of the rat optic nerve for a single process as 100 μm. The overall length of the processes is 400 μm, meaning that no significant portion of a current can cross into neighbouring glial cells. However, the length of the glial cell would be sufficient to redistribute K^+ from a site of maximal K^+ accumulation to a remote less active area.

Indirect measurements based on K^+ transport induced by an electric field esti- mated a length constant of around $200\,\mu m$ for the rat cerebral cortex (Gardner- Medwin 1983a). This study was based on observations that a steady current through a brain structure leads to changes in $[K^+]_e$ larger than expected from transport number (the portion of current transported by a given ion species in a given electrolyte which is dependent on relative concentration and mobility). Based on the assumption that glial cell membranes are only permeable for K^+ ions the average length constant was estimated. However, meanwhile, it was found that glial cells express a significant number of Cl^- channels and therefore the length constant of the glial syncytium was underestimated in the approach of Gardner-Medwin. Moreover, the length constant of a glial syncytium may also vary between species and may be longer in the more phylogenetically advanced mammals.

In Müller cells of the retina and astrocytes of the cerebral cortex, it has been shown that 90% of the ionic conductances are located at the end feet, and this might have led to the estimation of a smaller value of the length constant in acutely isolated astrocytes, since the length constant was measured along a pro- cess. Nevertheless, the available estimates of the glial length constant suggest that the depolarisation induced in the glial network at regions that experience elevated extracellular K^+ concentrations does not spread out over more than some $100\,\mu m$. The problem of length constants is far from being solved, since we do not have adequate information about the specific membrane resistances in mammalian glial cells in situ and its distribution along the geometry of these cells.

10.3 The Concept of a Spatial Buffering Function

The concept of the spatial buffer function and the contribution of its associated currents is illustrated in Fig. 10.1. It assumes a glial syncytium in which extra- cellular K^+ is increased at one region (in the left of Fig. 10.1). In a syncytium, the membrane of neighbouring cells has a tendency to stay iso-potential. Therefore the region experiencing an increased extracellular K^+ current will have a more positive K^+ equilibrium potential than the membrane potential. This leads to an inward driving force for K^+ and since the membrane is highly permeable to K^+, it will enter the cell via a passive current. This current loop has to be closed, of course, and the K^+ current will be distributed to the other parts of the syncytium via the gap junctions. In regions further removed from the high K^+ region, the K^+ equi- librium potential is more negative than the membrane potential and therefore there is a driving force for K^+ out of the cell. Thus the current into the cells (at high K^+ regions), inside the syncytium and out of the cells (at regions distant from high K^+ locations), is almost completely carried by K^+. The loop is closed by a return current in the extracellular space. This current is carried mainly by Na^+ and Cl^- (the bulk of the extracellular ions). Despite the closed current loop, K^+ does not circle but is passively transported from an extracellular location with high K^+ and dispersed to extracellular areas with low K^+. This original concept allowed for flexibility, since any part of the syncytium could be functionally exchangeable depending solely on the location of the raised extracellular K^+. Figure 10.1C shows the resulting extracellular potential changes along such a syncytium.

Since elevations in $[K^+]_e$ are never restricted to just one layer in a cortical structure, the problem of the restricted length constant of a glial cell syncytium is less severe than earlier discussed. For example, it is quite possible that a small cluster of glial cells may be depolarised at the point of maximal potassium accumulation and this depolarisation is spread over a given distance. Potassium released from active neurons will thus be redistributed in the less active surround. There, a new cluster of spatially extended glial and/or coupled glial cells could redistribute the potassium further into the surround. The different local currents gradients will then add and contribute to generation of slow potentials over the whole structure.

10.3.1 Spatial Buffer Function: Evidence from Mammalian Systems

Nicholson and Phillips (1981) studied ion diffusion in rat cerebellum using ion-selective micropipettes and iontophoretic point sources. They found that for a variety of cations and anions the laws of macroscopic diffusion were closely obeyed, assuming that the extracellular space occupies about 20% of the rat cerebellum. However, there is one ion that does not fit into this scheme. The movement of potassium in an electrical gradient behaves as if the extracellular space has a volume of more than 100% (Nicholson, Phillips and Gardner-Medwin 1979; Gardner-Medwin 1983a; Nicholson and Phillips 1981). The anomalous nature of K^+ migration can be solved by assuming that the ion does not remain in the extracellular space, but is in fact the major current carrier across cell membranes. Hounsgaard and Nicholson (1983) analysed this possibility in more detail. They measured changes in extracellular K^+ concentration in the vicinity of Purkinje cells in guinea-pig cerebellar slices. No extracellular K^+ changes were seen when the cells were hyperpolarised with current passage or during subthreshold depolarisations. Only during spike activity was there a rise in extracellular K^+. In the vicinity of glial cells, however, a hyperpolarising current injected into glia reduced extracellular K^+ concentration in a symmetrical manner, while depolarising current injection induced a rise in $[K^+]_e$. This experiment demonstrates that the K^+ ion is mainly using the glial cell membrane during its movement in an electrical gradient. It also provides additional evidence supporting the view that glial cells function as a spatial buffer for K^+. More recently, Schwindt and Nicholson have demonstrated that local K^+ injection into the extracellular space causes larger potassium signals when potassium uptake into glia is reduced due to blockade of inwardly rectifying channels by barium (Schwindt and Nicholson, personal communication).

10.3.2 Spatial Buffer Function: K^+ Siphoning in the Retina

Thanks to its easy accessibility and well layered structure, the retina is the part of the CNS that is best characterised in terms of spatial buffering. Chapter 4 in this book contains more specific information, therefore it will be only briefly described here. The major glial cell element of the retina stretches through all layers starting at the photoreceptors and ending with endfeet at the inner limiting membrane adjacent to the vitreous humor. The inner and outer plexiform layers are the areas of light-induced K^+ increases, this is where K^+ ions have to enter the Müller cells generating a current sink. The endfoot K^+ channel density is tenfold greater than in the other regions (Newman 1986a). Since the endfeet border at a large liquid reservoir, any K^+ released will quickly diffuse, keeping the extracellular K^+ concentration close to normal. If during light stimulation the plexiform layers accumulate high K^+ and the Müller cell parts in these regions are depolarised, there is a driving force for K^+ currents into the cell in these areas and toward the hyperpolarised endfeet where K^+ is released. Again, the return current will be carried by Na^+ and Cl^- ions (Newman 1995). This pattern is associated with negative extracellular potentials in the plexiform layers and a large positive potential at the endfeet–vitreous humor interface. This is the electroretinogram b-wave (Newman 1995). Since this mechanism is based on anatomically fixed loops due to the increased endfeet K^+ channel density, it is also called K^+ siphoning (Newman 1995). Whether such siphoning and special endfeet specialisation also applies to astrocytes in the cerebral cortex and other brain structures is still a matter of speculation.

10.3.3 Evidence for Spatial Potassium Buffering in Neocortical Structures

Four lines of evidence suggest that spatial buffering and generation of slow field potential occurs in the neocortex. Current transport experiments have shown both in intact cortex and in gliotic tissue that the transport number is much larger than expected from a pure extracellular current transport (Heinemann, Neuhaus and Dietzel 1983). It has been shown that focal iontophoretic application of K^+ induces slow negative potentials, both in gliotic tissue and in normal cortex. It is now widely accepted that the rises in $[K^+]_e$ induced by focal injections are smaller than expected from the diffusional properties of the extracellular space. Laminar profiles of changes in $[K^+]_e$ in relation to generation of slow negative field potentials have shown that negative potentials are always largest at the site of maximal rises in $[K^+]_e$ while positive field potentials occur attsi es where the rises in $[K^+]_e$ are smaller. Current source density analysis of slow potential changes has supported the conclusion that at sites of maximal rises in $[K^+]_e$ there is a large enough inward current into cellular compartments to limit rises in $[K^+]_e$ (Dietzel and Heinemann 1983, 1986; Lux, Heinemann and Dietzel 1986; Dietzel, Heinemann and Lux 1989). Moreover, it has been found that rises in $[K^+]_e$ are associated with a shrinkage of the extracellular space at sites of maximal $[K^+]_e$ accumulation, while at remote sites the extracellular space can get larger. This is presumably an effect of the spatial buffering, since at sites of maximal potassium accumulation there will be inward potassium currents into glia, while at remote sites there is outward current resulting in negative field potentials at the site of maximal K^+ accumulation and positive field potentials at remote sites where K^+ ions leave the glia. The compensating current through the extracellular space will be mostly carried by Na^+ and Cl^- because of their much higher concentration, with Na^+ movement to the site of current sink and Cl^- movement away from the current sink. As a result, osmotic inbalances occur which lead to water shifts into glia at sites of maximal K^+ accumulation and to a widening of the extracellular space at remote sites (see also Chapter 7). This could be shown to be the case for cat cortex while in rat cortex widening of the extracellular space was not observed, presumably due to a shorter length constant of the glial syncytium.

10.3.4 Evidence for Spatial K^+ Buffering in Relation to Generation of Slow Field Potentials in Rat Hippocampus

Based on such observations we, in Heinemann's laboratory, have recently begun a project where the changes in $[K^+]_e$ in relation to field potentials are studied in rat hippocampal slices. Because of its unique and very orderly organisation, this preparation offers some advantages over cortical structures. In area CA1, pyramidal cells are arranged in a parallel manner with their somatas all in the stratum pyramidale. The axons of the pyramidal cells project into the alveus while the dendrites extend into the stratum radiatum and the stratum moleculare. There is no projection from area CA1 to the neighbouring dentate gyrus. Only a few dendrites of granule cells and interneurons cross the fissure and expand into the neighbouring area CA1.

We have correlated maturation of astrocytes in this structure with rises in $[K^+]_e$ and associated slow field potentials evoked by stimulation of the alveus. In slices from adult rats the rises in $[K^+]_e$ are maximal in stratum pyramidale. In this layer, the slow field potentials are negative and also maximal. Rises in $[K^+]_e$ become smaller when the recording electrode is moved from the stratum pyramidale to the stratum radiatium or stratum oriens. The field potentials reverse polarity when they are recorded at a distance of more than 180 μm from the stratum pyramidale. The rises in $[K^+]_e$ vary with stimulus intensity, frequency and train duration. However, rises in $[K^+]_e$ are limited in adult tissue to about 12 mM. When recordings are performed on 2- to 3-week-old animals, the rises in $[K^+]_e$ are much larger and therefore can often induce spreading depression (Hablitz and Heinemann 1989; Heinemann, Albrecht and Ficker 1990). Studies on properties of these glial cells in the stratum radiatum had suggested that the glial cells in this layer do not yet all express mature densities of K^+ channels (Steinhäuser et al. 1992; Steinhäuser, Jabs and Ketternmann 1994; Kressin et al. 1995). Morphological examination also shows that it takes 3 weeks after birth to reach adult levels of GFAP positive astrocytes, with some remodelling of spatial orientation extending even further into adulthood (Nixdorf-Bergweiler, Albrecht and Heinemann 1994). Interestingly, in spite of the fact that rises in $[K^+]_e$ are larger in animals from a postnatal age of 2 and 3 weeks, the simultaneously recorded changes in slow field potentials are smaller when similar sized rises in $[K^+]_e$ are compared. A second argument for a contribution of astrocytes comes from studies where $[K^+]_e$ was simultaneously recorded in the stratum pyramidale and in the dentate gyrus (Albrecht, Rausche and Heinemann 1989). This was done under two conditions in slices from adult animals. In one condition, the alveus was stimulated. This resulted in large rises in $[K^+]_e$ in the stratum pyramidale and negative field potentials in this layer while in the dentate gyrus the stimulation induced small rises in $[K^+]_e$ associated with positive field potentials in the neighbouring leaflet of the dentate gyrus but not in the remote leaflet. A similar observation was made when low Ca^{2+} was applied to induce epileptiform discharges. Under these conditions, evoked chemical synaptic transmission was found to be blocked (Jones and Heinemann 1987). Small rises in $[K^+]_e$ and slow positive field potentials were observed to occur in the stratum moleculare of the dentate gyrus simultaneously with the larger rises in $[K^+]_e$ in the stratum pyramidale of area CA1. Moreover, also in the hippocampal slice preparation, rises in $[K^+]_e$ induced by its local iontophoretic application caused slow negative field potentials.

These observations encouraged us to study the relationship between rises in $[K^+]_e$ induced by stimulation of the alveus and the distribution of current sinks and sources of slow field potentials. We found two sinks to be associated with rises in $[K^+]_e$: one in the stratum pyramidale at the site of maximal rises in $[K^+]_e$ and one in the stratum radiatum. The latter disappeared when synaptic transmission was blocked by lowering $[Ca^{2+}]_e$ or by application of glutamate receptor antagonists. It was therefore of a presumably synaptic origin. In contrast, barium, which reduces potassium inward currents into glia, was shown to augment rises in $[K^+]_e$ while at the same time blocking the current sink during the stimulus train in the stratum pyramidale.

We also studied the relationship between elevations in $[K^+]_e$ and glial membrane potentials, both in the stratum pyramidale and in the stratum moleculare. While the relationship was sub-Nernstian in the stratum pyramidale, it was supra-Nernstian in the stratum moleculare. The current source density analysis revealed that at sites of sub-Nernstian depolarisation, there was maximal K^+ accumulation and a strong current sink indicating net inward current, while at remote layers the super-Nernstian depolarisation was associated with smaller and slower extracellular rises in $[K^+]_e$ and a current source indicating net outward currents into the extracellular space. These observations are fully compatible with the concept of spatial K^+ buffering and a role of glia in generation of slow field potential shifts.

10.3.5 *Neuronal Contribution to Generation of Slow Field Potential Shifts*

The available evidence supports the concept that glial cells can and do contribute to generation of slow field potentials. However, this does not exclude the likelihood that steady inward currents into neurons with a concomitant loss of positive charges in the extracellular space can also contribute to generation of slow negative field potentials. In fact, intracellular recordings from neurons during repetitive stimulation, seizures, spreading depression and anoxia all show that neurons display prolonged depolarisations during these phases which would be carried by net inward currents. Also, observations that glutamate does induce slow field potentials with both neuronal and glial depolarisation suggests a role of neuronal inward currents in the generation of slow negative field potentials. In fact, in a pure gliotic scar and in adult hippocampal slices where neurons have been destroyed by either hypoxia or hypoglycaemia, glutamate application no longer induces slow negative field potentials. Also, the studies in the hippocampus on stimulus-induced field potentials suggest that both neurons and glia contribute to the generation of slow field potentials, since one persistant sink is critically dependent on synaptic transmission. Thus at present, it would not be possible to state that slow potential shifts are exclusively due to spatial K^+ buffering and the involvement of glia in this process. Unfortunately, at present it is only in very few cases possible to state the relative contribution of glia and neurons to the generation of slow negative potentials, yet the evidence that glia are important players in the generation of slow potential shifts is gaining increasing support.

11

Acid/Alkaline Transients and pH Regulation by Glia

JOACHIM W. DEITMER

Summary

Glial cells provide an essential contribution to pH regulation and acid/base transients in nervous systems. The mechanisms of intracellular pH regulation and the transport of neurotransmitters and metabolites across the glial cell membrane also shape extracellular pH shifts. These pH transients can be very brief and local, and may constitute a proton-mediated signalling between glial cells and neurons. By modulating and shaping neuronal and synaptic processes, excitation and inhibition in nervous tissue may be affected, and hence potential shifts, which are associated with behavioural performances. Although our knowledge about a possible link between acid/base transients and electrical events recorded during behavioural tasks is virtually non-existent, such a link may be inferred by the fact that most neural processes are directly or indirectly influenced by changes in intra- and/or extracellular pH. This chapter summarises the mechanisms of acid/base transients and pH regulation, as far as they can be associated with glial cell activity and neuron–glial communication, without referring directly to certain behaviours.

11.1 Introduction

pH changes in nerve and glial cells and in the extracellular space in nervous systems can be evoked by neuronal activity, by neurotransmitters, by active cellular pH regulation and by metabolic processes. Rapid pH transients may actually be signals rather than only a result of inadequate homeostatic acid–base regulation. Analogous to the signalling pattern of other ions, such as, e.g. calcium and potassium, transient shifts of protons and bicarbonate, together with the gas carbon dioxide, may influence or initiate functional processes in the nervous system, including pH-induced changes of neuronal excitability, the modulation of gap junctions and thus of electrical synapses and the glial syncytium, and the control of enzyme activities. Proton signalling in cells and in local extracellular domains, as, e.g. in the vicinity of synapses, could well contribute to information processing in nervous systems (Deitmer and Rose 1996), and to slow potential shifts associated with neuronal activity (Chapters 10, 12, 13).

pH regulation in nervous systems is an essential homeostatic function of the cellular elements, glial cells and neurons. This is mainly achieved by transport of acid–base equivalents across the cell membranes. Substances transported out of the cells may be accumulated in the narrow spaces between nerve and glial cells – the extracellular or interstitial spaces – the third compartment in nervous tissue besides the two cellular elements (Chapter 7).

Extra- and intracellular pH, however, are not kept as tightly constant as often thought. In response to neuronal activity and cell activation by transmitters, hormones, growth factors or other messengers or receptor agonists, intra- and extracellular pH can rapidly and transiently change just like the activity of other ions, such as Ca^{2+} and K^+. However, while Ca^{2+} waves and Ca^{2+} transients are generally viewed as 'signals' serving in intra- and intercellular communication (Cornell-Bell and Finkbeiner 1991; Sanderson et al. 1994), pH transients have often only been considered as an 'unwanted interference' in homeostatic pH control, and explained by a limited buffering power and/or insufficient regulation in cells and tissues.

The most often used technique for direct measurement of pH in glial cells, neurons and extracellular spaces (ECS) has been pH-sensitive, neutral carrier microelectrodes (Ammann ct al. 1981), which are impaled into a cell or into a tissue and provide an 'on-line' recording of pH. The development of ion-sensitive fluorescent dyes (Heiple and Taylor 1982; Rink, Tsien and Pozzan 1982) has created another, very powerful, method to monitor intracellular pH (pH_i) directly and continuously. While the use of pH-sensitive microelectrodes is an 'invasive' technique, since the electrode has to be impaled into a cell or a tissue, pH-sensitive fluorescent dyes, such as BCECF (2′,7′-(bis carboxyethyl)-5,6-carboxyfluorescein), Me_2CF (4′,5′-dimethyl-5, 6-carboxyfluorescein), SNARF or SNAFL fluorophores can be loaded via their membrane-permeable acetoxymethyl ester (AM), which is cleaved off in the cell by intrinsic diesterases to trap the dye intracellularly.

Glial cells appear to contribute to the extracellular pH transients, and play a prominent role in overall H^+ homeostasis in nervous systems. While neuronal pH regulation has been extensively studied in the last 2 decades (cf. Roos and Boron 1981; Thomas 1984; Chcsler 1990), only in the last few years has special attention been given to glial pH regulation (cf. Deitmer and Rose 1996).

Apart from the recent rising interest in glial cells, new techniques for identifying glial cells and for measuring intracellular pH have allowed substantial progress in this field.

11.2 Intraglial pH and H^+ Buffering

Most living cells studied so far maintain an alkaline intracellular pH (pH_i) with respect to the H^+ electrochemical equilibrium. Therefore, cells must *actively* control their pH_i, which means that acid equivalents must be extruded out of the cells against an H^+/OH^- electrochemical gradient. Since the production of H^+ exceeds the H^+ consumption in most metabolic processes (Hochachka and Mommsen 1983), cells and tissues have to extrude acid constantly. In addition, any leak of acid–base equivalents across the cell membrane would lead to a flow of H^+ into, or OH^- and HCO_3^- out of the cell down their electrochemical gradient, which must be compensated by active transport in the opposite direction.

11.2.1 Electrochemical H⁺ Gradient

The H^+ equilibrium potential, at which H^+/OH^- and HCO_3^- are passively distributed across the cell membrane, is given by the Nernst equation

$$E_H = \frac{RT}{F} \ln \frac{[H^+]_e}{[H^+]_i} \qquad (11.1)$$

where $[H^+]_e$ and $[H^+]_i$ are the concentrations of intra- and extracellular H^+ concentration, R is the gas constant, T the absolute temperature and F the Faraday constant. This can be rewritten as

$$E_H = 58.5\,mV\,(pH_i - pH_e) \qquad (11.2)$$

where pH_i is the intracellular, and pH_e the external pH; T was assumed to be 295 K (22°C). Equation (11.2) predicts that at a pH_e of 7.4 (40 nM H^+) and a pH_i of 7.1 (80 nM H^+), the distribution of H^+ achieves an equilibrium at a cell membrane potential of $-18\,mV$. This is far more positive than the membrane voltage of most cells. Consequently, at potentials more negative than $-18\,mV$, H^+ must be actively extruded, although the intracellular H^+ concentration is twice that of the external fluid.

If a membrane potential of -75 mV is assumed for glial cells, a passive H^+ distribution at pH_e 7.4 would give a pH_i value of 6.1 (incidentally the pK' of carbonic acid). This, however, is far too acid for most living cells to survive for any length of time due to inhibition of major enzymes at this low pH. Hence, active pH_i regulation is essential also in glial cells, and can be predicted from these theoretical considerations alone. In the example given, H^+ efflux has to overcome an electrochemical gradient of 57 mV, equivalent to about 1 pH unit.

11.2.2 Intraglial pH Values

pH_i has been determined in a variety of glial cell types. The steady-state pH_i values obtained in different glial cells, either in intact tissue or in culture, ranged between 6.7 and 7.6, corresponding to 160–25 nM free H^+. In most glial cells, where pH_i

was measured in different buffer systems, pH_i was either the same (6.96; Brune et al. 1994), or significantly lower in HEPES-buffered salines (mean 7.02 ± 0.16) as compared to CO_2/HCO_3^--buffered salines (mean 7.17 ± 0.19). Only in salamander retinal Müller cells and in cultured rat Schwann cells was the pH_i reported to be higher in CO_2/HCO_3^--free salines (6.81, 7.08) than in CO_2/HCO_3^--buffered salines (7.02, 7.17, respectively) (Newman 1994; Nakhoul et al. 1994).

The mean pH_i values correspond to an average free H^+ concentration in glial cells of 95 nM and 68 nM, respectively. The H^+ equilibrium potentials (E_H) calculated from these values at an extracellular pH of 7.4 (equivalent to 40 nM H^+), are -21 mV for HEPES-buffered and -13 mV for CO_2/HCO_3^--buffered saline (at room temperature), while the membrane resting potential (E_m) is often more negative in CO_2/HCO_3^--buffered solutions (Astion and Orkand 1988; Deitmer 1991; Brune et al. 1994). The capability of maintaining a steeper H^+ gradient in the presence of CO_2/HCO_3^- indicates the importance of this buffer system for the maintenance of an alkaline steady-state pH_i. The electrochemical H^+ gradient, expressed as the difference between E_H and E_m, thus ranges between 40 and 70 mV, equivalent to a pH gradient of 0.7–1.2 pH units.

11.2.3 Intraglial Buffering

The intrinsic, intraglial buffering power (β_i) has only been determined in some studies; it varied between 12.8 and 37.7 mM. The value of β_i includes the cytoplasmic, physicochemical buffering as well as the 'organellar buffering power'. It can be measured as the 'instantaneous' change in pH_i in response to the addition of strong acid or base, in the absence of CO_2/HCO_3^- (for a more elaborate description of buffering, see Roos and Boron 1981; Deitmer 1995; Deitmer and Rose 1996).

The total intracellular buffering power (β_T) is the sum of β_i, and the CO_2/HCO_3^--dependent buffering power, β_{CO2}. The latter is negligible in the nominal absence of CO_2/HCO_3^-, but, in an open system, may add considerable intracellular buffer capacity in the presence of HCO_3^-. β_{CO2} depends upon the concentration of CO_2 and on pH_i, which determines the intracellular HCO_3^- concentration. The capacity of intracellular H^+ buffering by CO_2/HCO_3^- is matched by the amount of intracellular HCO_3^- used, and can be written as

$$\beta_{CO_2} = \Delta[HCO_3^-]_i / \Delta pH_i \qquad (11.3)$$

where $\Delta[HCO_3^-]_i$ is the change in intracellular HCO_3^- concentration, and ΔpH_i the change in pH_i. $[HCO_3^-]_i$ can be calculated by the modified Henderson–Hasselbalch equation

$$[HCO_3^-]_i = 10(pH_i - pH_e)[HCO_3^-]_e \qquad (11.4)$$

where $[HCO_3^-]_e$ is the external HCO_3^- concentration. Thus, equation (11.3) yields in first approximation

$$\beta_{CO_2} = 2.3[HCO_3^-]_i \tag{11.5}$$

For example, from a value of 7.2 for pH_i, measured in a saline buffered with 5% $CO_2/24$ mM HCO_3^- at pH 7.4, $[HCO_3^-]_i$ can be calculated to be 15.1 mM, which would add 34.8 mM buffering power to the cytoplasm. These are realistic values for glial cells, as well as for neurons and many other cell types; thus, the presence of CO_2/HCO_3^- can easily double or triple the buffering capacity provided by the intrinsic buffering power. In a cell with a steady-state pH_i of 7.2 in a CO_2/HCO_3^--buffered saline, the total buffering power may hence add up to 60 mM (given a β_i of 25 mM, and a β_{CO_2} of 35 mM, see above).

The buffering capacity of the narrow ECS in nervous tissue may have profound effects on pH_i and pH_i regulation (Pirttilä and Kauppinen 1993). The absolute buffering power of the ECS is expected to be limited by the small volume of the ECS, where buffering sites rapidly saturate upon an imposed pH change.

An attempt to estimate the intrinsic buffer capacity of the ECS by measuring pH_e changes at various buffer strengths of the bath saline gave a value of 5.2 mM in leech ganglia (Rose 1993). This value was determined after summing the effective buffering power of different salines and a calculated value in order to match stimulation-induced pH_e changes, and the produced acid or base equivalents in the different salines, respectively. However, this method did not take into account that buffering compounds, such as CO_2, HCO_3^- and organic acids, might be extruded from the cells during nerve stimulation, affecting the pH_e transients and hence the calculation of the intrinsic buffer capacity. Nevertheless, the results indicated that the extracellular intrinsic buffer capacity appears to be much lower than the cellular buffer capacity.

The presence of CO_2/HCO_3^- buffer not only increases the buffering capacity of the cells, but also that of the ECS. Experiments using weak acids and bases indicated an increase of the apparent extracellular buffer capacity in the presence of 2% $CO_2/11$ mM HCO_3 by a factor of 1.5–2.3 (Deitmer 1992a). Hence, CO_2/HCO_3^- seems to increase intra- and extracellular buffering power by a similar factor (see above).

The increase in extracellular buffer capacity was dependent on the presence of carbonic anhydrase (CA) activity, since it could be reversed by adding inhibitors of CA (acetazolamide, 100 µM, or ethoxyzolamide, EZA, 2 µM) (Thomas, Coles and Deitmer 1991; Deitmer 1992a). The rapid, reversible hydration of CO_2 catalysed by CA is obviously pivotal for rapid extracellular buffering by CO_2/HCO_3^-.

In nervous systems, this enzyme has been reported to be located most prominently in glial cells (Sapirstein, Strocchi and Gilbert 1984), except in the honeybee, where CA activity has been localised histochemically in brain glial cells, but not in retinal glial cells (Walz 1988).

In Müller glial cells of the salamander retina (Newman 1994), inhibition of CA reduced the initial rate of intracellular acidification upon addition of CO_2 as expected from reduction of CO_2 hydration. Newman (1994) suggested that Müller glial cells in the retina may help to regulate the level of CO_2, which may vary greatly in the metabolically active retina, by serving as CO_2 sinks, which would indeed require a high CA activity (see also below).

11.3 Acid–Base Transients

Acid and alkaline transients of up to several tenths of a pH unit can be recorded in the ECS during neuronal activity (for references see Deitmer and Rose 1996) or under pathophysiological conditions, such as anoxia or ischaemia, spreading depression or epileptiform activity. In the ischaemic brain, lactic acid levels may rise dramatically, leading to a severe acidification in the ECS; this lactacidosis may lead to glial cell swelling, impairment of synaptic transmission or even cell death (Lomneth, Medrano and Gruenstein 1990; Staub et al. 1990). It has been suggested that glial cells may help to control pH in the ECS (pH_e) by mechanisms which tend to damp large pH_e transients, and thereby play an important role in maintaining H^+ homeostasis in nervous tissue (Siesjö 1985; Deitmer 1992a; Ransom 1992). It was suggested that the pH_i regulation of astrocytes derived from jimpy mice, which carry a genetic disorder of myelination, is indeed abnormal, and the steady-state pH_i considerably higher than in normal astrocyte cultures (Knapp, Booth and Skoff 1993).

pH_e changes may well be physiologically important. The conductance and/or gating of many membrane channels and carriers may be modulated by pH_e. This has been shown for γ-aminobutyric acid (GABA) channels (Kaila, Saarikoski and Voipio 1990), for the N-methyl-D-aspartate (NMDA)-type glutamate channel (Tang, Dichter and Morad 1990; Traynelis and Cull-Candy 1990), and for Ca^{2+} channels (Konnerth, Lux and Morad 1987; Jarolimek, Misgeld and Lux 1990). This, in turn, may have severe consequences for neuronal excitability and information processing in the nervous system (see below).

There is also evidence that pH changes not only modify neuronal ion channels, but also channels in the glial membrane. In glial cells of an oligodendrocyte lineage, a rapid decrease of pH elicited large Na^+ currents (Sontheimer et al. 1989a), and in cultured Schwann cells (Hoppe et al. 1989) and in leech neuropil glial cells (Munsch and Deitmer 1991), the K^+ conductance was affected by pH.

11.3.1 Neuronal Activity-Induced pH Transients

Studies on central nervous systems of both vertebrates and invertebrates have shown that neuronal activity leads to defined extra- and intracellular pH changes

(Kraig, Ferreira-Filho and Nicholson 1983; reviewed by Chesler 1990, Chesler and Kaila 1992; Deitmer and Rose 1996). These consist of mono- or multiphasic pH shifts indicating that they might originate from multiple sources and/or via multiple pathways. It has to be emphasised, that not only experimental stimulation, but also neuronal activity under physiological conditions caused substantial pH changes (cf. Chesler 1990; Deitmer and Rose 1996).

Due to the increase in extracellular potassium activity, glial cells respond to the activity of neighbouring neurons by a depolarisation of their cell membrane. Electrical stimulation of the cortex, e. g. caused a K^+-induced glial depolarisation of 4–38 mV (Chesler and Kraig 1987). In the presence of Ba^{2+} to block K^+ channels, glial cells hyperpolarised during neuronal stimulation most likely due to electrogenic Na^+/K^+ pumping (Ballanyi, Grafe and Ten Bruggencate 1987).

In the cortex, the stimulus-evoked glial depolarisation was accompanied by an intracellular alkalinisation of astrocytes, the amplitude of which was dependent on the amplitude of the glial depolarisation (Fig. 11.1A; Chesler and Kraig 1989). A stimulus-induced depolarisation by 15 mV was associated with a mean alkaline shift of 0.19 pH units, indicating a slope of approximately 80 mV/pH unit. Qualitatively similar pH_i shifts were reported from glial cells in the medulla of cats (Fig. 11.1B; Ballanyi et al. 1994) and from leech neuropil glial cells (Fig. 11.1D; Rose and Deitmer 1995a).

Several lines of evidence suggest that the depolarisation-induced alkalinisation of glial cells in both vertebrate and invertebrate preparations is due to inward transport of bicarbonate via an electrogenic Na^+-HCO_3^- cotransport activated by the K^+-induced membrane depolarisation (Fig. 11.1C; Deitmer and Szatkowski 1990; Grichtenko and Chesler 1994a). In the cortex, the glial alkaline shift was partly inhibited in Na^+-free saline and turned into a small acidification during the application of Ba^{2+} (Chesler and Kraig 1989, Grichtenko and Chesler 1994a,b). The stimulus-induced alkalinisation of glial cells in the leech was turned into an acidification by all experimental protocols preventing the activation of Na^+-HCO_3^- cotransport: (1) by voltage-clamping the glial cell (Fig. 11.2A; Rose and Deitmer 1994), (2) in the presence of the stilbene DIDS and (3) in CO_2/HCO_3^--free saline (Fig. 11.1D; Rose and Deitmer 1995a,b). Suppressing the glial depolarisation during nerve root stimulation not only reversed the intraglial pH change, but also influenced the pH_e transient (Fig. 11.2B; Rose and Deitmer 1994). If a neuropil glial cell was voltage-clamped, nerve stimulation evoked an alkaline–acid shift in the ECS in the vicinity of the voltage-clamped glial cell instead of an acidification alone (J.W. Deitmer & H.P. Schneider, unpublished observation), just as in HCO_3^--free saline or in the presence of DIDS (Rose and Deitmer 1994, 1995b).

Other mechanisms proposed to be responsible for the depolarisation-induced alkalinisation (DIA) of vertebrate glial cells include an active acid secretion via outward transport of lactate (Walz and Mukerji 1988) or via a bafilomycin-sensitive H^+-adenosine triphosphate (ATP)ase (Pappas and Ransom 1993).

The intraglial alkalinisation might lead to an uptake of significant amounts of base equivalents from the ECS, supporting the idea that glial cells play a role in the regulation of extracellular pH (Deitmer 1992a). Observations on the developing rat optic nerve and spinal cord suggest that the glial alkalinisation might acidify the ECS, thereby leading to a dampening of the activity-induced extracellular alkalinisation (Ransom, Carlini and Connors 1986; Jendelová and Syková 1991). This was also demonstrated for the adult leech CNS, where blocking of the intraglial alkalinisation unmasked an extracellular alkalinisation at the beginning of the neuronal stimulation (Fig. 11.2B; Rose and Deitmer 1994).

Some studies suggested that a $GABA_A$-induced cellular efflux of HCO_3^-, a glutamate-mediated influx of H^+, and/or the activation of a Ca^{2+}/H^+-ATPase could partly be responsible for the extracellular alkalinisation observed during neuronal activity (Chen and Chesler 1992a,b; Kaila et al. 1992; see section 11.3.2). It should be emphasised, however, that glial cells are not likely to contribute to these neurotransmitter-mediated mechanisms to a great extent, since bath application of GABA or glutamate leads to an *acidification* of glial cells, whereas glial cells *alkalinise* during neuronal stimulation (Chesler and Kraig 1987; Ballanyi et al. 1994; Rose and Deitmer 1995a). Maybe a neurotransmitter-induced intraglial acidification is masked by the alkalinisation caused by inward going Na^+-HCO_3^- cotransport during neuronal activity. This was suggested for leech glial cells, where the stimulus-induced intraglial alkalinisation was converted to an acidification during inhibition of the Na^+-HCO_3^- cotransport (Fig. 11.2A; Rose and Deitmer 1994).

In the ECS, electrical stimulation elicits biphasic alkaline–acid shifts in most nervous systems, which could amount to several tenths of a pH unit (reviewed by Deitmer and Rose 1996). The extracellular alkalinisations are likely to emerge following neurotransmitter release. In the rat hippocampus, they are partly caused by a bicarbonate efflux through $GABA_A$ receptor channels (Kaila et al. 1992). A glutamate-dependent mechanism for the stimulus-induced extracellular alkalinisation has been proposed to involve either a direct proton influx into the cells through glutamate receptor-coupled cation channels (Chen and Chesler 1992a; Deitmer and Munsch 1992; Deitmer et al. 1995), uptake of excitatory amino acids into the glial cell (Bouvier et al. 1992; Deitmer and Schneider 1997), or the activation of a cellular Ca^{2+}/H^+-ATPase (Schwiening, Kennedy and Thomas 1993) subsequent to an increase of intracellular Ca^{2+} (Paalasmaa et al. 1994; Smith et al. 1994) (see above). In retinal slices of the honeybee drone, light-stimulated extracellular alkalinisations were associated with substrate transfer between photoreceptors and glial cells (Tsacopoulos et al. 1994; Coles et al. 1996b).

The stimulus-induced extracellular acidification has been mainly ascribed to metabolic production of acid and CO_2, and was, at least partly, blocked in a variety of preparations after application of amiloride, a blocker of Na^+/H^+-exchange (Chesler 1990; Voipio and Kaila 1993; Rose and Deitmer 1995b).

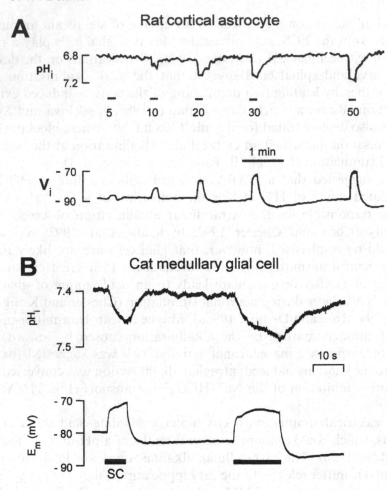

Fig. 11.1. Stimulation- and K^+-induced changes in intraglial pH and membrane potential of different glial cell types. (A) Increasing stimulation frequencies cause increasing membrane depolarisation and intracellular alkalinisation of rat cortical astrocytes in situ. (B) Repetitive electrical stimulation (100 Hz for 7 s) of the spinal cord (SC) causes glial depolarisation and alkalinisation in glial cells of the ventral respiratory group at a depth of 2.5–3.5 mm below the dorsal surface.

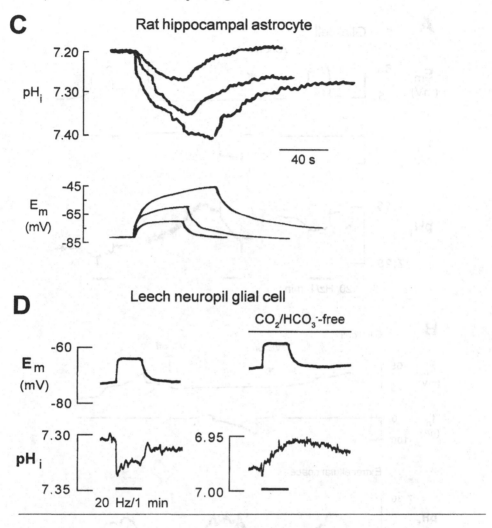

Fig. 11.1 (*cont.*). (C) K^+-induced membrane depolarisation and alkalinisation of astrocytes of rat hippocampal slices. (D) CO_2/HCO_3^- dependence of the stimulation-induced intracellular alkalinisation of leech neuropil glial cell: in CO_2/HCO_3^--free saline the alkalinisation reversed into an acidification, while the membrane depolarisation was unaffected. (A from Chesler and Kraig 1989; B from Ballanyi et al. 1994; C from Grichtenko and Chesler 1994a; D from Rose and Deitmer 1994.)

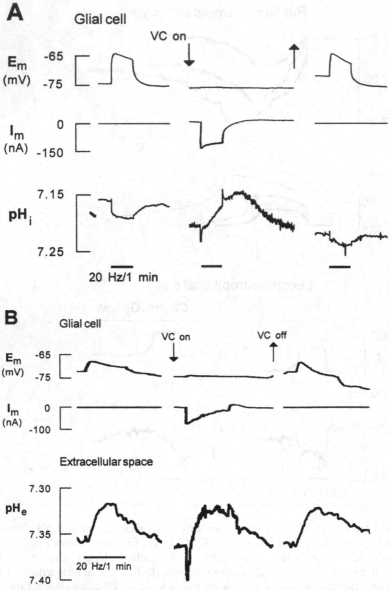

Fig. 11.2. Membrane potential (E_m) and membrane current (I_m), and pH transients in leech neuropil glial cell (A) and in the extracellular spaces of a leech ganglion (B) following side nerve stimulation. When the glial cell was voltage-clamped (middle columns in A and B), the intracellular alkalinisation was reversed into an acidification (A), and the extracellular acidification was preceded by a distinct alkaline transient (B). (From Rose and Deitmer 1994.)

Like the pH transients caused by neurotransmitter application (see below), the stimulus-evoked pH_e transients are sensitive to the inhibition of carbonic anhydrase. Benzolamide, a poorly membrane-permeable inhibitor, not only increased pH_e transients (Chen and Chesler 1992c; Gottfried and Chesler 1994), but also altered synaptic and neuronal activity in rat hippocampal slices (Taira et al. 1993; Gottfried and Chesler 1994). In the leech central nervous system, ethoxyzolamide, which reduces the effective extracellular buffering power (Deitmer 1992a), even reversed the stimulation-induced extracellular acidification to a prominent alkalinisation (Rose and Deitmer 1995b). In rat hippocampus, it was concluded that this was due to H^+ loss from the ECS, which was not compensated for fast enough by CA-associated buffering after CA-inhibition (Chen and Chesler 1992c). After the fast removal of H^+ from the ECS, presumably into the cells, at the onset of stimulation, the equilibrium of CO_2 hydration is shifted in favour of HCO_3^- and H^+. If CA is active, subsequent delivery of H^+ is very fast, and the initial H^+ loss would be quickly compensated. After inhibition of CA, however, the hydration reaction of CO_2 is too slow to compensate the H^+ loss, which results in an excess of base equivalents in the ECS, leading to a prominent stimulus-induced alkalinisation.

11.3.2 Neurotransmitter-Induced pH Transients

Glial cells have a variety of transmitter receptors coupled to ion channels (Hösli and Hösli 1993). The activation of these transmitter receptors can induce pH transients in nervous systems, which either emerge directly in response to the action of neurotransmitters themselves by both HCO_3^--dependent and independent mechanisms, or are secondary to membrane potential changes (Chesler and Kaila 1992; Deitmer and Munsch 1994). The majority of available data is on GABA- and glutamate-induced pH changes, while the effects of other transmitters, like acetylcholine or serotonin, on extra- or intracellular pH in the nervous system have been investigated in only a few reports. It has become clear, however, that there may be complex interactions between transmitter effects on both glial cells and neurons and extra- and intracellular pH changes, respectively.

11.3.2.1 GABA

It has been demonstrated in a variety of cells, such as crayfish muscle fibres or cortical neurons, that $GABA_A$ receptor-coupled chloride channels can possess considerable conductance for HCO_3^- ions (Kelly et al. 1969; Kaila and Voipio 1987). Due to the outwardly directed HCO_3^- gradient, the opening of these channels may lead to an efflux of HCO_3^- out of these cells, which becomes apparent as an intracellular acidification and an extracellular alkalinisation (Kaila, Saarikoski and Voipio 1990; Voipio et al. 1991).

Indeed, the $GABA_A$ receptor agonist muscimol caused a reversible, concentration-dependent acidification up to 0.15 pH units in cultured rat astrocytes (Kaila et al. 1991). This effect was only observed in CO_2/HCO_3^--buffered solution and was antagonised by elevating the bath K^+ concentration, suggesting that the muscimol-induced intraglial acidification was directly due to fluxes of acid–base equivalents through the $GABA_A$-gated ion channels. Kaila et al. (1991) suggested that glial cells, by contributing to the control of pH in the ECS, including that in the vicinity of GABAergic synapses, could modulate transmission at these synapses.

In leech giant glial cells, GABA sometimes produced a similar intracellular acidification, accompanied by a de- and hyperpolarising membrane response, both being dependent on the presence of extracellular CO_2/HCO_3^- (Deitmer and Rose 1996). This is in line with the study in cultured rat astrocytes (Kaila et al. 1991), indicating HCO_3^- efflux through GABA-gated receptor channels.

Extracellular alkalinisations occurred due to activation of $GABA_A$, but not of $GABA_B$ receptors, e.g. in the turtle cerebellum (Fig. 11.3A; Chen and Chesler 1990, 1991) and in the hippocampus (Jarolimek, Misgeld and Lux 1989; Kaila et al. 1992; reviewed by Kaila 1994). The GABA-induced pH_e shifts in the granular and molecular layers of the turtle cerebellum were partly transient and amounted to ca. 0.05 pH units. They were blocked by picrotoxin and mimicked by the $GABA_A$ agonists isoguvacine and muscimol (Chen and Chesler 1991). In rat hippocampus, $GABA_A$-induced extracellular pH shifts were blocked by both membrane-permeable and impermeable inhibitors of carbonic anhydrase (Chen and Chesler 1992a; Kaila et al. 1992), supporting the concept that they were due to HCO_3^- leaving the cells (Chesler and Kaila 1992).

11.3.2.2 Glutamate

The neurotransmitter glutamate and some of its agonists change the membrane potential and lead to substantial acidifications of both neurons (Endres et al. 1986; Hartley and Dubinsky 1993; Irwin et al. 1994) and glial cells. In glial cells, glutamate and its ionotropic agonists kainate and α-amino, 3-hydroxy, 5-methyl, 4-isoxazole proprionic acid (AMPA) evoked membrane depolarisations via receptors coupled to a non-selective cation channel.

The extracellular pH changes induced by glutamate agonists in both vertebrate and invertebrate preparations consisted of an alkalinisation followed by an acidification (e.g. Endres et al. 1986; Chen and Chesler 1992a; Rose and Deitmer 1995b). A sample recording from an intact leech ganglion is shown in Fig. 11.3B. The pH_e and pH_i responses to 500 μM glutamate were little affected by the ionotropic, non-NMDA receptor antagonist CNQX (Deitmer and Schneider 1997). The kainate-induced pH_e transients consisted of a small transient alkalinisation and a large, potentiating acidification (Fig. 11.3C), which were blocked by CNQX (Rose and Deitmer 1995b).

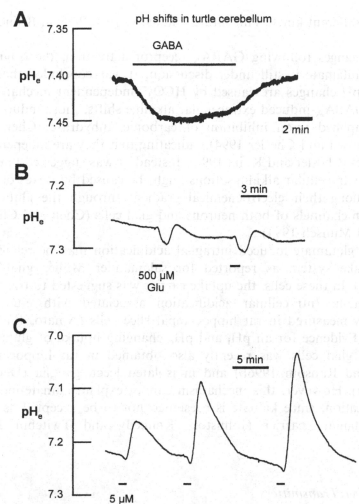

Fig. 11.3. Neurotransmitter-induced extracellular pH (pH$_e$) shifts. (A) Application of GABA induces a reversible alkaline shift in the granular layer of the turtle cerebellum. (B) Glutamate application causes an alkaline/acid shift in the neuropil of isolated leech ganglia. (C) The ionotropic glutamate agonist kainate evokes small alkaline transients followed by large, potentiating acid shifts in the extracellular spaces of a leech ganglion. (A from Chen and Chesler 1991; B and C from J.W. Deitmer and H.P. Schneider, unpublished.)

Activation of glutamate receptors of the kainate type led to a decrease in pH$_i$ of up to 0.3 pH units in cultured astrocytes (Plate 4; Brookes and Turner 1993; Brune and Deitmer 1995) and in leech neuropil glial cells (Deitmer and Munsch 1992, 1994). Glutamate itself caused a similarly large intracellular acidification in both glial cell types; the glutamate and the kainate-induced intracellular acidification, however, had quite different kinetics in cultured rat astrocytes (Plate 4; Brune and Deitmer 1995).

Unlike the pH changes following $GABA_A$ receptor activation, the origin of those induced by glutamate is still under discussion. It was concluded that the glutamate-induced pH changes are caused by HCO_3^--independent mechanisms. In contrast to the $GABA_A$-induced extracellular alkaline shifts, those induced by glutamate were amplified upon inhibition of carbonic anhydrase (Chen and Chesler 1992c; Gottfried and Chesler 1994), indicating that they are independent of bicarbonate fluxes (Chesler and Kaila 1992). Instead, it was suggested that the glutamate-induced extracellular alkalinisations might be caused by fluxes of H^+/OH^- equivalents along their electrochemical gradient through the glutamate receptor-coupled ion channels of both neurons and glial cells (Chen and Chesler 1992b; Deitmer and Munsch 1994).

Alternatively the glutamate-induced intraglial acidification may be related to the glutamate uptake system as reported for salamander Müller glial cells (Bouvier et al. 1992). In these cells, the uptake carrier was suggested to transport a pH_i-changing anion. Intracellular acidification associated with glutamate uptake was recently measured in rat hippocampal slice cells (Amato, Ballerini and Attwell 1994). Evidence for an pH_i and pH_e changing uptake of glutamate and aspartate into glial cells was recently also obtained in rat hippocampal astrocytes (Rose and Ransom 1996b) and in isolated leech ganglia (Deitmer and Schneider 1997). However, this mechanism cannot explain kainate-induced intracellular acidification, since kainate is presumed not to be accepted as substrate by the glutamate carrier (Johnston, Kennedy and Twitchin 1979; Kimelberg 1989).

11.3.2.3 Other Transmitters

Intraglial pH changes underlying a possible activation of acetylcholine receptors have not been subject to detailed investigations in the vertebrate CNS so far. In leech neuropil glial cells, the acetylcholine agonist carbachol (1 mM) induced an acid shift of 0.2 pH units in HEPES-buffered, CO_2/HCO_3^--free saline (Ballanyi and Schlue 1989; Deitmer 1995). The receptor was identified as a nicotinic ACh receptor-coupled to a cation channel, which is permeable to Na^+ and K^+ (Ballanyi and Schlue 1989). The extracellular pH changes induced by acetylcholine agonists in leech ganglia consisted of an alkalinisation followed by an acidification (Rose and Deitmer 1995b).

Noradrenaline, which causes a metabotropically mediated intracellular Ca^{2+} release, did not change the intracellular pH_i in cultured rat astrocytes (Plate 4; Brune and Deitmer 1995). Both activation of metabotropic receptors and intracellular Ca^{2+} release, have not yet been shown to be causally related to intracellular pH changes in glial cells.

11.4 pH Regulation

Like many other cell types, glial cells seem to use transport systems for their pH_i regulation. They share with most cells the use of a Na^+/H^+ exchanger and a Cl^-/HCO_3^- exchanger; with most epithelial cells they share a $Na^+\text{-}HCO_3^-$ cotransporter, which is absent in neurons and most non-epithelial cells. Recently, a bafilomycin-sensitive H^+ pump has been suggested in hippocampal astrocytes (Pappas and Ransom 1994). The steady-state pH_i and the pH_i changes in leech glial cells were unaffected by intracellular Ca^{2+} transients evoked by membrane depolarisation (Deitmer, Schneider and Munsch 1993), suggesting that the homeostasis of H^+ and Ca^{2+} is not interrelated in these glial cells.

Besides these transporters, the presence of a lactic acid carrier has been suggested in cultured astrocytes (Walz and Mukerji 1988; Staub et al. 1990), contributing to the transport of acid across glial cell membranes.

11.4.1 Na⁺/H⁺ Exchangers

A Na^+/H^+ exchanger has been found in all mammalian cells including various glial cell types, like cultured mammalian astrocytes, leech neuropil and connective glial cells, astrocytes of the optic nerve, cultured oligodendrocytes, cultured cat Schwann cells, and glial or glioma cell lines (cf. Deitmer and Rose 1996). The molecular structure and kinetic and pharmacological properties of this transporter and its different subtypes, have been well characterised and are the subject of several excellent reviews to some of which the reader is referred (Aronson 1985; Noel and Pouysségur 1995).

In glial cell lines (C6) the Na^+/H^+ exchanger was also inhibited by amiloride, Na^+ could be replaced by Li^+ to exchange with H^+, and increasing pH_e and decreasing pH_i increased the activity of the exchanger (Jean et al. 1986).

11.4.2 Cl⁻/HCO₃⁻ Exchangers

Cl^-/HCO_3^- exchangers across glial cell membranes, either Na^+-independent or Na^+-dependent, have been reported for cultured astrocytes, cultured oligodendrocytes, leech glial cells, and cultured rat Schwann cells (cf. Deitmer and Rose 1996). These exchangers are characterised by their dependence on Cl^- and HCO_3^-, and can be inhibited by the stilbene derivatives SITS and/or DIDS, known blockers of anion carriers in cell membranes (Cabantchik and Greger 1992).

It may be inferred by analogy from studies on other cell types that the Na^+-independent Cl^-/HCO_3^- exchangers primarily extrude HCO_3^- and thereby help to recover pH_i following an alkaline load. This was shown in leech connective glial cells, where a SITS-sensitive exchanger could induce a net acid load in the cells (Szatkowski and Schlue 1994). Since Cl^-/HCO_3^- exchangers are not known to use energy derived from ATP cleavage, active HCO_3^- extrusion is likely to occur only in cells with a Cl^- pump, keeping the Cl_i^- lower than expected from electrochemical equilibrium.

Evidence for a Na^+-dependent Cl^-/HCO_3^- exchanger is based on pH_i recovery from an acid load, which shows similar properties to the Na^+-independent Cl^-/HCO_3^- exchanger with the difference that it is dependent on the presence of external Na^+. This has been reported for different types of glial cells (e.g. Deitmer and Schlue 1987; Chow et al. 1991; Shrode and Putnam 1994). Using the large Na^+ gradients, it usually transports base equivalents into, and Cl^- out of, the cells.

11.4.3 Na^+-HCO_3^- Cotransporter

The first evidence for a Na^+-HCO_3^- cotransporter in glial cells was found in the giant neuropil glial cells of the leech (Deitmer and Schlue 1987, 1989), in astrocytes in the optic nerve of the mudpuppy *Necturus* (Astion and Orkand 1988; Astion, Chvátal and Orkand 1989) and in cultured mouse oligodendrocytes (Kettenmann and Schlue 1988). A large number of recent studies have contributed ample evidence for the existence of Na^+-HCO_3^- cotransport in a variety of other types of glial cells. A Na^+-HCO_3^- cotransporter was found in freshly dissociated Müller glial cells of the salamander retina, in cultured mouse and rat astrocytes, and in leech connective glial cells (cf. Deitmer and Rose 1996). The cotransporter was not found, however, in C6 glioma cells (Shrode and Putnam 1994) and has not been reported for neurons (Deitmer and Schlue 1987).

In most of these studies, the Na^+-HCO_3^- cotransporter was detected during addition or removal of CO_2/HCO_3^-. Addition of CO_2/HCO_3^- resulted in an intracellular alkaline shift and a rise in intracellular Na^+ (Na^+_i), while removal of CO_2/HCO_3^- reversed these pH_i and Na^+_i changes (Fig. 11.4A). Simultaneously, the glial membrane hyperpolarised and depolarised, respectively, during these buffer changes due to reversibility of this electrogenic cotransporter (Deitmer 1991). When voltage-clamped an outward and inward current, respectively, was recorded (Munsch and Deitmer 1994).

As in epithelial cells, the Na^+-HCO_3^- cotransporter in glial cells could be inhibited by stilbene derivatives, such as DIDS, SITS or DNDS, but was unaffected by amiloride. In cultured rat astrocytes DIDS was shown partly to block pH_i recovery and the CO_2/HCO_3^--dependent outward current (Brune et al. 1994) as has also been shown in leech glial cells (Deitmer and Schlue 1989; Deitmer 1991).

These CO_2/HCO_3^--dependent pH_i shifts and membrane potential changes were dependent upon the presence of external Na^+, but not on external or intracellular Cl^- concentrations. There was a reversible rise in Na^+_i during the exposure to

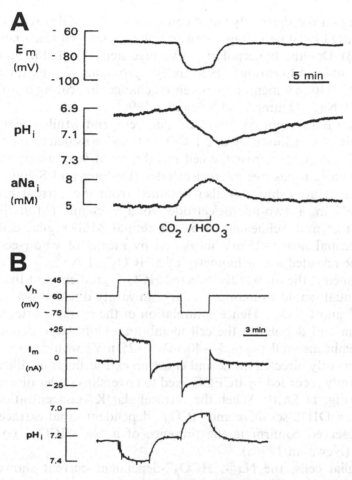

Fig. 11.4. Evidence for electrogenic Na^+-HCO_3^- cotransport in the leech giant glial cell: (A) Addition of CO_2/HCO_3^- hyperpolarises the membrane (upper trace), and induces an intracellular alkalinisation (middle trace) and a rise in intracellular Na^+ (lower trace), as recorded with a triple-barrelled ion-sensitive microelectrode. (B) De- and hyperpolarising voltage steps (upper trace) in a voltage-clamped cell evoke outward and inward currents, respectively (middle trace), with transient components, and intracellular alkalinisation and acidification, respectively (lower trace). (A and B modified from Deitmer and Rose 1996.)

CO_2/HCO_3^- in leech glial cells (Fig. 11.4A; Deitmer 1992b) and cultured rat hippocampal astrocytes (Rose and Ransom 1996a).

Reduction of the external pH by reducing the HCO_3^- concentration evoked an inward current in leech glial cells (Deitmer 1991; Munsch and Deitmer 1994) and rat astrocytes (Brune et al. 1994). This is consistent with activation of an outward-going electrogenic Na^+-HCO_3^- cotransport. The cotransporter could also be reversed in retinal Müller glial cells (Newman 1991), i.e. operating inwardly and outwardly, depending on the thermodynamic conditions. This is also reflected by the pH_i changes induced by slow voltage steps in voltage-clamped leech neuropil glial cells (Fig. 11.4B). De- and hyperpolarising voltage steps resulted in an intraglial alkalinisation and acidification, respectively, providing an extrapolated change of one pH unit/110 mV membrane potential change, indicating a stoichiometry of 2 HCO_3^- : 1 Na^+ (Deitmer and Schneider 1995).

The stoichiometry values reported for leech glial cells and Müller glial cells, however, are different. A stoichiometry of 2 HCO_3^- : 1 Na^+ was determined from the Na^+ and HCO_3^- gradients across the cell membrane of leech neuropil glial cells, as measured with ion-sensitive microelectrodes (Deitmer and Schlue 1989; Deitmer 1992b). This relationship was also obtained from the current reversal potential of -74 mV in a two-microelectrode voltage clamp (Munsch and Deitmer 1994; Deitmer and Schneider 1995). In retinal Müller glial cells the current reversal potential near -25 mV measured by means of whole-cell voltage-clamp technique revealed a stoichiometry of 3 HCO_3^- : 1 Na^+.

With this stoichiometry, the outwardly directed HCO_3^- gradient and the negative membrane potential would overcome the large inwardly directed Na^+ gradient and extrude Na^+ and HCO_3^-. Hence, stimulation of the cotransporter would acidify the cytoplasm and depolarise the cell membrane. Only large depolarisations of the cell membrane well beyond -40 mV (-25 mV) would reverse the cotransport to an inwardly directed mode and cause an extracellular acidification. Indeed, this was recently recorded by BCECF fixed to coverslips under dissociated retinal Müller cells (Fig. 11.5A,B). When the extracellular K^+ concentration was increased to 50 mM, a DIDS-sensitive and HCO_3^--dependent rapid extracellular acidification was observed confirming the presence of a Na^+-HCO_3^- cotransporter in these cells (Newman 1996a).

In these retinal glial cells, the Na^+-, HCO_3^--dependent current showed an inhomogeneous distribution (Fig. 11.5C; Newman 1991), suggesting a higher density of Na^+-HCO_3^- cotransporter molecules in the glial endfoot than in the rest of the cell membrane. It was postulated that this inhomogeneous distribution could serve to transport metabolically produced CO_2 out of the retina to the vitreous humor, which represents a sink for CO_2 (Newman 1991, 1994). Thus, the endfeet of retinal Müller glial cells could function as a CO_2 buffer system and the process was coined 'CO$_2$ siphoning' (Newman 1994), analogous to the 'K^+ siphoning' previously described for these cells (Newman, Frambach and Odette 1984).

11.4.4 H^+ Pumps

In addition to the pH regulating mechanisms presented in the preceding sections, hippocampal astrocytes have recently been reported to possess an acid extrusion mechanism that is neither dependent on the presence of Na^+, nor on the presence

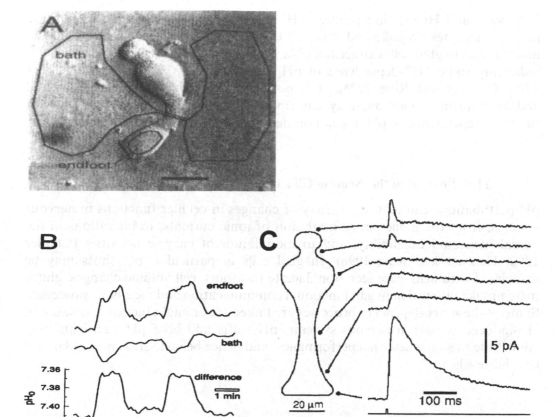

Fig. 11.5. Extra- and intracellular pH transients near or in isolated salamander retinal Müller glia cells. (A) Nomarski micrograph of a dissociated Müller cell with regions from which endfoot and bath extracellular pH (pH_o) were measured indicated. (B) Records of pH_o changes evoked by increasing the extracellular K^+ concentration from 2.5 to 50 mM. The corrected pH_o trace ('difference') is obtained by subtracting the 'bath' record from the 'endfoot' record, revealing the depolarisation-induced extracellular acidification. (C) Membrane currents evoked by local HCO_3^--ejection along a Müller cell (endfoot at bottom), showing the inhomogeneous distribution of the electrogenic Na^+-HCO_3^- cotransporter. (A and B from Newman 1996a; C from Newman 1991.)

of HCO_3^- (Pappas and Ransom 1993). This mechanism was observed in CO_2/ HCO_3^--free saline after blocking Na^+/H^+ exchange. Like the Na^+-independent acid extrusion mechanism observed in the kidney (Manger and Koeppen 1992), it could be blocked by either bafilomycin A_1 or N-ethylmaleimide, suggesting the presence of a vacuolar-type H^+-ATPase. Since the v-type H^+-ATPase is electrogenic, it is stimulated by membrane potential changes, and could hence contribute to the depolarisation-induced alkalinisation (DIA) of hippocampal astrocytes.

A Na^+- and HCO_3^--independent pH_i recovery was also observed in cultured mouse astrocytes (Wuttke and Walz 1990). It should be noted, however, that in most studies in glial cells extracellular Na^+ was necessary to observe pH_i recovery, indicating some Na^+-dependence of pH_i regulation in these cells (cf. Deitmer 1995; Deitmer and Rose 1996). It is not clear, whether different experimental and/or culturing conditions may contribute to the discrepancy with respect to the Na^+ dependence of pH_i regulation determined in the different studies.

11.5 Protons in the Neuron–Glia Dialogue

pH pertubations can induce a variety of changes in cellular functions in nervous systems, from the induction or inhibition of ionic currents, to alterations in the overall neuronal excitability, and to modulation of enzyme activities (Chesler 1990; Deitmer and Rose 1996). In glial cells in particular, pH shifts may be associated with acid–base secretion, lactate transport, cell volume changes, glutamate uptake, alteration in gap junctional communication and metabolic processes. Some of these pH-dependent processes are linked to, or might induce, a cascade of H^+-induced signals in nervous systems. pH shifts and brief pH transients may contribute to shape neuronal performance, and hence behaviour, at molecular and cellular levels.

11.5.1 Modulation of Gap Junctions

Glial cells of both invertebrates (Kuffler and Potter 1964) and vertebrates (Tang, Orkand and Orkand 1985; Kettenmann and Ransom 1988; Giaume et al. 1991) are often strongly coupled via gap junctions (Ransom 1995). These intercellular channels allow the passage and exchange of current and small molecules between cells. Cellular coupling may, e.g. play an essential role in the glial 'spatial buffering' of K^+ in the brain (Walz and Hertz 1983), and show potential changes across the glial syncytium. Moreover, propagation of Ca^{2+} waves may travel between astrocytes, which are believed to be mediated by the movement of IP_3 through gap junctions (Cornell-Bell and Finkbeiner 1991; Sanderson et al. 1994). These electrical potential and ionic shifts within the glial tissue and the ECS may well contribute to the slow EEG waves recorded under different behavioural states (see Chapters 12, 13).

Apart from its modulation by second messengers and high levels of intracellular Ca^{2+}, the conductance of gap junctions, and therefore the main channel of communication between coupled cells, is regulated by pH (Bennett et al. 1991). In several types of vertebrate glial cells, the gap junctional conductance was reduced by intracellular acidifications due to CO_2 or lactic acid (Connors, Benardo and Prince 1984; Anders 1988; Kettenmann, Ransom and Schlue 1990).

Due to this modulatory effect of protons on gap junctional conductance, reductions of pH are likely to reduce the exchange of molecules and diminish or even prevent intercellular communication between glial cells, whereas alkalinisations would support it. Changes in intracellular pH could thereby considerably change the functional syncytium formed by astrocytes and other glial cells in the brain.

11.5.2 pH Changes and Metabolism

A classical function ascribed to glial cells is that they might transfer metabolic substrates to neurons to support their metabolism during intense activity (cf. Schousboe 1981; Coles 1989; Lieberman, Hargittani and Grossfeld 1994; Chapter 5).

In contrast to neurons, glial cells are characterised by a high content of glycogen and few mitochondria (Pentreath et al. 1987; Tsacopoulos et al. 1988). Glial cells take up and phosphorylate glucose (Poitry-Yamate and Tsacopoulos 1991). Key enzymes of glycogenolysis and glucose degradation, e.g. the phosphorylase kinase, the phosphofructokinase or the pyruvate dehydrogenase multienzyme complex have been demonstrated to be highly pH sensitive, being activated by intracellular alkalinisations and suppressed by acidifications in the physiological pH range. Glial glycogenolysis can be stimulated by elevation of the extracellular K^+ concentration, as well as by neurotransmitter agonists, and neuronal activation (cf. Deitmer and Rose 1996). The activity-induced intraglial alkalinisation therefore would support glial metabolism.

In the honeybee retina, neither K^+ nor cyclic adenosine monophosphate (cAMP) mediated the effect of light stimulation on intraglial glucose metabolism (Evequoz-Mercier and Tsacopoulos 1991). Recent investigations indicate that alanine might be the metabolic substrate delivered from the glial cells which stimulate NH_3 release from the neighbouring photoreceptors. This NH_3, in turn, might partly cause the stimulation-induced extracellular alkalinisation observed in the drone retina and serve as a neuronal signal to glial cells (Tsacopoulos et al. 1994).

11.5.3 Neuronal Excitability

Due to the dependence on protons of many voltage-gated and transmitter-gated ion channels, both extra- and intracellular pH changes can significantly affect the overall neuronal excitability. Since protons can either induce or inhibit membrane conductances, the effects of pH changes strongly depend on the specific properties of the cell under study. This is evident in cell cultures or tissue preparations containing different types of cells. In cat spinal cord, it was reported that the activity of neurons was either depressed or enhanced by protons (Marshall and Engberg 1980). The same was true for cultured mammalian spinal neurons: iontophoretically applied protons evoked excitatory responses associated with an increase in membrane conductance in some neurons, whereas H^+ ions induced a hyperpolarisation associated with a decrease in membrane conductance in other neurons (Gruol et al. 1980). Moreover, protons appeared to elevate the threshold for spike generation, and caused a depression of the responses evoked by application of glutamate, glycine or GABA (Gruol et al. 1980).

The picture seems to be more uniform in brain regions like the hippocampus or the retina. In general, extracellular acidifications caused a decrease of compound action potentials and electrical excitability of central neurons, whereas alkalinisations led to their increase (Balestino and Somjen 1988; Jarolimek, Misgeld and Lux 1989). Pyramidal neurons in the hippocampus showed a hyperpolarisation, an increased threshold for action potential generation, a decrease in input resistance, and a reduction of the after-hyperpolarisation following intracellular acidification (Church and McLennan 1989; Church 1992). A depressing effect of protons on overall neuronal activity was confirmed in epileptiform tissue: extracellular acidification reduced or abolished epileptiform discharges, whereas extracellular alkalinisation tended to induce it (Aram and Lodge 1987).

Another system, in which the modulatory effects of protons on neuronal excitability are documented, is the retina. Light transmission in the retina is critically dependent on pH: an intracellular acidification depressed the cyclic guanosine monophosphate (cGMP) content and the light sensitivity of rod photoreceptors, while extracellular acidification hyperpolarised retinal horizontal cells, reduced light-sensitive postsynaptic currents in horizontal and bipolar cells, depressed the non-inactivating voltage-sensitive K^+ current, and affected the dopamine-modulated gap junctions between horizontal cells (cf. Takashi and Copenhagen 1996). In contrast, increased Ca^{2+} influx and transmitter release, and larger postsynaptic currents were facilitated by alkalinisations (Barnes, Merchant and Mahmud 1993).

The pH dependence of neuronal excitability can also alter functional properties of whole neuronal networks. In the mollusc eye, low intracellular pH abolished the circadian rhythm in the optic nerve compound action potentials (Khalsa, Ralph and Block 1991). In the stomatogastric ganglion of the crayfish, a change in intraganglionic pH induced by NH_4^+/NH_3 influenced the frequency of rhythmically active neurons, while changing the bath pH did not (Golowasch and Deitmer 1993). It was concluded that glial cells may help to protect neurons from pH changes in the haemolymph, and that inert gases such as NH_3 which usually pass cell membranes without hindrance, are needed to shift the intraganglionic pH.

In contrast to the systems discussed above, where acidification leads to a reduction of neuronal excitability, the number of discharges of the ventral medulla oblongata increased at lower, and decreased at higher, pH values (Jarolimek, Misgeld and Lux 1990), indicating the existence of a central chemoreceptor excited by increasing P_{CO_2} and/or decreasing pH (Fukuda and Loeschke 1977). Single neurons of the medulla oblongata increased their firing rate with increasing

P_{CO_2} (Richerson 1995). Rat ventral medullary neurons responded transiently to relatively small changes in extracellular pH between 7.2 and 7.4 with an altered discharge frequency (Jarolimek, Misgeld and Lux 1990). The pH-induced response was stronger when increasing P_{CO_2} than when reducing the HCO_3^- concentration, and was amplified during hypoxia; this was interpreted as being due to intrinsic properties of these neurons in the medulla oblongata.

11.5.4 Synaptic Transmission

Protons not only modulate the conductance of voltage-gated channels, they can also significantly influence synaptic transmitter release and the conductance of transmitter-coupled ion channels. In general, acidifications seem to depress synaptic transmission, whereas alkalinisations tend to increase its efficacy.

A pH dependency of synaptic transmitter release influencing miniature endplate current and endplate current fluctuations was reported from cholinergic synapses at the frog neuromuscular junction (Landau et al. 1981). This effect was probably due to protonation of the receptor molecules. In presynaptic terminals from rat brain, vesicular release of dopamine was directly stimulated by cytoplasmic acidification to pH 5.8. In contrast, extracellular acidification inhibited the release of dopamine by blocking voltage-gated Ca^{2+} channels (Drapeau and Nachshen 1988).

At the postsynaptic side, a strong pH dependency of NMDA-gated glutamate receptor channels and $GABA_A$ receptor-gated chloride channels was observed. Several groups showed that NMDA-induced currents were reduced by small extracellular acidifications and increased by alkalinisations (Tang, Dichter and Morad 1990; Vyklický, Vlachová and Kruse 1990; Traynelis and Cull-Candy 1991) with half maximal inhibition at pH 7.1–7.3. It is thought that this effect is due to a proton-induced inhibition of the conformational changes which normally lead to the opening of the channel (Cull-Candy, Wyllie and Traynelils 1991). The H^+ interaction with the NMDA receptor channel was recently localised at the exon 5 of the NR1 subunit (Traynelis, Hartley and Heinemann 1995).

It is noteworthy that the steep pH dependence of the channel conductance occurred in the physiological pH range (pH 6.8–7.5). It was suggested that the H^+ modulation of the NMDA-receptor channel would serve as an intrinsic protective mechanism by which calcium influx into neurons is regulated, particularly in hypoxic and/or ischaemic conditions (Tang, Dichter and Morad 1990). On the other hand, alkalosis-induced epileptiform activity could be blocked by NMDA-receptor antagonists (Aram and Lodge 1987), linking H^+ modulation of glutamatergic neurotransmission via NMDA receptors to pathological phenomona observed during stroke, epilepsy and seizures.

Due to the high H^+-sensitivity of NMDA receptor gated channels, neuronal excitability in the hippocampus could even be influenced by rather small pH shifts such as those occurring during repetitive stimulation of the Schaffer collaterals. It was demonstrated recently that the conductance of NMDA-gated ion channels, and therefore the efficacy of excitatory synaptic transmission, was critically dependent on the fast buffering of activity-induced pH shifts for carbonic anhydrase (Taira et al. 1993; Gottfried and Chesler 1994). An amplification of the stimulus-induced extracellular alkaline transients by application of the CA inhibitor benzolamide considerably increased the duration of excitatory postsynaptic currents (Gottfried and Chesler 1994). This may also be relevant to forms of long-term potentiation (LTP) that have been linked to NMDA receptor activation, and in general to learning and memory (Bliss and Collingridge 1993).

In contrast to their influence on glutamatergic transmission, extracellular acidifications led to an increase in the conductance of $GABA_A$-activated chloride channels of crayfish muscle and neurons from cat dorsal root ganglia fibres, whereas alkalinisation decreased it (Takeuchi and Takeuchi 1967; reviewed by Kaila 1994). It was suggested that these effects might be due to a proton-induced increase in channel lifetime (Onodera and Takeuchi 1979), or to a decrease in its desensitisation (Pasternack et al. 1992). These opposing effects of protons on excitatory and inhibitory synaptic transmission could partly explain the depressing effects of acidification on neuronal excitability observed, e.g. in the hippocampus (Balestino and Somjen 1988; Jarolimek, Misgeld and Lux 1989).

11.6 Conclusions

Protons are diverse modulators and mediators of many neural functions. They can be regarded as signalling molecules themselves. Glial cells possess an array of mechanisms (Fig. 11.6) which regulate and change intraglial pH as well as the pH in the ECS. Most of these pH transients are anticipated to be very discrete transients, i.e. very brief and local pH changes, under normal physiological conditions. They may also be considerably larger in amplitude in vivo as compared to those recorded with invasive recording techniques. The largest, and probably most significant pH_i changes appear to be contributed by the neurotransmitters, by Na^+/H^+ exchange and by the reversible, electrogenic Na^+-HCO_3^- cotransporter as well as by organic acid transporters and metabolic processes. With respect to the action of neurotransmitters on pH_i and most pH_i regulating mechanisms, glial cells appear to resemble neurons, while the electrogenic Na^+-HCO_3^- cotransporter, reminiscent of epithelial cells, exists exclusively in glial cells in nervous systems.

The action of neuronal electrical activity, neurotransmitters and the H^+/HCO_3^--transporting carriers in the cell membranes produce pH shifts in neurons, ECS and glial cells. It often seems necessary to monitor pH in all three compartments in order to understand the mechanisms of the acid and alkaline transients. Often, the pH shifts in the ECS are mirror images of intracellular pH changes; however,

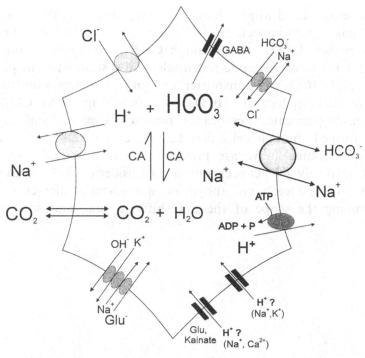

Fig. 11.6. Schematic summary of membrane channels and carriers relevant for pH_i assumed for a hypothetical glial cell. The carbonic anhydrase (CA) catalyses a fast equilibrium between $H^+ + HCO_3^-$ and $CO_2 + H_2O$, to which the cell membrane is permeable. An ATP-driven proton pump has been suggested, and the H^+ permeability of glutamate and acetylcholine receptor channels still need to be shown more directly (hence marked with question mark). The glutamate uptake carrier can acidify a glial cell. The steady-state pH_i, at least in some glial cell types, appears to be dominated by electrogenic Na^+-HCO_3^- cotransport, which may operate as a voltage-dependent pH_i clamp. For further details see text. (Modified from Deitmer 1995.)

different kinetics and spatial extents of intra- and extracellular pH transients can make it difficult to match, e.g. intracellular acidosis with extracellular alkalosis. In addition, we still know little about intracellular processing of H^+ or about the significance, capacity and time course of organellar H^+ sequestration and storage. Although we have long accepted that most biological processes display some pH dependence, we know much less about the involvement of H^+ than about, e.g. the role of Ca^{2+}, in initiating and shaping signalling cascades in and between cells.

We have begun to learn some of the mechanisms of the diverse and multiphasic, extra- and intracellular pH changes. It is clear that glial cells regulate their pH_i, and make a significant contribution to the pH_e shifts, which feed back on neuronal and glial cell functions. Thus, pH transients have characteristics of signals, analogous to Ca^{2+} transients.

For nearly all events related to pH changes in nervous tissue, the presence of CO_2 and HCO_3^- has a great impact. HCO_3^- determines the buffering power to a large extent, it enables HCO_3^- flux through $GABA_A$ receptor channels and thereby modifies the inhibitory synaptic potentials, and it stimulates the powerful glial electrogenic Na^+-HCO_3^- cotransporter and other carriers such as Na^+-dependent and Na^+-independent Cl^-/HCO_3^- exchange (Fig. 11.6). CO_2, as an inert gas, which easily permeates membranes, rapidly dissipates from any location where it is formed through cells and tissues, and together with a high enzyme activity of carbonic anhydrase provides an effective and high buffer capacity even at relatively low concentrations. Considering H^+ transients as signals, CO_2, HCO_3^- and carbonic anhydrase are essential elements in this signalling, determining the shape of the pH shifts in time and space within nervous systems.

12

Intracranial Slow Potential Shifts and Behavioural State

PETER R. LAMING, ALISTER U. NICOL and
JOHN V. ROUGHAN

Summary

Slow or sustained potential shifts (SPSs) are long-lasting changes (from ca. 0.5 to tens of seconds) in the direct current (DC) recorded potential of a region of nervous tissue. Intracranially recorded slow potentials occur in the brains of all vertebrates thus far studied in response to trains of electrical pulses applied to the brain or to sensory stimuli. At the site of stimulation or sensory input, SPS responses are negative and reflect neuronal activity, extracellular potassium ($[K^+]_e$) and glial depolarisation.

Slow potential shift responses are of greater amplitude in mammals and birds than in fish and amphibians. However, in all species they seem to reflect the biological relevance of a stimulus, whether this be a consequence of novelty, learning or motivational state.

In brain regions distant from the site of initial excitation, SPS waveforms may be negative, positive or have several polarity phases, presumably reflecting alternating or multiple sinks and sources of spatial buffering currents. At these sites remote from the source of the evoking stimulus or in cases of 'spontaneous' shifts, local neuronal activity and the local SPS amplitude and duration may be dissociated from each other, suggesting some degree of independence of the eliciting mechanisms and hinting at an active role for glia. These situations arise during changes in motivation and in certain learning paradigms. They can also result from surgery, drug treatments and anaesthesia.

The amplitudes of SPSs reflect the level of behavioural arousal of an animal as measured by changes in heart rate in fish or behavioural activity in gerbils. Prior to development of drug-induced seizures in fish or in seizure prone gerbils, (whilst not expressing seizures), SPS amplitudes and these measures of arousal are elevated.

Apart from the SPS, there are long lasting, apparently tonic, DC changes in the brain associated with profound behavioural change, such as from wakefulness to sleep or anaesthesia, which may also have ionic fluxes as a component of their origin. During induction of anaesthesia, large DC oscillations indicate disruption of mechanisms which normally regulate extracellular ionic movements.

The SPS reflects ionic movements within the brain and between the brain and other fluid compartments, movements largely controlled by glia. The long phylogenetic association between these shifts and changes in behavioural state, combined with their ability to be dissociated from local neuronal activity, suggests that they comprise an important component of the mechanisms by which behaviour is adaptively modified.

12.1 Introduction

Caton in 1875 first described the 'steady cortical current voltage' and the much smaller ($< 100\,\mu V$) oscillations of potential known as the electroencephalogram (EEG). The EEG attracted much more interest than the SPS, even though the latter may reach amplitudes in the order of millivolts.

Little subsequent progress in SPS recording occurred until the middle of this century. Apart from an apparent lack of interest, there were at least two technical reasons for this. Firstly, early DC amplifiers exhibited considerable drifts in potential, making the biological component difficult if not impossible to interpret. Secondly, metal electrodes demonstrate polarisation when immersed in electrolyte and therefore generate their own potential, difficult to distinguish from those of biological origin. The development of stable transistorised DC amplifiers and non-polarisable electrodes during the last 50 years has greatly improved these recordings and enhanced interest in their relationships both with behaviour and the underlying cellular events. Thus, research into intracranial SPSs was regenerated in the 1950s when Arduini et al. (1957) first elicited a cortical, surface-negative potential change following stimulation of the reticular formation in the cat.

Since the early recordings made by Caton, similar duration changes of potential have been recorded extracranially from mammals including humans and the description of 'contingent negative variation' (CNV) by Walter et al. (1964) generated interest amongst behaviourists and psychologists. The progress in that area of research is described in the following chapter; it is mentioned here because those shifts are considered likely to reflect intracranial shifts. Both types of study have continued at a moderate pace since that time.

This brief historical statement has been made to illustrate the development of two lines of SPS research, both showing links with behavioural phenomena. However, until recently, neither has yielded evidence as to the origin of these slow shifts, or the relationships between intra- and extracranial events. Evidence was presented in the last two chapters, that intracranial SPSs are largely a reflection of redistribution of extracellular ions, especially K^+, via the glial syncytium. This concept is supported by findings presented here, derived from a behavioural rather than a neuroscience perspective.

12.2 Origins of SPS Responses

The vast majority of slow potential recordings from behaving animals have until recently been derived from the cortex of mammals. This has given rise to the perhaps erroneous conclusion that they are only related to behaviour in corticate vertebrates. The ancient phylogeny of the vertebrate SPS is evidenced by recent findings in fish and amphibia which also display SPS responses, albeit with a much lesser amplitude (30–300 µV) than those of mammals (mV). This difference may reflect the phylogenetic increase in glial number and differentiation (Chapter 2). In the sections that follow, the conditions with which intracranially recorded SPSs have been commonly associated are described, with a greater stress on phylogenetic comparisons than has been possible hitherto.

12.2.1 SPS Responses to Direct Electrical Stimulation

Electrical stimulation of the mammalian cortex with a short (0.2–0.8 ms) square wave pulse induces a brief (20–30 ms) negative wave at the cortical surface. This is known as the dendritic response (Chang 1951), as it represents the excitatory postsynaptic potentials (EPSPs) of apical dendrites. Such responses can be induced regardless of the polarity of stimulation (Roitbak and Fanardjian 1981). As the strength of the stimulating current is increased, the amplitude of the dendritic response increases proportionally, and a second, longer duration (250 ms) negativity develops (Chang 1951; Goldring et al. 1959). The intensity required to provoke the secondary negativity is close to that required to induce depolarisation of deeply situated glial cells identified by their high resting potential and their lack of either spike activity or activity within the EEG range (Roitbak and Fanardjian 1981). Increasing the frequency of the applied pulses to the cortical surface causes prolonged negativity, associated with summation of the secondary negativity (O'Leary and Goldring 1964) and glial depolarisation (Karahashi and Goldring 1966; Ransom and Goldring 1973a,b; Roitbak and Fanardjian 1981; Roitbak et al. 1987). The latter paper suggested that the SPS can be almost entirely accounted for by glial depolarisation, except for the first 300 ms to which inhibitory post synaptic potentials (IPSPs) make a major contribution. It is probable that events occurring in the first 500–700 ms after stimulation include elements of both neuronal and glial, event-related depolarisations.

Generation of SPSs also occurs with stimulation of the optic tectum of conscious but immobilised anuran amphibia (frogs and toads). The optic tectum is the main integrative region of the brains of these animals and its electrical stimulation to single stimuli provokes dendritic responses (Fig. 12.1A). The initial negativity of these dendritic responses declines on repeated stimulation, and is replaced by an SPS (Fig. 12.1B) (Laming, Ocherashvili and Nicol 1992) which, as in mammals, outlasts the stimulus by seconds (Roitbak and Fanardjian 1981). The amplitude of

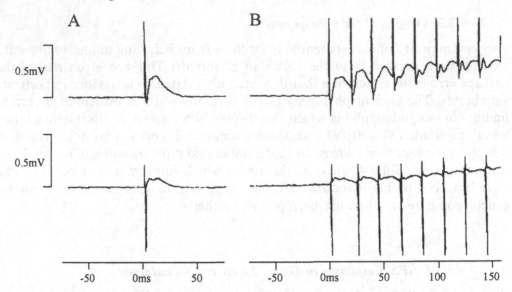

Fig. 12.1. (A) Dendritic response to a 600-μs, 100-μA pulse to the surface of the optic tectum. Note that the artifact changes polarity with polarity of the stimulus (upper compared to lower trace). (B) With repetition of a 500-μs, 100-μA stimulus at 50-Hz for 1 s, the dendritic responses decline, superimposed on a generated SPS. (After Laming, Ocherashvili and Nicol 1992.)

SPSs so generated reflect the 'strength' of the stimulus, whether this be measured by pulse duration, current or frequency (Fig. 12.2).

It thus appears that slow negativity of the cortical surface of mammals and of the similarly laminate, yet also radially organised tectum of amphibia can be induced by electrical stimulation, which also induces glial depolarisation. A number of studies have also demonstrated a close association between glial depolarisation and the elevated extracellular potassium ion concentrations ($[K^+]_e$) resulting from neuronal activation in both mammalian (Ransom and Goldring 1973b; Somjen and Trachtenberg 1979; Heinemann et al. 1979; Roitbak et al. 1987) and non-mammalian (Kuffler, Nicholls and Orkand 1966; Roitbak et al. 1992) vertebrates. At the site of electrical stimulation, the induced SPS negativity closely paralleled the rise in $[K^+]_e$ and therefore has been considered to reflect activation of a region of nervous tissue (Fig. 12.3). This relationship is not constant with depth of recording (Fig. 12.4), as in amphibia the SPS is maximal at the tectal surface (0–200 μm), to invert at depth (450 μm), perhaps as the electrode encounters the optic ventricle. In comparison, $[K^+]_e$ rises were maximal at 200 μm and declined to zero at 550 μm (Roitbak et al. 1992). The cause of the SPS is probably K^+ released from unmyelinated optic nerve fibres in the upper two-fifths of the tectum, depolarising the radial glial elements and initiating the electric currents seen as the SPS, with a current source in the periventricular regions.

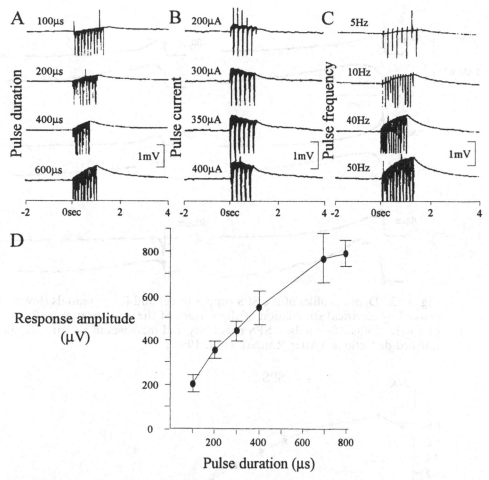

Fig. 12.2. SPS response amplitude changes with differing characteristics of a 1 s pulse train, delivered by paired stimulating electrodes, ca. 1 mm distant from the recording electrode on the tectal surface. Amplitude increases with pulse duration (A), current (B) and frequency (C). Results from four frogs with directly comparable recording situations are presented (mean ±SEM) in (D). Up is negative, down positive, with respect to an extra-cerebral reference. (After Laming, Ocherashvili and Nicol 1992.)

Similar relationships between SPSs and $[K^+]_e$ have been described for cortical and transcallosal stimulation in the cat, where the relationship between SPS and $[K^+]_e$ can be disturbed, as the SPS tends to decline before $[K^+]_e$ returns to normal. This has been ascribed to a more generalised elevation of $[K^+]_e$, causing a similarly widely distributed glial depolarisation (Ocherashvili and Roitbak 1992).

The fact that the depth profiles of the SPS are similar in the radially organised tectum of amphibia (Laming, Ocherashvili and Nicol 1992) and teleost fish (Nicol, Savage and Laming 1993), as well as the cortex of mammals (Ocherashvili and

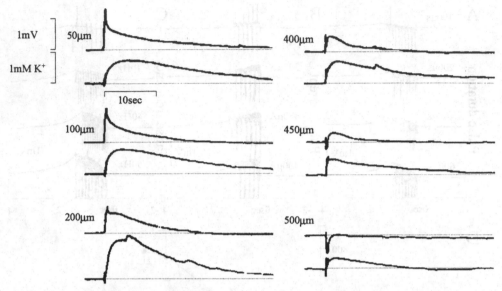

Fig. 12.3. Depth profiles of the SPS (upper trace) and K^+ potentials (lower trace) evoked by electrical stimulation of the surface of the optic tectum by 0.4-s trains of 50-Hz, 50-μs, 40-V pulses. SPS negativity and increases in K^+ are revealed by upward deflections. (After Roitbak et al. 1992.)

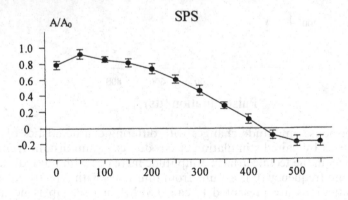

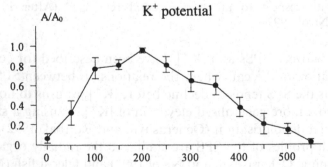

Fig. 12.4. Plot of mean ±SEM ($n = 10$) of changes in SPS and K^+ potential to electrical stimulation of the frog tectal surface. Note that the SPS is maximal at 50 μm, the K^+ potential at 200 μm. (After Roitbak et al. 1992.)

Roitbak 1992), may demonstrate similar source and sink relationships in these tissues. In the lower vertebrates, the tectum is characterised by primarily radial, sensory processing fibres and radial glia. In the mammalian cortex, a similar arrangement of radially oriented neurons is present and astrocytes may also be radially oriented (Colombo et al. 1995).

Studies on electrically induced SPS activity have revealed that they represent extracellular ionic fluxes which depolarise glia. However, such studies have described little of their relationships with behaviour, those on mammals employing anaesthetised animals or isolated brain preparations. To examine the relationships between SPSs and behaviour effectively, more biologically normal preparations are necessary.

12.2.2 Reactive Responses to Sensory Stimuli

To record SPSs in relation to behaviour, natural stimuli and unanaesthetised preparations are required. In unrestrained animals, movement can produce artifactual contamination of recordings, or SPSs induced by the central motor command centres themselves may render interpretation of the sensory response component difficult (see later section). Averaging techniques may overcome some of these problems if the response is resistant to habituation (Roughan and Laming 1998). There has, nevertheless, developed a quite substantial literature on mammalian 'reactive' SPS responses to sensory stimuli (Rowland et al. 1985), which may have a general distribution in the cortex or may be localised.

In unrestrained cats, Gumnit (1961) recorded SPS responses to acoustic stimuli in the auditory cortex. Lickey and Fox (1966), using a muscle relaxant to immobilise the animal, similarly found surface negative SPS responses to visual, auditory and peripheral electroshock stimuli, localised in the primary sensory region for the stimulus modality used. This SPS could extend, with reduced amplitude, to other cortical regions or could appear in other regions as positivity. However, the relationship between the sensory significance of the response and its polarity, may not be a simple one, as Rowland (1968), using cortical, bipolar recordings from a reference electrode and one 1.5 mm sub-surface, found a negative shift to light onset and a positive one to offset. The duration of the response could be prolonged, raising the possibility that the presence of visual stimulation is associated with negativity and its absence with positivity. In general, however, negativity of the SPS has been associated with activation of a region of brain tissue. Positivity of the SPS may reflect inhibition, or a passive source of current in responses to negativity in an active region. The occurrence of SPS responses in the mammalian cortex has led many to assume that it is a strictly cortical phenomenon, yet SPSs in response to visual stimulation have been recorded from the hyperstriatum of pigeons, a region lacking a laminated cortical structure (Durkovic and Cohen 1966, 1968). This led to the proposal that a radially organised structure was not necessary for the expression of SPSs. This concept might be supported by recordings of SPSs from apparently non-radially organised or laminated regions of the fish brain, such as the telencephalon and medulla (Nicol and Laming 1992).

Evidence has accumulated to emphasise that the SPS recorded intracranially is a general expression of sensory activity in vertebrates as a whole. In response to direct electrical stimulation, or sensory stimuli, the negative SPS reflects the strength of the stimulus or the activity of local neurons, respectively. Thus, in anurans, the SPS amplitude is correlated with visual unit activity at the tectal surface, where it is presumably the retinal ganglion cell input that releases K^+ and thus generates the SPS (Laming and Ewert 1984). In response to the onset of illumination, the tectal surface SPS also closely reflects changes in $[K^+]_e$ (Roitbak et al. 1992). In mammals also, the reactive SPS to sensory stimulation is fairly closely correlated with the neuronal activity (Rowland 1968).

Reactive SPSs are always negative at the source of their generation, but may be reflected elsewhere in the brain by either positivity or negativity. In the teleost, *Carassius auratus* (goldfish), a negative SPS is evoked in the midbrain in response to visual or pressure-wave stimuli, whilst in the fore and hind brain regions, the SPS is initially positive (Quick and Laming 1990). In the common toad, *Bufo bufo,* SPS responses were first recorded in conscious but immobilised animals in response to stimuli which emulated natural prey objects (Laming and Ewert 1984). In the optic tectum, these stimuli caused activation of visual units, an increase in EEG frequency and amplitude and a monophasic negative SPS, these being recorded with the same electrode. At the tectal surface, the region of retinal fibre input, the unit activity preceded EEG changes and the SPS, but in deeper layers of the sensory processing system, the SPS marginally preceded the EEG change but significantly pre-empted the activity of local units. This led to the suggestion that the radial glial potassium buffering currents were acting to translocate K^+ to deep layers of the sensory processing system prior to the onset of activity in the neurons themselves (Laming 1989a; Fig. 12.5). A system of this nature is made possible by the lack of synaptic delay in the glial syncytium, and would be adaptive, in that it would 'prime' neurons likely to be imminently in receipt of visual input. The release of $[K^+]_e$ in reponse to sensory stimulation, as implied by this hypothesis, is evidenced by SPSs and changes in $[K^+]_e$ recorded in response to a visual stimulus in frogs. These have a similar depth profile to that induced by tectal electrical stimulation (Roitbak et al. 1992; Fig. 12.2).

The toad tectum derives much of its ability to discriminate prey from non-prey from inhibitory projections arising from the pretectal thalamus that are activated by non-prey stimuli. If appropriately positioned small lesions are made in the pretectal thalamus, the toad will treat almost any moving object as prey (Ewert 1989). In an immobilised animal, a similar lesion causes enhanced neuronal responses to visual stimuli, and the selectivity of units for the configuration of the stimulus is lost. In spite of the greatly enhanced neuronal activity in the tectum, the SPS is considerably attenuated (Laming and Ewert 1983). In contrast,

Sensory input

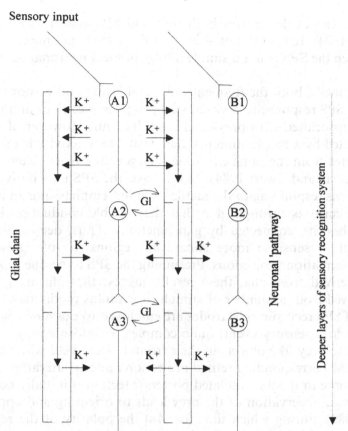

Fig. 12.5. A mechanism by which glia may sensitise neurons by relocation of potassium in a radially organised sensory system, like the toad tectum. On arrival of the sensory input, active neurons, e.g. A1, release K^+ which is translocated to the regions of A2 and A3, which are therefore partially depolarised prior to the specific neuronal activity being conducted through the A1/A2 and A2/A3 synapses. Spatial buffering would make this sensitisation mechanism passive, but could be more dramatic as glia have active uptake of K^+ and participate in glutamate metabolism. In sensory systems that are organised topographically to represent spatial sensory experience, like the visual system, neurons in areas close to the part of the sensory map being stimulated would also be sensitised (B1, B2, B3) and responses to moving objects would be enhanced. (After Laming 1989a.)

telencephalic ligature causes declines in both unit and SPS responses (Laming, Ewert and Borchers 1984). It would thus seem that there are experimentally contrived conditions when the SPS is not a simple mirror of local neuronal activity in toads.

In freely behaving toads, both the frequency of tectal visual unit responses and the amplitude of the SPS response to a visual stimulus is greater than in immobilised animals and is associated with prey-catching behaviour. However, if defensive behaviour is elicited by a tactile stimulus, then visual unit activity is minimal, whilst the SPS recorded from the same electrode is larger than from visual stimulation (Laming, Borchers and Ewert 1984). In this case, the SPS may derive from deeper midbrain regions responding to the tactile stimulus, emphasising an important aspect of ionic currents through glia: that they enable conduction in any direction in which they are connected by gap junctions. Thus, deep activation could potentially act to sensitise more superficial regions, a role previously ascribed to reticular formation projections. Presuming the SPS to be due to spatial buffering currents derived from glia, these results suggest that glia may act to integrate effects derived from a number of stimuli or stimulus modalities.

When a number of SPS recording electrodes are employed to examine responses of behaving animals to a sensory event, quite complex waveforms may emerge. Thus, toads respond to prey-like objects in their frontal visual field with an initially negative SPS in the corresponding retinal projection (antero–lateral) region of the tectum. The response in the unstimulated posterior tectum is initially positive. In the behaving animal, observation of the prey leads to orienting and approach behaviour (Ewert 1989), during which time (ca. 4 s) the polarity of the regional waves becomes reversed. If the same animals are immobilised, they still exhibit anterior negativity and posterior positivity in tectal SPS responses to the prey stimulus. However, under such conditions these responses are monophasic, suggesting that some aspect of the behaviour itself might explain 'rebound' in SPS polarity. One explanation is that the movement of the toad causes visual input to the whole tectum to be activated and thus causes many different sources and sinks to be generated (Laming et al. 1995).

Of perhaps greater interest was the finding that in immobilised animals with no visual stimulation of the posterior tectal projection region, a positive SPS was recorded which mirrored the negative SPS in the stimulated region of the anterior tectum. This implies that sinks and sources for current may be present across the surface of the tectum as well as through its depth. If the conduction pathway through the depth of the optic tectum is via radially oriented glia, then that across the surface may be via tangentially oriented glia. Glial processes are often tangentially oriented at the brain surface, which itself is comprised of a sheet of glial cells or radial glial endfeet as part of the pia limitans, which separates cerebrospinal fluid (CSF) of the subarachnoid space from the fluid of the extracellular space (ECS) of the brain (Chapters 1 and 4). The apparent separations between sources and sinks found in these immobilised animals of (1 mm), would suggest a low resistance pathway for current spread (potentially available through the CSF). It would be interesting to determine whether the movement of ions, especially K^+, between ECS and CSF has the buffering properties ascribed to similar K^+ movements in the retina, between vitreous humor and Müller cells (Newman 1986b) and whether such properties might form part of a mechanism for controlling ECS constituents (Chapter 7).

12.2.3 SPS Responses During Arousal and Attention

The reactive responses of animals to sensory input, as described above, vary in association with behavioural state. This may provide clues to the origin of that state.

Animals are not in a constant state of alertness. Even when awake, there are periods when neural activity and the behaviour of the animal are increased. The animal may be described as being 'aroused'. External factors which induce arousal are stimuli which have biological relevance because they are novel, or stimuli which are relevant either due to an endogenous trigger (food, mate) or have acquired relevance through experience. The response to such relevant stimuli is the 'orientation reaction' (Sokolov 1963), initially comprising a non-directed alerting response (arousal) associated with generalised increases in neuronal activity, changes in EEG frequencies and amplitudes, a general reduction in sensory thresholds, SPSs and changes in measures of peripheral physiology such as heart and ventilatory rate. This initial generalised response is brief, especially in mammals, and is followed by a more directed behaviour towards the source of the stimulus and a reduction in the expression of the responses in those regions of the brain not associated with further assessing the stimulus. This secondary phase may be described as 'attention' and includes behavioural orienting towards the stimulus source (Laming 1989a,b). The magnitude of the SPS (in terms of amplitude and/or duration) appears to reflect the level of arousal or activation of the brain (Rowland 1968).

In fish, a bradycardia (a transient reduction in heart rate) provides a quantifiable measure of the arousal response to a novel stimulus and the decline of that response with repetition of the stimulus (Laming and Savage 1980). Situations that evoke a bradycardia, like the onset of increased illumination, also induce SPSs, recorded with implanted electrodes in the midbrain, hindbrain and forebrain (Quick and Laming 1990). These 4–8 s SPSs were predominently negative in the midbrain, positive in the forebrain and mildly positive in the hindbrain in response to a moving visual stimulus, the onset of illumination or a tap to the side of the aquarium. During early presentations of the tap stimulus, when cardiac arousal responses were large, these responses were strongly related, by regression analysis, to the amplitude of the midbrain SPS response to the tap stimulus.

A. Optic Tectum (anterior)

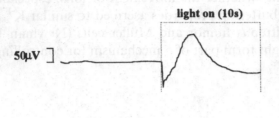
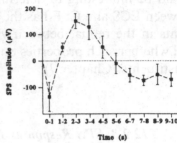

B. Telencephalon (dorsal central)

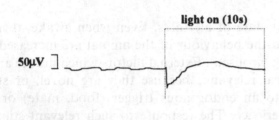
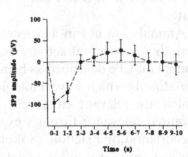

C. Medulla (octavolateralis)

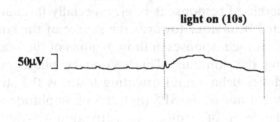
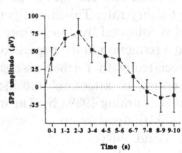

D. Cerebellum (dorsal medial)

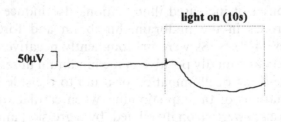
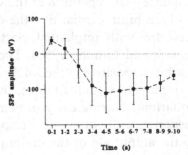

Interest in this relationship provoked further studies of cardiac arousal and SPS responses, this time with Ag/AgCl electrodes on the telencephalic, anterior tectal, cerebellar and medullary surfaces (Nicol and Laming 1992). Initial presentation of the onset of illumination to fish in a darkened enclosure evoked a bradycardiac arousal response accompanied by a predominantly positive SPS on the medullary surface, one predominantly negative on the cerebellum and an SPS that was initally negative (1–2 s), then positive and returning to negativity on the anterior tectal and the telencephalic surfaces (Nicol and Laming 1992, Fig. 12.6). An SPS response to an arousing stimulus can thus be recorded in many regions of the fish brain, not only those most directly involved in processing the primary stimulus input, though such regions are associated with SPS responses of greatest amplitude.

During arousal, it is considered that all brain responses are amplified, whereas during attention there is selective response inhibition (Lynn 1966). In rabbits, visual evoked potentials are enhanced in amplitude if preceded by cortical negativity (Richter et al. 1992). We have performed studies on fish to determine if evoked potentials to a relatively neutral stimulus (sound) were affected by the prior presentation of an arousing, SPS-evoking stimulus. Presentation of a non-acoustic stimulus to fish may cause an increase or a decrease in the brainstem acoustic evoked potential (AEP) response to subsequently presented 'click' stimuli (Laming and Brooks 1985). When more localised recordings are made it has been found that it is the peak to peak amplitude that is most affected by the preceding stimulus (Laming and Bullock 1991). Although tenuous relationships have been found between the broad-band increase in EEG power in response to the non-acoustic stimulus and the change in the AEP, these were stimulus-specific and could not alone account for the change in sensory evoked activity (Laming, Bullock and McClune 1991a). Sustained potential shift responses and changes in AEP amplitude were thus simultaneously recorded in the midbrain tectum and torus semicircularis in response to water or saline applied to the flank of carp. A 4-s negative SPS wave was followed by a positive one in response to both stimuli (Laming Bullock and McClune 1991b). Trains of six clicks delivered in the absence of a priming stimulus showed that the highest amplitude AEP was that evoked by the first click in the train. With a priming stimulus, this AEP was the most attenuated, indicating an attentional rather than an arousal response type, arousal being associated with increased evoked potential amplitudes (Lynn 1996). These changes in AEP amplitude did not relate to the SPS in the region

---

Fig. 12.6. Examples of SPSs on the left and on the right, mean ±SEMs of amplitudes recorded from the surface of (A) the tectum ($n = 13$); (B) the telencephalon ($n = 13$); (C) the medulla ($n = 12$); and (D) the cerebellum ($n = 12$) of a goldfish in response to a visual stimulus (the onset of illumination for 10 s). (After Nicol and Laming 1992.)

where these were recorded. Rather, they showed relationships with the SPS in the other region from which recordings were made (i.e. torus or tectum). Although these studies suggested links between mechanisms generating the SPS and mechanisms causing changes in sensory evoked responses, they were not shown to be causally related and were coincidentally timed so that the SPS was going from negative to positive at a time when the AEP was attenuated.

Further experiments were therefore performed in which the fish was subjected to continuous background auditory stimulation (clicks delivered at 1 click/s), with averaging of AEP response changes, subsequent to the induction of SPSs on the telencephalic, posterior tectal and medullary surfaces in response to the onset of illumination. The posterior midbrain response was similar to that of the cerebellum reported previously, i.e. a largely monophasic, 10 s duration negative wave; the medulla gave a small positive wave and that on the telencephalic surface was smaller still, and positive (Nicol and Laming 1993). Attenuation of AEPs was again recorded in response to illumination onset as the priming stimulus, again suggesting an attentional response. However, least attenuation was associated with large cardiac responses, indicating that both facilitatory and inhibitory (arousal and attention) mechanisms might be simultaneously active. Again, the amplitudes of these SPSs were closely related across the different regions. Correlations were also found between stimulus-evoked changes in AEP amplitude and simultaneously recorded SPSs during initial presentations of the stimulus: in the telencephalon SPS amplitude and changes in AEP amplitude were significantly correlated, and changes in midbrain AEP amplitude were significantly correlated with SPS amplitudes in the telencephalon and the medulla. These studies on fish have revealed that many modalities of naturalistic stimuli induce SPS responses in most regions of the brains of fish. These responses are often related to cardiac (arousal) responses, but also share features of attention in that they accompany regional attenuation of sensory evoked neuronal activity.

12.3 Arousal and Seizures

The association of large SPS responses with behavioural and cardiac expressions of arousal, led to speculation as to whether elevated neuronal activity, expressed in seizure tendency, was associated with heightened arousal and accordingly with heightened SPS responses. This hypothesis would suggest that seizures should occur during the aroused state. Although this may often be the case in mammals, they also occur during sleep, albeit in the waking phase (Niedermeyer 1982). They are, however, associated with massive SPSs (e.g. Swann and Brady 1983). In the present discussion, however, we confine our interest to those periods when animals with seizure tendencies are behaving relatively normally.

12.3.1 Seizures in Fish

To establish whether there are links between seizure propensity and arousal, experiments were initially performed on fish, in spite of the fact that seizures are rare and chemical seizure induction thresholds are high in less phylogenetically advanced vertebrates (Servit 1977). Teleost fish are among the simplest vertebrates to express arousal responses to novelty or to respond to epileptogenic agents with seizures. Seizures can be initiated in fish by applying aluminium hydroxide topically to the brain surface or by intramuscular injection of sodium penicillin (Laming, Rooney and Ferguson 1987). Roach *(Rutilus rutilus)* with either treatment, prior to seizure development, consistently took more presentations of 'tap' or 'light on' stimuli for habituation of behavioural arousal responses than controls. Subsequently seizures developed with an increase in maximum EEG amplitude from $70 \mu V$ to over 1 mV. Seizures initially involved an abnormal 'weaving' movement of the body; later, they comprised violent, uncoordinated muscular activity. Goldfish (*Carassius auratus*) with electrodes for monitoring cardiac activity and treated with topically applied aluminium hydroxide, exhibited cardiac arousal responses to a 'light on' stimulus of over twice the normal value, prior to seizure development. This latter study, using heart rate changes as a quantifiable measure of arousal, would suggest that the delay in habituation found in both studies was a consequence of heightened arousal, rather than intervention in the process of habituation.

These results demonstrate links between arousal and seizures and arousal and SPSs but further work has also implicated glutamate in arousal. Both glutamatergic over-activity and γ-aminobutyric acid (GABA)ergic under-activity are candidates for seizure induction. Experiments were therefore performed to determine the effects of topically applied glutamate or GABA on arousal responses of fish. The brain of teleosts occupies less than 50% of the cranial cavity, so perfusion of this cavity with fluid is a simple operation. Perfusion with glutamate at physiological levels or above gave a dose related increase in cardiac arousal responses to a novel stimulus. GABA at even higher levels had no such effect (Laming and Lenke 1991). These results and those of Jasper, Khan and Elliot (1965), which indicated that glutamate was present at a higher concentration in the aroused state compared to ambient wakefulness, and in ambient wakefulness compared with sleep, implicate glutamate in the regulation of levels of neuronal activity. Such increased activity is also evident during epileptogenesis in carp *(Cyprinus carpio)*, as acoustic evoked responses in the torus semicircularis are approximately doubled in amplitude 5 h after the topical application of aluminium hydroxide to the brain and prior to seizure genesis (Laming, Bullock and McClune 1991b). A similar treatment also elevates motor output, like the electric organ discharge of the mormyrid electric fish (*Gnathonemus petersii*), which reaches a maximum just prior to EEG seizures and then becomes silent prior to recovery or death (Laming, Rooney and Szabo 1991).

All these experiments loosely link arousal, seizures, SPSs, enhanced sensory and motor responsiveness and glutamate in regulation of CNS activity and behaviour in fish. The method of seizure genesis was unlikely to reflect 'natural' mechanisms of seizure genesis, however, so further experiments were performed on gerbils.

12.3.2 Seizures in Gerbils

Established laboratory colonies of the Mongolian gerbil (*Meriones unguiculatus*) usually have some individuals which will exhibit seizures when confronted with a novel situation like an 'open field' (Thiessen, Lindzey and Friend 1968). These seizures can be quantified on a numerical scale, ranging from 0 to 5.5, depending on how many seizure-related behavioural activities are performed. Individuals scoring more than 2 on this scale are considered seizure-prone (SP), those scoring zero, non-seizure prone (NSP). On repeated presentation to the 'open field' arena SP animals cease to have seizures but ambulate more than NSP individuals. SP animals also show less attentive 'rearing' behaviour. As ambulation is considered a measure of arousal in these animals (Nauman 1968), these experiments indicate that seizure-prone gerbils are also more 'arousable' than NSP animals which show more attentional behaviour (Laming, Elwood and Best 1989).

A link between glial activity, arousal and seizures in gerbils has been established by the finding that SP individuals have a deficiency in glutamine synthetase (GS) activity in the frontal cerebral cortex (Laming, Cosby and O'Neill 1989), though the posterior cortex seems to be the EEG-determined site of origin of seizures in these animals (Majkowski and Donadio 1984). Glutamine synthetase is a glutamate deactivating enzyme of almost purely glial origin (Shousboe 1981) and its lack accounted for 40% of the variance of seizures in regression analysis. Statistical (principal components) analysis (PCA) also revealed direct relationships between seizure expression, ambulation and glial cell count and an inverse relationship between seizure score and GS activity. Further examination of brain amino acid levels have indicated elevated glutamine and arginine in SP animals. Levels of glutamate, aspartate, glycine, citrulline and cysteine were, in contrast, reduced (Gardiner, Laming and Blumson 1993). Subsequent studies have revealed that SP animals have elevated brain and plasma ammonia levels and by artificially elevating intraventricular ammonia seizures are induced by lower doses in SP compared to NSP animals (Gardiner and Laming unpublished results). This research has implicated ammonia and amino acid metabolism in the expression of seizures in gerbils. Perhaps more importantly, they also suggest that similar mechanisms operating at less extreme levels, may be responsible for changes in brain activity associated with behavioural arousal.

The apparent involvement of glial enzymes important in metabolism of neurotransmitter amino acids, in the expression of seizure propensity in gerbils has prompted an examination of spontaneous SPSs during ambulatory (arousal-related) and rearing (attention-related) behaviours.

Average calculations of behavioural tendency for seizures, ambulatory activity and rearing behaviour were derived by testing 50 animals in an 'open field' arena (a 1 m × 1 m × 0.25 m high black box), for five 3-min periods (trials) with inter-trial intervals of 3-min periods of rest in their home cage (Laming, Elwood and Best 1989). Seizure prone animals displayed seizures, mainly during trial 1, which was used to derive the seizure score. Behaviour during trials 3–5 was used to derive measures of ambulatory and rearing tendency. During these trials, SP animals made significantly more ambulations than were expressed by NSP animals, and less high rearing behaviour. As in previous studies, the results showed that SP animals exhibit a greater level of arousal, and less tendency to express attentional behaviour.

Two weeks after behavioural testing, 12 of the NSP animals with a seizure score of zero and 12 of the SP animals with seizure scores ranging from 2.0 to 5.0 were prepared by implantation of Ag/AgCl ball (0.5 mm diameter) electrodes, positioned 1 mm anterior to (anterior), 1.8 mm posterior to (mid) and 4.5 mm posterior to (posterior) the bregma on each cortical hemispere, 2 mm lateral to the sagittal suture. Subjects were gently introduced to a reduced arena (0.4 × 0.4 m × 0.5 m high black box) and SPSs were recorded simultaneously from each recording site for 10 × 16 s epochs whilst the animal was not performing active behaviours. Animals that exhibited seizures were excluded from further recordings. Subsequently, > 15 SPS recordings were taken during ambulatory and rearing behaviours; these recordings incorporated 5 s preceding the moment of onset of behaviour and for the subsequent 11 s.

Fifteen recordings of the SPS for each of the three behavioural categories (control periods, ambulation and rearing) were sampled via a laboratory interface (Cambridge Electronic Design, Ltd, UK), stored on a computer and averaged using signal averaging software (Cambridge Electronic Design). The data were then further reduced by measuring the average amplitude of the averaged waveform during each of eight 2-s periods during the 16-s recording period giving a total of eight measures of the SPS over time.

Statistical (PCA) analyses showed that ambulatory and seizure tendencies were positively related, agreeing with previous findings (Laming, Elwood and Best 1989) and that during ambulatory behaviour both are related to overall SPS positivity across the right anterior cortical surface and negativity across the opposite posterior cortical surface (Fig. 12.7, factor 2). Ambulatory tendency was also related to mid-cortical positivity of the surface SPS (Fig. 12.7, factor 1). It was thus apparent that the positivity of the right anterior cortex was associated with the exhibition of ambulatory behaviour, i.e. behaviour which was enhanced in SP animals.

Previous work has shown a negative relationship between attentive rearing and 'aroused' behaviour (Laming, Elwood and Best 1989). It is therefore perhaps surprising that the positivity of the SPS on the right anterior cortex of SP animals

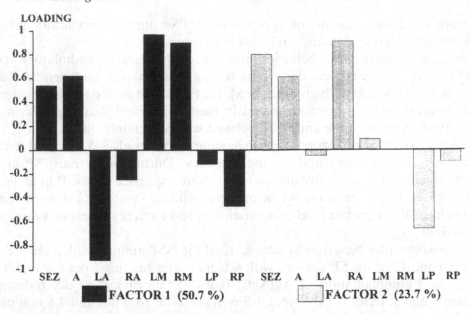

Fig. 12.7. A Varimax rotated principal components analysis (PCA) to find any relationships between behavioural tendencies (seizure score, ambulations) and the averaged SPS activity (pooled for all time periods) recorded subsequent to behavioural testing, during normal ambulation. PCA divides the total variability into factors, within which are common sources of variability. Loadings for variables > 0.6 are considered important. Percentage figures denote the proportion of variability accounted for by each factor. SEZ = seizure score; A = ambulatory tendency. Electrode positions are given by LA (left anterior cortex); RA (right anterior cortex); LM (left mid-cortex); RM (right mid-cortex); LP (left posterior cortex); and RP (right posterior cortex). Note that seizure scores, ambulatory tendency and right posterior SPS positivity are related (factor 2), as are ambulatory activity, left anterior SPS negativity and midbrain positivity (factor 1).

occurred with rearing as well as with ambulatory behaviour. The relationships between the initial quantitative measures of behaviour (the ambulatory and rearing tendencies and seizure scores) and the SPS pooled for all time periods at each recording site were therefore examined using PCA. In this analysis, rearing tendency and seizure scores were associated with different factors; seizure score was associated with ambulatory tendency and with right anterior positivity and left posterior negativity of the SPS, and rearing tendency was associated with bilateral mid-cortical SPS negativity.

These results indicate that (a) regionally specific SPS responses are associated with ambulatory and rearing behaviour, and (b) the right anterior and left posterior cortical SPS responses are associated with a gerbil's tendency to express seizure-related behaviour. Previous EEG studies have suggested that seizures in gerbils may have a focal origin in the cortex (Loskota and Lomax 1975; Suzuki and Nakamoto 1978), although others suggest a contribution by sub-cortical regions, especially the hippocampus (Peterson, Ribak and Oertel 1985; Peterson and Ribak 1987). The association of left posterior SPS responses with ambulatory and rearing behaviour may support the suggestion that seizures are initiated in the occipital cortex (Majkowski and Donadio 1984). That of the right anterior SPS response might be related to the aforementioned deficiency in glutamine synthetase in that cortical region of SP gerbils (Laming, Cosby and O'Neill 1989).

From these data, it is difficult to determine whether temporally associated opposite polarity effects, such as those between the left anterior and mid-cortices during ambulation, represent a single source-sink distribution of current flow between recording sites. Indeed, it is unlikely that intra-cortical spatial buffering could act by direct glial connections over the distances involved, to produce the observed surface polarity effects. It is possible that many behaviourally associated dipoles (Geddes 1972) are simultaneously active within each region of the cortex, or that extra-cortical current flow through the CSF may occur, as suggested earlier for toads.

These results indicate that SPSs, assumed to reflect activities of cellular populations, differ regionally in magnitude, time course and even polarity between SP and NSP gerbils. That this was not just a group-based difference is apparent from PCA analysis, which identifies common sources of variance between animals. This suggests that the SPS difference reflects quantitative differences in cellular (glial?) activity, related to seizure tendency.

12.4 Plasticity of SPS Responses to Stimuli

One of the features of arousal and attentional responses is that they are responses to biologically relevant stimuli, like a novel event, one with learnt relevance or one with motivational significance. The biological relevance of an initially novel stimulus alters with experience of that stimulus. The amplitudes and waveforms of SPSs evoked by novel stimuli also change with experience of such stimuli.

12.4.1 Changes in the SPS During Habituation

Simple repetition of an initially novel sensory experience may result in a decline in the amplitudes of SPS responses evoked by that stimulus. This was demonstrated for SPS responses to acoustic stimuli in the auditory cortex of the unrestrained cat (Gumnit 1961), and for auditory, visual and peripheral electroshock stimuli in immobilised cats (Lickey and Fox 1966). Similar observations have been made in rats (Caspers 1963; Rowland 1968).

During habituation to a variety of arousing stimuli, the decline in the cardiac arousal response of fish to all types of stimuli used has been found to be related to a decline in the positivity of SPS responses in the telencephalon (Quick and

Laming 1989). This is of interest because of the considerable body of evidence linking telencephalic regions (posterior dorso–central) with habituation of arousal responses in fish (Laming 1981b; Laming and Ennis 1981; Laming and Hornby 1981; Laming and McKee 1981; Rooney and Laming 1986, 1988). Nicol and Laming (1992) found that during the period of habituation of the cardiac arousal response in goldfish to the onset of illumination, SPSs recorded from the telence-phalic, tectal and medullary surfaces in response to the same stimulus also declined in amplitude. In a further study (Nicol and Laming 1993), it was found that such changes in the amplitudes of SPS responses to this stimulus are related to con-current changes in the modulatory effects of the presentation of such stimuli on the amplitudes of AEPs evoked by continuous background auditory stimulation. This was particularly apparent in the telencephalon (Fig. 12.8). In this region, over successive presentations of the visual stimulus, the visually-induced attenuation of AEPs declined, and this decline was related to the change, over the same series of presentations, in the amplitudes of SPSs recorded from the same site. Nicol and Laming (1992) also reported that, once the cardiac arousal response had fully habituated (i.e. when the presentation of the light-on stimulus no longer elicited

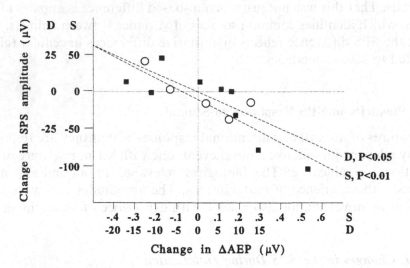

Fig. 12.8. The relationship between SPS responses to a visual stimulus and the acoustic evoked response to a click during response habituation. A 10-s onset of illumination induces an SPS both on the surface and at depth in the telencepha-lon. Telencephalic evoked responses to a continuous train of clicks are attenuated during this SPS. Both the change in acoustic response and the overall SPS response to the visual stimulus change in a significantly related manner during habituation to the visual stimulus over an initial set of four stimuli compared to the four subsequent (probabilities from regression analysis, $n = 7$). The relation-ship existed for both surface (S) recording sites (■) and for those made at depth (D) in the region of the dorsal central nucleus (○). (After Nicol and Laming 1993.)

a bradycardia), the SPS response, having also habituated, returned to the amplitude and polarity evoked by the initial presentation of the arousing stimulus, and, over subsequent presentations of the stimulus, this response was maintained (Fig. 12.9).

A response to an arousing stimulus, having habituated, may return after a period of time during which the stimulus is withdrawn. However, during a series

A. Telencephalic SPS during trial 1

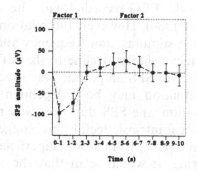

B. SPS amplitudes during trials 1-24

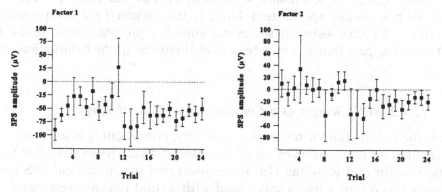

Fig. 12.9. (A) The second by second amplitude (mean ±SEM) of the SPS response recorded from the telencephalic surface of goldfish ($n = 10$) during the first of 24 presentations of a visual stimulus (10 s of illumination). A principal components analysis had identified two factors, accounting for 62% and 18% of the variability respectively, which contributed to this waveform. (B) When examined individually, the component of the waveform attributed to factor 1 declined in amplitude on stimulus repetitions 1–11, when the cardiac arousal response habituated. However, subsequent to trial 12, this early component of the SPS waveform returned to the negativity seen prior to habituation. The later part of the waveform, attributed to factor 2, also exhibited greater negativity after trial 11. (After Nicol and Laming 1992.)

of presentations of such a stimulus subsequent to the initial series, habituation occurs more rapidly (Thompson and Spencer 1966). Thus, habituation has both a transient, short-term component and a long-term component. One might speculate that the sustained return, following habituation, of the SPS response to the initially arousing stimulus in the telencephalon, a region crucially involved in habituation, may reflect long-term changes in glial physiology in that region.

In toads (*Bufo bufo*), intrinsic tectal visual unit activity frequency and burst duration habituate on repeated presentation of a prey-like object to immobilised but conscious animals. This habituation may reflect the unobtainability of the simulated prey. SPS amplitude and duration and the duration of characteristics associated with arousal in the EEG recorded with the same electrode, similarily decline (Laming and Ewert 1984). However, the relationship is not a simple one. Over 20 presentations of the stimulus, unit frequency and burst duration declined to 50% of the original value; a similar decline to that of the duration of SPS and EEG responses. The decline in SPS amplitude was much larger, in the order of 70%, suggesting its habituation may be independent of the decline in unit responses. During habituation, the SPS duration was reduced to closely match that of the bursts of the local intrinsic tectal unit, suggesting that initially it was deriving some of its source $[K^+]_e$ from more superficial (retinal input) regions, perhaps by spatial buffering. It would seem that the spatial buffering currents decline in magnitude disproportionately to the decline in neuronal activity. This may be due to passive build up of $[K^+]_e$ over the repeated stimuli, or to an experiential decline in potentially sensitising, spatial buffering currents. If the former, then it would appear that 1 min is insufficient time for potassium to equilibriate (the time between successive stimulus presentations), if the latter, then it would appear that glia may be actively involved in the habituation process.

12.4.2 SPS Changes as a Consequence of Conditioning

As with the habituation of responses to novelty, conditioning is a situation when there is apparent dissociation of neural activity from activity expressed in the SPS. In cats, Shaefor and Rowland (1974) demonstrated that a cortical SPS could be conditioned to a tone when it was paired with a food reward presented 5 s later. Simultaneously recorded massed action potentials revealed that these were not associated with the SPS response to the tone, though they were correlated with that generated in response to the reward. Irwin and Rebert (1970) have also recorded conditioned SPSs in the motor cortex, hypothalamus and amygdala in response to a tone in cats anticipating a food reward. Rebert, Diehl and Matteucci (1993) and Bauer and Rebert (1990) have since stressed the importance of evocation of sub-cortical SPSs in the learning process. Most other workers have concentrated on cortical, intra-cranial SPS responses for comparison with those recorded epicranially, especially in humans (Chapter 13).

Rowland et al. (1985) refer to an SPS occurring in response to the conditioned stimulus as the proactive SPS. Such SPSs occur prior to the reward and are not correlated with massed action potentials. These proactive SPSs may be similar to the CNV which occurs in the fore-period of a reaction time task in humans (Walter et al. 1964). Although the experimental paradigms are not identical to those used to elicit an epicranially recorded CNV in humans, many have tried to emulate their expression in experimental animals.

Pirch, Corbus and Rigden (1983) paired a tone with rewarding medial forebrain bundle (MFB) stimulation to induce a frontal lobe, CNV-like SPS in rats. They also simultaneously recorded frontal lobe unit activity, which increased at the cortical surface on pairing of the tone with the reward. They interpreted the SPS as reflecting the increased neuronal excitation. Rowland et al. (1985) performed similar experiments using a combined light/tone conditioned stimulus with MFB stimulation as the reward. Again, they reported a negative anticipatory potential in the visual cortex, associated with increased multiple unit activity. In this case, unlike with the food reward, the unit activity and the SPS were associated.

Pirch (1977) and Pirch (1980) have studied the effects of amphetamines on conditioned SPS responses in rats and found differential dose and regional changes in the amplitude of the conditioned SPS, suggesting complex actions of the drug on brain cellular constituents. Acetylcholine, applied iontophoretically to the cortex enhanced neural responses to a conditioned stimulus but left the SPS unaffected (Pirch, Turco and Rucker 1992), again implying dissociation of neural and glial activity. Evidence for a link between SPS responses and inactivation of second messenger molecules has derived from experiments with rats repeatedly given cutaneous 'startling' shocks. An SPS in response to the shock was accompanied by rapid elevation of cyclic adenosine monophosphate (AMP). The subsequent decline in the amplitude of the SPS was related to the decline in cyclic AMP (Skinner et al. 1978).

Several workers have described negative cortical shifts in the period between a conditioned stimulus and a motor response neccessary to obtain a reward. Monkeys were trained to respond to a warning stimulus by pressing a key and holding it down until a second stimulus was given. A transcortical negative variation occurs whilst the animal waits for the second stimulus (Donchin et al. 1971).

The SPS associated with movements might reflect potentials associated with motor cortex activity. Indeed, a surface negative SPS wave preceeds voluntary hand movements in premotor and motor cortices of monkeys (Hashimoto, Gemba and Sasaki 1979). However, Donchin et al. (1971) reported a negative CNV-like wave in animals not required to press the key, indicating that only part of the conditioned SPS could be so explained.

It has become increasingly apparent that the conditioned anticipatory epicortically recorded SPS in animals bears similarities to the human epicranially recorded CNV and is comprised of at least two components. The early component reflects the sensory response to a warning stimulus and anticipation of the imperative stimulus which requires a motor response. The second component of the SPS is the preparative phase, especially in motor cortex, associated with movement. These components have been recognised not only in monkeys (Gemba, Sasaki and Tsujimoto 1986), but also in rats (Nakamura et al. 1993 and Chapter 13).

12.5 SPS Responses Associated with Changes in Motivation

In mammals, large (mV) and often sustained (min) shifts occur in response to consummatory stimuli in animals in a highly motivated state. Perhaps the best examples are those during food intake in hungry cats.

Rowland et al. (1967) recorded shifts in the millivolt range in hungry cats during lapping of a fish/milk homogenate. A large part of the shift was lost if the oral cavity was anaesthetised, suggesting that the response was, in part, a sensory one; however, the shift magnitude was related also to the degree of motivation as greater deprivation enhanced it and feeding caused its decline (Rowland 1968). On satiation, the cats rejected food and the polarity of the SPS was reversed, usually from negative to positive depending on the recording site. Further studies have shown unconditioned SPS responses to food in motor cortex, hypothalamus and amygdala which increased in magnitude with the palatability of the reward. SPS responses in the midbrain reticular formation did not show this relationship (Irwin and Rebert 1970).

Most female mammals show regular periods of sexual activity (oestrus) which can be experimentally induced by hormone treatment. The degree of sexual responsiveness was measured behaviourally in cats, by Rowland (1968), and found to correspond to the magnitude of negative, cortically recorded SPS responses to vaginal stimulation. The SPS to vaginal stimulation continued during the subsequent rolling and rubbing after-response of the animal, but did not occur during equivalent magnitude motor activities not related to sexual behaviour.

Most of the motivational studies of SPS responses in mammals have used the motivational state of the animal to condition SPS and behavioural responses. These have used food or rewarding electrical self-stimulation as positive reinforcement or peripheral electrical stimulation as an aversive stimulus.

In toads, the feeding motivational state of the animal can be tested and quantified by the number of times the animal will perform the behavioural components of the prey catching sequence when presented with a simulated prey object. The 'prey' is an elongate piece of black card moving in its long axis against a contrasting background, i.e. a 'worm'. The behaviours are categorised as 'orient', 'approach', 'fixate' and 'snap' (Ewert 1989). After testing for the motivational state, animals were prepared for recording SPSs during subsequent stimulus presentation. Ag/AgCl 0.5 mm ball electrodes were placed bilaterally on the anterior, mid- and posterior tectal surfaces through small apertures in the cranium and fixed in place before leaving the animal 24 h to recover. Testing with the simulated prey showed that orientation to prey was associated with a negative shift on the anterior tectal surface , the retinal projection region of the frontal visual field. This negative shift was followed by a positive wave after ca. 4 s. On the surface of the posterior tectum, the reverse occurred, i.e. a positive shift was followed by negativity (Laming et al. 1995). The amplitude of these shifts was related to the prey catching motivation prior to the operation. Animals were then re-anaesthetised and immobilised and retested to the 'worm' stimulus. The SPS response now was a monophasic negative wave in the anterior tectum and a monophasic positive wave in the posterior tectum. Again their amplitudes were related to the previously recorded motivational state. In order to determine if the motivational state had been affected by the operation and subsequent testing, animals were again anaesthetised to allow them to recover from the muscle relaxant and they were then tested again. They demonstrated no change in prey catching activity from that exhibited prior to the experiment (Laming et al. 1995). Current experiments indicate that administration of glucose to the stomach of toads eliminates prey catching motivation in 15 min and also causes suppression of both visual unit and SPS responses to 'prey' stimuli (Lewers et al., unpublished). These changes in SPS, reported above, might just reflect overall activation of the brain in response to a stimulus that has acquired significance because of the motivational state of the animal. Whether the change in responsiveness, e.g. due to hunger is initially mediated by changing neuronal and/or glial functions has yet to be determined. (but see Chapters 5, 14, 15).

12.6 DC Changes During Sleep, Wakefulness and Anaesthesia

Although sleep is perhaps the most profound behavioural change exhibited by animals, it has been little explored with respect to a possible glial contribution to its onset and maintenance. In 1961, Caspers reported that the 'tonic' (durations of minutes to hours) DC potential of the rat cortical surface shifted towards negativity on awakening from sleep and towards positivity on sleep onset (Caspers 1961). Several subsequent studies have shown a shift towards negativity during paradoxical sleep (Kawamura and Sawyer 1964; Wurtz 1965), in rabbits and rats, respectively, which in mammals is often equated to dreaming sleep in humans, where cortical activation occurs without behavioural activity. The shift from negativity to positivity in correlation with high to lowered brain activity would accord with negativity in association with activation in the waking state, though whether this involves a glial mechanism has not yet been directly explored. The gross changes in extracellularly recorded 'tonic' DC levels in the brain presumably indicate changes in the ionic balance of ECS, either shunting through the blood–brain or brain–CSF glial interfaces. This possibility deserves future examination.

Other reasons to suspect a glial involvement in sleep–wakefulness regulation relate to correlated changes in brain glutamate levels and brain metabolism. Overactivity of glutamatergic systems or underactivity of GABAergic systems have been implicated in the sleep–wakefulness cycle. Glutamate levels in the brain appear to be elevated during wakefulness and lowered during sleep. The converse is true for GABA (Jasper, Khan and Elliot 1965). As glia, especially astrocytes, are intimately involved in glutamate metabolism, this may be further evidence for their involvement in sleep and wakefulness.

Sleep involves a reduction in neuronal activity and brain metabolism engendered by an endogenous humoral agent which may be a peptide or hormone (Inoue 1989) or uridine or glutathione (Inoue 1993) among others. Glutathione is largely synthesised in astrocytes, but even if the sleep promoting factor itself is not of glial origin, glia are obvious targets for reducing the availability of metabolic substrates for neurons (see Chapter 5).

Anaesthesia may be considered as an imposed state of sleep, lacking the cortical activation which accompanies paradoxical (dreaming) sleep. It has generally been accepted that the principal target site for general anaesthetics is the synapse (Somjen 1967). At this region, the effects are thought to be mediated by an increase in presynaptic inhibitory transmitter release, a reduction in excitatory transmitter release, a change in the sensitivity of postsynaptic terminals to these transmitters, or a combination of these influences (Pocock and Richards 1991). Although there is no doubt that reduced synaptic excitatory transmission could account for the abolition of behaviour that occurs during anaesthesia, it may not necessarily follow that synapses are the principal target sites for general anaesthetics.

General anaesthetics suppress neuronal activity, yet appear to eliminate SPS responses entirely after a period of oscillatory activity in the DC recording (O'Leary and Goldring 1964). Preliminary experiments on gerbils in our laboratory have confirmed that visual evoked potentials are attenuated by ca. 50% during halothane anaesthesia, whilst spontaneous SPS responses disappeared. Experiments were therefore performed to examine the time-course of SPS activity during anaesthesia induction and recovery in NSP and SP gerbils.

Twelve NSP animals with a seizure score of 0.0 and 12 SP animals with seizure scores of not less than 4.5 were selected from categorised groups for implantation of electrodes as described earlier. Animals were then allowed 24 h to recover in their home cages prior to recording. The SPS simultaneously occurring at each electrode location was sampled continuously for 20 consecutive 16-s periods for animals in the experimental arena and not exhibiting overt behaviour. These were used as controls for later comparison with continuous recordings of spontaneously occurring SPS activity during induction of anaesthesia.

The animal was then placed in a $0.2 \times 0.3 \times 0.2$ m high perspex induction chamber placed in the centre of the recording arena. The induction chamber was initially flushed with a 50% mixture of O_2 and air and 4% halothane was subsequently provided at a constant flow of 4 l/min. When all the animal's movement had ceased, the halothane concentration was reduced to 2% for the remainder of the recording period. A continuous recording of 70 × 16 s samples of the SPS at each electrode position began immediately after placement of the subject into the induction chamber. After completion of these recordings, the halothane supply was terminated and animals received only oxygen. The recovery period was noted, this corresponding to the duration of a supply of 100% oxygen necessary for the resumption of ambulations and the animal traversing at least one of the four 20 cm squares marked on the floor of the experimental arena.

The criteria used to define the SPS-like waveforms were frequency and the maximum and minimum amplitudes of the slow oscillatory DC changes observed in preliminary studies. In addition, the overall DC level of the brain at each recording site was calculated for each 80 s of the continuous recording during anaesthesia in comparison to that in the non-behaviour periods prior to anaesthesia. Frequency (*C/16S*) was the number of oscillations during each 16 s of recording in which the DC oscillation amplitude was greater than 50 µV. Maximum and minimum values (mV) were the largest positive and negative deflections in the SPS within each 16-s epoch of the total recording.

Due to variation in times of immobilisation between animals, the data for anaesthesia was pooled for blocks of 5 × 16 s epochs. This gave 10 time periods (blocks), one from the onset of recording, one prior to immobilisation, followed by eight consecutive periods constituting the remainder of the continuous recording.

During the first minute of induction, there was an increase in behavioural activity, including frantic ambulatory and rearing behaviour with repeated escape attempts. The second minute was dominated by disorientated ambulations, often accompanied by loss of balance. Ambulations subsequently ceased and only limb movements were apparent before complete immobilisation. The times for immobilisation and for recovery of mobility did not differ between SP and NSP animals.

During the early phase of anaesthesia, large amplitude DC-recorded oscillations occurred, illustrated in Fig. 12.10 in a recording from preliminary experiments of an animal artificially ventilated and immobilised with succinyl choline to remove any trace of movement artifacts. In non-immobilised animals, the oscillations in the left anterior cortex of SP animals had a higher frequency (ca. 3.5 *C/16S*) than in NSP animals (ca. 1 *C/16S*). This was the only difference in oscillation frequency between SP and NSP animals. The early oscillation frequencies of recordings from anterior and posterior cortical sites ranged from 2 to 4-*C/16S*, those from mid-cortical regions from 2 to 3-*C/16S*. In all regions, there was a decline in the frequency of DC oscillations which was evident both before (< 80 s) and subsequent to immobilisation (> 160 s).

The DC oscillation amplitudes about the average baseline potential, recorded prior to anaesthesia, initially ranged from an average per animal of 500 µV to 2.7 mV. These oscillations were consistently larger in SP compared to NSP animals. In both groups, they were most pronounced in the right anterior and

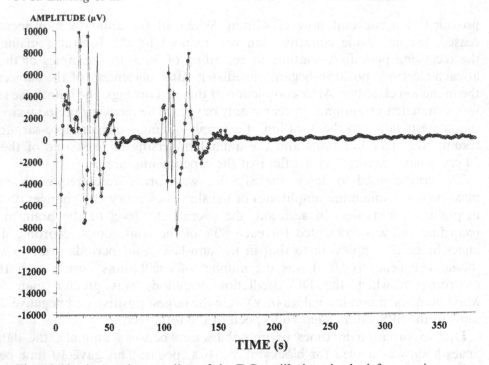

Fig. 12.10. A sample recording of the DC oscillations in the left posterior cortex of an immobilised and artificially ventilated non-seizure prone gerbil during Halothane induced anaesthesia (initially 4%, then 2%). Note the large amplitude oscillations which occurred during the early induction phase of anaesthesia which persisted after 120 s, the normal time of immobilisation in freely behaving animals.

left posterior cortices of SP animals. In both groups, and in all regions, there was a rapid decline in amplitude during the first three periods of 80 s recording both before and after immobilisation was achieved. Subsequent to ca. 400 s after induction commenced, the DC changes rarely exceeded $200 \pm 100 \, \mu V$.

The average SPS baseline determined for each 80 s, compared to that in the pre-anaesthesia period, showed that a shift occurred during the first 160 s of recording at all electrode locations, which was more variable in SP than in NSP animals. During the phase of induction of anaesthesia (t = 0–240 s), in SP animals, the left cortex showed a negative DC baseline change while the reverse was true for the right cortex. This result just failed significance.

The large, slow oscillations in DC potentials during anaesthesia would suggest that large ionic fluxes are occurring in ECS, the ionic constituents of which are normally regulated by glia (Chapters 7 and 10). These fluxes may be due to changes in neuronal synaptic excitatory activity. Thus, glutamate responses are decreased in lamprey (Yamamura et al. 1993), mice (Perouansky et al. 1995) and rats (McFarlane, Warner and Dexter 1995), whilst those in rats to GABA seem to be increased (Longoni, Demontis and Olsen 1993) during halothane anaesthesia. However, others report a general decrease in both excitatory and inhibitory amino acid neurotransmitter synthesis in mice (Watanabe et al. 1993). These effects are not restricted to amino acid neurotransmitters, as striatal dopamine is increased in rats (Miyano, Tanifuji and Eger 1993), whilst acetylcholine release is decreased in the pontine reticular formation of cats (Keifer et al. 1994) or the rat cortex (Griffiths et al. 1995).

An alternative to reduced chemical synaptic activity for induction of anaesthesia is that ion channel conductance is affected by the anaesthetic agent. In skeletal muscle, Ca^{2+}-activated K^+ channels have a decreased open-state probability (Beeler and Gable 1993) and K^+ channels from oocytes are less conductive (Zorn et al. 1993; Kulkarni et al. 1996) under the influence of halothane. Halothane not only affects K^+ channels, but also decreases Ca^{2+}-ATPase activity in synaptic membranes (Franks et al. 1995) and glioma cell membranes (Singh et al. 1995). Halothane has also been found to inhibit Ca^{2+} currents in pituitary cells (Herrington et al. 1991) and sensory neurons (Takenoshita and Steinbach 1991).

The effects of halothane on glial cells are not clear, although blockage of gap junctions between astrocytes in culture (Dermietzel and Spray 1993; Finkbeiner 1992), may prevent the normal movement of Ca^{2+} through the glial syncitium (Cornell-Bell et al. 1990). If a similar effect occurred in vivo, gap-junction closure may have important implications for the effectiveness of glia as regulators of the ionic constituents of the ECS, especially with regard to spatial redistribution of potassium. The possible reduction in ECS potassium regulation might account for the loss of spontaneous SPS responses after a period of large oscillations, found in the study described here. However, Ransom et al. (1977) obtained electrically-induced shifts under barbiturate and procaine anaesthesia in cats. They concluded that a large component of the shift under barbiturate anaesthesia was due to summated IPSPs and not to glial depolarisation in response to elevated $[K^+]_e$. Similarily, conditioned SPS responses to environmental stimuli have been obtained with rats under urethane anacsthesia and with rewarding brain electrical stimulation (Pirch and Corbus 1985; Rucker, Corbus and Pirch 1986).

The above quoted evidence might mitigate against a glial role in general anaesthesia or may be restricted to the anaesthetic agents or species used. However, it seems unlikely that the initially large and widespread oscillations in DC recorded potentials in the brain reported here would not involve or be a result of changes in glial participation of ionic regulation of the ECF. That the effect is more dramatic in SP animals may reflect the increased volatility of these regulatory mechanisms in these animals, evidenced by their expression, when conscious, of enhanced SPS responses and behavioural arousal.

12.7 General Discussion

The SPS to electrical stimulation of the brain or in regions of primary afferent sensory activity reflects the local neuronal activity and $[K^+]_e$ presumably because it is a response to glial spatial buffering of the neuronally released potassium. This could be considered a passive phenomenon and would suggest that SPS neuronal response relationships would be consistent. This is not the case during surgical or drug induced changes in neuronal activity, or more normally during habituation or changes in motivation. The data presented here indicate that throughout phylogeny SPS activity is correlated with behavioural state changes from sleep through wakefulness to arousal and attention. SPS amplitude changes reflect changes in motivation and plastic changes associated with at least the simplest forms of learning. With the likelihood that SPS changes reflect to a large degree the activity of glial cells and the growing realisation that these cells are crucial for neural activity, the real possibility exists that these cells modulate the activity of neurons. This would be enabled by their reception and subsequent integration of information from neurons about the sensory environment, information from 'homeostatic' systems by, e.g. hormones, glucose levels, tonicity etc. In order to determine the involvement of glial cells in behaviour, experiments will have to be carried out to target specific glial activities and monitor the behavioural and physiological (SPS) outcome.

13

Slow Scalp Recorded Brain Potentials, Sensory Processing and Cognition

HERBERT BAUER, NIELS BIRBAUMER and
FRANK RÖSLER

Summary

Slow brain potentials, although first described by Caton (1875), did not gain proper attention until the mid-1960s when Walter et al. (1964) reported on the scalp recorded 'CNV (contingent negative variation)' and Kornhuber and Deecke (1965) on the readiness potential (RP) (Bereitschaftspotential). Due to the temporal extension of these negative going slow potential shifts (SPSs), an additional or alternative (glial) origin has since been discussed.

Both SPSs accompany the kinds of preparatory and/or attentional processes that can be seen as localised threshold regulations of cortical excitability. Attempts to train subjects to gain operant control of these processes via biofeedback have led to successful therapeutic applications.

Although it was known from the very beginning of electroencephalography that SPSs accompany actual cortical processing (enhanced cellular activity within a circumscribed cortical segment), this fact has not attracted much attention until recently. Since the late 1980s, slow potential topography has evolved and is gaining substantial influence in cognitive neuroscience.

13.1 Introduction

As far as the generators of slow shifts in scalp-recorded brain potentials are concerned, two aspects have to be considered, the *what* and the *where*, i.e. what are the generators made of, electrically and structurally, and where within the brain they are located.

13.1.1 Generating Units

Scalp-recorded brain potentials and their changes (shifts) originate from extracellular ionic currents within the brain tissue. Such extracellular currents are maintained by ionic concentrations and potential gradients of different origin that have a tendency towards reduction. According to the generally accepted model (see reviews by Caspers 1974; Creutzfeldt and Houchin 1974; Goff et al. 1978; Vaughan and Arezzo 1988), it is, firstly, the neurons that boost up ionic gradients when they become active. Whenever an action potential arrives at a presynaptic terminal, synaptic processes become activated and subsequently lead to post-synaptic potentials: to EPSPs, which might culminate in action potentials with temporal or spatial summation, in the case of excitatory synapses, or to IPSPs due to inhibitory synaptic activity (Eccles 1964). Both are changes in the membrane potential of postsynaptic cells. With excitatory synaptic activity a net inflow of cations occurs at the subsynaptic membrane producing an extracellular current sink and an ionic current develops extra- and intracellularly in the opposite direction along the neuronal membrane, where extracellularly the ionic flux aims toward the synaptic area. Similarly, during IPSP generation an influx of anions and/or an efflux of cations takes place which again establish extra- and intracellular ionic fluxes but in the opposite direction. These processes are one major source in the generation of extended extracellular field potentials (cf. Creutzfeldt, Watanabe and Lux 1966; Caspers, Speckmann and Lehmenkühler 1984; Speckmann, Caspers and Elger 1984).

However, neurons are not the only type of brain cells that can generate extra-cellular ionic currents. Glial cells respond to the extracellular potassium concentration in various ways, depending on their bioelectric membrane properties (cf. Roitbak 1965, 1983; Kuffler and Nicholls 1966; Kuffler, Nichols and Orkand 1966; Roitbak and Fanardjian 1973; Somjen 1973, 1975; Somjen and Trachtenberg 1979; Nicholson 1980; Kettenmann 1987; Roitbak et al. 1987; Chapters 10 and 12). Local elevation of extracellular potassium due to repetitive firing of adjacent neurons, for example, initiates a local potassium influx into glia along its electrochemical gradient and an efflux in cell regions where potassium is low extracellularly (Dietzel et al. 1980, 1989; Coles and Orkand 1983; Gardener-Medwin 1983a; Syková 1983). Due to widespread processes of the glial cells and their interconnections via gap junctions (the functional syncytium), spatially extended currents develop which 'amplify' neuronally generated field potentials but possibly also modify their shape because of the different time course of glial membrane processes (see Chapter 10). To what extent mere potassium redistribution within the extracellular space (without any intracellular bypass) contributes to long lasting steady potentials has not yet been thoroughly investigated (but see Chapter 7).

13.1.2 Spatial Prerequisites

If the generating units for ionic fluxes were spatially randomly oriented, the extra-cellular currents they evoke would cancel each other out and no volume conducted field potential would be recordable on the scalp. It is the columnar structure perpendicular to the cortical laminae that makes summation possible and leads to oriented currents strong enough to produce recordable differences in scalp potential. In these cortical columns, pyramidal cells with their deeply situated somata have dendrites arborising towards the cortical surface and thus have an elongated shape suitable for generating spatial ionic currents. Another crucial aspect is the question of where an extracellular current originates, whether at the apical dendrites or at the soma, and in which direction it flows, since these factors determine the polarity of surface potentials. To illustrate this, Fig. 13.1 shows calculated extracellular fields with depolarisation of different parts of a pyramidal cell (Creutzfeldt and Houchin 1974).

Investigating the laminar current density distribution in the cortex, Mitzdorf (1985) described the main types of cortical activation and resultant currents in extracellular space as illustrated in Fig. 13.2.

Based on such data, excitatory activities within the apical dendrites seem to be the most probable candidates for DC potential initiation, since their temporal extension is sufficient to make summation possible and lead to volume conducted, surface negative, going slow potential changes. In terms of temporal extension and amplitude, there was no synaptically controlled intracortical current to generate

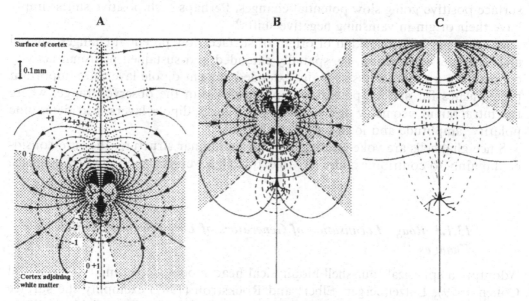

Fig. 13.1. Theoretical extracellular fields generated by depolarisation of different parts of a pyramidal cell. (A) Depolarisation of somatic region; (B) Depolarisation of the middle region of the apical dendrite; (C) Depolarisation of the distal end of the apical dendrite. Solid lines are current flow lines; arrows indicate the direction of the flow of positive charges; the density of flow lines indicates the density of current. Broken lines are voltage contours numbered on an arbitrary but linear scale with reference to the potential at a distant point. Shading indicates negative potential. (From Creutzfeldt and Houchin 1974.)

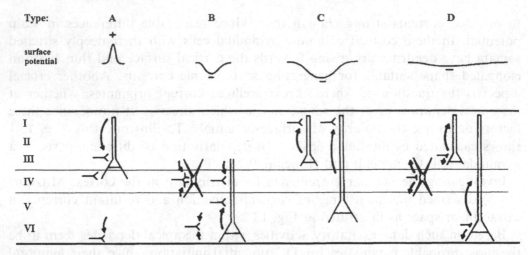

Fig. 13.2. Schematic diagram of four main types of cortical activation and their reflection in surface potential (or EEG). Cell types, synaptic contacts, and currents in extracellular space (arrows) are indicated. (From Mitzdorf 1985.)

surface positive going slow potential changes. Perhaps such positive shifts simply have their origin in vanishing negative shifts?

In any case, with that kind of origin of surface slow potential changes, spatial and temporal summation, i.e. spatially extended and sustained neuronal activity constituting a more or less spatially extended current dipole layer, are important prerequisites for surface potential amplitudes within the observed range, where the intracranial geometry and orientation of such dipole layers also determine polarity, amplitude and localisation of changes.

Since glial cells are yoked elements of this columnar structure, they are considered mainly to contribute additively to extracellular currents initiated by neurons.

13.1.3 Rough Localisation of Generators of Large Scalp Potential Changes

Adopting a spherical four-shell biophysical head model (according to Cuffin and Cohen 1979), Lutzenberger, Elbert and Rockstroh (1987) exemplify the surface potential distributions of various intraspherical dipoles and dipole fields of different location, strength, and size. It can be shown, firstly, that the maximal surface amplitudes generated by a superficial dipole become reduced by a factor of 7 when the same dipole is moved to the centre. Secondly, the size of a calotte-shaped dipole layer (field) is the prominent factor for surface potential amplitude, e.g. a dipole field of a diameter of 1.6 cm contributes only 4% of a larger layer of about 14 cm. Combining these two aspects, the authors give another example:

Even if a large portion of the thalamus were synchronously active, the active area would not exceed 0.8 cm in radius. Since its position more distant to the surface would diminish the potential at the surface by at least a factor of 4, its relative small size would reduce potential amplitudes by another 25 times . . . . Altogether this amounts to a reduction of amplitudes by 100. This is the reason why an intracranial polarisation of 100 μV might produce a scalp potential of more than 20 μV when it is generated in extended cortical areas, but will produce only 0.2 μV when focal and arising from deep structures.

In general, we may therefore assume that scalp recorded slow potentials of large amplitudes are most likely of cortical origin.

13.1.4 Types of Slow Potential Shifts

Scalp recorded slow potential changes are observable whenever cortical structures alter their state of activity phasically or tonically; depending on the amount of this shift, the aforementioned generator substrates and processes will contribute according to their temporal characteristics. On this basis, two kinds of SPSs can be distinguished, namely spontaneous and event related ones. Spontaneous SPSs (sSPSs) have been observed and described by several researchers (Aladjalova 1964; Bauer and Nirnberger 1980, 1981; Stamm 1984) and have been used to define experimental conditions in order to identify the functional role of cortical areas (for details see section 13.2.3).

SPSs that exhibit distinctly different topographical distribution on the scalp and coincide with behavioural events (overt or covert behaviour) are manifold: Gradually increasing negativities such as the readiness potential (RP) accompany the intention to act, negativities such as the contingent negative variation (CNV) coincide with preparatory activities evoked by announced information delivery, DC potentials accompany the perception of long lasting sensory stimuli (David et al. 1969), and negative SPSs also accompany temporally extended (in the range of seconds) cognitive processing (Lang W. et al. 1988, 1989; McCallum, Cooper and Pocock 1988; Rösler et al. 1993; Bauer et al. 1995).

When investigating changes in the time range of up to several hours, very slow changes can be observed that are closely linked to those just mentioned. Negative SPSs that accompany information processing decline slowly after processing ceases; therefore, if processing continues before the resolution of such SPSs is complete, new negative going SPSs start from more negative baselines, and if this continues, resolution deficits accumulate over time amounting to baseline shifts with amplitudes of up to several 100 μV. This has been shown by Bauer, Korunka and Leodolter (1993), using a simple CNV paradigm and recently also by means of topographic representation during spatial processing (Vitouch et al. 1997); for details see Fig. 13.3.

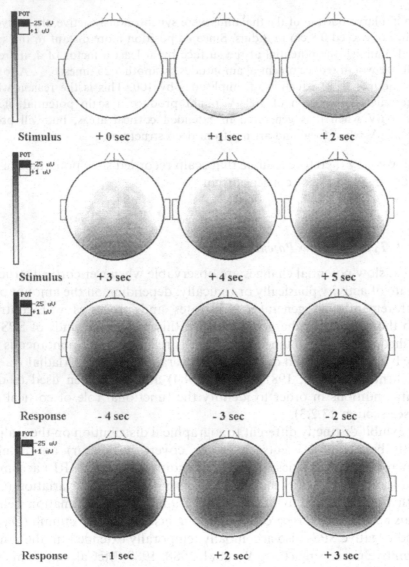

Fig. 13.3. Maps of grand mean SPSs accompanying spatial processing ($n = 400$) that lasted for a median duration of about 13 s per trial. Gradually mounting SPs are obvious in occipito–right–parieto–temporal cortices that decrease after response. It is unlikely that this mirrors a gradual recruiting of neurons involved in solving the task; it most probably indicates an alternative non-neuronal generator (e.g. glial depolarisation or mere K^+ redistribution within the extracellular space) that becomes gradually excited with tonic focal neuronal activity.

13.2 SPSs and Performance

Since the beginning of slow potential research, the relationship between SPSs and performance has been one of its main focuses. It started out with various aspects of motor activities and eventually extended to correlations observed with complex cognitive processing employing variants of the basic experimental paradigms that evoke RPs and CNVs.

13.2.1 Readiness Potentials (RPs)

This SP was originally described by Kornhuber and Deecke (1964) as a gradually mounting negative potential ($-10\,\mu V$ on average) that starts some 700–1000 ms before simple self-initiated and self-paced (voluntary) motor activity. Meanwhile, it is apparent that it presumably precedes any intentional motor activity such as eye movements (Becker et al. 1972), writing and drawing (Deecke et al. 1986), speech production (Grözinger et al. 1972) and piano playing (Kristeva 1984), to give just a few examples. The RP does not seem to be a unitary phenomenon: Deecke et al. (1984) distinguished an early and a late part. The latter is characterised by a steeper slope starting at around -500 ms. It also manifests a contralateral dominance that demonstrates a closer relationship to the behavioral action planned. The early part of the RP is referred to as the true readiness potential and shows a symmetric precentral localisation. The amplitude of RPs is correlated with intentional and behavioral demands and the initial conditions of the processing system:

Amplitudes are directly related to the strength, velocity, complexity and precision demands of motor activities (e.g. Grünewald et al. 1979; Becker and Kristeva 1980; Kristeva and Kornhuber 1980; Kristeva 1984; Freude and Ullsperger 1987; Trimmel et al. 1989).

Similarly there is a direct relationship to the intentional engagement, concentration, motivation and behavioural significance of the intended action – fatigue also seems to be compensated for by enhanced preparatory activity, i.e. larger amplitudes (e.g. Kornhuber and Deecke 1965; Kristeva 1977; Freude and Ullsperger 1987).

Repetition of actions leads to amplitude reduction (Kristeva 1977) as does switching from controlled to automatic processing (or mode of operation) (Tayler 1978; Cooper, McCallum and Papakostopoulos 1978; Kristeva and Cheyne 1990).

Based on the overall empirical result, the common aspect of brain activities accompanied by RPs seems to be their preparatory purpose.

13.2.2 Contingent Negative Variation (CNV)

In predominantly externally controlled behavioural situations cortical activities are likewise accompanied by slow negative potentials: whenever an event (warning stimulus; WS or S1) announces another event (imperative or informational stimulus; IS or S2) that occurs within a predictable time window, we observe a negative going SPS – the CNV originally described by Walter et al. (1964). Using inter-stimulus intervals longer than 1 s, it became apparent that this negative potential had an early and a late component that vary independently and have different topographies; they were termed the O-wave (orienting wave) and E-wave (expectancy wave), respectively, by Loveless and Sanford (1973, 1974). To avoid these narrow interpretative designations, Rockstroh et al. (1989) introduced the neutral terms initial and terminal CNV (iCNV, tCNV), but evidently the iCNV is more closely related to the information delivery by the S1 whereas the tCNV amplitude varies with the kinds of responses demanded or the information delivered by the S2.

Since the relationship between CNV amplitudes and various behavioural aspects has been investigated by innumerable studies, only a summarising conclusion will be given here (for details see, for example, McCallum 1988; Rockstroh et al. 1989).

Taking the S1–S2 stimulus pair as a solid complex event, we can adopt a model originally designed by Johnson (1986) to summarise variables that determine the P300 amplitude (positive component of the sensory evoked potential with a latency of about 300 ms), and observe CNV amplitudes as directly related to subjective probability (Rebert 1985; 'the oddball CNV' – Bauer et al. 1992) and meaning of the stimulus in an independent and additive way, whereas the quality of information transmission has an equal but multiplicative influence on both of these factors (Bauer 1993). As far as responses are concerned, there is a positive correlation between their difficulty and complexity and the CNV amplitude.

In addition, the initial conditions of the cortical structures involved seem to exert a prominent influence; amplitudes of CNVs that were recorded in a time locked manner with spontaneous slow potential shifts (sSPSs) are inversely related to the amplitude of these sSPSs (Bauer et al. 1986; Korunka et al. 1990).

Employing the S1–S2 paradigm, it was also possible to demonstrate clearly that preparatory SPs do not depend exclusively on motor responses. Imagining, rather than really giving, a motor response to the S2 leads to even larger CNV amplitudes (Bauer 1968). Even if no motor activity at all is requested, CNV-like SPSs can be observed when signals are to be anticipated, e.g. stimulus preceding negativity (Damen and Brunia 1987; Brunia and Damen 1988; Chwilla and Brunia 1989).

In sum, it is the preparatory and anticipatory aspect of the brain processes that is common to these widely varying experimental conditions where CNVs or CNV-like SPSs are observed. This points to a global organising system that oversees all the ongoing cortical activities such as sensory processing, memory retrieval and the actual activity state of functional cortical units, and is able to control these processes according to the momentary demands. An essential part of such a system seems to be the so-called 'medio–thalamo–fronto–cortical' system (MTFC-system) that regulates specific and unspecific neuronal input to the cerebral cortex via the nucleus reticularis thalami (NRT) (Skinner 1978, 1984). This model has been extended to a threshold regulation model of cortical excitability by including a cortico–thalamic feedback loop via the basal ganglia (Elbert and Rockstroh 1987). Experimental support for such a system will be given in section 13.4.

13.2.3 *Rough Localisation of Cortical Functions Using the CNV*

If CNVs indicate a tuning of cortical excitability for anticipated tasks, their amplitude distribution should allow a rough localisation of functions that will become active with task execution. This has actually been demonstrated for arithmetic processing (larger CNVs in left temporal recording sites) and pattern matching (dominance of right temporal CNVs) by Birbaumer et al. (1981b), but only with 'easy' and not with 'difficult' tasks. Signalling an upcoming left or right hand response using complex tactile S1–S2 pairs also led to CNV dominance contralateral to the responding hand (Rockstroh et al. 1988).

Trying to specify cognitive functions of circumscribed parts of the monkey's cortex, Stamm (1979) also used SPS recordings, but in addition developed an ingenious procedure for testing results based merely on correlations. During the early intratrial delay epoch, he first observed a surface-negative SPS in the prefrontal cortex that was related to the level of correct delayed response (DR) performance. In order to check whether this SPS can be used to speed up the monkey's learning rate, he then reversed his experimental task design and initiated trials only when a spontaneous SPS was observed in the very same cortical region. In this way, the SPS became converted from a dependent to an independent variable allowing a much more unequivocal interpretation. The finding of faster/(slower) learning rates with leading negative/(positive) prefrontal SPSs not only confirmed the original interpretation, but also suggested employing this potential related event (PRE) procedure in human experimentation.

Independently, an essentially identical procedure, the so-called 'brain trigger design (BTD)', was developed for human learning experiments (Bauer and Nirnberger 1980, 1981). Paired associate learning as well as concept identification (learning) were significantly faster/(slower) with spontaneous negative/(positive) going pretrial SPSs at left central recording sites. Significant localised effects have also been found with tasks involving frontal lobe function (choice reaction task for differing geometric configurations; Born, Whipple and Stamm 1982; Stamm 1984) and parietal lobe function (semantic discrimination between synonyms and unrelated word-pairs; Stamm 1984) when task presentation was synchronised to frontal and parietal pretrial SPSs. In Vienna we are continuing this kind of experimentation, now using more precisely localised shifts. This requires good cooperation on the part of the subjects, since the spontaneous rate of such shifts is low, which necessarily leads to very long experimental sessions.

More efficient in this respect is the localisation of cortical functions as well as a description of their specific characteristics and ways of interaction by analysing the topography of those SPSs that actually accompany temporally extended cognitive processing using genuine DC-recording.

13.3 Slow Potential Topography and Cognition

Classic examples of performance related slow negative shifts in the EEG are the contingent negative variation (CNV) (Walter et al. 1964), the readiness potential (RP) (Kornhuber and Deecke 1965), and the processing negativity (Nd) (Hansen and Hillyard 1983). From the very beginning, it was assumed that these negativities are correlates of specific cognitive processes. They were associated with the state of event anticipation (CNV), motor preparation (RP), and selective attention (Nd), respectively. Other 'early' studies claimed the existence of relationships between negative SPSs and mental computation (Ruchkin et al. 1988; Rösler, Schumacher and Sojka 1990; Rösler and Heil 1991), visual monitoring and/or scanning of short-term memory (Horst, Ruchkin and Munson 1987; Looren de Jong, Kok and van Rooy 1987; Wijers et al. 1989a,b), imagery and mental rotation (Farah and Peronnet 1989; Wijers et al. 1989c; Rösler, Schumacher and Sojka 1990), concept formation (Delisle, Stuss and Picton 1986; Lang M. et al. 1987b; Uhl et al. 1990), and planning and execution of motor responses (Deecke et al. 1987; Lang W. et al. 1988; Lang et al. 1989).

These more or less unsystematic observations suggested that negative SPSs are a general phenomenon which accompany all types of information processing and whose characteristic features – topography, amplitude and duration – reflect the particular task demands. In the studies mentioned, the location of the amplitude maximum of a negative SPS was quite often found exactly over that part of the scalp where, according to neurological evidence, cortical structures are located which are essential for a particular task performance (e.g. the somatosensory, visual, or motor projection areas). Moreover, the amplitude of negative SPSs was found to covary with the amount of effort that has to be invested in order to solve a task and the duration of a SPS pattern was found to be related to the duration of a specific mental state or processing episode.

These preliminary observations motivated us to study negative SPSs systematically with genuine DC-recording equipment and full 10–20 electrode system montages (Jasper 1958) in a variety of processing conditions. All cognitive tasks were constructed such that processing episodes prevailed for several seconds and that the demands imposed on the system could be varied systematically.

13.3.1 Memory Retrieval

To study SPSs during memory retrieval, we used an experimental task which allowed us systematically to vary the type and the number of representations which had to be reactivated (Heil, Rösler and Hennighausen 1994). In this task, subjects had to learn new associations between so-called target items and mediators and later they were tested on their knowledge about these experimentally established links. In one study, the target items were line drawings of real objects (e.g. dogs, ships, airplanes, trees etc.) and the mediators were either words or spatial positions in a grid. In order to manipulate task complexity, different target items became associated with a different number of mediators by training; e.g. some target items (say a drawing of a German shepherd or a sailing boat) were always presented with only one mediator-word, other target items (the drawing of a beagle or a steamer) with two mediator-words and a third group of target items was always delivered together with three different mediator-words. These mediator-words were not semantically associated with the target drawings because verbal concepts like 'school', 'station', 'restaurant', 'bar', 'church', etc. served as mediators. In another experimental condition, the same target items (German shepherd, beagle, and terrier, or sailing boat, steamer, and warship) were linked to either one, two or three spatial positions in a grid. These associations were trained until the subject knew them by heart. In each condition they had to learn associations between 54 target items and 18 different mediators. In the retrieval test, the subject saw two target items and he or she had to decide if these two shared a common mediator or not. To come up with an answer, the subject had to reactivate the mediators in any case, irrespective of whether the answer was yes or no. As the mediators were varied systematically, it was possible to study the reactivation of different types of memory representations (verbal concepts or spatial positions). Moreover, since the number of associations was also varied systematically, it was possible to study the effect of retrieval effort. With more associations linked to a target the retrieval task becomes more difficult. This becomes manifest as a monotonic increase of decision times and is known in the literature as the 'fan-effect' (Anderson 1974). In our studies, the average response times amounted to about 4, 6 and 8 s for conditions fan 1, fan 2, and fan 3, respectively.

The findings in this experimental setup concerning negative SPSs are quite impressive (see Fig. 13.4 and for more details, Rösler, Heil and Glowalla 1993; Rösler, Heil and Hennighausen 1995a,b; Heil, Rösler and Hennighausen 1996). Contingent to the presentation of the retrieval cues (the two target items) a very pronounced negative SPS is evoked in the EEG which may prevail for 6 or more seconds depending on the difficulty of the task. The maximum of this negative SPS peaks at different locations over the scalp depending on the type of representation which has to be reactivated. The maximum is found over left frontal areas when words serve as mediators, over central parietal areas with spatial positions as mediators, and over occipital to right posterior temporal areas with colour patches as mediators, respectively. Moreover, the difficulty of the retrieval task becomes manifest as an amplitude variation. The amplitude increases systematically from the easiest (fan 1) to the most difficult condition (fan 3). However, most important

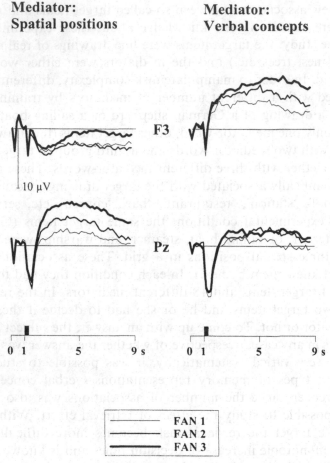

Mediator:
Spatial positions

Mediator:
Verbal concepts

F3

10 µV

Pz

0 1   5   9 s   0 1   5   9 s

————— FAN 1
————— FAN 2
————— FAN 3

Fig. 13.4. SPS effects in a memory retrieval experiment in which either spatial positions or verbal concepts had to be reactivated contingent to a cue presented at time 1 s. The negative SPS reaches its maximum amplitude over the left-frontal cortex in the verbal and over the parietal cortex in the spatial condition. Increasing difficulty of the retrieval task (fan 1, 2, 3) is reflected as an amplitude increase at those electrodes where the maximum negativity is observed for a particular type of representation (spatial or verbal). (Data from Heil, Rösler and Hennighausen 1996.)

is that this amplitude modulation is restricted to those scalp locations where the maximum of the SPS pattern appears anyway.

These findings agree with the assumption that negative SPSs are specifically related to the retrieval process. Their topography reflects which code has to be reactivated and their amplitude the extensiveness of the memory search. It is interesting to notice that the maximum of these SPSs peaks exactly over those cortical areas which are known from lesion studies to be important for the processing of the respective code, i.e. verbal = left frontal, spatial = parietal, and colour = occipital to posterior temporal. This SPS topography is also congruent with that recently observed in PET scans with a similar memory retrieval situation (Martin et al. 1995).

In a recent study, Heil, Rösler and Hennighausen (1996) showed that the SPS pattern is not only evoked if overlearned representations have to be reactivated. If targets and mediators are presented one after another in an anticipation learning task, the specific topography develops contingent to a target as soon as the subject has acquired some knowledge which can be used to anticipate the mediator. The topographic differentiation between spatial and verbal concepts is then also seen in a within subject design, in which the type of mediator changes from trial to trial.

13.3.2 Sensory Processing and Mental Imagery

A standard task to study mental imagery is the so-called mental rotation paradigm (Shepard and Cooper 1982). In one variant of this paradigm the subject sees an object (a letter or a line drawing) which has to be stored in working memory. After this, an instruction stimulus is presented which informs the subject mentally to transform the object representation. For example, the stimulus may tell that the image of the object has to be rotated clockwise for a certain angle. At the end of the trial, a comparison stimulus will be presented and the subject has to decide, if the mentally transformed stimulus and the comparison stimulus are identical or not. Behavioural studies show that the time which is needed to transform the mental representation increases monotonically with the rotational angle.

In two different studies, we achieved this task with visual and haptic (tactile) stimuli, respectively. In the visual condition (Rösler et al. 1995) different star-like figures were presented on a computer display. In each trial, one figure was visible for 3 s and it had to be stored in working memory. After this, a tone of different pitch informed the subject either to keep the image as it was (0°-condition) or to rotate it clockwise for either 60° or 120°. Ten seconds later, a comparison stimulus was presented for 2 seconds which comprised a subset of the stored and possibly rotated image elements. The decision whether the comparison stimulus formed a match with the stored image or not had to be given within these two seconds of stimulus presentation.

In the haptic condition (Röder, Rösler and Hennighausen 1997), the setup was by and large the same. Instead of visual figures, pixel patterns were presented on a specially constructed tactile display (91 pixels arranged as a hexagon of 2 cm diameter). These stimuli were present for 5 s and had to be scanned with the index finger of the dominant hand. After haptic encoding of the pattern, a tone informed the blindfolded subject to keep the image (0°-condition) or to rotate it either 60° or 120°. Finally, after a delay of 7 s a comparison stimulus was presented which could be the same pattern as the image or a mirror version of it, thus a parity judgement was required.

Visual Mental Rotation

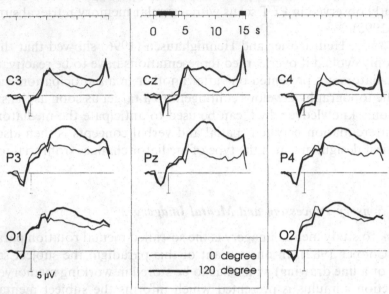

Haptic Mental Rotation

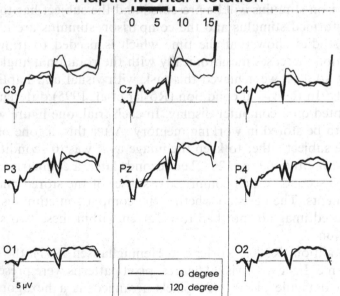

On the basis of pilot work, the two tasks were equalised with respect to processing times and error rates (This is the reason why the events – stimulus on- and offset, comparison stimulus – were timed differently in the two versions of the task). Processing times were estimated in a condition in which the subjects had the option to trigger the comparison stimulus as soon as they had finished the mental transformation. In this situation the response times in both the visual and the haptic version amounted to about 2, 4 and 5 s for the 0°, 60°, and 120° condition, respectively.

In both tasks, the experimental setup allowed separation of three cognitive states, that of image encoding (i.e. the first epoch while the stimulus is presented on the display), that of image storage in working memory (i.e. the epoch after the instruction stimulus in the 0°-condition), and that of mental transformation (i.e. the epoch after the instruction stimulus in the 60°- and 120°-rotation condition proper).

Figure 13.5 summarises the SPS pattern observed over the central and posterior part of the scalp. During encoding negative SPSs emerge with a maximum over the modality specific projection areas, i.e. over the occipital cortex (electrodes O_1 [left], O_2 [right] occipital cortex; all following electrode names are given according to the 10–20 electrode system) in the visual and over the left central cortex (electrode C_3) in the haptic condition (subjects were right handers and scanned the tactile display with their dominant hand). This SPS pattern continues largely unchanged after the instruction stimulus, if the image had just to be kept unchanged (0°). In the 120°-rotation condition (and also in the not shown 60°-condition), however, an additional negativity develops over the parietal cortex. This holds for both versions, the visual and the haptic one. The topographic difference between encoding and storage on one side and mental transformation on the other becomes even more impressive in the topographic maps which were computed from average amplitudes (see Fig. 13.6). The top two maps show very clearly that the maximum negativity during encoding is located over the somatosensory and the visual projection areas, respectively. The bottom two maps show the pure rotation effect, i.e.

Fig. 13.5. Main findings of two mental rotation studies with visual or tactile information input. Top: visual condition. Presentation of the visual stimulus and maintaining a visual image is accompanied by a substantial negative potential over the posterior part of the scalp with the maximum amplitude at occipital electrodes O_1, and O_2 (0°-condition). Transformation of an image as it is required in the 120°-condition is accompanied by an additional negativity peaking over the parietal cortex. Bottom: haptic condition. The negativity due to stimulus processing and image storage peaks is now over the left central cortex (0°-condition). The additional negativity evoked by the rotation activity in the 120°-condition has again its maximum over the parietal cortex. (Data from Röder, Rösler and Hennighausen, submitted; Rösler et al. 1995, with kind permission from Elsevier Science-NL, Amsterdam, The Netherlands.)

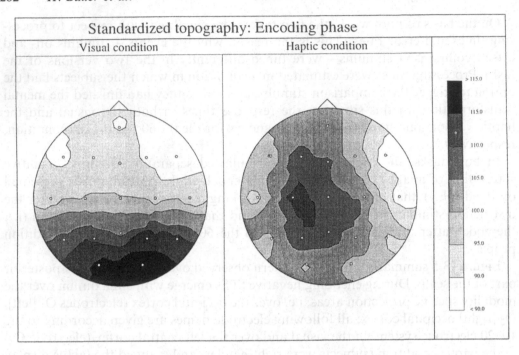

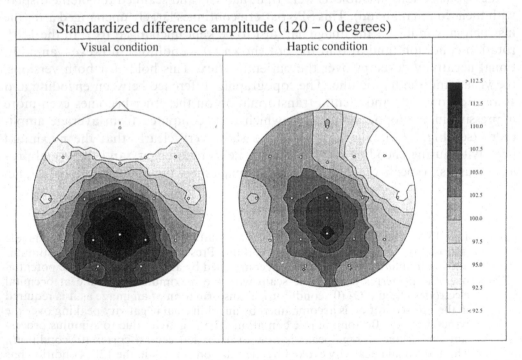

the difference amplitude between the 0° and the 120° condition. There, the maximum is found over the parietal cortex (electrode P_z) in both experiments. Comparable results about the topography of SPSs during image transformation were reported by Bauer et al. (1997).

These results are compatible with the idea that mental images are held in code- or modality-specific buffers while mental transformations of these images are performed by one and the same processing module which is located in the parietal cortex. Again, these findings are well in line with findings from lesion studies which suggest that there exist modality specific working memories located in the respective primary and secondary projection areas and modality unspecific processors which handle spatial representations (e.g. Kosslyn 1987; Kosslyn and Koenig 1992).

13.3.3 Cortical Plasticity

Recently, Röder and coworkers (Rösler et al. 1993; Röder et al. 1996; Röder, Rösler and Hennighausen, 1997) investigated if the SPS topography reveals functional changes of cortical plasticity in congenitally and adventitiously blind subjects. Among others, subjects were tested with tactile and auditory stimuli in a sensory discrimination or odd ball task and also with a haptic version of the mental rotation task as outlined above. In these tasks, blind and blindfolded sighted subjects showed by and large the same task specific overall patterns of negative SPSs. However, an additional, general finding was that blind subjects always showed an enlarged occipital negativity (see Fig. 13.7). The amplitude of this occipital negativity was also modulated by factor task difficulty. For example, in the haptic mental rotation paradigm blind subjects showed, as did sighted subjects, an increasing negativity over the parietal cortex with increasing rotational angle, but in addition, they also showed an increasing negativity with increasing rotational angle over the occipital cortex.

For the time being, it is not completely clear what these findings imply for cortical plasticity. It could be that the negativity over the occipital cortex in blind subjects is in fact specifically related to tactile information processing. It is conceivable that such modality specific activities are taken over by the otherwise

Fig. 13.6. Top: standardized topography during the encoding phase of the mental rotation task (left visual, right haptic condition.) Bottom: standardized topography of the rotation effect (120°–0° condition) in the transformation phase (left visual, right haptic condition.) Larger scores (darker shading) indicate relative more negativity. (Data from Rösler et al. 1995, with kind permission from Elsevier Science-NL, Amsterdam, The Netherlands; Röder, Rösler and Hennighausen, 1997.)

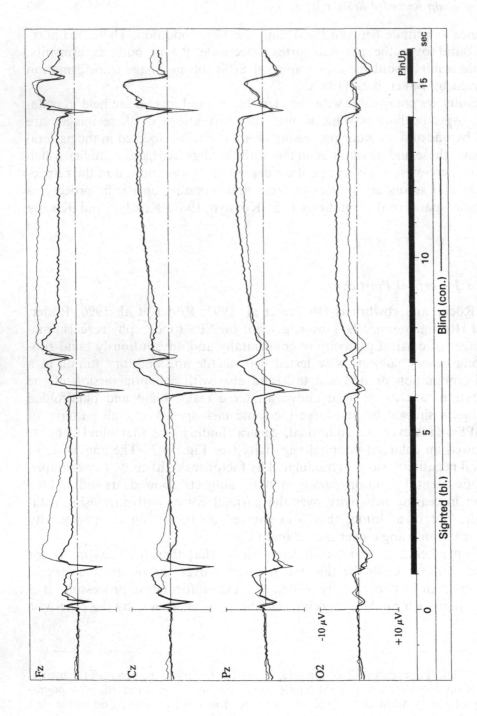

Fig. 13.7. Negative SPSs recorded in a haptic mental rotation task with sighted and blind subjects. Subjects inspected two successively presented tactile stimuli and indicated whether the second stimulus was a mirror image of the first. The second stimulus could be rotated and reflected in relation to the first. The thick and thin lines represent the grand means of blind and sighted subjects, respectively. (Data from Rösler et al. 1993.)

idle visual projection areas due to rewiring effects in subcortical structures, e.g. in the thalamus. A less specific hypothesis states that the occipital negativity is simply due to a coactivation of the idle visual projections areas whenever other cortical areas are busy with specific tasks. Such a spill-over of activation could be due to the fact that intracortical inhibitory mechanisms are less well developed in cortices in which modality specific input is missing (Röder, Rösler and Hennighausen, submitted).

13.3.4 Conclusions About Cognitive SPSs

A principal finding in all of our (Rösler and co-workers) studies was that slow negative potentials emerged in parallel to specific processing episodes, i.e. the amplitude raised and dropped rather sharply at the beginning and the end of a trial, respectively. These negative SPSs had a task specific topography and an amplitude which reflected the amount of load which was imposed on the system in a particular processing episode. All these features suggest that negative SPSs reflect the activation of restricted cortical areas while the subject is engaged in specific episodes of information processing.

With respect to the physiological basis of these negative SPSs we believe that our results fit nicely into the theoretical framework outlined in the introduction. Accordingly we assume that performance related slow negative potentials reflect the activation of localised cortical cell assemblies. This functional interpretation of negative SPSs is corroborated by studies in which scalp recorded event-related negative DC potentials and regional cerebral blood flow (SPECT) were measured in the same group of subjects and in the very same task. This approach revealed that in a given task condition the maximum of the negative DC potential emerged exactly over that area of the cortex where also the highest metabolic rate was recorded (Lang M. et al. 1987a, 1988).

Taken together, negative SPSs seem to reflect subtle changes of localised cortical activation and may be used as a tool to monitor the functional topography of the cortex. Compared to other brain imaging methods such as positron emission topography (PET) and functional magnetic resonance imaging (fMRI), negative SPSs have several advantages. First of all, they have a much greater temporal resolution. As shown above, topographic changes of a SPS pattern can be observed already within one short trial (see the topographic shift between storage and transformation of an image). Moreover, SPSs reflect subtle differences in the level of area specific activation. Minor and moderate differences in task difficulty become apparent as reliable amplitude changes. And last but not least, the method can be used with much less design restrictions than PET and fMRI. For one thing, SPSs can be observed directly. To record them it does not need a subtraction design nor an integration over longer processing epochs. Moreover, the recording technique does not impose any restrictions on the subject. There is neither a high noise level, nor a potentially claustrophobic tube, nor any radioactivity.

13.4 Self-Regulation of Slow Potential Shifts

13.4.1 Instrumental Learning of SPSs and its Effects on Behaviour: The Pioneering Studies

In 1979, two studies were published independently, one by Bauer and Lauber (1979) and the other by Lutzenberger et al. (1979). A year before, the dissertation of Elbert (1978) had already appeared and was followed by a paper of Elbert et al. (1980), the latter receiving more widespread attention. Although the Bauer and Lauber paper reported changes of SPSs in positive and negative directions after positive reinforcement (points), Elbert et al. informed their subjects about SPS amplitude by providing them with feedback of their own SPS changes over 6 s by means of the outline of a rocket ship moving toward two goals, one for cortical positivity, the other for negativity (see Fig. 13.8). Subjects were reinforced after each 6-s trial by points exchangeable for money.

An on-line control algorithm compensated for eye movement artifacts and excluded the manipulation of baseline DC shifts. Most importantly, the

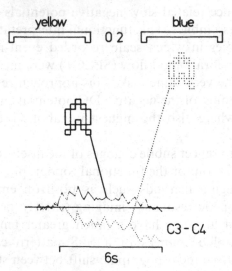

Fig. 13.8. Feedback display to train amplitude differences of SPSs between right (C$_4$) and left (C$_3$) premotor cortices. Subjects observe the difference between C$_3$ and C$_4$ for 6 s: EEG is represented as a rocket-ship moving toward one of two goals. If C$_3$ is more positive relative to C$_4$ the rocket moves toward the right goal, if C$_3$ is more negative relative to C$_4$ the rocket moves toward the left goal. Points are used as reinforcer for each successful trial. Discriminative stimuli (SD) indicating the direction of the required SPS polarity are tones or letters.

Viennese (Bauer and Nirnberger 1980, 1981) as well as the Tuebingen group (Lutzenberger et al. 1979) reported a strong positive relationship between the achieved cortical negativity and reaction time, signal detection and short-term memory performance. Self-induced cortical positivity consistently reduced cognitive and motor performance (see Birbaumer et al. 1981b for an early summary). The effects of self-regulation of SPSs on behaviour were in perfect accordance with neurophysiological facts, demonstrating that cortical negative SPSs in the EEG lasting more than 300 ms reflect widespread depolarisation of apical dendrites, partly dependent upon glial K^+ influx (see above). A critical argument which hampered biofeedback research from its beginnings in the seventies was the unspecific nature of the physiological effects: self-achieved cortical negativity and positivity may be the result of unspecific autonomic or somatic whole body activation and deactivation. This problem of somatic 'mediation' cannot be solved conclusively in human subjects, and animal curarisation during instrumental learning of autonomic responses produced equivocal results (Dworkin et al. 1984). Birbaumer et al. (1981a) demonstrated that improving self control of SPSs led to decreased covariation of electromyographic (EMG) activity, heart rate and skin conductance with the achieved SPS amplitudes.

In addition, during transfer trials in which subjects received no feedback at all, highly successful subjects did suppress peripheral covariations such as muscle tension, respiration and blood pressure, while unsuccessful subjects showed high correlations of SPSs and autonomic–somatic measures (Rockstroh et al. 1989). Birbaumer et al. (1988) even instructed subjects to use mental imagery of arm–hand movements which were accompanied by actual EMG changes to manipulate the cortical changes (Birbaumer et al. 1988). No significant difference for SPS control between the instructed group and a muscularly 'silent' group was found. Finally, in a totally paralysed patient ('locked-in', see below), an equivalent of curarisation, significant self-control of SPSs was possible (Kotchoubey et al. 1997). Taken together, these results provide strong, albeit not conclusive evidence for specific, non mediated self-control of SPSs.

13.4.2 The Specificity of Learned SPS-Control

Because SPSs exhibit topographical differences on the scalp according to the sensory, cognitive and motor function employed (Birbaumer et al. 1981b) regional self-control of SPSs should be possible. Several studies have established that healthy subjects could learn to change SPS amplitudes in an area-specific manner. The easiest task is to manipulate SPSs at the mid-central cortical area (C_z). However, to achieve control of the potential difference between left (C_3) and right (C_4) central areas, a minimum of five sessions is necessary and only half of the subjects achieve reliable control with specific behavioural consequences: after learned increase of unilateral negativity response speed, tactile performance and willingness to respond were improved at the contralateral hand (Rockstroh et al. 1990). To push the SPS-learned specificity towards its limits, subjects learned to differentiate SPS amplitude at mid-frontal (F_z) or mid-central (C_z) or mid-parietal (P_z) locations on 3 consecutive days (Birbaumer et al. 1992). Despite significant differences between the three groups (electrode locations) in SPS-control, complex cognitive tasks, presumably specific for the local SPS amplitude change, did not improve. The achieved differentiation was too fragile and broke down during task presentation; subjects used motor imagery strategies to manipulate F_z and C_z and attentional (non-motor) strategies for P_z.

In a more recent version of the feedback task, subjects had to manipulate right (C_4) minus left (C_3) SPSs simultaneously with C_z negativity-positivity in a fast 2-s rhythm which was paced by two tones of different pitch; one tone signalled the 2-s baseline interval, the other tone the 2-s feedback interval. During the 2-s feedback interval one of four goals (Fig. 13.9) was illuminated, indicating the required SPS-shift. Only after extended training of more than 10 sessions were some subjects able to achieve significant self-control on this extremely demanding task. Figure 13.10 gives an example (see Kotchoubey et al. 1997).

A further and final argument for the learned specificity of SPS control can be derived from fMRI of highly successful subjects. With fMRI, local cortico–subcortical blood flow changes can be recorded non-invasively (for a description of

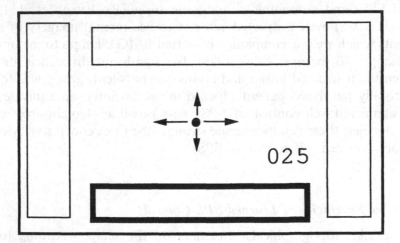

Fig. 13.9. Four goal display to train two-dimensional SPS changes: The 'ball' in the centre indicates actual SPS changes from a 2-s baseline. Beginning of baseline recording is indicated to the subject by a high pitched tone ('tic'). After 2-s, a low pitched tone ('tac') indicates 2-s feedback interval. Subjects have to move the ball (SPS change) toward one of the four goals during the feedback interval. The required goal-direction lights up. Right goal indicates that the subject has to achieve SPS negativity at C_4, left goal at C_3, upper goal negativity at C_z, and lower goal positivity at a very lateral location of the left hemisphere's central region C_7.

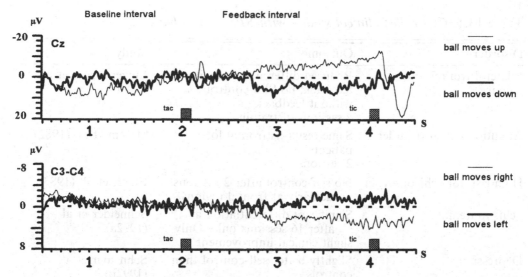

Fig. 13.10. SPSs of one subject after training of negativity-positivity at C_z (upper panel) and SPS differences between C_3 and C_4 (lower panel) using the feedback display of Fig. 4.2 and the described 2-s rhythmic baseline-feedback intervals.

the technology see Birbaumer and Schmidt 1996). Plate 5 shows an MRI slice at the level of the thalamus, encompassing frontal and occipital as well as temporal cortices. Colour coding indicates significantly increased blood flow during self-produced cortical negativity (blue) or positivity (red). No overlap in brain regions involved during self-induced negativity and positivity exists. Secondly, during self-induced negativity, brain structures responsible for the regulation of attention are primarily involved: right dorsomedial prefrontal cortex, bilateral anterior prefrontal cortex, bilateral thalamus and right parieto–occipital cortex. During positivity, the inferior right dorsolateral prefrontal cortex and left occipital region (the visual discriminative stimulus for required EEG polarity was presented during fMRI recording) are primarily involved. These data together with the clinical results (see below) provide conclusive support of the CNS-origin of learned cortical self-regulation (Birbaumer et al. 1998) and strengthens the threshold regulation model of SPS function formulated earlier (Birbaumer et al. 1990).

13.4.3 Applications of SPS Biofeedback

Age (15–70 years, see Kotchoubey et al. 1997), sex and IQ (from 65 to 140, Rockstroh et al. 1989) do not influence SPS biofeedback. Table 13.1 constitutes a summary of published studies with clinical groups. It is evident from this table that disorders characterised by attentional dysfunctions involving prefrontal functions such as brain lesions, attention decificit disorders, subjects with a high risk for schizophrenia and schizophrenics do not learn the task or need extensive training.

Table 13.1. *Controlled clinical studies with SPS-biofeedback*

Disorder	Outcome	Study
Bilateral frontal lobe damage	Reduced differentiation with feedback, no SPS-control without feedback 2 sessions of training	Lutzenberger et al. (1980)
Attention deficit disorder	Same result as frontal lobe patients 2 sessions	Stamm et al. (1982)
High-risk for schizophrenia	No self-control after 2 sessions, particularly at frontal regions	Elbert et al. (1983)
Schizophrenia	Significant differentiation at C_z after 16 sessions only. Only slight clinical improvement	Schneider et al. (1992a)
Depression	Slightly better self-control than controls	Schneider et al. (1992b)
Alcohol dependence	No self-control 2 weeks after withdrawal, normal 4 months after withdrawal	Schneider et al. (1993)
Psychosomatic disorder (migrain, hypertension)	Improved SPS self-control after 2 sessions compared to normals	Haag et al. (1981)
Drug-resistant epilepsy (mostly temporal lobe)	Two thirds of patients achieved self-control after 20 sessions. Significant clinical improvement after 28 to 40 sessions	Birbaumer et al. (1991) Rockstroh et al. (1993) Daum et al. (1993) Kotchoubey et al. (1997)
Complete motor paralysis ('locked-in')	Extended training led to improved communication	Birbaumer et al. (1994, 1996)

Behavioural disorders with a heightened sensitivity for autonomic processes and excessive cognitive self-perception show improved performance in SPS-control (such as in depression and psychosomatic disturbances). Clinically relevant therapeutic improvements were achieved for drug resistant epilepsy and total motor paralysis. Overall, basic and clinical research on SPS-self-regulation over the past 20 years constitutes an impressive example of the usefulness of this applied psychophysiological approach guided by a neurophysiological theory of SPS function.

Acknowledgements

This research was supported by the Austrian Scientific Research Fund (FWF) and the German Research Foundation (DFG).

14

Recent Evidence from Around the Brain for Structural Plasticity of Astrocytes in the Adult CNS

ADRIENNE K. SALM, NICHOLAS HAWRYLAK,
JOANNA B. BOBAK, GLENN I. HATTON and
CHIYE AOKI

Summary

Evidence that structural plasticity of astrocytes accompanies neuronal activation in the normal adult central nervous system (CNS) is now available in a number of diverse neural systems, including several hypothalamic nuclei, the hippocampus, and neo- and cerebellar cortices. For each of these regions we ask the following: What is the evidence for astrocytic structural plasticity? What is the nature of this plasticity? What behaviors could be associated with each of these regions? We conclude this chapter by briefly discussing how structural plasticity of astrocytes might be induced.

14.1 Introduction

Little is known about what determines the physical configuration of neurons and astrocytes in the adult CNS. It is often thought that astrocytes simply conform themselves to fill up otherwise empty spaces in the CNS. However, rigorous morphometric measures indicate that astrocytic processes contact other astrocyte processes only randomly in the neuropil, whereas they appear to have a preferential affinity for contacting neuronal surfaces (Wolff 1970). Current evidence also indicates that astrocytes alter their physical relationships with neurons, termed structural plasticity, to regulate neuronal communication. This is thought to be accomplished by astrocytes rearranging their processes to modulate synaptic contacts (Hatton and Tweedle 1982; Garcia-Segura, Baetens and Naftolin 1986; Meshul, Seil and Herndon 1987, Olmos et al. 1989) and through the establishment and maintenance of neuronal subgroupings (Cooper and Steindler 1986; Tolbert and Oland 1990). In each region where astrocytic structural plasticity has been documented in the normal adult CNS, the commonality is that a fairly discrete group of neurons is challenged to adapt to a changing internal or external milieu. Below, we review a number of these regions where evidence for structural plasticity of astrocytes has accumulated. In keeping with the overall theme of this volume, we speculate as to the possible impact of astrocytic structural plasticity on behaviour.

14.2 Structural Plasticity of Hypothalamic Astrocytes

14.2.1 Structural Plasticity of Astrocytes Associated with Neuroendocrine Neurons: The Hypothalamo-neurohypophysial Neurosecretory System

It has been 20 years since Tweedle and Hatton (1976, 1977) first published their observations that stimulation of the hypothalamic supraoptic nucleus (SON) and nucleus circularis of rats by water deprivation resulted in a profound remodelling of these nuclei, seemingly brought about by a de-ensheathment of magnocellular neuroendocrine cells (MNCs) by their neighbouring astrocytes. Theodosis and colleagues thereafter described similar observations in the SON of lactating animals (Theodosis, Poulain and Vincent 1981). This work was soon extended with the finding that astrocytes of the posterior pituitary, pituicytes, also change their ensheathment of neurosecretory axons with stimulation (Tweedle and Hatton 1980).

Since these seminal observations, the hypothalamo-neurohypophysial neurosecretory system (HNS) has served as a powerful model for the study of structural plasticity of neurons and associated astrocytes in the adult nonpathological brain. The HNS, consisting primarily of the SON (Fig. 14.1), the paraventricular nucleus, nucleus circularis and the posterior pituitary, responds to a variety of stimuli by activating MNC's to synthesize and/or release their neuropeptides oxy-

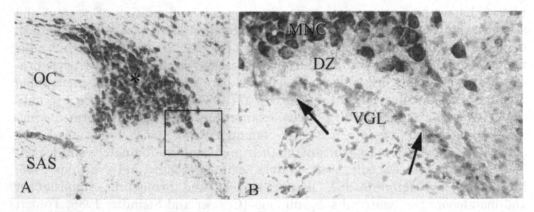

Fig. 14.1. Light micrograph of a pyronine Y stained section through the hypothalamus of a rat showing the location and organisation of the SON. (A) Low power image showing the SON (asterisk) adjacent to the optic chiasm (OC). (B) Higher power view of enclosed area in (A), showing the location of the ventral glial limitans (VGL), dendritic zone (DZ) and magnocellular neuroendocrine cell (MNC) somata. Arrows in (B) point to a row of astrocyte nuclei in the VGL. SAS, subarachnoid space.

tocin, vasopressin, or both. These stimuli include parturition, lactation, and dehydration brought about by 2% saline substitution for drinking water, intraperitoneal injection of hypertonic saline, or water deprivation. Structural changes of the SON have also been observed in virgin female rats induced to behave maternally by exposure to rat pups (Salm, Modney and Hatton 1988), behaviours known to be associated with oxytocin (Fahrbach, Morrell and Pfaff 1984).

14.2.2 The Glial Retraction Hypothesis

From electron microscopic studies showing an absence of astrocyte processes where they were normally seen, Tweedle and Hatton postulated (1976, 1977) that HNS astrocytes and pituicytes (Tweedle and Hatton 1980) actively retract their processes from between MNCs and posterior pituitary axons, respectively, concurrent with stimulation. Further observations also indicated that retraction of astrocytic processes leads to an 'uncovering' of postsynaptic sites and the establishment of additional synaptic contacts (Theodosis, Poulain and Vincent 1981; Hatton and Tweedle 1982) in the form of novel 'multiple' synapses (one pre-synaptic profile in synaptic contact with two or three postsynaptic elements) in both the somatic and dendritic zones (Perlmutter, Tweedle and Hatton 1984; Theodosis and Poulain 1984). The absence of glial processes was thereafter implicated in the formation of dendritic bundles (Perlmutter, Tweedle and Hatton 1984, 1985; Salm, Modney and Hatton 1988) and gap junctions (Andrew et al. 1981; Cobbett and Hatton 1984). With the cessation of stimulation, most of these changes are entirely reversed (Hatton et al. 1984), with astrocytes apparently reinserting their processes around neighbouring neuronal structures. Analogously, in the posterior pituitary, the resident pituicytes re-envelop neurosecretory axon terminals, again segregating them from the fenestrated capillaries there and hampering peptide release.

Thus, the accumulated evidence indicates that HNS astrocytes are inextricably involved with events of neurosecretion. The original observations and their functional import have been recent subjects of extensive reviews (Hatton 1990, 1997; Theodosis and Poulain 1993). The reader is referred to these articles for in-depth discussion.

14.2.3 Quantitation and Three-Dimensional Imaging of GFAP Immunoreactivity

To assess further the possible active rearrangement of SON astrocytic processes, we (Salm, Smithson and Hatton 1985) earlier investigated immunoreactivity for a major astrocytic cytoskeletal constituent, glial fibrillary acidic protein (GFAP; Uyeda, Eng and Bignami 1972), reasoning that changes in GFAP might accompany gross structural changes of these cells. GFAP immunoreactivity in the SON of lactating rats was reduced in the SON, relative to control rats in the oestrous phase of their cycle. These results are consistent with the notion that astrocyte processes retract. Recently, we have assessed whether the stimulus of dehydration would also have the same effect on GFAP immunoreactivity, and whether the reduction in staining was reversible (Hawrylak, Fleming and Salm 1998). As expected, the GFAP immunoreactivity of the SON significantly decreased in the dehydrated group compared to controls and subsequently returned to control levels with rehydration. Again, these reversible changes in a cytoskeletal protein are consistent with reversible morphological changes of the resident astrocytes.

Examination of this material with three-dimensional microscopy (Edge Scientific Instrument Corporation, Santa Monica, CA, USA) also revealed that, in normally hydrated animals, the astrocyte processes present in the SON appeared to delineate the spaces that, we believe, are occupied by MNCs (Fig. 14.2). With dehydration, there was significantly less GFAP immunoreactivity as determined by densitometry, and the apparent delineation of MNCs was less visible. With rehydration, the original organisation was re-established.

While changes in GFAP immunoreactivity are consistent with the idea of morphological remodelling, they are not entirely irrefutable evidence for active structural plasticity (Salm, Smithson and Hatton 1985). The changes in GFAP immunoreactivity might simply reflect slight modifications in the GFAP epitope that render the protein differently visible to GFAP antibodies. Moreover, since GFAP may or may not be distributed throughout an entire astrocyte, immunostaining may be inadequate to visualise changes in fine, GFAP immunonegative processes, where astrocyte process motility could be greatest, as is suggested by observations made in vitro (Cornell-Bell, Thomas and Smith 1990).

14.2.4 Direct Light and Electron Microscopic Evidence of Structural Plasticity of Son-VGL Astrocytes

We have recently carried out direct electron and light microscopic measures of astrocytes in the ventral glial limitans subjacent to the SON (son-*VGL*). These son-*VGL* astrocytes send exceptionally long GFAP- and vimentin-immunoreactive processes dorsally into the SON, where they surround and ensheathe magnocellular neuronal somata and dendrites (Yulis, Peruzzo and Rodriguez 1984; Bonfanti, Poulain and Theodosis 1993). We observed that the thickness of the son-*VGL* was significantly decreased in 9-day dehydrated animals when compared with controls (Figs 14.3, 14.4, and 14.5; Bobak and Salm 1996). This reversed toward control levels with rehydration. An electron microscopic evaluation of individual astrocytes in the same material revealed that a reversible overall reorientation of astrocyte cytoplasm, from a direction perpendicular to the pial surface to one parallel to the pial surface also occurred with stimulation. The orientation of individual astrocytes was much more likely to be vertical in control animals.

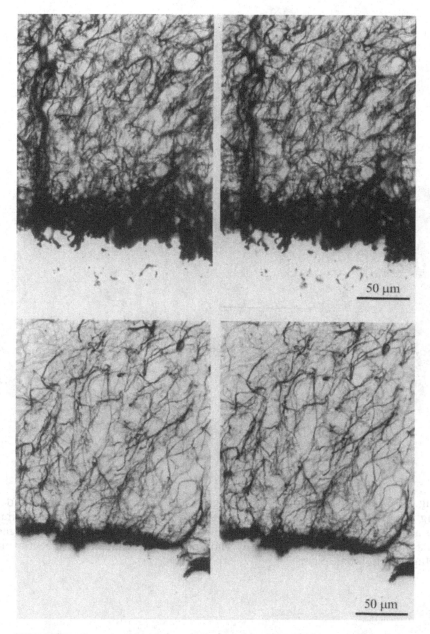

Fig. 14.2. Stereo pair micrographs showing GFAP immunoreactivity in the SON. (Top) Hydrated control and (bottom) 6-day dehydrated rats. Stereo viewing reveals a highly organised arrangement of astrocyte processes in the SON of the hydrated rat. This organisation is lost in the dehydrated rat. (Stereo viewers available from Reel 3-D Enterprises, Inc., Culver City, CA, or from many electron microscopy vendors.)

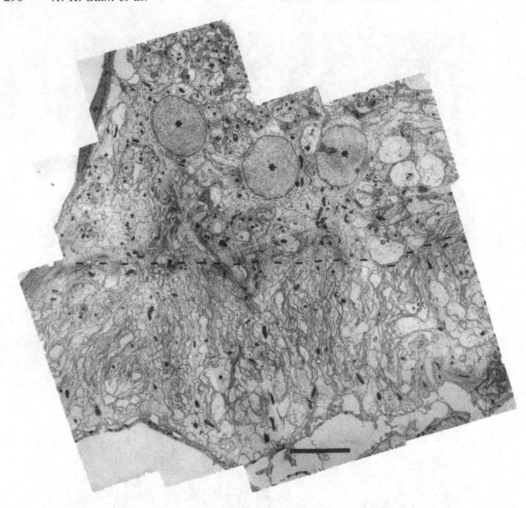

Fig. 14.3. Electron micrograph montage of the VGL of a control animal depicting vertically oriented palisading processes (below the dashed line), contributing to a thick VGL subjacent to the SON. SAS is located ventrally. The magnocellular neurons are located dorsally (not pictured.) Asterisks, astrocytic nuclei. Magnification bar, 5 μm.

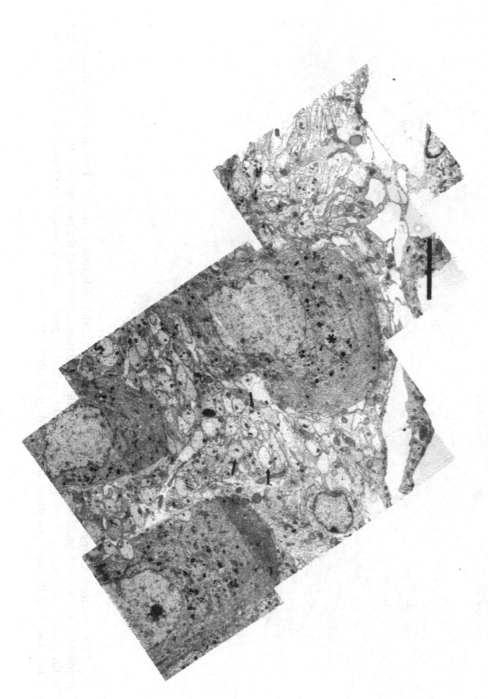

Fig. 14.4. Electron micrograph montage of the VGL of a 9-day dehydrated animal. Note the relative absence of glial processes, resulting in a very thin VGL. SAS is located ventrally. Note the close proximity of a magnocellular neuron (asterisk), and many dendritic profiles (arrows) to the subjacent SAS. Magnification bar, 5 μm.

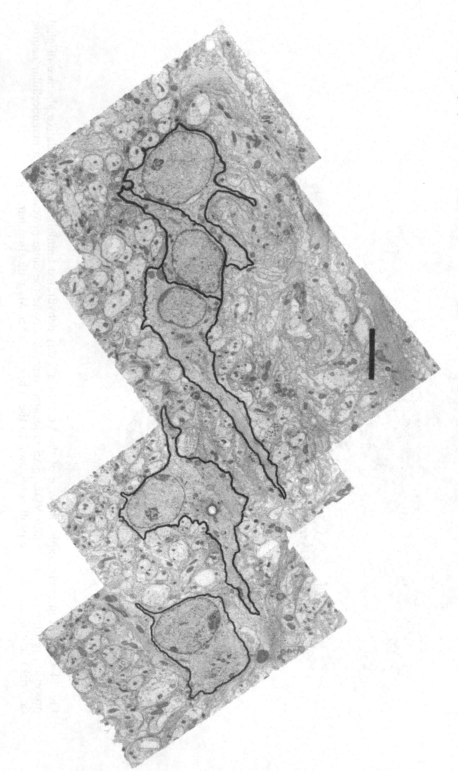

Fig. 14.5. Electron micrograph montage of astrocytes in a 2-day dehydrated animal. This montage depicts astrocytes (outlined in black) with predominantly intermediate orientations, relative to the pial surface. We postulate that they were in the process of changing from a predominantly vertical to predominantly horizontal orientation when the animal was killed. The dendritic zone is located dorsally. Magnification bar, 5 μm.

Conversely, astrocytes with a horizontal orientation were significantly greater in number in 9-day dehydrated animals. It appears that astrocytes in the son-*VGL* have a preferred orientation, depending on hydration state. A regression analysis revealed that astrocytes were predominantly oriented in horizontal or vertical orientations and that a non-oriented state was not favoured by astrocytes. Since cells with no orientation were included in this analysis, this indicates that son-*VGL* astrocytes have a propensity to be polarised in relation to the pial surface. As to how these changes might come about, it may be that cells achieve reorientation by 'pinwheeling' 90° around a somatic axis without radically changing their overall configuration. Alternatively, a similar result could occur if astrocyte cytoplasm flows, amoeboid-like, from one part of the cell to another. Either type of motion could conceivably result in a removal of fine processes from between neuronal somata and dendrites in the SON, i.e. glial retraction (Fig. 14.6).

As to the possible functional significance of astrocyte reorientation, we speculate that it could contribute to the clearance of extracellular potassium from the SON to the cerebrospinal fluid (CSF) of the subarachnoid space (SAS). Coles and Poulain (1991) found an increase in K^+ in the SAS at the inferior limit of the SON during antidromic stimulation of the pituitary stalk and suggested that K^+ clearance occurs through spatial buffering by glial cells to the SAS during stimulation of the SON. Astrocyte reorientation may enhance K^+ clearance by increasing the astrocytic surface area interfaced between the SON and SAS, or by otherwise making an existing astrocytic syncytium more efficient. As to possible functional consequences of decreased son-*VGL* thickness, one hypothesis is that thinning may facilitate increased CSF–SON communication. It is known that diffusible molecules may pass into the parenchyma from the CSF (Wagner, Pilgrim and Brandl 1974; Davson 1989) or vice versa. Given that peptides are released by exocytosis from SON dendrites (Pow and Morris 1989), a thinner son-*VGL* might enable peptide release directly into the CSF. This may provide a means of communication between the two supraoptic nuclei, as well as other circumventricular structures (see Summy-Long et al. 1994, for discussion) and explain, at least in part, how neurohypophysial peptides get into the CSF (Robinson and Coombes 1993). A second possibility is that a thinner VGL enables an osmotic signal contributed by a hyperosmotic CSF (Pape and Katzman 1970; Pullen, DePasquale and Cserr 1987) to reach osmosensitive magnocellular neurons in the SON (Oliet and Bourque 1994).

14.2.5 *A Possible Role for Pituicyte Proliferation in Structural Plasticity of the Neurohypophysis*

It has been known for a long time that there is significant proliferation of astrocytes in the SON and posterior pituitary of very young rats when the HNS is stimulated by dehydration (Murray 1968; Paterson and LeBlond 1977).

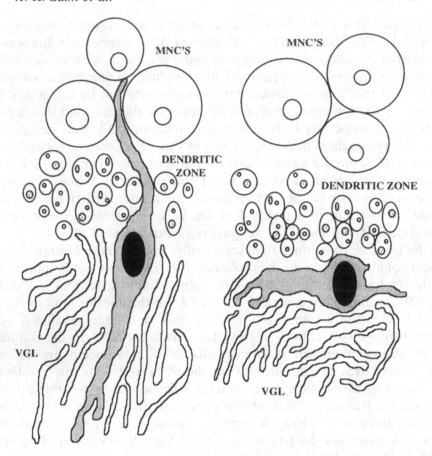

Fig. 14.6. Hypothetical schematic demonstrating how astrocyte reorientation may lead to glial retraction in the SON. The figure on the left demonstrates a control animal, while that on the right depicts a 9-day dehydrated animal. Note the thinner VGL and astrocyte reorientation to a horizontal orientation with dehydration.

Observations of astroglia in vitro, which often lose their processes prior to cell division, suggested that re-entry into the cell cycle may account, in part, for the changes seen in pituicyte ensheathment of axons in response to stimulation. We quantified proliferation of pituicytes in tissue sections obtained from fully adult hydrated, dehydrated, and rehydrated rats (Murugaiyan and Salm 1995; Fig. 14.7). Marked proliferation began within three days of dehydration and continued thereafter, even in animals allowed to rehydrate. After 9 days of dehydration, approximately 35% of identified pituicytes had participated in mitosis. While cell density remained constant across conditions, a reversible increase in posterior pituitary area was seen, suggesting that some cell death may occur simultaneously.

With respect to a relation between pituicyte proliferation and structural plasticity of pituicytes, we observed that cells well-stained for the proliferation marker bromodeoxyuridine (BrdU) often did not display arrays of well-differentiated processes as seen by GFAP immunocytochemistry. In these cases, nuclei were more often surrounded by only a thin rim of GFAP+ cytoplasm from which few, if any, processes projected. In tissue from rehydrated animals, pituicytes frequently had thick perinuclear, GFAP+, cytoplasm, as well as long, thick processes. We propose that this proliferative response is related to the morphological changes previously reported for these cells under activating conditions, although a direct test of this hypothesis will prove a challenge.

14.2.6 A Possible Role of Glycoconjugate Molecules in SON Plasticity

The plasticity observed in the stimulated SON may also involve tenascin (Erickson and Bourdon 1989; see Singleton and Salm 1996, for review), a molecule thought to influence the direction of outgrowing axons and dendrites and, ultimately, determine specific cell–cell interactions. Tenascin has been shown to both inhibit or facilitate neurite outgrowth (Grumet et al. 1985) and neural pattern formation during development. In the normal adult CNS, tenascin expression generally has been reported to be minimal with a few exceptions (see Singleton and Salm, 1996, for discussion). In tissue sections from control adult rats, the tenascin antibody stained the son-*VGL* and dendritic zone subjacent to the SON (Fig. 14.8). This staining was absent in tissues obtained from dehydrated rats. Likewise, Coomassie stained mini-gels of son-*VGL* tissues revealed a decrease in the 210–220 kD tenascin band after prolonged dehydration (Fig. 14.8). An increase in tenascin expression back to, or beyond, control levels was also repeatedly observed with rehydration.

Since immunocytochemistry of tissue sections revealed this protein to be predominantly present in the son-*VGL* itself and in the dendritic zone of the SON, through which son-*VGL* astrocytes project, its effects are probably limited to dendrites, their associated synapses, and local astrocytes. One major impact of its decrease in the son-*VGL* with dehydration might be to enable dendritic bundling (Perlmutter, Tweedle and Hatton 1985) and gap junction formation (Cobbett and Hatton 1984). Both are thought to enhance neurosecretory activity of magnocellular neurons. In this regard, it has been shown that, with stimulation, gap junctions form only between dendrites of like peptide containing neurons (Cobbett, Smithson and Hatton 1985; Hatton, Yang and Cobbett 1987). Similarly, at least for oxytocinergic somata, it has also been reported that direct membrane appositions usually occur only with other oxytocinergic somata or dendrites (Chapman et al. 1986). It may be that the disappearance of tenascin from the son-*VGL* is related to selective alliances between cells. Further support for this idea comes from Grierson et al. (1990), who found that neonatal

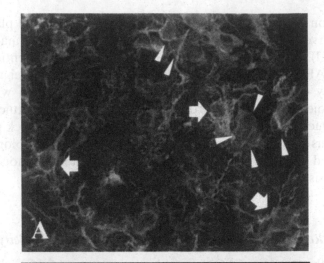

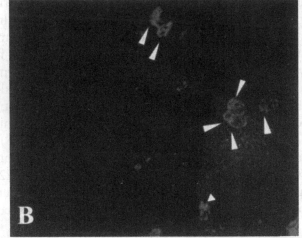

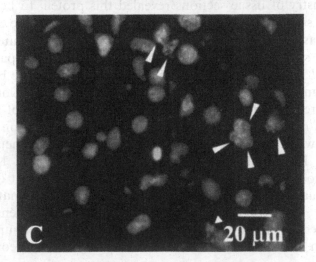

hypothalamic neurons were loath to come into contact with a subpopulation of underlying 'rocky' astroglia that were also immunoreactive for tenascin.

Other investigators have suggested a role for cell-surface-associated molecules in the HNS. Most notably, Theodosis, Rougon and Poulain (1991) have described the presence of the polysialic acid-linked form of the neural cell adhesion molecule, PSA-NCAM, in the adult HNS. We find it of interest that the deposition of PSA-NCAM is very similar to that of tenascin, being distributed most heavily in the son-*VGL* and dendritic zone. Although these authors did not report variations in PSA-NCAM expression with changes in stimulus conditions, it is possible that PSA-NCAM, tenascin, and perhaps other extracellular matrix molecules work together to regulate plasticity in the SON. Kiss et al. (1993) have also reported PSA-NCAM on both neurosecretory axons and pituicytes of the posterior pituitary. PSA-NCAM expression by pituicytes was dependent on intact neurosecretory axons: stalk transection led to its disappearance from the neural lobe, and suggests that extracellular matrix molecules can be regulated by neuronal signals from adjacent axons (see Chapter 15).

Before leaving the HNS, we should note that despite similar observations made under dissimilar stimulus conditions in various parts of the HNS, we do not believe that all astrocytes are the same, even within the individual nuclei of the HNS. In the SON alone, the data indicate that son-*VGL* astrocytes are a different population to those in the nucleus proper. First, SON-proper astrocytes proliferate readily when the nucleus is activated (Murray 1968; Paterson and LeBlond 1977), whereas son-*VGL* astrocytes do not (Salm and Moats, unpublished observations). In addition, son-*VGL* astrocytes express relatively high levels of vimentin (Bonfanti, Poulain and Theodosis 1993) and tenascin (Singleton and Salm 1996), whereas SON-proper astrocytes do not. This suggests that there are at least two functionally and phenotypically distinct populations of astrocytes serving the SON.

Fig. 14.7. Triple-labelled section through the posterior pituitary showing proliferating and non-proliferating pituicytes in a 9-day dehydrated rat. (A) GFAP immunostaining, (B) immunostaining for the proliferation marker bromodeoxyuridine (BrdU), and (C) labelling of all cell nuclei with DAPI. A number of well differentiated pituicytes can be seen (large arrows in A) with clear perinuclear cytoplasm and well developed processes. Such cells were never seen to be labelled with BrdU. Also a number of BrdU + cells are visible in (B) (large carets), all except one are also GFAP + (small caret.) Two cells in the act of dividing can be seen in the top centre field. These cells display only a thin rim of perinuclear cytoplasm and two short processes. Dehydration was induced by substitution of 2% saline for drinking water. (After Murugaiyan and Salm 1995.)

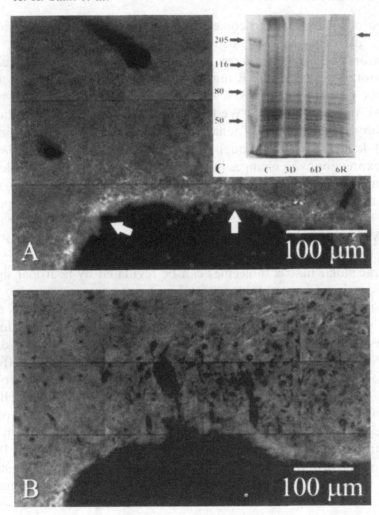

Fig. 14.8. Computer generated montages of the son-*VGL*. (A) Tenascin immunostaining in the son-*VGL* in a normally hydrated rat. (B) Montage of an identically processed tissue section from a 6-day dehydrated rat. No tenascin immunostaining in the son-*VGL* is evident. (Inset) Coomassie-Blue-stained protein gel of the combined bilateral SONs dissected from control (C), 3-day dehydrated (3D), 6-day dehydrated (6D), and 6-day rehydrated (6R) rats. Total protein was 18.2 μg loaded in each lane. The 210–220 kD tenascin bands are indicated by the arrow on the right. A consistent decrease in this band was seen following dehydration with an increase back toward control levels with rehydration. (After Singleton and Salm 1996.)

14.2.7 *Evidence for Structural Plasticity of Astrocytes in Hypothalamic Regions Involved with Reproduction*

A number of investigators have examined the arcuate nucleus and median eminence of rodents and the preoptic area, mediobasal hypothalamus, and infundibular areas of primates as models to study gonadal steroid influences on brain plasticity (Garcia-Segura, Baetens and Naftolin 1986; Garcia-Segura et al. 1996), and have found evidence for structural plasticity of astrocytes. Olmos et al. (1989) examined synaptic remodelling in the arcuate nuclei of the rodent over the oestrous cycle. By electron microscopy, they determined that the percentage of neuronal membrane covered by synapses, as well as the number of synapses per 1000 μm of membrane decreased at oestrus, a time of high plasma oestrogen. This change occurred quickly, within the 24-h period between pro-oestrus and oestrus. Concurrently, they also observed an increase in the percentage of neuronal membranes ensheathed by glial processes.

Witkin and colleagues (1991) pursued these observations in their study of whether gonadal steroids affect synapses and glial appositions onto immunocytochemically identified gonadotrophin releasing hormone (GnRH) neurons in the mediobasal hypothalamus and preoptic area of Rhesus monkeys. These areas are somewhat analogous to the rodent arcuate, although the latter does not contain GnRH neurons. Ovariectomised animals demonstrated an increase in glial ensheathment in both the preoptic area and mediobasal hypothalamus, relative to animals receiving silastic implants with steroids or intact animals. This was concomitant with a decrease in synaptic density in both regions. While these results are consistent with the idea that glial ensheathment and synaptic coverage are inversely related, as also determined by Olmos et al. (1989), the impact of oestrogen appears to be opposite in the two experimental systems.

Naftolin et al. (1993) also investigated the astrocyte ensheathment/synapse relationship in the African green monkey and found that ovariectomised animals had significantly more synapses and less glial ensheathment of hypothalamic infundibular neurons (equivalent to arcuate neurons in the rat) than did ovariectomised animals that had received intramuscular injections of 1 mg/kg oestradiol valerate 3 days before sacrifice. Their results were the same as in the rat arcuate: oestrogen replacement led to an increased ensheathment of infundibular neurons and a concomitant decrease in synaptic density.

In a recent study, Garcia-Segura et al. (1994) re-examined astrocyte structural plasticity and its relationship to synaptic ensheathment in the rat arcuate nucleus. Using modern stereological methods, this group again reported an increase in the neuronal membrane coverage by astrocytic profiles on the afternoon of pro-oestrus/morning of oestrus. As seen by glial fibrillary acid protein (GFAP) immunoreactivity, they found that there was a simultaneous, reversible, increase in the surface density (amount of astrocyte surface in the neuropil) of astrocytic processes during the afternoon of pro-oestrus and the morning of oestrus. These then declined to baseline for the rest of the cycle. With electron microscopy, they further measured the incidence and size of filament bundles. Somewhat paradoxically, they found that the size of filament bundles decreased on the afternoon of pro-oestrus and morning of oestrus, whereas the number of astrocyte profiles containing filament bundles increased at the same time. Since filament bundles decreased, but the number of glial profiles containing filament bundles increased, we can surmise that new GFAP is being assembled into nascent, smaller, filament bundles on the afternoon of pro-oestrus. Kohama et al. (1995) and Chowen et al. (1995) have shown that GFAP messenger ribose nucleic acid (mRNA) increases on the afternoon of pro-oestrus and in response to injections of oestradiol into ovariectomised female rats, confirming that changes of GFAP immunoreactivity are related to alterations in GFAP mRNA synthesis.

While these data are nicely complementary, in an earlier study, Tranque et al. (1987) found an increased astrocytic surface density in the globus pallidus and hippocampus, but not in the arcuate nucleus after oestradiol valerate injections. The reason for this disparity is not clear, but may be related to the relatively high dose of oestrodial (s.c. 20 mg/kg) used in this study.

Recently, confocal microscopic imaging has demonstrated a dynamic relationship between luteinising hormone releasing hormone (LHRH) immunoreactive axon terminals and vimentin+ tanycytes (astrocytes) in the median eminence during the preovulatory surge of LHRH (King, Ronsheim and Rubin 1995). This change in tanycyte ensheathment appears similar to the structural plasticity of pituicytes observed in the posterior pituitary.

While it is significant that another neural system, in addition to the HNS, undergoes changes that seem dependent on structural plasticity of astrocytes, the identity of the neurons that are the recipients of changing synaptic input, at least in the rodent, has to our knowledge not yet been established. Neither is it clear if the physiology of these neurons is altered in any significant way from pro-oestrus to oestrus, concurrent with the changing synaptic input, reduction in astrocyte coverage or both. Thus, it is not possible to determine the consequences of changing synaptic input to these neurons beyond speculating that these changes are somehow involved in the hormonal changes that precede oestrus. Since the rodent arcuate nucleus does not contain GnRH neurons, it is likewise difficult to speculate on the behavioural significance of astrocyte de-ensheathment and increased synaptic input to arcuate neurons.

14.2.8 Studies of Astrocyte Plasticity in a Hypothalamic Region that Controls Circadian Rhythms: The Suprachiasmatic Nucleus

Another area of the hypothalamus where the activity of the resident neurons must vary in a matter of hours for the nucleus to perform its function is the suprachiasmatic nucleus (SCN). Here it has been shown that neurons in this region are responsible for encoding photic information and entraining circadian rhythms in rodents (Miller 1993). Rhythms in glucose consumption, electrical activity and peptide synthesis have been documented for this nucleus. Furthermore, many of these rhythms are maintained when the nucleus is placed in explant cultures. Hence, the diurnal 'clock' is contained in the SCN and determining its mechanism has been the subject of much interest (see Miller 1993, for review). Although relative numbers of astrocytic cell bodies per neuron in the SCN proper are a great deal lower than in surrounding areas of the anterior hypothalamus (van den Pol 1980), the SCN is heavily invested with extensive astrocytic processes. Recently, evidence has been presented that GFAP immunoreactivity in the SCN is cyclic in Syrian hamsters, reaching a nadir approximately 2 h after activity onset (2 h after 'lights off'; Lavialle and Serviere 1993). At this time, immunoreactivity was seen only in isolated stellate astrocytes, rather than spread in a complex meshwork throughout the SCN. Interestingly, this pattern persisted in animals who had been exposed to 8 days of constant darkness. Lu et al. (1996) have also shown by GFAP immunocytochemistry that SCN astrocytes are larger during oestrus, relative to pro-oestrus in two strains of hamsters. They postulated that this 'glial swelling' acted to block electrotonic coupling between SCN neurons because a light pulse given to animals after 2 weeks of constant darkness induced a much larger phase-shift in their activity rhythms when administered during oestrus versus pro-oestrus.

These data offer the tantalising possibility that SCN astrocytes might be involved with very profound aspects of behaviour: regulation of diurnal activities. However, it should be noted that electron microscopic investigations in the rat failed to detect any changes in the amount of astrocytic coverage of SCN neurons over the circadian cycle (Elliot and Nunez 1994). Hence, the significance and interspecies prevalence of these observations have yet to be determined.

14.2.9 Structural Plasticity of Hypothalamic Astrocytes and Behaviour

To summarise, regions of the hypothalamus where structural plasticity of astrocytes may ultimately prove to influence behaviour are the HNS, the arcuate nucleus and median eminence (rodents), preoptic area, infundibular nucleus, and mediobasal hypothalamus (primates) and the suprachiasmatic nucleus. The overall function of the hypothalamus, that of integrating sensory, endocrine, visceral, and internal metabolic signals to maintain homeostasis, is accomplished in part by adjusting motivational states and resultant overt behaviours. This includes ingestive behaviours necessary to maintain the internal milieu, i.e. feeding and drinking. It also applies to reproductive and parenting behaviours, including parturition and lactation, lordosis, crouching, nest building, pup retrieval and nursing, and overall activity levels. We speculate that these are some of the behaviours that could ultimately prove to be influenced by structural plasticity of astrocytes.

14.3 Structural Plasticity of Hippocampal, Neo- and Cerebellar Cortical Astrocytes

14.3.1 Correlation of Astrocytic Structural Plasticity with Long-Term Potentiation (LTP) and Kindling: Hippocampus

Hippocampal long-term potentiation (LTP) has become the best model for a cellular explanation of biological information storage, i.e. memory (see Baudry and Davis 1991, for review). Kindling, a technique whereby hippocampal tissue is rendered seizure-prone, shares many similarities with LTP (see Cain 1989; Wallace, Hawrylak and Greenough 1991). A dynamic correlation of astrocytic structural changes with synaptic plasticity has been demonstrated with both LTP and kindling (Cain 1989; Wallace, Hawrylak and Greenough 1991). An increase in the number of synapses in the hippocampus is a feature of both LTP (Lee et al. 1980; Chang and Greenough 1984) and kindling (Hawrylak, Chang and Greenough 1993). In rat, hippocampal dentate gyrus potentiations resulted in increased astrocytic coverage of dendritic buttons and spines compared to controls (Wenzel et al. 1991). Similar ultrastructural changes of astrocytic processes occurred in the hippocampal CA1 region when rats were kindled to five generalised seizures (Hawrylak, Chang and Greenough 1993). In addition, the kindled rats demonstrated an increase in the density of synapses on dendritic shafts simultaneously with an increase in the volume fraction of astrocytic processes (a measure of how much of the neuropil is composed of astrocytes).

The profound effects of oestrogen on hypothalamic tissues, discussed above, are also seen in the hippocampus. Electrophysiological studies of the hippocampus have demonstrated that neuronal excitability increases with the rising levels of oestrogen that occur during the afternoon of pro-oestrus. Seizure threshold is lowered during pro-oestrus (Teresawa and Timiras 1968), and female rats examined during the afternoon of pro-oestrus demonstrated the greatest degree of LTP compared to male rats and female examined at each phase of the oestrous cycle either in the morning or afternoon (Warren et al. 1995). Anatomically, the number of dendritic spines and axo–spinous synapses in the hippocampus fluctuates across the rat oestrous cycle, being high on pro-oestrus and low on oestrus (Woolley et al. 1990; Woolley and McEwen 1992). Interestingly, the volume fraction of astrocytic processes, as estimated in electron micrographs, also fluctuates across the estrous cycle, being significantly lower on the afternoon of pro-oestrus than on the afternoon of oestrus (Klintsova, Levy and Desmond 1995).

14.3.2 Experience Induces Structural Plasticity of Astrocytes: Visual Cortex

Unlike LTP and kindling, the use of the 'enriched' or 'complex' environment procedure, originated by Hebb (1947) and extensively used by Rosenzweig, Bennett and Diamond (1972) and Greenough (1988) permits the assessment of structural plasticity of all cortical neural elements in relation to an animal's interaction with the environment. The work of Hebb first demonstrated that rats reared with the opportunity for a variety of behavioural experiences outperformed standard laboratory reared animals on learning tasks, thus providing a rationale for using this paradigm in studying the mechanisms of memory.

Neurons in the visual cortex of rats raised in enriched conditions (EC) have increased dendritic arborisation, greater numbers of synapses per neuron and greater lengths of synaptic contact zone, compared to individually caged (IC) rats (reviewed Greenough and Chang 1988). These neuronal changes are paralleled by an increased volume fraction of glial nuclei (Turner and Greenough 1985) and a time-dependent increase in the surface density (the amount of astrocyte surface in the neuropil) and number of astrocytes positive for GFAP (Sirevaag and Greenough 1991). Recent findings also demonstrate that astrocytic processes directly apposed to synapses are, in fact, altered by experience. EC rats have a greater surface area of astrocytic processes surrounding synapses than the IC rats (Jones and Greenough 1996). This greater astrocytic ensheathment of synapses in EC rats is even more interesting if one considers that astrocytic processes were not significantly different in EC and IC rats, as indicated by measures of overall astrocytic growth: surface density, volume fraction and average area per process. These data suggest that astrocytes are not just filling up the extra volume like glue or packing material, but appear to be selectively participating in synaptic formation and plasticity.

Time-course work suggests that the response of astrocytes in EC rats appears to be two-phased: a period of astrocyte growth, followed by one of astrocyte proliferation. GFAP immunoreactive astrocytes grew larger in the EC rats over the first month of exposure. With an additional month of EC exposure, the relative size of the astrocytes decreased while the number of GFAP-positive cells increased (Sirevaag and Greenough 1991). Similar to astrocytes in the activated HNS, the postnatal proliferation of visual cortical astrocytes appears to be greatly influenced by environmental complexity; a consistent result from a number of laboratories is an increase in the number of glial cells in EC rats compared to those raised in standard conditions (Altman and Das 1964; Diamond et al. 1966; Szeligo and LeBlond 1977). Because the visual cortex of young-adult rats exposed to complex environments shows dendritic growth and synaptogenesis, events that parallel those of development, it is possible that the proliferation of astrocytes provides a transient population of 'young' cells that recapitulate the conditions necessary for early developmental levels of neuronal plasticity (see Chapter 3).

14.3.3 Motor Learning Induces Synaptogenesis and Astrocytic Structural Plasticity: Cerebellum

As we have seen in the visual cortex and hippocampus, astrocytic volume fraction and process surface density increases in association with the addition of synapses.

In these cases, the additional synapses are associated with a presumed increase in the average amount of synaptic activity as well as an increase in peak activity levels (and synchronous discharge in the case of kindling). Thus, the increased astrocytic parameters could reflect responses to either increased synaptic activity, synapse number, or both. A paradigm that allows these two influences to be separated is to subject a 'learning' group of rats to daily practice on a series of difficult motor tasks. Two 'activity' control groups are additionally subjected to either forced exercise on a treadmill or voluntary exercise in a running wheel attached to the home cage. Black et al. (1990) found that, in the cerebellar paramedian lobule, the exercise group had a higher density of capillaries relative to both a third, 'inactive' control and the learning group, indicating that the exercise manipulation placed increased metabolic demands on the tissue. In the learning group, synapse number per neuron was increased relative to all other groups, suggesting that synapse addition corresponds specifically to learning. Subsequently, using the same tissue, Anderson et al. (1994) found that an increased volume of astrocytic processes per Purkinje cell occurred only in the learning animals. Hence, in this case, structural plasticity of astrocytes appeared to correspond with learning-related synaptogenesis rather than to a general increase in metabolic or synaptic activity, as reflected by the angiogenesis seen in the vasculature.

With respect to dynamic astrocyte–neuron interactions in the cerebellum, in vitro evidence indicates that cerebellar astrocytes act to modulate synaptic density. Purkinje cells in glia-free cultures form aberrant synapses with their own somata and dendrites. When cerebellar astrocytes were added to these cultures, the number of synapses decreased and the number of noninnervated spines increased (Meshul, Seil and Herndon 1987; Seil, Meshul and Herndon 1988). Astrocyte-conditioned medium, similarly, increased the number of noninnervated spines, apparently by proliferation of spines in the absence of presynaptic innervation (Seil, Eckenstein and Reier 1992).

The cerebellum is important for the control and fine tuning of movements that appear to occur through a motor learning process involving both synaptogenesis and astrocytic structural change. A critical role for astrocytes in motor learning is further suggested by the fact that mutant mice lacking GFAP display specific deficiencies in eyeblink conditioning (a form of discrete motor learning involving the cerebellum) and long term depression, a putative synaptic mechanism for eyeblink conditioning (Shibuki et al. 1996).

14.3.4 Possible Mechanisms for Inducing Structural Changes of Astrocytes: Lessons from the Developing and Adult CNS

Given the diversity of the regions where structural plasticity of astrocytes has been documented, there are undoubtedly multiple signalling pathways that can bring it about. It is likely accomplished in different brain regions by the stimulation of astrocyte receptors for locally available neurotransmitters, for example noradrenaline and/or adrenaline in the SON (McNeill and Sladek 1980; Beagley and Hatton 1994) and epinephrine in the posterior pituitary (Beagley and Hatton 1994). In the SCN, glutamate would appear to be a good candidate as it is released from the retinohypothalamic afferents that entrain the SCN clock and is known to influence the motility of astroglial filopodia (Cornell-Bell, Thomas and Caffrey 1992; van den Pol and Dudek 1993). As we have seen, in the rodent arcuate, median eminence, globus pallidus, and hippocampus as well as the primate mediobasal hypothalamus and infundibular nucleus, oestrogen is a likely stimulus for astrocytic structural plasticity. At the moment, perhaps the most complete case can be made for stimulation of β-adrenergic receptors (β-ARs) as a means of inducing structural plasticity of astrocytes.

It has been known for a decade that astrocytes grown in culture or freshly dissociated from neonatal cortical tissue exhibit β-adrenergic receptor-type radioligand binding activities and coupling to second messenger systems. Further it has been known that activation of astroglial β-ARs in vitro results in morphological changes of these cells (see Salm and McCarthy 1992, for review). There is now also ample evidence that adult astrocytes in situ express these receptors (Salm and McCarthy 1989, 1992; Aoki and Pickel 1992a), and, by immunoelectron microscopy, these receptors on astrocytes have been demonstrated to be localised immediately adjacent to catecholaminergic axons (Aoki 1992; Aoki and Pickel 1992a; Fig. 14.9A and B). Based on fluorocitrate studies, Stone and colleagues (Stone, Sessler and Weimin 1990) have argued that astrocytes, in fact, are the primary recipients of adrenergic input to the cortex.

Studies of β-AR expression in the developing cerebral cortex also offer clues about possible mechanisms of astrocyte plasticity in adults. Receptive field properties of primary sensory cortical neurons in adulthood reflect, in specific ways, the sensory experience received during early postnatal life, i.e. during the critical period (Movshon and Van Sluyters 1981). The critical period is a relatively brief time when the cortical environment is exceptionally permissive for the formation and elimination of synaptic connections. Immunoelectronmicroscopy has now provided evidence that β-adrenergic receptors on astrocytic processes in the visual cortex are developmentally regulated during the critical period (Aoki 1992; Aoki and Venkatesan 1997). For example, within layer 1, the layer exhibiting the earliest maturation, β-adrenergic receptors became readily apparent in astrocytes by postnatal day 10, but were rare at younger ages. Within the visual cortex of kittens, where the critical period for cortical plasticity begins later (ca. 1 month of age), astrocytic β-adrenergic receptors were rare prior to the first postnatal month (Fig. 14.9C and D) but become readily apparent thereafter. Hence, the appearance of β-ARs on astrocytes is correlated with the onset of the critical period. It is perhaps significant, then, that plasticity of the type, measurable during the critical period, can be regained in adulthood by stimulation of the locus coeruleus (where noradrenergic axons arise) or by the administration of exogenous noradrenaline,

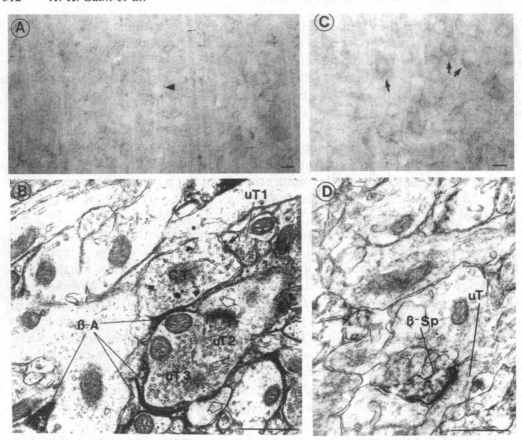

Fig. 14.9. Electron micrographs of β-AR + astrocytic processes in adult and postnatal day 11 cortex. Cortical tissue of adult (A, B) and postnatal day 11 (C, D) rats that was incubated together in immunoreagents to achieve immunoperoxidase labelling for β-adrenergic receptors. (A) Immunoperoxidase labelling is associated with small particles that are distributed throughout the neuropil. Many perikarya (e.g. arrowhead) and apical dendrites (small arrows) are revealed by the absence of labelling; bar, 10 μm. (B) Astrocytic processes exhibit immunoreactivity for β-adrenergic receptors along the plasma membrane (β-A, asterisks point to unlabelled cytoplasm.) These astrocytic processes surround many unlabelled axon terminals (μT1, μT2, μT3) that form asymmetric junctions with unlabelled spines. This micrograph was obtained from a Vibratome section that was labelled for β-adrenergic receptors together with tyrosine hydroxylase by the immunogold method. The presence of silver–gold particles indicates that CT is a catecholaminergic axon terminal. However, the spine that is postsynaptic to CT is not labelled (arrow points to the postsynaptic density.) CT also is juxtaposed to an astrocytic process with β-adrenergic receptor immunoreactivity bar, 0.5 μm. (C) Immunoperoxidase labelling appears diffusely distributed within the cytoplasm of several perikarya (arrows.) Their nuclei remain unlabelled. Numerous punctate labelling is apparent in the neuropil; bar, 10 μm. (D) Electron micrograph of the same area reveals that immunolabelling is discretely associated with plasma membranes, including those of a dendritic spine (β-Sp.) β-Sp is postsynaptic to an unlabelled axon terminal (μT) containing a cluster of vesicles. No labelling of astrocytic processes is evident; bar, 0.5 μm.

β-adrenergic agonists or of a membrane-permeable cyclic adenosine monophosphate (cAMP) analog (Kasamatsu 1991).

Several lines of evidence also suggest that astrocytic β-ARs in adulthood regulate structural plasticity in selected populations of astrocytes. The son-*VGL*, predominantly astrocytic, receives a dense catecholaminergic innervation (McNeill and Sladek 1980) and β_2-ARs on son-*VGL* astrocytes are upregulated in response to dehydration (Lafarga et al. 1992). Further, in the posterior pituitary, structural changes of pituicytes have been induced in explanted pituitaries by incubation in β-AR agonists (Smithson, Suarez and Hatton 1990). Also, structural changes of pituicytes and SON astrocytes after a hypertonic intraperitoneal saline injection are blocked by ablation of the adrenal medulla (Beagley and Hatton 1994), suggesting that these cells need an adrenergic signal to alter their shapes.

Recently, it has been observed also that monocular enucleation in adulthood causes upregulation of β-adrenergic receptor immunoreactivity in the corresponding cortical column. This change is evident more than a year after deafferentation and without apparent changes in GFAP levels indicative of gliosis (Aoki, Lubin and Fenstemaker 1994). It is possible that the observed change serves to help conserve glutamate released from the remaining few glutamatergic inputs arriving at the deprived columns. This could be accomplished by decreasing glutamate uptake into local astrocytes (Hansson and Rönnbäck 1992), particularly during alert behavioural states when glial β-ARs would be activated following firing of locus coeruleus neurons. As we have seen, this could also be brought about by changing the configuration of astrocytic processes near individual synapses.

Many events are known to follow activation of astrocytic β-adrenergic receptors. These involve mobilisation of a carbohydrate localised almost exclusively to astrocytes, i.e., glycogen and cAMP production (Stone and Ariano 1989 and Chapter 5). Since noradrenaline would be expected to be released when an animal is brought to a vigilant or aroused state by sensory stimulation (Aston-Jones, Chiang and Alexinsky 1991), glycogenolysis during this behavioural state could provide ATP and metabolic substrates useful for the cortical neuropil's enhanced activity. Elevation of cAMP, in turn, has been linked to reorganisation of the actin protein (Goldman and Abramson 1996) and phosphorylation of GFAP (McCarthy et al. 1985) that, in turn, could result in changes of astrocyte morphology.

14.4 Functional Significance of Structural Changes of Astrocytes: Some Caveats

In our work in the HNS we have made the assumption that the HNS is a 'dedicated system' where astrocytic structural plasticity is readily apparent, but that similar processes occur elsewhere in the activated CNS. This assumption is now supported by evidence gained from elsewhere in the hypothalamus and cortical regions discussed in this chapter. It is tempting to closely compare the form and dynamics of this plasticity in these different systems. For example, in the HNS and the rodent arcuate nucleus and hippocampus across the oestrous cycle, an inverse relation between glial coverage and synapse formation is evident. However, in the kindled CA1 region, the cerebellum after motor learning, and in the visual cortex of EC animals, astrocytic coverage and/or volume fraction vary together. These differences are not surprising, given the evidence that astrocytes can be as hetero- geneous as neurons in some characteristics (McCarthy and Salm 1991). We expect that structural plasticity of astrocytes is not stereotypic, i.e. it will likely prove to be individualised in form and dynamics, depending on the functional demands of the particular brain region. With respect to stimuli necessary to elicit such changes, it is probably relevant that the time points examined vary widely in the diverse systems discussed in this chapter, from minutes or hours in the HNS and rodent arcuate, to weeks in the visual cortex.

Currently, it seems reasonable to speculate that astrocytic structural plasticity acts to enhance communication in the CNS. By altering coverage of neuronal elements astrocytes may diversely inhibit or facilitate the formation of synapses. By selectively associating with synaptic complexes, astrocytes may be in a position to modulate synaptic physiology through their well-known abilities to regulate the extracellular ionic environment or to take up and metabolise neurotransmitters (see Chapters 10, 11 and 6, this volume). Nevertheless, to determine ultimately the functional significance of such changes, it will first be necessary experimentally to verify that astrocytic structural changes are indeed necessary or sufficient for neuronal changes to occur or for the smooth functioning of the nervous system to proceed, perhaps with the aid of gene 'knockout' technology.

15

Astrocytic Involvement in Learning

KIM T. NG, CIARAN REGAN and BRONA O'DOWD

Summary

Recent evidence from studies with neonate chicks, trained on a single trial passive avoidance task, unequivocally point to a central role for astrocytes in learning and memory formation as part of a broader picture of astrocytic involvement in regulating neural activity and neuroplasticity. This role is played out in a temporally well-defined sequence during early stages of memory formation following learning, at least in this species with the learning task used, and implicates astrocyte–neuron interactions in the release, uptake and synthesis of glutamate, the most abundant of the brain's excitatory amino acids, and in brain energy metabolism. Glutamate, released immediately following training, activates NMDA and metabotropic glutamate receptors associated with the induction of long-term potentiation-related memory consolidation processes. The released glutamate is taken up rapidly by both neurons and astrocytes, but more efficiently by the latter. Blockade of glutamate uptake mechanisms results in immediate loss of memory, probably as a result of massive cellular depolarisation. However, subsequent replenishment of transmitter glutamate appears to be essential both for sustaining intermediate-term memory processes and for activation of AMPA glutamate receptors linked to the maintenance and expression of long-term potentiation. This appears to be accomplished by astrocytic conversion of glutamate to non-neuroactive glutamate in the glutamate–glutamine cycle, by the astrocyte specific enzyme, glutamine synthetase, since inhibition of this enzyme abolishes memory formation within minutes after application of the inhibitor, with a narrow window of effective time of administration. Cellular activity underlying memory processing up to this point, in both neurons and astrocytes, seems to be sustained by energy derived from oxidative metabolism in the TCA cycles of these cells and to be depleted by these processes. Memory processing beyond this point is probably dependent on astrocyte-specific glycogenolysis, stimulated by a reinforcement-dependent release of noradrenaline. Blockade of β-adrenergic receptors or of astrocytic glycogenolysis (as well as neuronal and astrocytic glycogenolysis, which do not generate as much ATP sufficiently rapidly), abolishes memory at the same time after learning.

The results reported in this chapter represent the first direct evidence for the direct involvement of astrocyte–neuron interactions in memory processes.

15.1 Introduction

It is generally assumed that the brain processes associated with learning and memory occur exclusively in nerve cells, and there is no a priori reason to believe otherwise. However, the recent discovery and characterisation of unique biochemical and biophysical properties of glial cells in the central nervous system (Hertz 1989; Laming 1989a; Barres 1991; Hertz and Peng 1992b; Schousboe et al. 1992; Smith 1992; Hertz et al. 1992, 1996; Hertz, O'Dowd and Ocherashvili 1994) have led to speculation that disruption of functional and metabolic interactions between neurons and astrocytes may be implicated in a number of pathological conditions, such as Alzheimer's disease and clinical depression, in which behavioural dysfunctioning is a symptom. Evidence for an interaction between neurons and glia during information processing by the brain is accumulating (Roitbak 1993; Hertz, O'Dowd and Ocherashvili 1994). Processes such as glycogenolysis and glutamine synthesis, which in normal brains occur exclusively in astrocytes, have been shown to play a crucial role in central nervous system (CNS) consolidation of memory (O'Dowd et al. 1994a,b; Gibbs et al. 1996). In this chapter, we explore possible roles of neuron–glia interactions in learning and memory processing, primarily within the framework of a model of memory based on single trial discriminative passive avoidance conditioning of day-old chicks.

15.2 General Aspects of Learning and Memory

15.2.1 Forms of Learning

Learning is the process by which an experience leads to a relatively permanent change in behaviour. Memory is the ability to recall the experience, thereby effecting the behavioural change. Memory presupposes some form of neural representation of the experience. What and where this representation is and the processes by which the brain goes about establishing this representation define the essence of the relationship between learning, memory and neuroplasticity. What little we know about this relationship has been achieved mainly through the use of animal models involving a wide range of species and learning tasks.

Non-associative learning, in the form of habituation and sensitisation, has been studied extensively in invertebrates such as the *Aplysia* (see, for example, Castelluci and Kandel 1974), but occurs in almost all species. It has been reported even in animals without a 'nervous system', such as the paramecium. The course of habituation appears to be similar in all species studied. In contrast, associative learning, such as classical and operant conditioning, depends on the existence of a nervous system. However, the same brain mechanisms may not underpin different types of learning and learning in different species. Not all stimuli are alike for all species for purposes of learning, with some stimuli more compelling than others for a given species. The rapidity of learning a given response also varies enormously across species. The presence of species-specific learning renders generalisations difficult for any model of learning and memory formation. The investigation of a particular learning experience in a particular species may only isolate *a* mechanism for learning or memory, rather than *the* mechanism. Nonetheless, it can provide a sound basis for inferences about what *might* work (Kalat 1992) and generate testable hypotheses for investigation with other species and other tasks. This is the essential rationale for the model-systems approach to investigating memory (see Hoyenga and Hoyenga 1988), exemplified in the use of brain slices for studying long-term potentiation (Bliss and Lomo 1973), and the simpler neuronal networks in *Aplysia* (see, for example, Kandel 1983) and *Hermissenda* (see, for example, Alkon 1984) for studying synaptic events in memory processing.

15.2.2 *Reinforcement and Selectivity in Information Processing by the Brain*

In any learning situation *contextual stimuli*, such as background noise, odour and lighting, as well as the internal stimuli present at the time of learning, form part of the stimulus complex to which the organism is exposed. It is reasonable to suppose that organisms have a limited capacity for processing information at any given time and must have attentional mechanisms, innate or otherwise, which allow them to focus on a limited number of stimuli. Selectivity may be with respect to the stimuli that are encoded or registered (Broadbent 1958). Alternatively, all stimuli may in fact be registered but, given limited processing resources, a choice may have to be made between processing all inputs to a small degree and selecting some inputs for a greater degree of processing at the expense of others (Kahneman 1973).

The psychology of motives is concerned with the arousal, energisation and choice aspects of behaviour. Motives induce both behavioural arousal and energisation, in the form of the probability, intensity and vigour of behaviour, and neural arousal and energisation, in the form of changes in neural activity. Deprivation, pain or any unpleasant emotional state is arousing and forms the basis for negative reinforcement. Stimuli from some types of goal objects, such as food to a hungry animal, are also arousing and underpin positive reinforcement. Both forms of arousal give rise to selective attention and direct behaviour. Thus, reinforcement may alter internal states of the organism, including brain states, to determine what stimuli are attended to, what information is processed and how far the processing goes. This may extend to the broader choice of what learning experiences are to be encoded into long-term neural representation, if the reasonable assumption is made that not all learning experiences are permanently encoded. The choice may depend on the saliency or significance of the experience with respect to acquired or innate mechanisms of adaptation and survival (Kety 1972; Matthies 1989; McGaugh 1990).

15.3 Brain Neuroplasticity

15.3.1 Neurons as Information Processing Units

Neurons and glia are the two unique classes of cells existing in the nervous system. The neuronal cell body receives signals from the dendrites and transmits these in a polarised manner to the postsynaptic cell by means of the axon. Multipolar neurons predominate in the CNS. These have a single axon and one or more dendritic branches which emerge from all parts of the cell body. The critical signalling functions of the brain are carried out by interconnecting sets of neurons. Neuronal signalling depends on rapid changes in the electrical potential difference across nerve cell membranes which are modulated by allosteric ion channels. Channel function may be activated or repressed by chemical transmitters which bind directly or indirectly via a receptor which stimulates an intracellular enzyme cascade system to elicit inhibitory or excitatory actions. Long-term potentiation (LTP) is an example of neurotransmitter-mediated synaptic plasticity which can induce synaptic facilitation or depression. Application of trains of high frequency stimulation of afferent excitatory pathways can result in long-lasting changes to the strength and efficacy of synaptic transmission. The potentiation effect is synapse specific and develops and stabilises within one to two minutes. LTP occurs in many brain regions but is studied most widely and best understood in the hippocampus where it has been used as a model for the early stages of memory formation and learning. Both pre- and postsynaptic mechanisms are implicated and many mechanisms potentially capable of re-setting the synaptic apparatus may play a role. Although no detailed analysis of LTP can be developed in this chapter, induction requires depolarisation, most likely by the action of glutamate at co-localised α amino, 3-hydroxy, 5-methyl, 4-isoxazole proprionic acid (AMPA) and kainate receptors of the postsynaptic cell and activation of postsynaptic N-methyl-D-aspartate (NMDA) receptors. The presynaptic element of this process may involve increased quantum release of glutamate. This coincidence of pre- and postsynaptic activity provides a formalism for the first direct evidence of Hebbs' (1949) rule on the cellular basis for associative memory.

Nerve cells are surrounded by glia, an unfortunate term derived from the Greek for 'glue'. The two major classes of glia are microglia and macroglia. The former are activated to remove debris following injury to the CNS. Oligodendrocytes and Schwann cells are macroglia which insulate neurons by forming myelin sheets. Astrocytes, the third glass of macroglia, are the most numerous and characterised by the presence of markers such as glial fibrillary acidic protein (GFAP) and glutamine synthetase. These induce the formation of the impermeable tight junctions of the blood–brain barrier, which suggests that they may have a nutritive role. Those which surround synaptic regions terminate transmitter action by high affinity uptake mechanisms (see Chapter 6). Furthermore, their high permeability regulates neuronal depolarisations by removal of excess K^+ accumulation released by repetitive neuronal firing. As they form syncytia by connecting cytoplasmic bridges the excess K^+ can be redistributed (see Chapters 10 and 12). This also provides a mechanism for autoregulation of potassium-dependent control of artery and arteriole diameter within the vasculature in a manner which provides adequate blood flow and oxygen supply in pace with neuronal activity. The above issues are discussed in greater detail in Kandel, Schwartz and Jessell (1991).

15.3.2 Organisation of the Central Nervous System

Information coming from peripheral receptors that sense the environment give rise to perceptions, some of which are stored as memory. On the basis of this information the brain commands co-ordinated responses by neural cells with basically similar properties. The component neurons of the cortex have been suggested to be vertically organised into interconnected functional units termed columns, each containing 10^3–10^4 cells, which may serve as devices by which information may be equivalently distributed. This concept is somewhat idealised, as no compelling anatomical or functional evidence can be adduced for the idea that a subdivision exists as a general organising property of the cortex. Such columns exist as the barrel fields of the somatosensory cortex and, in the visual cortex, these functional columns (the ocular dominance columns) have a diameter of approximately 400 µM. Columnar organisation has likewise been found outside the sensory area of the cortex, notably in the prefrontal cortex. As the organisation of the developing cortex is primarily mediated by radially distributed glia, this has led to the conjecture that the cortical units are derived from proliferative units in a manner which is intimately dependent on glia. A review of the above may be found in Squire (1987) and Chapter 3.

15.3.3 Neuroplasticity

Recent research has shown that the brain has a remarkable capacity for immediate functional plasticity coupled with long-lasting structural change and to retain a repair capability following cell loss due to injury or neurodegenerative disease. The nervous system exhibits both subtle and specific neural changes in response to stimuli such as learning a new task, environmental enrichment or cycles in hormonal levels. Rats living in complex environments exhibit several plastic changes including expanded cortical thickness, greater cell body size, more complex dendritic branching and an increased number of glial cells (see Chapter 14). The earliest indication that remodelling of these nerve endings occurs among neuronal targets was the observation that axonal branches sometimes appeared to be degenerating or growing (Sotelo and Palay 1971). An additional example is provided by the mammalian primary somatosensory cortex. When arrangements of peripheral targets are perturbed in adult animals by amputation or nerve section, the cortical representation of the body undergoes substantial reorganisation (Merzenich et al. 1983). It is not clear whether these changes depend on actual axonal growth of synaptic terminals into new zones or whether a large number of potential synaptic connections exist from the beginning.

Epigenetic influences which control plasticity arise within the organism and from the external environment. The former involve intracellular signals that consist of diffusible factors and surface molecules. The latter provide nutritive factors, sensory and social experiences, and learning, which mediate their effects through changes in neural activity. Cellular signalling associated with neuroplasticity can be mediated by direct cellular contact through the apposition of specific membrane-bound cell-surface molecules. Many of the glycoproteins involved in the adhesion of neural cells belong to one of three major structural families – the immunoglobulin superfamily, cadherins and integrins. The latter additionally mediate interactions between the cell surface and extracellular matrix. Members of these three families of glycoproteins are expressed at high levels on both neurons and non-neuronal cells.

The neural cell adhesion molecule (NCAM) is one of the most abundant adhesion molecules on the surface of neural cells. It is derived from a single gene but exists in multiple protein forms derived from extensive post-translational modifications. Two of the major forms are transmembrane glycoprotein; a third is attached to the membrane via a glycosylphosphatidyl inositol anchor. All these forms have a conserved extracellular region with five domains which fold in a manner similar to those found on immunoglobulins. NCAM is modified by glycosylation. The structure of this carbohydrate is unusual and consists of long chains of $\alpha2,8$-linked polysialic acid (PSA). The molecular mechanisms by which NCAM regulates neural structuring remain to be established; however, evidence exists to suggest an important role for NCAM prevalence and polysialylation in neuritogenesis and neurite path finding (Doherty, Cohen and Walsh 1990; Doherty et al. 1990; Tang, Landmesser and Rutishauser 1992). Recent evidence suggests that modulation of NCAM prevalence and polysialylation continues in defined brain regions in the adult (Rougon 1993). The number of immunoglobulin structural motifs varies between molecules in this superfamily. The L1 member contains six domains, whereas Thy-1, the smallest member, contains a single domain.

Over 10 cadherin molecules have been characterised in vertebrates. Unlike NCAM, related cadherins derive from different genes. *N*-Cadherin is a major form in the CNS. It is found on most neural cells, both glia and neuron, and, unlike NCAM, binds in a calcium-dependent manner. The cytoplasmic domain binds to a family of proteins called catenins which interact with the cytoskeleton which appears to be important for the adhesive functions of these molecules. A third major family of glycoproteins involved in adhesion are the integrins. These consist of non-covalently linked subunits, termed α and β. Different α and β subunits are expressed by distinct cell types. The particular combination of subunits defines which of the extracellular matrix proteins will be recognised by each integrin. Fibronectin and laminin are the two most prominent extracellular matrix glycoproteins that interact with integrins. Laminin is a large protein of 10^6 kDa composed of three subunits, designated, α, β and γ. Other subunits have been identified, suggesting that there may be a family of laminins. Fibronectin is composed of two disulphide-linked subunits, each of which has many distinctive binding sites. An overview of the above cell recognition systems may be found in Kandel, Schwartz and Jessell (1991).

15.3.4 Learning-Associated Neuroplasticity

Behaviour emerges gradually as the brain develops. Initially, this is under the control of genetic and developmental programmes. Influences of the environment begin to exert their effect in utero and become of prime importance after birth. Although the literature on the neurobiology of memory is extensive, much of what is known can be summarised to suggest that memory has stages and is continually changing, and that long-term memory may be represented by plastic changes localised in multiple brain regions. Thus, the current consensus for information storage is that long-term memory is stored in the brain in terms of changes in synaptic connectivity within ensembles of neurons, brought about by cellular and molecular mechanisms which have much in common with those of developmental neural plasticity (Bailey and Kandel 1993). The fundamental concept that neuronal growth and change occur during the formation of permanent memory brings the neurobiological study of memory into contact with developmental neurobiology.

Intraventricular administration of the radio-labelled sialic acid precursor (pulse-chase) combined with anti-NCAM immunoprecipitation studies have demonstrated that animals trained in a passive avoidance task exhibit a transient time-dependent increase in hippocampal NCAM polysialylation at 12–24 h following the initial learning trial (Doyle et al. 1992a). This is restricted to the 180 kDa isoform which is associated with post-mitotic neurons and enriched in the synaptic structure. On the basis of antibody interventive studies, it has been suggested that memory-associated NCAM polysialylation plays a role in the selective stabilisation of synaptic contacts transiently overproduced in the learning process (Doyle et al. 1992b,c). Intracerebroventricular administration of anti-NCAM, at a discrete 6-h post-training time-point, results in amnesia at a 48-h recall time but not at 24 h, when NCAM sialylation is maximal. Thus, the novel synaptic contacts/ modifications, widely believed to underlie the memory process, would appear to be preserved at 24 h but fail to compete or mature and an ensuing amnesia results. The idea that the principle of neuronal competition for functional connectivity is relevant to learning and memory comes from the fact that competition not only occurs during normal development; it also occurs after birth as a result of an individual animal's experience.

Immunohistochemical studies using a monoclonal antibody which specifically recognises polysialic acid have demonstrated the learning-associated change in NCAM polysialylation to be localised to a defined population of granule-like cells at the border of the granule cell layer of the adult rat dentate gyrus (Fox, Kennedy and Regan 1995). This is not task-specific as precisely the same transient and temporal changes occur following Morris water maze and passive avoidance training, which are spatial and non-spatial forms of learning, respectively. In water maze studies, increased NCAM polysialylation occurs in response to repetitive learning trials on subsequent days; however, the magnitude of the response remains constant despite improved task performance, suggesting that activation of NCAM-dependent events is required for processing information in response to task-associated environmental stimuli rather than retrieval from or contribution to previously stored, task-associated memory (Murphy, O'Connell and Regan 1996). These results are consistent with observations which show mice homozygous for disrupted NCAM gene function fail to exhibit spatial learning (Cremer et al. 1994), an effect consistent with lack of polysialic acid (PSA) modulation, since NCAM is the major carrier in the CNS (Rougon 1993). NCAM has also been demonstrated to be critical in establishing long-term potentiation (LTP), a phenomenon accepted widely as a model of learning (Luthi et al. 1994; Ronn et al. 1995).

15.4 Astrocytic Contributions to Neuroplasticity

Whereas the roles of glial cells are usually described as limited to maintenance of the ionic environment, recent evidence indicates additional functions that give glial cells a greater role in the regulation of neural activity and plasticity (for reviews see Kettenmann and Ransom 1995). Unlike neurons, glial cells do not produce action potentials. However, they share with neurons more functional characteristics than was previously thought. Glial cells carry a multiplicity of voltage-gated ion channels and receptors for transmitters; and they store and release messenger substances. Thus they are not an electrically passive element. Despite this, typical synaptic contacts on the surface of glial cells or morphologically specialised sites of glial messenger release are not evident.

15.4.1 Regulation of Neurotransmission

Glial cells are involved in the synthesis and uptake of neurotransmitters and can respond to many of the same communication factors as neurons (see Chapter 6). Astrocytes express high affinity for the amino acids that are either neurotransmitters or neuromodulators in their own right, or serve as precursors for these substances (Schousboe et al. 1992). Since astrocytes are in close anatomical contact with synapses, it is very likely that these cells serve important roles with regard to supply of transmitter precursors to neurons and, with respect to the excitatory amino acids, the maintenance of a low extracellular concentration which is of utmost importance for protection of neurons against their cytotoxic actions. Since these roles are primarily associated with astrocytes, these cells are of fundamental importance for metabolic regulation and the supply of precursors for synthesis of neurotransmitters. The supply of glutamate is an example. Glutamine synthetase (GS) catalyses the conversion of glutamate to glutamine in the presence of adenosine triphosphate (ATP) and ammonia and therefore, is a pivotal enzyme in nitrogen metabolism. In the central nervous system the enzyme has the dual function of disposing of the neurotoxic substances glutamate and ammonia and providing glutamine as a substrate for neuronal glutaminase as well as for further utilisation in protein synthesis and oxidative metabolism. GS modulates not only the activity of glutamate neurons but also plays a role in the metabolism of the inhibitory transmitter γ-aminobutyric acid (GABA), the transamination of which furnishes glutamate as one of the products. A compartmentation of GS (glial cells) and glutaminase (neurons) with cycling of the respective substrates between the two cell types has been proposed (Kvamme 1983).

15.4.2 Role in Metabolism

The major energy source required to maintain this neural homeostasis are the oxidative substrates of glucose and oxygen. It has been suggested that astrocytes rely more strongly on glycolysis whereas neurons preferentially produce their energy by oxidative phosphorylation (see Chapter 5). Glycogen is located in astrocytes and tends to be metabolised during acute changes in regional energy demands at the start of neuronal activity, or under conditions of substrate deprivation (Siesjö 1978; Swanson 1992). Its breakdown in primary astrocyte cultures can be induced by adenosine, histamine, noradrenaline, vasoactive intestinal peptide and serotonin, which elevate levels of cyclic adenosine monophosphate (cAMP) (see Hertz and Peng 1992b; Magistretti, Sorg and Martin 1993).

Glycogen phosphorylase and fructose-1,6-biphosphatase (the enzymes responsible for glycogen breakdown and the resynthesis of glycogen from 3-carbon compounds such as lactate, respectively) co-localise with GFAP positive astrocytes in the brain (Schmoll et al. 1995b). Surprisingly, the glycosyl residues do not appear as glucose but are released as lactic acid and may subsequently be taken up into neurons, suggesting these cells to be a store of lactic acid (Hamprecht et al. 1993; Tsacopoulos and Magistretti 1996). Consistent with the localisation of fructose-1,6-biphosphatase in these cells, astroglia in the brain are gluconeogenic (Dringen, Gebhardt and Hamprecht 1993) and may rapidly switch between production and consumption of lactic acid, depending on the activities and needs of neighbouring neurons. This points to a crucial role for astrocytes in the energy metabolism of the brain.

15.4.3 Structural Plasticity

Given that glial cells are closely associated with synapses, it is likely that transmitters may serve as signals to regulate glial cell plasticity. In culture, neurotransmitters have been shown to influence glial process growth. Glial cell filopodia in culture grow in the direction of glutamate and β-adrenergic receptor activation changes a neuroepithelial morphology to a stellate morphology (Shain et al. 1987; Cornell-Bell Thomas and Smith 1990). There is also evidence of a close association between synaptic numbers and glia. Internal states such as dehydration affect glial process growth and retraction. Neuropeptidergic neurons in the supraoptic nucleus increase direct cell–cell apposition, via glial process retraction (Tweedle and Hatton 1977 and Chapter 14). Astrocytes may similarly regulate synaptic numbers in cerebellar cultures. Purkinje cells in glial-free cell cultures form synapses with Purkinje cell somata and dendrites. Astrocytes added to the culture decrease the number of synapses and increase the number of non-innervative spines (Meshul, Seil and Herndon 1987; Meshul and Seil 1988). Glial conditioned medium similarly increases the number of non-innervative spines, apparently by proliferation of spines in the absence of presynaptic innervation (Seil, Eckenstein and Reier 1992).

Evidence from intact animals undergoing behavioural treatment also reveals a close association between neuronal and glial morphological plasticity. Sirevaag and Greenough (1987) have shown that, when the number of synapses per neuron is increased in the visual cortex following exposure to a complex environment, there is also an increase in supportive elements such as glia and blood vessels. Rats maintained in an enriched environment have 20–25% more synapses (Turner and Greenough 1985) and a greater ratio of glial cell surface area to neurons than those maintained in an impoverished environment (Diamond et al. 1966; Sirevaag and Greenough 1991). A similar glial hypertrophy is associated with the synaptogenesis related to kindling and the induction of LTP in the hippocampus (Wenzel et al. 1991; Hawrylak, Chang and Greenough 1993).

15.4.4 Role of Cell Recognition Systems

Despite convincing ultrastructural evidence for the involvement of glia in adult neuroplastic remodelling, there is little evidence to demonstrate their underlying molecular mechanisms, such as the relative contributions of cell recognition systems to this process. Although the activity-dependent expression of polysialylated NCAM with neurons and astrocytes in the supraoptic and paraventricular nuclei of the hypothalamus (Theodosis, Rougon and Poulain 1991; Kiss, Wang and Rougon 1993) is consistent with their capacity for structural plasticity in adulthood, studies on induced modulation of astrocytic NCAM polysialylation remain equivocal. Following lesions to the entorhinal cortex, a transient increase in NCAM polysialylation has been associated with axonal sprouting and synaptogenesis in the denervated molecular layer of the dentate gyrus but not on GFAP-labelled astrocytes (Miller et al. 1994). This contrasts with the profound and persistent activation of astroglial polysialylation observed in the hippocampus following kainate-induced sprouting in the hippocampal formation (Le Gal La Salle, Rougon and Valin 1992) and the transient upregulation of NCAM messenger ribose nucleic acid (mRNA) in hippocampal astrocytes following entorhinal cortex lesions (Jucker et al. 1995). In the adult hippocampus, polysialylated radial astrocytes have been observed to traverse the dentate granule cell layer and to be in close association with the dendrites of the learning-associated PSA-positive neurons located at the granule cell layer/hilar border (Fox et al. 1995). These PSA-positive neurons and radial glia decline dramatically with age and are virtually absent in the 1.5-year-old animal. Based on the strict numerical ratio between neuronal and glial numbers that is maintained during ageing, the PSA-positive neurons and radial astroglia processes have been suggested to form 'plastic units' traversing the granule cell layer. Double immunofluoresence studies employing anti-PSA and anti-GFAP have shown the radial glia processes to exhibit apparent points of cell and/or dendritic contact, providing further support for this concept. These may serve to augment the observed transient increase in neuronal NCAM polysialylation in the 12-h time point following passive avoidance training, as the radial glia become significantly activated within this period, suggesting a learning-associated role for these 'plastic units' (Fig. 15.1). Whether the glial response is a consequence of or a contributing factor to neuronal activation still remains to be established.

Thy-1, which is the smallest member of the immunoglobulin superfamily, also has received considerable attention in memory-associated neuroplastic responses. It is a major cell surface component expressed by several tissues. It is highly expressed in nervous tissue, where it appears on neurons after the cessation of axonal growth. In the chick model of avoidance conditioning, intracranial administration of anti-Thy-1 just prior to training results in an amnestic effect which is observed in the early post-training period (Bernard et al. 1983). The underlying molecular mechanism remains to be elucidated but may relate to Thy-1-mediated

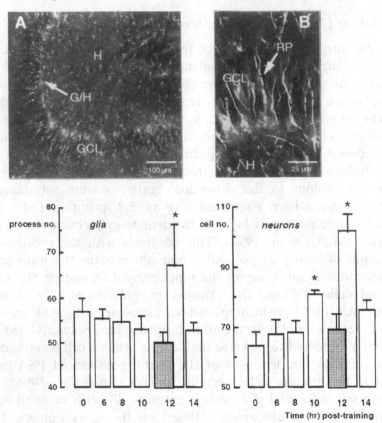

Fig. 15.1. Activation of astroglial NCAM polysialylation in the rat dentate gyrus following acquisition of a passive avoidance response. (A) PSA-immunopositive astroglia associated with the hilar region (H) and granule cell layer (GCL.) In (B) the radial processes (RP) traversing the granule cell layer are demonstrated (adapted from Fox et al. 1995). The time-dependent activation of polysialylated astroglia and neurons at the granule cell layer/hilar border (G/H) following passive avoidance training are illustrated in the accompanying histograms. (Unpublished observations of G. B. Fox and adapted from Fox, Kennedy and Regan 1995, respectively.) All values are the mean ±SEM ($n = 3$) and those significantly different from animals rendered amnesic with scopolamine (shaded columns) are indicated with an asterisk. For details of the training protocols and immunohistochemical procedures employed refer to Fox, Kennedy and Regan (1995).

regulation of learning-associated neuritic elaboration in a manner which is astrocyte-dependent. Neural cells transfected with Thy-1 exhibit a profound reduction in neurite outgrowth when cultured on astrocytes as compared to plastic surfaces (Tiveron et al. 1992). Blocking with Thy-1 antibodies restores neurite outgrowth, suggesting a receptor-mediated mechanism (Tiveron et al. 1992; Dreyer et al. 1995). This does not appear to occur by a homophilic interaction on the apposing cells as neurite extension is unaffected when non-astrocytic Thy-1-positive cells are employed. Thus, inactivation of Thy-1 with the antibody may pre-empt an astro-cyte growth inhibitory signal across neural membranes coincident with final synaptic elaboration. This is consistent with the unimpaired water maze perfor-mance in mice with inactivated Thy-1 gene function (Nosten-Bertrand et al. 1996). However, these mice exhibit region specific abnormalities in the generation of LTP, being normal following stimulation of the Schaeffer-commissural input to pyramidal cells of the CA1 area but defective following stimulation of the perfor-ant path input to granule cells of the dentate.

15.5 Memory Formation

15.5.1 Memory Formation and Neuroplasticity

From the time of the pioneering work of Hebb (1949), investigations into how the brain forms memories have been shaped by the hypothesis that long-term memor-ial representation of an experience involves increases in synaptic efficacy brought about by relatively permanent changes to neuronal connectivity in a network activated by the experience, possibly in the number and properties of synapses (Matthies 1989). Such a network would yield a preferred pathway for subsequent stimulation by both internal and external stimuli associated in the course of the learning experience. Since the consolidation of such a network would be time-consuming, transient representations of the experience during the consolidation process are necessary for purposes of short-term recall. The dominant view is that memory formation proceeds in multiple stages involving multiple memory traces (see, for example, McGaugh 1966; Atkinson and Schiffrin 1968; Gibbs and Ng 1977; Matthies 1989), although there have been alternative theories (see, for exam-ple, Craik and Lockhart 1972; Gold and McGaugh 1975).

Matthies (1989) has argued that detection of the general mechanisms of memory formation is enhanced by the use of tasks which entail learning at a relatively high level of complexity and neuronal organisation, given that the 'real carrier of information' in the CNS can be said to be found at the systemic level of neuronal structures rather than at the molecular level of membrane processes and intra-neuronal mechanisms. However, activity at the molecular level ultimately deter-mines changes to the connectivity and functional structure of the neuronal assemblies which define memory traces. Tracking cellular events at the molecular level during the course of memory formation may provide a more complete under-standing of *how* a memory is formed and *why* at least some failures in memory occur. Furthermore, if memory is formed in stages, isolation of the stages and identification of the neural mechanisms underlying each stage are more easily achieved with a learning task which allows a relatively precise determination of the time of acquisition and generates a single sequence of memory formation processes. Single-trial tasks are ideal for this purpose.

15.5.2 A Three-Stage Model of Memory Formation

A one-trial passive avoidance learning task in day-old chicks, adapted from Cherkin (1971), has been widely used for isolating the cascade of time-dependent and stage-specific cellular events underlying memory formation (Gibbs and Ng 1977; Patterson et al. 1986; Andrew 1991; Ng and Gibbs 1991; Rose 1991). The paradigm has considerable ecological validity, since the neonate chick is precocially prepared to peck at shiny objects and to discriminate very quickly between edible and inedible, and pleasant and unpleasant tasting, objects (Gibbs and Ng 1977; Andrew 1991). In a discrimination version of the task, 1- to 2-day-old chicks are trained on a single 10-s trial to discriminated between a small red glass bead coated with an unpleasant tasting chemical, methylanthranilate (MeA), and a non-aversive blue glass bead of the same size. A discrimination response is clearly evident within 5 min after the training trial, and persists for at least several days.

Memory for the passive avoidance learning experience in the chick appears to develop in three sequentially dependent stages, inferred both from purely behavioural (Gibbs and Ng 1979) and from pharmacological intervention studies (Gibbs and Ng 1977, 1984; Ng and Gibbs 1991; see also Patterson et al. 1986). A short-term (STM) stage, formed by 5 min post-training and decaying after 10 min post-training, is followed by an intermediate-term (ITM) stage, expressed between 20 and 50 min post-training, and a long-term (LTM) stage formed by 60 min after training. Behaviourally, the stages are shown to be separated by transient retention deficits at 15 and 55 min post-training. Pharmacologically, the stages are distinguished by their differential susceptibility to abolishment by different classes of pharmacological agents. Inhibition of any given stage results in the loss of all stages thereafter, suggesting a sequential dependence across stages.

Formation of the STM stage in the chick is prevented by depolarising treatments with isotonic (154 mM) KCl or a low concentration (4 mM) of monosodium glutamate (Gibbs and Ng 1977). Formation of STM may depend upon an initial phase of neuronal hyperpolarisation mediated by K^+ conductance changes following neural input and dependent on $[Ca^{2+}]_e$ (see Jansen and Nicholls 1973), since this stage is also abolished by the Ca^{2+} channel blocker lanthanum chloride and its duration is extended by increased extracellular Ca^{2+} (Gibbs, Gibbs and Ng 1979). Formation of the ITM stage is prevented by inhibition of Na^+/K^+-ATPase activity with ouabain and the astrocytic $Na^+/K^+/Cl^-$ cotransport system with ethacrynic acid (Gibbs and Ng 1977). ITM formation is thought to involve a second phase of neuronal hyperpolarisation brought about by the coupled action of the electrogenic sodium pump and the astrocytic cotransport system (see Jansen and Nicholls 1973). Finally, formation of LTM is prevented by protein synthesis inhibitors such as cycloheximide, anisomysin and emetine (Gibbs and Ng 1977; Patterson et al. 1986).

The ITM stage itself consists of two phases: ITMA (approximately 20–35 min) and ITMB (approximately 35–50 min). These phases are uniquely distinguished by the ability of the uncoupler of oxidative phosphorylation 2,4-dinitrophenol (DNP) to abolish ITMA but not ITMB. Furthermore, while all three stages are formed when the chicks are trained with concentrated MeA, reducing the intensity of this reinforcer by dilution to 20% in alcohol results in the formation of STM and ITMA, but not ITMB or LTM (Crowe et al. 1989), with normal retention levels observed only until about 35–40 min post-training. However, both ITMB and LTM are reinstated in the presence of adrenocorticotrophic hormone $(ACTH)_{1-24}$ or noradrenaline (NA) (Crowe et al. 1991a).

15.5.3 Active Ion Transport and Memory Formation

Matthies (1989), from studies of shock-based brightness discrimination learning in rats, has suggested that a short-term memory stage, lasting from seconds to minutes, may be induced after learning by translocation of ions resulting from extensive or repetitive synaptic activity, leading to a transient change in synaptic efficiency as a result of alterations in transmitter release and/or synthesis. A second, intermediate, memory stage, lasting minutes to hours, is postulated also to be induced by translocation of ions and by receptor site occupation, leading to longer lasting transient increases in synaptic strength through second messenger-mediated modifications of pre-existing receptor, enzyme or structural proteins. Some indirect evidence for an involvement of active ion transport in memory formation comes from the chick studies.

Stimulation of the CNS leads to an elevation of $[K^+]_e$ (see, for example, Syková 1983 and Chapters 7, 10 and 12), which can result in prolonged changes in neuronal excitability, synaptic transmission and glial cell function by altering neuronal and glial cell membrane potentials and transmitter release (Syková 1983, 1987). In untrained anaesthetised chicks, stimulation of the beak with methylanthranilate results in a prolonged increase in $[K^+]_e$ in the neostriatal/hyperstriatal region of the forebrain (Syková et al. 1990), a region shown to be metabolically active during memory formation (Rose and Csillag 1985; Sedman et al. 1992). Local application of 4 mM monosodium glutamate to this forebrain region also results in significant increases in $[K^+]_e$ (Ng et al. 1991). Clearance of accumulated extracellular K^+ involves astrocytic uptake of K^+, glial spatial buffering, and activity of the electrogenic Na^+/K^+ pump and an electroneutral $Na^+/K^+/Cl^-$ cotransport system (Syková 1992). Blockade of one or more of these systems can lead to a conductance block in neurons and consequential amnesia.

Na^+/K^+-ATPase activity is present in both neurons and astrocytes (Sweadner 1992; Huang et al. 1994b). In both cell types, the enzyme activity increases with an increase in $[K^+]_e$ up to the normal extracellular concentration (Huang et al. 1994b). However, in astrocytes, but not in neurons, there is a further stimulation of the enzyme when $[K^+]_e$ rises above normal levels (Huang et al. 1994b). In addition, an ionic cotransport system in astrocytes, but probably not in neurons, accumulates one K^+ ion, one Na^+ ion, and two Cl^- ions. Once inside the cell, the accumulated Na ions will stimulate Na^+/K^+-ATPase activity at sodium sensitive sites, resulting in an active energy-dependent extrusion of Na^+ ions and a concomitant uptake of K^+ ions (Walz 1992). The joint operation of the Na^+/K^+ pump and the cotransport system in astrocytes will result, therefore, in an uptake of K^+ and Cl^- ions from the interstitial space without any net movement of Na^+ ions. The intensity of the K^+ transport mechanisms operating across the astrocytic membrane and the absence of any net movement of Na^+ ions during the operation of these mechanisms may result in the $[K^+]_e$ returning to normal before the $[Na^+]_e$ is normalised. Continued stimulation of Na^+/K^+-ATPase beyond this point may lead not only to Na^+ extrusion from neurons and glia but also to a coupled active uptake of K^+ ions, resulting in an $[K^+]_e$ 'undershoot'. This could lead to the neuronal hyperpolarisation postulated to be associated with the formation of ITM and may account for the amnestic effects of ouabain and ethacrynic acid.

15.5.4 Transient Membrane Modifications in Early Stages of Memory Formation

As discussed earlier, not all learning experiences lead to the laying down of permanent memory. Reversibility in synaptic plasticity is essential if current network models of learning and memory are to possess sufficient flexibility to serve as information storage devices that are capable of allowing some pieces of information to proceed to long-term storage and others not (Laboritt and Zerbib 1987). Protein phosphorylation is a dynamic and inherently reversible process which is ideally suited to the role of regulating the transient changes in synaptic efficacy that are presumed to characterize pre-long-term memory processing. Both protein phosphorylation and dephosphorylation can change the structure and function of membrane proteins. For example, phosphorylation of channel proteins via G-protein-coupled second messenger activation can open or close synaptic ion channels that were closed or open at resting membrane potential. Protein phosphorylation can exert a modulatory effect on neurotransmission by altering the sensitivity of postsynaptic receptors, such as occurs in receptor desensitisation. Second messenger systems also can mediate the longer term effects of extracellular signals by inducing transcription of 'immediate early genes', such as c-*fos*, and the nuclear translation of their mRNAs to regulatory proteins which can initiate 'late gene' expression (see, for example, Matthies 1989).

Protein kinase activity has been implicated in memory processing in *Aplysia* (Dash, Hochner and Kandel 1990), *Drosophila* (Drain, Folkers and Quinn 1991), mutants flies deficient in learning and memory (Buxbaum and Dudai 1989), *Hermissenda* (Lester and Alkon 1991), rabbit (Olds et al. 1989), rat (Paylor, Rudy and Wehner 1991), and transgenic flies possessing an inducible peptide inhibitor of the Ca^{2+}/calmodulin-dependent kinase CaMK-II, once expression of the gene is induced (Griffith et al. 1993). There is increasing evidence from chick studies linking specific aspects of phosphorylative activity to specific stages in memory formation. Inhibition of protein kinase C (PKC) activity in the left, but not the right, hemisphere induces amnesia for the passive avoidance task from 25 min post-training (Rose 1991; Zhao et al. 1994a), during the ITMA phase of the intermediate memory stage. This effect is prevented by phorbol 12-myristate 13-acetate (PMA), an activator of PKC. Significant changes in the phosphorylation state of the PKC substrate protein GAP-43 have been reported to occur by 30 min post-training (Ali, Bullock and Rose 1988; Zhao, Ng and Sedman 1995b). This change is absent in weakly reinforced chicks but recovers when the training is augmented with ACTH (Zhao et al. 1994b). Rose (1991) also reported increased translocation of the Ca^{2+}/phospholipid-dependent kinase, PKC, presynaptic phosphorylation of the PKC substrate GAP43, and c-*fos* and c-*jun* expression within minutes following passive avoidance training. Neurogranin, a PKC substrate similar to GAP43 but located postsynaptically, shows increased phosphorylation following induction of LTP (Ramakers et al. 1995). Phosphorylation of the myristoylated alanine-rich C-kinase substrate (MARCKS), a calmodulin-binding substrate protein of PKC in presynaptic terminals which is phosphorylated when synaptosomes are depolarised, has been reported following imprinting in chicks (Sheu et al. 1993). Inhibition of CaMK-II in the *left* hemisphere also abolishes memory from ITMA onwards, but inhibition in the *right* hemisphere blocks memory formation from STM onwards (Zhao et al. 1996). Inhibition of the cAMP-dependent protein kinase A (PKA) results in memory loss in the chick from 60 min post-training when administered into either hemisphere (Zhao et al. 1995). Synapsin 1, a substrate for both PKA and CaMK-II located in presynaptic terminals, is involved in transmitter release (Greengaard 1987), including glutamate (Nichols et al. 1992), from nerve terminals. Much more salient, from the point of view of PKA activity, is CREB, a transcriptional activator binding protein which binds to a gene promoter and regulates gene transcription following phosphorylation by PKA. CREB phosphorylation, through modulation of protein synthesis, has been implicated in long-term memory formation in a variety of species (Yin et al. 1995).

Taken together, the above results suggest a cascade of kinase activity associated with the various stages of memory formation, with CaMK-II activation necessary for STM, CaMK-II and PKC activation for ITM, and PKA activation for LTM. Furthermore, the results point to the possibility that there may be hemispheric specialisation for STM and ITM. The observed increase in forebrain noradrenaline (NA) levels by 30 min post-training, the amnestic effects of β-adrenergic receptor blockade, and the known relationship between GAP-43 phosphorylation and NA release (Dekker et al. 1990; De Graan et al. 1991), suggest a consistent interpretation of the results. This is that PKC activity is mandated before formation of the ITMB phase of the Gibbs–Ng intermediate memory stage, with formation of this phase triggered by NA released as a consequence of reinforcement.

Direct evidence implicating phosphatase activity in memory formation per se is much less extensive (Bennett et al. 1996; Zhao, Bennett and Ng 1995; see also Asztalos et al. 1993). In passive avoidance training in the chick, okadaic acid, which preferentially inhibits protein phosphatase 1 (PP1) and protein phosphatase 2A (PP2A), abolishes ITMB and the subsequent LTM stage (Zhao et al. 1995a). It is unclear as to which protein phosphatase is involved. The immunosuppressant cyclosporin A (CyA), in contrast to okadaic acid, induces retention deficits only after 85 min post-training (Bennett et al. 1996), well after formation of the anti-biotic-sensitive LTM stage. This phosphatase inhibitor appears to exert its effects on calcineurin (CaN), the Ca^{2+}/calmodulin-dependent protein phosphatase 2B (PP2B) (Schwaninger et al. 1993). CaN is the only phosphatase known to be activated in direct response to second messengers thought to mediate signal trans-duction processes (Klee, Draetta and Hubbard 1988) and dephosphorylates a range of neuronal substrates including, in particular, NMDA channels, MARCKS, and GAP43, as well as the endogenous PP1 inhibitors inhibitor-1 and DARPP-32 (dopamine- and cAMP-regulated phosphoprotein). However, cyclosporin A also inhibits the peptidyl-prolyl *cis/trans* isomerase activity of cyclo-philins. Non-immunosuppressive analogues of CyA, which do not bind to and inhibit CaN, also induce amnesia at the same time as CyA (unpublished data). Since translation appears to be required for long-term memory formation and since cyclophilins and fuskolin binding protein (FKBP) are ubiquitously distrib-uted in the brain, a role for the protein phosphate inhibitors (PPI)ases in long-term memory formation is possible.

15.5.5 Long-Term Potentiation, Long-Term Depression and Memory Formation

Kinase and phosphatase activities, and protein phosphorylation and dephosphor-ylation, have been implicated in both long-term potentiation (LTP) and long-term depression (LTD) (see, for example, Malenka et al. 1989; Gianotti et al. 1992; Fukunaga, Soderling and Miyamoto 1992; Matthies and Reymann 1993; Abeliovich et al. 1993; Funauchi, Haruta and Tsumoto 1994;). LTP has been widely accepted as providing a suitable neuronal model for memory representation in the CNS (Bliss and Collingridge 1992). However, LTD is thought to be a necessary adjunct to LTP in any LTP-related memory model (Linden 1994). It has been suggested that the synaptic efficacy of mammalian hippocampal path-ways may depend on an intricate network of interacting kinase and phosphatase activities (see, for example, Artola and Singer 1993), with a kinase cascade increas-ing synaptic strength via LTP and a phosphatase cascade decreasing synaptic strength via LTD. Induction and maintenance of LTP and LTD are mediated by the activation of ionotropic NMDA and AMPA receptors, as well as metabo-tropic glutamate receptors (mGluR). Hypotheses linking these synaptic phenomena to memory processing are particularly persuasive in the light of many studies implicating NMDA, AMPA and mGluR receptor activation in several forms of memory (see Advocat and Pellegrin 1992; Holscher 1994; Rickard, Ng and Gibbs 1994; Rickard and Ng 1995). Phosphorylation of the microtubule associated protein, tau, has been linked to NMDA receptor and PKA activation in rat brain slices (Fleming and Johnson 1995). The guanosine $3'5'$-cyclic monophosphate (cGMP)-dependent protein kinase (PKG) appears to play a central role in cerebellar LTD, possibly through a nitric oxide/cGMP/PKG cascade. It has been proposed that activation of PKG phosphorylates AMPA glutamate receptors such that synaptic responsivity is reduced (Haley and Schuman 1994). There appears to be no direct evidence linking PKG activity to memory processing, although the PKC inhibitor H-7, which also inhibits PKG, induces amnesia in chicks.

In chicks trained on the passive avoidance task, blockade of NMDA receptors by AP5, AMPA receptors by DNQX, and mGluRs by MCPG all yielded retention deficits around 80–85 min post-training (Rickard, Ng and Gibbs 1994; Rickard and Ng 1995). Significantly, however, the NMDA and mGluR antagonists have to be administered within 5 min following training to produce their amnestic effects. In contrast, the effective time-of-administration window for the AMPA antagonist is between 15 and 25 min post-training, during the ITMA phase of the intermediate memory stage. These results would seem to suggest two periods of glutamate release critical to long term memory consolidation, one immediately after learning, binding to NMDA and mGluR receptors, and one during ITMA, binding to AMPA receptors. Moreover, if the amnestic actions of these drugs are in fact due to interference with LTP- and/or LTD-related memory processes, the memory consequences of these processes are not expressed until after formation of a distinct protein synthesis-dependent LTM stage.

15.6 Astrocytic Processes and Memory Formation

We have already seen above that formation of the early stages of memory may involve astrocyte–neuron interactions in processes associated with the re-establishment of resting ion distribution following extracellular ionic perturbations consequent on neural activity. There is now evidence also that astrocytic regulation of glutamate synthesis, uptake and release and astrocyte–neuron interactions in energy metabolism may be implicated in early memory processes.

15.6.1 Astrocytic Regulation of Glutamate Synthesis, Uptake and Release, and its Role in Memory Formation

While there is no evidence from direct measurements of extracellular glutamate levels that glutamate is released during memory formation following passive avoidance learning in the chick, the fact that blockade of NMDA receptors by AP5 and of AMPA receptors by DNQX must occur at different times after training to induce amnesia (Rickard, Ng and Gibbs 1994) suggests strongly that extracellular glutamate concentrations must be elevated at these two time points.

Extracellular glutamate is preferentially taken up into astrocytes (Hertz et al. 1992; Schousboe et al. 1992) where it is partly converted to non-neuroactive glutamine by the glial-specific enzyme glutamine synthetase (Norenberg and Martinez-Hernandez 1979), in the so-called 'glutamate–glutamine cycle'. Glutamine is released into the extracellular space, where it is partly re-accumulated into glutamatergic neurons to be used as a glutamate precursor and into GABAergic neurons where decarboxylation of glutamate yields GABA. Although astrocytically generated glutamine is a suitable precursor for neuronal glutamate (see Pow and Robinson 1994), a substantial amount of the glutamate taken into astrocytes is not converted to glutamine but used as a metabolic fuel (Hertz, Drejer and Schousboe 1988; Hertz et al. 1992; Schousboe et al. 1992; Sonnewald et al. 1993). Since glutamate does not cross the blood–brain barrier, there must be additional glutamate precursors to make up for the net loss of this transmitter. Astrocytes, but not neurons, can readily synthesise the citric acid intermediate oxaloacetate through condensation of pyruvate, a reaction catalysed by pyruvate carboxylase (Kaufman and Driscoll 1992; Sonnewald et al. 1993; Huang et al. 1994b). Oxaloacetate can then be oxidatively metabolised in the citric acid cycle to α-ketoglutarate. Neurons lack pyruvate carboxylase activity and cannot, therefore, carry out net synthesis of citric acid cycle constituents and their metabolites from pyruvate to replenish released transmitters, including glutamate and GABA. But neurons can utilise *exogenous* α-ketoglutarate to synthesise glutamate in the presence of a suitable amino group donor, such as alanine which is formed in large amounts in astrocytes from pyruvate (Yudkoff et al. 1992), although the process is relatively slow (Peng, Schousboe and Hertz 1991) and may not alone supply sufficient glutamate. Astrocytic metabolism in the citric acid cycle, therefore, can play a central role in the *net* synthesis of transmitter glutamate and GABA for glutamatergic and GABAergic neurons activated in learning and memory processing.

The glial specific inhibitor of the citric acid cycle, fluoroacetate (FA), inhibits de novo astrocytic formation of glutamine from glutamate and α-ketoglutarate with little, if any effect, on ATP content (Swanson and Graham 1994). In contrast, neurons do not readily oxidise glutamate or glutamine as metabolic fuels. Astrocytic conversion of glutamate to glutamine can also be blocked by methionine sulphoximine (MSO), an inhibitor of glutamine synthetase activity. MSO abolishes memory in day-old chicks trained on the passive avoidance task by 20 min post-training, provided it is administered shortly before the training trial (Gibbs et al. 1996). MSO would appear to abolish memory from the ITMA phase of the intermediate memory stage onwards. A similar effect is observed with FA (O'Dowd et al. 1994b). Unlike MSO, however, FA can be administered slightly later. This may not be too surprising, since MSO affects synthesis of glutamine directly from glutamate accumulated into astrocytes immediately upon release while FA affects de novo glutamine synthesis from glucose. It is interesting, too, that blockade of glutamate uptake (into both glia and neurons) by L-aspartic acid β-hydroxamate induces amnesia only if the drug is given within the first few seconds following training (Ng et al. 1996). If the amnestic effects of MSO are indeed due to restricted replenishment of neuronal glutamate, they should be challenged by alternative supplies of precursors and perhaps by glutamate itself. Extracellular glutamine, glutamate or a combination of α-ketoglutarate and alanine effectively overcomes MSO-induced amnesia (Gibbs et al. 1996; Ng et al. 1996). Alpha-ketoglutarate or alanine alone had little or no effect. The amnestic effects of FA are also successfully challenged by extracellular glutamine. Since FA also inhibits energy production in astrocytes, it is possible that this counteractive effect of glutamine may be attributed to its acting as a metabolic fuel. However, FA toxicity appears to derive mainly from its inhibition of synthesis of glutamate/glutamine precursors rather than from interference with astrocytic energy production (Swanson and Graham 1994). Finally, the fact that interference with glutamate production results in loss of memory from the ITMA phase (20 min post-training) onwards strongly suggests that glutamate may play a role in intermediate memory processing (Ng et al. 1996) in addition to its role in inducing and sustaining LTP- and LTD-related memory processes, since blockade of glutamate receptors associated with LTP and LTD did not yield amnesia until some 85 min following training.

15.6.2 Astrocyte–Neuron Interactions in Energy Production and Memory Formation

All CNS function is abolished within minutes in the absence of glucose, transported across the blood–brain barrier by specific glucose carriers. Not all cells metabolise glucose completely to carbon dioxide and water. Glucose metabolism begins with glycolysis, resulting in the formation of pyruvate. Under anaerobic conditions, pyruvate can be reduced to lactate and, in astrocytes, transaminated to alanine. Pyruvate, lactate and alanine can exit across cell membranes, although it is not known to what extent they can be used for further metabolism in adjacent neurons and astrocytes (see Hamprecht et al. 1993; Tsacopoulos and Magistretti 1996). Glycolysis occurs at a very high rate in astrocytes, although neurons are also capable of metabolising glucose to pyruvate/lactate (Hertz and Peng 1992).

Glycolysis results in the production of ATP, but with a much smaller yield per molecule of glucose than oxidative metabolism. Nonetheless, glycolytically derived energy is essential for certain energy-requiring processes in astrocytes, including uptake of glutamate and potassium (Kauppinen et al. 1988; Huang, Shuaib and

Hertz 1993). In contrast, potassium uptake in neurons depends on oxidative metabolism (Kauppinen et al. 1988; Rosenthal and Sick 1992). Glycogen, a high-molecular carbohydrate synthesised from glucose, is a suitable substrate for glycolysis (glycogenolysis) (Peters, Palay and Webster 1991). Glycogenolysis occurs very rapidly in astrocytes, giving rise to a large amount of energy production within a short time. The pyruvate/lactate produced by astrocytic glycolysis may be available for further metabolism in the astrocytes themselves or in adjacent neurons, but glycogenolytically derived energy can only be used by the astrocytes themselves. Pyruvate and lactate can also be used to resynthesise glycogen in astrocytes (Dringen, Gebhardt and Hamprecht 1993; Huang et al. 1994). In the presence of oxygen, pyruvate formed during glycolysis can be further metabolised via acetylcoenzyme A in the mitochondrial citric acid cycle to carbon dioxide and water to produce a large amount of ATP by oxidative phosphorylation.

The inhibitor of oxidative phosphorylation dinitrophenol (DNP) abolishes the ITMA phase of the intermediate memory stage in chicks trained on the passive avoidance task, but has no direct effect on the succeeding ITMB phase (Gibbs and Ng 1984). Since glycolysis and oxidative metabolism occur in both neurons and astrocytes (Hertz, Drejer and Schousboe 1988), it is unclear as to whether the amnestic effects of DNP are due to inhibition of neuronal or glial metabolism. Neuronal metabolism must be involved since astrocytes survive (Sochocka et al. 1994) and accumulate glutamate on glycolysis alone. The possibility that astrocytic metabolism also may be involved cannot be ruled out, since fluoroacetate has the same effect as DNP. However, as argued earlier, this effect of FA is likely to be due to interference with glutamate/glutamine synthesis rather than astrocytic energy production. It is reasonable to conclude that the energy demands of at least some of the cellular processes underlying ITMA are met by neuronal and astrocytic oxidative metabolism. However, memory processing during ITMB appears to be able to proceed in the absence of oxidative metabolism, such as would occur in the presence of DNP. Glycogenolysis in astrocytes may be a sufficient alternative source of energy. This is supported by the finding that iodoacetate (IO), which inhibits glycolysis in both neurons and astrocytes, has no effect on ITMA but abolishes ITMB, with significant retention losses appearing after 30 min post-training (O'Dowd et al. 1994a,b). The use of IO does not distinguish between neuronal glycolysis, astrocytic glycolysis, astrocyte-specific glycogenolysis or any combination of these. However, a significant increase in uptake of 2-deoxyglucose has been observed during ITMB (Sedman et al. 1992). Moreover, the mean forebrain level of glycogen in the chick shows a rapid reduction beginning 30 min post-training, reaching a nadir by 55 min and recovering quickly to untrained levels by 65 min post-training (O'Dowd et al. 1994a). A number of other findings are also pertinent.

The appearance of ITMB is preceded by a significant increase in whole forebrain NA levels by 30 min post-training (Crowe, Ng and Gibbs 1991b). β-adrenergic blockers, such as propranolol (Crowe, Ng and Gibbs 1991a) and sotalol (Stephenson and Andrew 1981), abolish ITMB but not ITMA. These findings suggest that consolidation of memory traces beyond ITMA may depend upon adequate reinforcement promoting sufficient arousal mediated by increased nor-adrenergic activity. Both NA and the β-adrenergic agonist isoproterenol have been shown to amplify glycogen turnover and glycolysis in mouse astrocytes (Cambray-Deakin et al. 1988; Subbarao and Hertz 1991), and propranolol inhibits this stimulation (Subbarao and Hertz 1990a). These findings are consistent with increasing evidence for a β-receptor-mediated metabolic response to NA in mammalian glia, but perhaps not in neurons (Stone and Ariano 1989; Sorg and Magistretti 1991; Sokoloff 1992).

Mammalian astrocytes express large numbers of β-adrenergic receptors (Stone and Ariano 1989) and compared to neurons show particularly marked rises in cAMP if these receptors are stimulated (Stone and Colbjornsen 1989; Stone et al. 1992a,b). Glycogen levels in the chick brain peak at the time of hatching (Edwards and Rogers 1972). In 10- to 12-day-old chick primary astrocyte cultures (corresponding approximately to hatching age), glycogenolysis is stimulated by NA, as is cAMP formation (O'Dowd 1995; O'Dowd et al. 1995). We have preliminary evidence that NA, isoprenaline, and the β_3-adrenergic agonist BRL37344A, but not the α_1-adrenergic agonist phenylephrine or the α_2-adrenergic agonist clonidine, stimulate glycogenolysis in 21-day chick primary astrocyte cultures, and that the glycogen content in the forebrains of day-old chicks is depressed by intracerebral injections of NA (unpublished data). It seems reasonable to suggest that NA released by neurons, in response to adequate reinforcement before the transition from ITMA to ITMB, may act as a metabolic signal that stimulates astrocytic glycogenolysis, and possibly neuronal and astrocytic glycolysis, to provide energy or substrates (alanine, pyruvate or lactate) required to drive the cellular processes underlying the expression and maintenance of ITMB. The finding that inhibition of the activity of the cAMP-dependent protein kinase A results in memory loss only after 50 min post-training (Zhao et al. 1995) is consistent with this view.

15.7 Concluding Remarks

The evidence reviewed above makes a persuasive case for the involvement of glial cells in neural information processing in general and memory formation in particular. The evidence is as yet coarse and fragmented, based primarily as it is on pharmacological studies (see Fig. 15.2). Most of the more direct evidence comes from studies with the chick, within the framework of the Gibbs–Ng memory model.

Further systematic research, with more specific and selective probes and with other species and other learning tasks, is needed to provide a comprehensive and

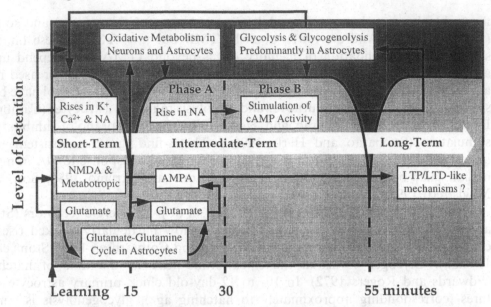

Fig. 15.2. Schematic diagram of the Gibbs–Ng three-stage model of passive avoidance memory formation in the day-old chick showing astrocyte–neuron interactions in glutamate turnover and in energy metabolism. Glutamate is released from neurons immediately after training (stimulating NMDA and metabotropic receptors), and during phase A of the intermediate memory stage (stimulating AMPA receptors.) This glutamate may activate LTP/LTD-like mechanisms related to long-term memory, and some other glutamate-sensitive process operating during phase A of intermediate memory. The glutamate–glutamine cycle in astrocytes is involved in the restocking of neuronal glutamate supplies following release. The rise in forebrain noradrenaline (NA) during phase A of intermediate memory may stimulate glycolysis and the astrocyte-specific process of glycogenolysis via the cAMP second messenger system, providing energy or substrates necessary to drive the memory-related mechanisms active during phase B of this stage. The release of K^+, Ca^{2+} or NA following training may also stimulate glycolysis and glycogenolysis in astrocytes. Finally, neuronal and astrocytic oxidative metabolism energises memory-related processes necessary for phase A of intermediate memory.

generalisable understanding of the cascade of cellular events which form the biological basis for information processing and storage by the brain. The cascade unquestionably involves a complex interaction of neuronal and glial mechanisms and processes extending far beyond the essentially homeostatic roles traditionally assigned to the latter. The research enterprise will be of necessity interdisciplinary, involving sophisticated behavioural, ultrastructural, biochemical, and biophysical techniques.

References

Abbott, N. J. (1995). Morphology of non-mammalian glial cells: functional implications. In *Neuroglia*, eds H. Kettenmann and B. R. Ransom, pp. 97–116. New York and Oxford: Oxford University Press.

Abbott, N. J., Lieberman, E. M., Pichon, Y., Hassan, S., and Larmet, Y. (1988). Periaxonal ion regulation in the small squid *Alloteuthis*: studies on isolated and in situ axons. *Biophys. J.*, **53**, 275–279.

Abbott, N. J., Brown, E.R., Pichon, Y., and Kukita, F. (1995). Electrophysiology of squid Schwann cells. In *Cephalopod Neurobiology*, eds N. J. Abbott, R. Williamson and L. Maddock, pp. 197–212. Oxford: Oxford University Press.

Abeliovich, A., Chen, C., Goda, Y., Silva, A. J., Stevens, C. F., and Tonegawa, S. (1993). Modified hippocampal long-term potentiation in PKC-mutant mice. *Cell*, **75**, 1253–1262.

Advokat, C., and Pellegrin, A. I. (1992). Excitatory amino acids and memory: evidence from research on Alzheimer's disease and behavioural pharmacology. *Neurosci. Biobehav. Rev.*, **16**, 13–24.

Aladjalova, N. A. (1964). Slow electrical processes in the brain. *Prog. Brain Res.* (Vol. 7 pp. 1–243). Amsterdam: Elsevier.

Albrecht, D., Rausche, G., and Heinemann, U. (1989). Reflections of low calcium epileptiform activity from area CA1 into dentate gyrus in the rat hippocampal slice. *Brain Res.*, **480**, 393–396.

Ali, S. M., Bullock, S., and Rose, S. P. R. (1988). Phosphorylation of synaptic proteins in chick forebrain: Changes with development and passive avoidance training. *J. Neurochem.*, **50**, 1579–1587.

Alici, K., Gloveli, T., Schmitz, D., and Heinemann, U. (1996). Various glutamate receptor agonists reduce presynaptic Ca^{2+} influx in hippocampal area CA1 and CA3. *Pflug. Arch. Eur. J. Phys.*, **431**(Suppl.), R80–R86. (Abstract)

Alkon, D. L. (1984). Calcium-mediated reduction in ionic currents: A biophysical memory trace. *Science*, **226**, 1037–1045.

Allen, T. J. A., and Rouot, B. (1995). Cyclic nucleotide homeostasis and axonal G proteins in the squid *Loligo forbesi*. In *Cephalopod Neurobiology*, eds N. J. Abbott, R. Williamson and L. Maddock, pp. 35–52. Oxford: Oxford University Press.

Altman, J., and Das, G. D. (1964). Autoradiographic examination of the effects of enriched environment on the rate of glial multiplication in the adult rat brain. *Nature*, **204**, 1161–1163.

Alvarez-Buylla, A., Buskirk, D. A., and Nottebohm, F. (1987). Monoclonal antibody reveals radial glia in adult avian brain. *J. Comp. Neur.*, **264**, 159–170.

Alvarez-Buylla, A., Kirn, J. R., and Nottebohm, F. (1990). Birth of projection neurons in adult avian brain may be related to perceptual or motor learning. *Science*, **249**, 1444–1446.

Amato, A., Ballerini, L., and Attwell, D. (1994). Intracellular pH changes produced by glutamate uptake in rat hippocampal slices. *J. Neurophysiol.*, **72**, 1686–1696.

Amedee, T., Ellie, E., Dupouy, B. and Vincent, J. D. (1991). Voltage-dependent calcium and potassium channels in Schwann cells cultured from dorsal root ganglia of the mouse. *J. Physiol.*, **441**, 35–56.

Ames, A., and Nesbett, F. B. (1981). In vitro retina as an experimental model of the central nervous system. *J. Neurochem.*, **37**, 867–877.

Ames, A., Li, Y.-Y., Heher, E. C., and Kimble, C. R. (1992). Energy metabolism of rabbit retina related to function: high cost of Na^+ transport. *J. Neurosci.*, **12**, 840–853.

Ammann, D., Lauter, F., Steiner, R. A., Schulthess, P., Shijo, Y., and Simon, W. (1981). Neutral carrier based hydrogen ion selective microelectrode for extra- and intracellular studies. *Anal. Chem.*, **53**, 2267–2269.

Amoroso, E. C., Baxter, M. I., Chiqudine, A. D., and Nisbet, R. H. (1964). The fine structure of neurons and other elements in the nervous system of the giant African land snail, *Archachatina marginata*. *Proc. R. Soc. Lond. B.*, **160**, 167–180.

Amundson, R. H., Goderie, S. K., and Kimelberg, H. K. (1992). Uptake of [^{3}H]serotonin and [^{3}H]glutamate by primary astrocyte cultures II. Differences in cultures prepared from different brain regions. *Glia*, **6**, 9–18.

Anders, J. J. (1988). Lactic acid inhibitors of gap junctional intercellular communication in in vitro astrocytes as measured by fluorescence recovery after photobleaching. *Glia*, **1**, 371–379.

Anderson, B. J., Li, X., Alcantara, A. A., Isaacs, K. R., Black, J. E., and Greenough, W. T. (1994). Glial hypertrophy is associated with synaptogenesis following motor-skill learning, but not with angiogenesis following exercise. *Glia*, **11**, 73–80.

Anderson, D. H., Guèrin, C. J., Erickson, P. A., Stern, W. H., and Fisher, S. K. (1986). Morphological recovery in the reattached retina. *Invest. Ophthalmol. Vis. Sci.*, **27**, 168–83.

Anderson, J. R. (1974). Retrieval of propositional information from long-term memory. *Cog. Psychol.*, **6**, 451–474.

Andrew, R. D., MacVicar, B. A., Dudek, F. E., and Hatton, G. I. (1981). Dye transfer through gap junctions between neuroendocrine cells of the rat hypothalamus. *Science*, **211**, 1187–1189.

Andrew, R. J., ed. (1991). *Neural and Behavioural Plasticity: The Use of the Domestic Chick as a Model*, pp. 17–18. Oxford: Oxford University Press.

Antonini, A., and Stryker, M. P. (1993). Rapid remodelling of axonal arbors in the visual cortex. *Science*, **260**, 1819–1821.

Aoki, C. (1992). β-Adrenergic receptors: astrocytic localization in the adult visual cortex and their relation to catecholamine axon terminals as revealed by electron microscopic immunocytochemistry. *J. Neurosci.*, **12**, 781–792.

Aoki, C., and Pickel, V. M. (1992a). Ultrastructural relations between β-adrenergic receptors and catecholaminergic neurons. *Brain Res. Bull.*, **29**, 257–263.

Aoki, C., and Pickel, V. M. (1992b). C-Terminal tail of β-adrenergic receptors: immunocytochemical localization within astrocytes and their relation to catecholaminergic neurons in N. tractus solitarii and area postrema. *Brain Res.*, **571**, 35–49.

Aoki, C., and Venkatesan, C. (1997). Differential timing for the appearance of neuronal and astrocytic β-adrenergic receptors in the developing rat visual cortex as revealed by light and electron microscopic immunocytochemistry. *Visual Neurosci.*, **14**, 1129–1142.

Aoki, C., Kaufman, D., and Rainbow, T. C. (1986). The ontogeny of the laminar distribution of beta-adrenergic receptors in the visual cortex of cats, normally reared and visually deprived. *Dev. Brain Res.*, **27**, 109–116.

Aoki, C., Joh, T. H., and Pickel, V. M. (1987). Ultrastructural localization of immunoreactivity for beta-adrenergic receptors in the cortex and neostriatum of rat brain. *Brain Res.*, **437**, 264–282.

Aoki, C., Milner, T. A., Berger, S. B., Shea, K. F., Blass, J. P., and Pickel, V. M. (1987). Glial glutamate dehydrogenase: ultrastructural localization and regional distribution in relation to the mitochondrial enzyme, cytochrome oxidase. *J. Neurosci. Res.*, **18**, 305–318.

Aoki, C., Zerncik, B. A., Strader, C. D., and Pickel, V. M. (1989). Cytoplasmic loop of beta-adrenergic receptors: synaptic and intracellular localization and relation to catecholaminergic neurons in the nuclei of the solitary tracts. *Brain Res.*, **493**, 331–347.

Aoki, C., Kaneko, T., Starr, A. and, Pickel, V. M. (1991). Identification of mitochondrial and non-mitochondrial glutaminase within select neurons and glia of rat forebrain by electron microscopic immunocytochemistry. *J. Neurosci. Res.*, **28**, 531–548.

Aoki, C., Lubin, M., and Fenstemaker, S. (1994). Columnar activity regulates astrocytic β-adrenergic receptor-like immunoreactivity in V1 of adult monkeys. *Visual Neurosci.*, **11**, 179–187.

Aoki, C., Go, C-G.,Venkatesan, C., and Kurose, H. (1994). Perikaryal and synaptic localization of α$_{2A}$-adrenergic receptor immunoreactivity in brain as revealed by light and electron microscopic immunocytochemistry. *Brain Res.*, **650**, 181–204.

Aoki, C., Venkatesan, C., Go, C-G., Mong, J. A., and Dawson, T. M. (1994). Cellular and subcellular localization of NMDA-R1 subunit immunoreactivity in the visual cortex of adult and neonatal rats. *J. Neurosci.*, **14**, 5202–5222.

Aram, J. A., and Lodge, D. (1987). Epileptiform activity induced by alkalosis in rat neocortical slices: block by antagonists of *N*-methyl-D-aspartate. *Neurosci. Lett.*, **83**, 345–350.

Arduini, A., Mancia, M., and Mechelse, K. (1957). Slow potential changes elicited in the cerebral cortex by sensory and reticular stimulation. *Arch. Ital. Biol.*, **95**, 127–138.

Armett, C. J., and Ritchie, J. M. (1961). The action of acetylcholine and some related substances on conduction in mammalian non-myelinated nerve fibres. *J. Physiol.*, **155**, 372–384.

Aronson, P. S. (1985). Kinetic properties of the plasma membrane Na$^+$/H$^+$ exchanger. *Annu. Rev. Physiol.*, **47**, 545–560.

Artola, A., and Singer, W. (1993). Long-term depression of excitatory synaptic transmission and its relationship to long-term potentiation. *TINS*, **16**, 480–487.

Aschner, M., and LoPachin, R. M. (1993a). Glial-neuronal interactions: relevance to neurotoxic mechanisms. *Toxicol. Appl. Pharm.*, **118**, 141–158.

Aschner, M., and LoPachin, R. M., Jr (1993b). Astrocytes: targets and mediators of chemical-induced CNS injury. *J. Toxicol. Environ. Health*, **38**, 329–342.

Astion, M. L., and Orkand, R. K. (1988). Electrogenic Na$^+$/HCO$_3^-$ cotransport in neuroglia. *Glia*, **1**, 355–357.

Astion, M. L., Coles, J. A., Orkand, R. K. and Abbott, N. J. (1988). K^+ accumulation in the space between giant axon and Schwann cell in the squid *Alloteuthis*: effects of changes in osmolarity. *Biophys. J.*, **53**, 281–285.

Astion, M. L., Chvátal, A., and Orkand, R. K. (1989). Na^+/H^+ exchange in glial cells of *Necturus* optic nerve. *Neurosci. Lett.*, **107**, 167–172.

Aston-Jones, G., Chiang, G., and Alexinsky, T. (1991). Discharge of noradrenergic locus coeruleus neurons in behaving rats and monkeys suggests a role in vigilance. *Prog. Brain Res.*, **88**, 501–519.

Asztalos, Z., Wegerer, J., Wustmann, G., Dombradi, V., Gausz, J., Spatz, H-C., and Friedrich, P. (1993). Protein phosphatase 1-deficient *Drosophila* is affected in habituation and associative learning. *J. Neurosci.*, **13**, 924–930.

Atkinson, R. C., and Shriffin, R. M. (1968). Human memory: A proposed system and its control processes. In *The Psychology of Learning and Motivation: Advances in Research and Theory,* Vol. 2, eds K. W. Spence and J. T. Spence, pp. 89–105. New York: Academic Press.

Attwell, D., Brew, H., and Mobbs, P. (1986). Electrophysiology of the Müller cell network in the isolated axolotl retina. *J. Physiol. (Lond.)*, **369**, 33P.

Attwell, D., Barbour, B., and Szatkovski, M. (1993). Nonvesicular release of neurotransmitter. *Neuron*, **11**, 401–407.

Ayala, G. F., Dichter, M., Gumnit, R. J., Matsumoto, H., and Spencer, W. A. (1973). Genesis of epileptic interictal spikes. New knowledge of cortical feedback systems suggest neurophysiological explanation of brief paroxysms. *Brain Res.*, **52**, 1–17.

Bach-y-Rita, P. (1993). Neurotransmission in the brain by diffusion through the extracellular fluid: a review. *NeuroReport*, **4**, 343–350.

Bailey, C. H., and Kandel, E. R. (1993). Structural changes accompanying memory storage. *Annu. Rev. Physiol.*, **55**, 397–426.

Baker, M., Bostock, H., Grafe, P. and Martius, P. (1987). Function and distribution of three types of rectifying channel in rat spinal root myelinated axons. *J. Physiol.*, **383**, 45–67.

Balestino, M., and Somjen, G. G. (1988). Concentration of carbon dioxide, interstitial pH and synaptic transmission in hippocampal formation of the rat. *J. Physiol.*, **396**, 247–266.

Ballanyi, K. (1995). Modulation of glial potassium, sodium, and chloride activities by the extracellular milieu. In *Neuroglia*, eds H. Kettenmann and B. R. Ransom, pp. 289–298. New York and Oxford: Oxford University Press.

Ballanyi, K., and Schlue, W. R. (1989). Electrophysiological characterization of a nicotinic acetylcholine receptor on leech neuropile glial cells. *Glia*, **2**, 330–345.

Ballanyi, K., Grafe, P., and Ten Bruggencate, G. (1987). Ion activities and potassium uptake mechanisms of glial cells in guinea-pig olfactory cortex slices. *J. Physiol.*, **382**, 159–174.

Ballanyi, K., Mückenhoff, K., Bellingham, M. C., Okada, Y., Scheid, P., and Richter, D. W. (1994). Activity-related pH changes in respiratory neurons and glial cells of cats. *NeuroReport*, **6**, 33–36.

Banker, G. A. (1980). Trophic interactions between astroglial cells and hippocampal neurons in culture. *Science*, **209**, 809–810.

Barbour, B., Szatkowski, M., Ingledew, N., and Attwell, D. (1989). Arachidonic acid induces a prolonged inhibition of glutamate uptake into glial cells. *Nature*, **342**, 918–920.

Barbour, B., Brew, H., and Attwell, D. (1991). Electrogenic uptake of glutamate and aspartate into glial cells isolated from the salamander (*Ambystoma*) retina. *J. Physiol. (Lond.)*, **436**, 169–193.

Barnes, S., Merchant, V., and Mahmud, F. (1993). Modulation of transmission gain by protons at the photoreceptor output synapse. *Proc. Natl Acad. Sci. USA*, **90**, 10081–10085.

Barnett, N. L., and Osborne, N. N. (1995). Redistribution of GABA immunoreactivity following central retinal artery occlusion. *Brain Res.*, **677**, 337–340.

Barnett N. L., Pow, D. V., Plenderleith, M. B., and Robinson, S. R. (1996). Inhibition of glutamine synthetase suppresses the electroretinogram B-wave in the rat. *Soc. Neurosci. Abstr.*, **22**, 121.

Barres, B. A. (1991). New roles for glia. *J. Neurosci.* **11**, 3684–3695.

Barres, B. A., Chun, L. L. Y., and Corey, D. P. (1990). Ion channels in vertebrate glia. *Annu. Rev. Neurosci.*, **13**, 441–474.

Barres, B. A., Koroshetz, W. J., Swartz, K. J., Chun, L. L., and Corey, D. P. (1990a). Ion channel expression by white matter glia: the O-2A glial progenitor cell. *Neuron*, **4**, 507–524.

Barres, B. A., Koroshetz, W. J., Chun, L. L. Y., and Corey, D. P. (1990b). Ion channel expression by white matter glia: the type-1 astrocyte. *Neuron*, **5**, 527–544.

Barrett, E. F., and Barrett, J. N. (1982). Intracellular recordings from vertebrate myelinated axons: mechanism of the depolarizing after-potential. *J. Physiol.*, **323**, 117–144

Baudry, M., and Davis, J. L. (1991). *Long-term Potentiation. A Debate of Current Issues.* Cambridge: MIT Press.

Bauer, H. (1968). Corticale evozierte Potentiale als Auswirkung von Aktion und Reaktion des Menschen. Doctoral Thesis, University of Vienna.

Bauer, H. (1993). Determinants of CNV Amplitude. In *Slow Potentials in the Brain,* eds W. Haschke, A. I. Roitbak, E.-J. Speckmann, pp. 45–61. Boston: Birkhäuser.

Bauer, H., and Lauber, W. (1979). Operant conditioning of brain steady potential shifts in man. *Biofeedback Self-Regul.*, **4**, 145–154.

Bauer, H., and Nirnberger, G. (1980). Paired associate learning with feedback of DC potential shifts of the cerebral cortex. *Arch. Psychol.*, **132**, 237–239.

Bauer, H., and Nirnberger, G. (1981). Concept identification as a function of preceding negative or positive spontaneous shifts in slow brain potentials. *Psychophysiology*, **18**, 466–469.

Bauer, H., and Rebert, C. S. (1990). Preliminary studies on subcortical slow potentials related to the readiness potential in the monkey. *Int. J. Psychophysiol.*, **9**, 269–278.

Bauer, H., Guttmann, G., Weber, G., and Trimmel, M. (1986). The brain-triggered CNV: Baseline effects on CNV and P300. In *Cerebral Psychophysiology: Studies in Event-Related Potentials,* eds W. C. McCallum, R. Zappoli and F. Denoth, pp. 232–243. Electroencephalography and Clinical Neurophysiology, Suppl. 38. Amsterdam: Elsevier.

Bauer, H., Rebert, C. S., Korunka, Ch., and Leodolter, M. (1992). Rare events and the CNV – the oddball CNV. *Int. J. Psychophysiol.*, **13**, 51–58.

Bauer, H., Korunka, Ch., and Leodolter, M. (1993). Possible Glial Contribution in the Electrogenesis of SPs. In *Slow Potential Changes in the Human Brain,* eds W.C. McCallum and S. H. Curry, pp. 23–34. New York: Plenum Press.

Bauer, H., Vitouch, O., Gittler, G., Leodolter, M., and Leodolter, U. (1995). Topography of slow cortical potentials evoked by spatial and verbal processing. *Brain Topography*, **7**, 343.

Bauer, H., Vitouch, O., Leodolter, M., and Leodolter, U. (1997). Topography of phasic and tonic steady potential changes evoked by spatial processing. *Brain Topography*, **9**, 51.

Beagley, G. H., and Hatton, G. I. (1994). Systemic signals contribute to induced morphological changes in the hypothalamo-neurohypophysial system. *Brain Res. Bull.*, **33**, 211–218.

Becker, W. and Kristeva, R. (1980). Cerebral potentials prior to various force deployments. In *Motivation, Motor and Sensory Processes of the Brain: Electrical Potentials, Behaviour and Clinical Use*, eds H. H. Kornhuber and L. Deecke, pp. 189–194. Progress in Brain Research Vol. 54. Amsterdam: Elsevier.

Becker, W., Hoehne, O., Iwase, K., and Kornhuber, H. (1972). Bereitschaftspotential, prämotorische Positivierung und andere Hirnpotentiale bei sakkadischen Augenbewegungen. *Vision Res.*, **12**, 421–436.

Beeler, T., and Gable, K. (1993). Effect of the general anaesthetic, halothane on the activity of the transverse tubule Ca^{2+} activated K^+ channel. *FEBS Lett.*, **331**, 207–210.

Behrens, U. D., Kadner, A., and Wagner, H.-J. (1996). Double labelling of zinc and GFAP-immunoreactivity in Müller cells of cyprinid retinae. *Invest. Ophthalmol. Vis. Sci.*, **37**, S1041.

Bennett, M. V. L., Verselis, V., White, R. L., and Spray, D. C. (1991). Gap junctional conductance: gating. In *Gap Junctions*, eds E. L. Hertzberg and R. Johnson, pp. 287–304. New York: Alan R. Liss.

Bennett, P. C., Zhao, W-Q., Lawen, A., and Ng, K. T. (1996). Cyclosporin A, an inhibitor of calcineurin, impairs memory formation in day-old chicks. *Brain Res.*, **730**, 107–117.

Bernard, C. C. A., Gibbs, M. E., Hodge, R. J., and Ng, K. T. (1983). Inhibition of long-term memory formation in the chick by anti-chick Thy-1 antibody. *Brain Res. Bull.*, **11**, 111–116.

Berthold, C. H., and Rydmark, M. (1983). Electron microscopic serial section analysis of nodes of Ranvier in lumbosacral spinal roots of the cat: ultrastructural organization of nodal compartments in fibres of different sizes. *J. Neurocytol.*, **12**, 475–505.

Berthold, C., and Rydmark, M. (1995). Morphology of normal peripheral axons. In *The Axon; Structure, Function and Pathophysiology*, eds S. G. Waxman, J. D. Kocsis and P. K. Stys, pp. 13–50. New York: Oxford University Press.

Bevan, S. (1990). Ion channels and neurotransmitter receptors in glia. *Semin. Neurosci.*, **2**, 467–481.

Bevan, S., Chiu, S. Y., Gray, P. T. A., and Ritchie, J. M. (1985). The presence of voltage-gated sodium, potassium and chloride channels in rat cultured astrocytes. *Proc. Roy. Soc. (Lond.)*, **225**, 299–313.

Biedermann, B., Eberhardt, W., and Reichelt, W. (1994). GABA uptake into isolated retinal Müller glial cells of the guinea pig detected electrophysiologically. *NeuroReport*, **5**, 438–440.

Biedermann, B., Fröhlich, E., Grosche, J., Wagner, H.-J., and Reichenbach, A. (1995). Mammalian Müller (glial) cells express functional D_2 dopamine receptors. *NeuroReport*, **6**, 609–612.

Bignami, A., Hosley, M., and Dahl, D. (1993). Hyaluronic acid and hyaluronic acid-binding proteins in brain extracellular matrix. *Anat. Embryol.*, **188**, 419–433.

Bignami, A., Perides, G., Asher, R., and Dahl, D. (1992). The astrocyte–extracellular matrix complex in CNS myelinated tracts: a comparative study on the distribution of hyaluronate in rat, goldfish and lamprey. *J. Neurocytol.*, **21**, 604–613.

Billups, B. and Attwell, D. (1996). Modulation of glutamate release by pH. *Nature*, **379**, 171–174.

Birbaumer, N., and Schmidt, R. F. (1996). *Biologische Psychologie [Biological Psychology]*. Berlin, Heidelberg, New York: Springer-Verlag.

Birbaumer, N., Elbert, T., Rockstroh, B., and Lutzenberger, W. (1981a). Biofeedback of event-related slow potentials of the brain. *Int. J. Psychol.*, **16**, 389–415.

Birbaumer, N., Elbert, T., Lutzenberger, W., Rockstroh, B., and Schwartz, J. (1981b). EEG and slow cortical potentials in anticipation of mental tasks with different hemispheric involvement. *Biol. Psychol.*, **13**, 251–260.

Birbaumer, N., Lang, P., Cook, E., Elbert, T., Lutzenberger, W., and Rockstroh, B. (1988). Slow brain potentials, imagery and hemispheric differences. *Int. J. Neurosci.*, **39**, 101–116.

Birbaumer, N., Elbert, T., Canavan, A. G. M., and Rockstroh, B. (1990). Slow potentials of the cerebral cortex and behavior. *Physiol. Rev.*, **70**, 1–41.

Birbaumer, N., Elbert, T., Rockstroh, B., Daum, I. Wolf, P., and Canavan, A. (1991). Clinical psychological treatment of epileptic seizures: a controlled study. In *Perspectives and Promises of Clinical Psychology*, ed. A. Ehlers, pp. 81–96. New York: Plenum Press.

Birbaumer, N., Roberts, L. E., Lutzenberger, W., Rockstroh, B., and Elbert, T. (1992). Area specific self-regulation of slow cortical potentials on the sagittal midline and its effects on behavior. *Electroenceph. Clin. Neuropsychol.*, **84**, 353–361.

Birbaumer, N., Lutzenberger, W., and Schleichert, H. (1994). Think to move – and move! *Soc. Neurosci. Abstr.*, **154**, 18

Birbaumer, N., Lutzenberger, W., Schleichert, H., Kotchoubey, B., and Anokhin, A. (1996). Think to move and move: biofeedback in severe motor paralysis. *Proc. Ass. Applied Psychophysiol.*, p. 12.

Birbaumer, N., Pulvermueller, F., Preissl, H., Heinze, H-J., Tempelman, J., Schleichert, H. (1998). Self-regulation of slow cortical potentials changes regional blood flow in the brain. Submitted.

Bjelke, B., England, R., Nicholson, C., Rice, M. E., Lindberg, J., Zoli, M., Agnati, L. F., and Fuxe, K. (1995). Long distance pathways of diffusion for dextran along fibre bundles in brain. Relevance for volume transmission. *NeuroReport*, **6**, 1005–1009.

Black, J. A., Sims, T. J., Waxman, S. J., and Gilmore, S. A. (1985). Membrane ultrastructure of developing axons in glial cell deficient rat spinal cord. *J. Neurocytol.*, **14**, 79–104.

Black, J. A., Waxman, S. G., and Hildebrand, C. (1985). Axon-glial relations in the retina–optic nerve junction of the adult rat: freeze-fracture observations on axon membrane structure. *J. Neurocytol.*, **14**, 887–907.

Black, J. A., Yokoyama, S., Waxman, S. G., Oh, Y., Zur, K. B, Sontheimer, H., Higashida, H., and Ransom, B. R. (1994a). Sodium channel mRNAs in cultured spinal cord astrocytes: in situ hybridization in identified cell types. *Mol. Brain Res.*, **23**, 235–245.

Black, J. A., Westenbroek, R., Ransom, B. R., Catteral, W. A., and Waxman, S. G. (1994b). Type II sodium channels in spinal cord astrocytes in situ: immunocytochemical observations. *Glia*, **12**, 219–227.

Black, J. E., Isaacs, K. R., Anderson, B. J., Alcantara, A. A., and Greenough, W. T. (1990). Learning causes synaptogenesis, whereas motor activity causes angiogenesis, in cerebellar cortex of adult rats. *Proc. Natl Acad. Sci. USA*, **87**, 5567–5572.

Blakemore, W. F., and Crang, A. J. (1985). The use of cultured autologous Schwann cells to remyelinate areas of demyelination in the central nervous system. *J. Neurol. Sci.*, **70**, 207–223.

Blakemore, W. F., and Patterson, R. C. (1978). Suppression of remyelination in the CNS by X-irradiation. *Acta Neuropath.*, **42**, 105–113.

Blight, A. R. (1985). Delayed demyelination and macrophage invasion: a candidate for secondary cell damage in spinal cord injury. *CNS Trauma*, **2**, 299–314.

Blight, A. R. (1989). Effect of 4-AP on axonal conduction block in chronic spinal cord injury. *Brain Res. Bull.*, **22**, 47–52.

Bliss, T. V. P., and Collingridge, G. L. (1993). A synaptic model of memory: long-term potentiation in the hippocampus. *Nature*, **361**, 31–39.

Bliss, T. V. P., and Lomo, T. (1973). Long-lasting potentiation of synaptic transmission in the dentate area of the anaesthetized rabbit following stimulation of the perforant path. *J. Physiol.*, **232**, 331–356.

Bobak, J. B., and Salm, A. K. (1996). Plasticity of astrocytes of the ventral glial limitans subjacent to the supraoptic nucleus. *J. Comp. Neurol.*, **376**, 188–197.

Bock, E. (1978). Nervous system specific proteins. *J. Neurochem.*, **30**, 7–14.

Boison, D., and Stoffel, W. (1989). Myelin-deficient rat: a point mutation in exon III (A–C, Thr75–Pro) of the myelin proteolipid protein causes dysmyelination and oligodendrocyte death. *EMBO J.*, **8**, 3295–3302.

Bolwig, T. G., and Quistorff, B. (1973). In vivo concentration of lactate in the brain of conscious rats before and during seizures: a new ultra-rapid technique for the freeze sampling of brain tissue. *J. Neurochem.*, **21**, 1345–1348.

Bondareff, W., and Pysh, J. J. (1968). Distribution of extracellular space during postnatal maturation of rat cerebral cortex. *Anat. Rec.*, **160**, 773–780.

Bonfanti, L., Poulain, D. A., and Theodosis, D. T. (1993). Radial glia-like cells in the supraoptic nucleus of the adult rat. *J. Neuroendocrinol.*, **5**, 1–5.

Bonhoeffer, F., and Huf, J. (1982). In vitro experiments on axon guidance demonstrating an anterior-posterior gradient on the tectum. *EMBO J.*, **1**, 427–431.

Borgula, G. A., Karwoski, C. J., and Steinberg, R. H. (1989). Light-evoked changes in extracellular pH in frog retina. *Vision Res.*, **29**, 1069–1077.

Bormann, J., and Kettenmann, H. (1988). Patch clamp study of GABA receptor Cl⁻ channels in cultured astrocytes. *Proc. Natl Acad. Sci. USA*, **85**, 9336–9340.

Born, J., Whipple, S. C., and Stamm, J. (1982). Spontaneous cortical slow-potential shifts and choice reaction time performance. *Electroenceph. Clin. Neurophysiol.*, **54**, 668–676.

Boss, V., and Conn, P. J. (1992). Metabotropic excitatory amino acid receptor activation stimulates phospholipase D in hippocampal slices. *J. Neurochem.*, **59**, 2340–2343.

Bouvier, M., Hausdorff, W. P., De Blasi, A., O'Dowd, B. F., Kobilka, B. K., Caron, M. G., and Lefkowitz, R. J. (1988). Removal of phosphorylation sites from the β2–adrenergic receptor delays onset of agonist-promoted desensitization. *Nature*, **333**, 370–373.

Bouvier, M., Szatkowski, M., Amato, A., and Attwell, D. (1992). The glial cell glutamate uptake carrier countertransports pH-changing anions. *Nature*, **360**, 471–474.

Bowman, C. L., and Kimelberg, H. K. (1984). Excitatory amino acids directly depolarize rat brain astrocytes in primary culture. *Nature*, **311**, 656–659.

Bowman, C. L., and Kimelberg, H. K. (1988). Adrenergic-receptor-mediated depolarization of astrocytes. In *Glial Cell Receptors,* ed. H. K. Kimelberg, pp. 53–76. New York: Raven Press.

Brattstrom, B. H. (1978). Learning studies in lizards. In *Behaviour and Neurology of Lizards*, eds N. Greenberg and P. D. MacLean, pp. 173–181. DHEW Publication, US Government.

Brew, H., and Attwell, D. (1987). Electrogenic glutamate uptake is a major current carrier in the membrane of axolotl retinal glial cells. *Nature*, **327**, 707–709.

Brew, H., Gray, P. T. A., Mobbs, P., and Attwell, D. (1986). Endfeet of retinal glial cells have higher densities of ion channels that mediate K^+ buffering. *Nature*, **324**, 466–468.

Brill, M. H., Waxman, S. G., Moore, J. W., and Joyner, R. W. (1977). Conduction velocity and spike configuration in myelinated fibers: computed dependence on internode distance. *J. Neurol. Neurosurg. Psychiat.*, **40**, 769–774.

Broadbent, D. E. (1958). *Perception and Communication*. Oxford: Pergamon Press.

Brockes, J. P., Fields, K. L., and Raff, M. C. (1979). Studies on cultured rat Schwann cells. I. Establishment of purified populations from cultures of peripheral nerve. *Brain Res.*, **165**, 105–118.

Brodersen, P., Paulson, O. B., Bolwig, T. G., Rogan, Z. E., Rafaelsen, O. J., Lassen, N. A. (1973). Cerebral hyperemia in electrically induced epileptic seizures. *Arch. Neurol.*, **28**, 334–338.

Broide, R. S., Robertson, R. T., and Leslie, F. M. (1996). Regulation of alpha 7 nicotinic acetylcholine receptors in the developing rat somatosensory cortex by thalamocortical afferents. *J. Neurosci.*, **16**, 2956–2971.

Brookes, N., and Turner, R. J. (1993). Extracellular potassium regulates the glutamine content of astrocytes: mediation by intracellular pH. *Neurosci. Lett.*, **160**, 73–76.

Brown, E. R. (1993). K^+ accumulation around the giant axon of the squid; comparison of electrical and morphological studies. *Jpn. J. Physiol.*, **43**, S279–284.

Brown, E. R., and Abbott, N. J. (1993). Ultrastructure and permeability of the Schwann cell layer surrounding the giant axon of the squid. *J. Neurocytol.*, **22**, 283–298.

Brown, E. R., and Kukita, F. (1996). Coupling between giant axon Schwann cells in the squid. *Proc. Roy. Soc. Lond. B.*, **263**, 667–672.

Brown, E. R., Bone, Q., Ryan, K. P., and Abbott, N. J. (1991). Morphology and electrical properties of Schwann cells around the giant axon of the squids *Loligo forbesi* and *Loligo vulgaris*. *Proc. Roy. Soc. Lond. B.*, **243**, 255–262.

Brown, E. R., Inoue, I., and Tsutsui, I. (1996). Voltage-activated ionic currents from isolated squid giant axon Schwann cells. *J. Physiol. (Lond.)*, **495**, P34–P35.

Brune, T., and Deitmer, J. W. (1995). Intracellular acidification and Ca^{2+} transients in cultured rat cerebellar astrocytes evoked by glutamate agonists and noradrenaline. *Glia*, **14**, 153–161.

Brune, T., Fetzer, S., Backus, K. H., and Deitmer, J. W. (1994). Evidence for electrogenic sodium-bicarbonate cotransport in cultured rat cerebellar astrocytes. *Pflügers Arch.*, **429**, 64–71.

Brunet, P. C., and Jirounek, P. (1994). Long-range intercellular signalling in glial cells of the peripheral nerve. *NeuroReport*, **5**, 635–638.

Brunia, C. H. M., and Damen, E. J. P. (1988). Distribution of slow potentials related to motor preparation and stimulus anticipation in a time estimation task. *Electroenceph. Clin. Neurophysiol.*, **69**, 234–243.

Buchheit, T. E., and Tytell, M. (1992). Transfer of molecules from glia to axons in the squid may be mediated by glial vesicles. *J. Neurobiol.*, **23**, 217–230.

Bullock, T. H., and Horridge, G. A. (1965). *Structure and Function in the Nervous Systems of Invertebrates*. 2 vols. San Francisco: Freeman.

Bunt-Milam, A. H., and Saari, J. C. (1983). Immunocytochemical localization of two retinoid-binding proteins in vertebrate retina. *J. Cell Biol.*, **97**, 703–712.

Burnard, D. M., Crichton, S. A., and MacVicar, B. A. (1990). Electrophysiological properties of reactive glial cells in the kainate-lesioned hippocampal slice. *Brain Res.*, **510**, 43–52.

Burnashev, N., Khodorova, A., Jonas, P., Helm, P. J., Wisden, W., Moyner, H., Seeburg, P. H., and Sakmann, B. (1992). Calcium-permeable AMPA-kainate receptors in fusiform cerebellar glial cells. *Science*, **256**, 1566–1570.

Butt, A. M., and Jennings, J. (1994a). Responses of astrocytes to γ-aminobutyric acid in the neonatal rat optic nerve. *Neurosci. Lett.*, **168**, 53–56.

Butt, A. M., and Jennings, J. (1994b). The astrocyte response to γ-aminobutyric acid attenuates with age in the rat optic nerve. *Proc. Roy. Soc. Lond. B.*, **258**, 9–15.

Butt, A. M., and Tutton, M. (1992). Response of oligodendrocytes to glutamate and γ-aminobutyric acid in the intact mouse optic nerve. *Neurosci. Lett.*, **146**, 108–110.

Buxbaum, J. D., and Dudai, Y. (1989). A quantitative model for the kinetics of cAMP-dependent protein kinase (type 11) activity. *J. Biol. Chem.*, **264**, 9344–9351.

Byrne, T. N., and Waxman, S. G. (1990). *Spinal Cord Compression*. Philadelphia: F. A. Davis Co.

Cabantchik, Z. I., and Greger, R. (1992). Chemical probes for anion transporters of mammalian cell membranes. *Am. J. Physiol.*, **262**, C803–827.

Cain, D. P. (1989). LTP and kindling: How similar are the mechanisms? *Trends Neurosci.*, **12**, 6–10.

Cambray-Deakin, M., Pearce, B., Morrow, C., and Murphy, S. (1988). Effects of extracellular potassium on glycogen stores in astrocytes in vitro. *J. Neurochem.*, **51**, 1846–1851.

Cameron, R.S., and Rakic, P. (1994). Polypeptides that comprise the plasmalemmal microdomain between migrating neuronal and glial cells. *J. Neurosci.*, **14**, 3139–3155.

Campagnoni, A. T. (1995). Molecular biology of myelination. In *Neuroglia*, eds H. Kettenmann and B. R. Ransom, pp. 555–570. New York and Oxford: Oxford University Press.

Canady, K. S., and Rubel, E. W. (1992). Rapid and reversible astrocytic reaction to afferent activity blockade in chick cochlear nucleus. *J. Neurosci.*, **12**, 1001–1009.

Cardinaud, B., Coles, J. A., Perrottet, P., Spencer, A. J., Osborne, M. P., and Tsacopoulos, M. (1994). The composition of the interstitial fluid in the retina of the honey bee drone: Implications for the supply of substrates of energy metabolism from blood to neurons. *Proc. Roy Soc. Lond. B.*, **257**, 49–58.

Carlson, S. D. (1987). Ultrastructure of the arthropod neuroglia and neuropil. In *Arthropod Brain: Its Evolution, Development, Structure, and Functions*, ed. A. P. Gupta. New York: Wiley & Sons.

Caroni, P., and Schwab, M. E. (1988). Two membrane protein fractions from rat central myelin with inhibitory properties for neurite growth and fibroblast spreading. *J. Cell Biol.*, **186**, 1281–1288.

Caspers, H. (1961). Changes of cortical DC potentials in the sleep-wakefulness cycle. In: *Ciba Foundation Symposium on the Nature of Sleep*, eds G. E. W. Wolstenholme and M. O'Connor, pp 237–253. London: Churchill.

Caspers, H. (1963). In *Brain function, Proceedings of the First Conference, Cortical Excitability and Steady Potentials*, ed. M. A. Brazier. Berkeley, California: UCLA Press.

Caspers, H. (1974). DC potentials recorded directly from the cortex. Preface. In *Handbook of Electroencephalography and Clinical Neurophysiology,* ed. A. Remond, Vol. 10, Part A. Amsterdam: Elsevier.

Caspers, H., and Speckmann, E.-J. (1969). DC potential shifts in paroxysmal states. In *Basic Mechanisms of the Epilepsies,* eds H. H. Jasper, A. A. Ward, and A. Pope, pp. 375–388. Boston: Little, Brown and Company.

Caspers, H., Speckmann, E.-J., and Lehmenkühler, A. (1980). Electrogenesis of cortical DC potentials. *Prog. Brain Res.,* **54,** 3–15.

Caspers, H., Speckmann, E.-J. and Lehmenkühler, A. (1984). Electrogenesis of slow potentials of the brain. In *Self-Regulation of the Brain and Behavior,* eds T. Elbert, B. Rockstroh, W. Lutzenberger and N. Birbaumer, pp. 26–41. Berlin: Springer-Verlag.

Castelluci, V. F., and Kandel, E. R. (1974). A quantal analysis of the synaptic depression underlying habituation of the gill-withdrawal reflex in *Aplysia. Proc. Natl Acad. Sci.,* **71,** 5004–5008.

Caton, R. (1875). The electric currents of the brain. *Br. Med. J.,* **2,** 278.

Caviness, V. S., and Rakic, P. (1978). Mechanisms of cortical development: a view from mutations in mice. *Annu. Rev. Neurosci.,* **1,** 297–326.

Cesar, M., and Hamprecht, B. (1995). Immunocytochemical examination of neural rat and mouse primary cultures using monoclonal antibodies raised against pyruvate carboxylase. *J. Neurochem.,* **64,** 2312–2318.

Chalmers, D. J. (1995). The puzzle of conscious experience. *Sci. Am.,* **273,** 80–86.

Chamak, B., Fellons, A., Glowinski, J., and Prochiantz, A. (1987). MAP2 expression and neuritic outgrowth and branching are coregulated through region-specific neuro-astroglial interactions. *J. Neurosci.,* **7,** 3163–3170.

Chan, P. H., and Chu, L. (1989). Ketamine protects cultured astrocytes from glutamate-induced swelling. *Brain Res.,* **487,** 380–383.

Chang, F.-L. F., and Greenough, W. T. (1984). Transient and enduring morphological correlates of synaptic activity and efficacy change in the rat hippocampal slice. *Brain Res.,* **309,** 35–46.

Chang, H. T. (1951). Dendritic potentials of cortical neurons produced by direct electrical stimulation of the cerebral cortex. *J. Neurophysiol.,* **14,** 1–21

Chao, T. I., Henke, A., Reichelt, W., Eberhardt, W., Reinhardt-Maelicke, S., and Reichenbach, A. (1994a). Three distinct types of voltage-dependent K^+ channels are expressed by Müller (glial) cells of the rabbit retina. *Pflüger's Arch.,* **426,** 51–60.

Chao, T. I., Skatchkov, S. N., Eberhardt, W., and Reichenbach, A. (1994b). Na^+ channels of Müller (glial) cells isolated from retinae of various mammalian species including man. *Glia,* **10,** 173–185.

Chapman, D. B., Theodosis, D. T., Montagnese, C., Poulain, D. A., and Morris, J. F. (1986). Osmotic stimulation causes structural plasticity of neurone-glia relationships of the oxytocin but not vasopressin secreting neurones in the hypothalamic supraoptic nucleus. *Neuroscience,* **17,** 679–686.

Charles, A. C., Merrill, J. E., Dirksen, E. R., and Sanderson, M. J. (1991). Intercellular signaling in glial cells: calcium waves and oscillations in response to mechanical stimulation and glutamate. *Neuron,* **6,** 983–992.

Chebabo, S. R., Hester, M. A., Jing, J., Aitken, P. G., and Somjen, G. G. (1995). Interstitial space, electrical resistance and ion concentrations during hypotonia of rat hippocampal slices. *J. Physiol. (Lond.),* **487,** 685–697.

Chen, J. C., and Chesler, M. (1990). A bicarbonate-dependent increase in extracellular pH mediated by $GABA_A$ receptors in turtle cerebellum. *Neurosci. Lett.,* **116,** 130–135.

Chen, J. C. T., and Chesler, M. (1991). Extracellular alkalinization evoked by GABA and its relationship to activity-dependent pH shifts in turtle cerebellum. *J. Physiol.*, **442**, 431–446.

Chen, J. C. T., and Chesler, M. (1992a). Modulation of extracellular pH by glutamate and GABA in rat hippocampal slices. *J. Neurophysiol.*, **67**, 29–36.

Chen, J. C. T., and Chesler, M. (1992b). Extracellular alkaline shifts in rat hippocampal slice are mediated by NMDA and non-NMDA receptors. *J. Neurophysiol.*, **68**, 342–344.

Chen, J. C. T., and Chesler, M. (1992c). pH transients evoked by excitatory synaptic transmission are increased by inhibition of extracellular carbonic anhydrase. *Proc. Natl Acad. Sci. USA*, **89**, 7786–7790.

Chen, Y. (1995). Effects of selected transmitters on free cytosolic calcium concentration and pyruvate dehydrogenation in primary cultures of mouse astrocytes. PhD thesis, University of Saskatchewan.

Chen, Y., Peng, L., Zhang, X., Stolzenburg, J.-U., and Hertz L. (1995). Further evidence that fluoxetine interacts with a $5-HT_{1C}$ receptor. *Brain Res. Bull.*, **38**, 153–159.

Cheng, H.-J., Nakamoto, M., Bergemann, A. D., and Flanagan, J. G. (1995). Complementary gradients in expression and binding of ELF-1 and Mek4 in development of the topographic retinotectal projection map. *Cell*, **82**, 371–381.

Cherkin, A. (1971). Biphasic time course of performance after one-trial avoidance training in the chick. *Commun. Behav. Biol.*, **5**, 379–381.

Chesler, M. (1990). The regulation and modulation of pH in the nervous system. *Prog. Neurobiol.*, **34**, 401–427.

Chesler, M., and Kaila, K. (1992). Modulation of pH by neuronal activity. *TINS*, **15**, 396–403.

Chesler, M., and Kraig, R. P. (1987). Intracellular pH of astrocytes increases rapidly with cortical stimulation. *Am. J. Physiol.*, **253**, R666–R670.

Chesler, M., and Kraig, R. P. (1989). Intracellular pH transients of mammalian astrocytes. *Neuroscience.*, **9**, 2011–2019.

Chiu, S. Y. (1991). Functions and distribution of voltage-gated sodium and potassium channels in mammalian Schwann cells. *Glia*, **4**, 541–558.

Chiu, S. Y. (1995). Schwann cell functions in saltatory conduction. In *Neuroglia*, eds H. Kettenmann and B. R. Ransom, pp. 777–792. New York and Oxford: Oxford University Press.

Chow, S. Y., Yen-Chow, Y. C., White, H. S., and Woodbury, D. M. (1991). pH regulation after acid load in primary cultures of mouse astrocytes. *Dev. Brain Res.*, **60**, 69–78.

Chowen, J. A., Busiguina, S. and Garcia-Segura, L. M. (1995). Sexual dimorphism and sex steroid modulation of glial fibrillary acidic protein messenger RNA and immunoreactivity levels in the rat hypothalamus. *Neuroscience*, **69**, 519–532.

Christensen, O. (1987). Mediation of cell volume regulation by Ca^{2+} influx though stretch-activated channels. *Nature*, **330**, 66–68.

Church, J. (1992). A change from $HCO_3^- - CO_2^-$ to Hepes-buffered medium modifies membrane properties of rat CA1 pyramidal neurons in vitro. *J. Physiol.*, **455**, 51–71.

Church, J., and McLennan, H. (1989). Electrophysiological properties of rat CA1 pyramidal neurons *in vitro* modified by changes in extracellular bicarbonate. *J. Physiol.*, **415**, 85–108.

Chvátal, A., Jendelová, P., Kříž, N., and Syková, E. (1988). Stimulation-evoked changes in extracellular pH, calcium and potassium activity in the frog spinal cord. *Physiol. Bohemoslov.*, **37**, 203–212.

Chwilla, D. J. and Brunia, C. H. M. (1989). Slow negative potentials in anticipation of sensory input. *J. Psychophysiol.*, **3**, 200–201.

Clark, B. A. and Mobbs, P. (1992). Transmitter-operated channels in rabbit retinal astrocytes studied in situ by whole-cell patch clamping. *J. Neurosci.*, **12**, 664–673.

Clark, B. A. and Mobbs, P. (1994). Voltage-gated currents in rabbit retinal astrocytes. *Eur. J. Neurosci.*, **6**, 1406–1414.

Clarke, P. B. S., Schwartz, R. D., Paul, S. M., Pert, C. B., and Pert, A. (1985). Nicotinic binding in rat brain: autoradiographic comparison of [^{3}H]acetylcholine, [^{3}H]nicotine and [^{125}I]alpha-bungarotoxin. *J. Neurosci.*, **5**, 1307–1315.

Clasen, T., Jeserich, G., and Krüppel, T. (1995). Glutamate-activated ionic currents in cultured astrocytes from trout: evidence for the occurrence of non-N-methyl-D-aspartate receptors. *J. Neurosci. Res.*, **40**, 632–640.

Cobbett, P. and Hatton, G. I. (1984). Dye coupling in hypothalamic slices: dependence on *in vivo* hydration state and osmolality of incubation medium. *J. Neurosci.*, **4**, 3034–3038.

Cobbett, P., Smithson, K. G. and Hatton, G. I. (1985). Dye-coupled magnocellular peptidergic neurons of the rat paraventricular nucleus show homotypic immunoreactivity. *Neuroscience*, **16**, 885–895.

Coles, J. A. (1989). Functions of glial cells in the retina of the honeybee drone. *Glia*, **2**, 1–9.

Coles, J.A. and Abbott, N. J. (1996). Signalling from neurones to glial cells in invertebrates. *TINS*, **19**, 358–362.

Coles, J. A., and Orkand, R. K. (1983). Modification of potassium movement through the retina of the drone (*Apis mellifera*) by glial uptake. *J. Physiol.*, **340**, 157–174.

Coles, J. A., and Poulain, D. A. (1991). Extracellular K$^+$ in the supraoptic nucleus of the rat during reflex bursting activity by oxytocin neurones. *J. Physiol.*, **439**, 383–409.

Coles, J. A., and Tsacopoulos, M. (1979). Potassium activity in photoreceptors, glial cells and extracellular space in the drone retina: changes during photostimulation. *J. Physiol. (Lond.)*, **290**, 525–549.

Coles, J. A., and Tsacopoulos, M. (1981). Ionic and possible metabolic interactions between sensory neurones and glial cells in the retina of the honeybee drone. *J. Exp. Biol.*, **95**, 75–92.

Coles, J. A., Marcaggi, P., Véga, C., and Cotillon, N. (1996a). Effects of photoreceptor metabolism on interstitial and glial cell pH in bee retina: evidence of a role for NH^{4+}. *J. Physiol. (Lond.)*, **495**, 305–318.

Coles, J. A., Thwaites, D. T., Marcaggi, P., and Deitmer, J. W. (1996b). Ammonium causes acidification of glial cells isolated from drone retina. *J. Physiol.*, **491P**, 147P.

Colombo, J. A., Yanez, A., Puissant, V., and Lipina, S. (1995). Long, interlaminar astroglial cell processes in the cortex of adult monkeys. *J. Neurosci. Res.*, **40**, 551–556.

Conn, P. J., and Desai, M. A. (1991). Pharmacology and physiology of metabolic glutamate receptors in mammalian central nervous system. *Drug Dev. Res.*, **24**, 207–229.

Connors, B. W., Benardo, L. S., and Prince, D. A. (1984). Carbon dioxide sensitivity of dye coupling among glia and neurons of the neocortex. *J. Neurosci.*, **4**, 1324–1330.

Constanti, A., and Galvan, M. (1978). Amino acid evoked depolarization of electrically inexcitable (neuroglial?) cells in the guinea pig olfactory cortex slice. *Brain Res.*, **153**, 183–187.

Conti, F., Minelli, A., and Brecha, N. C. (1994). Cellular localization and laminar distribution of AMPA glutamate receptor subunits mRNAs and proteins in the rat cerebral cortex. *J. Comp. Neurol.*, **350**, 241–259.

Conti, F., DeBiasi, S., Minelli, A., and Melone, M. (1996). Expression of NR1 and NR2A/B subunits of the NMDA receptor in cortical astrocytes. *Glia*, **17**, 254–258.

Cooper, A. J. L., and Plum, F. (1987). Biochemistry and physiology of brain ammonia. *Physiol. Rev.*, **67**, 440–519.

Cooper, N. G. F., and Steindler, D. A. (1986). Monoclonal antibody to glial fibrillary acidic protein reveals a parcellation of individual barrels in the early postnatal mouse somatosensory cortex. *Brain Res.*, **380**, 341–348.

Cooper, R., McCallum, W. C., and Papakostopoulos, D. (1978). Bimodal slow potential theory of cerebral processing. In *Multidisciplinary Perspectives in Event-Related Brain Potential Research*, ed. D. A. Otto, pp. 651–656. Washington, DC: U.S. Environmental Protection Agency.

Coopersmith, R., and Leon, M. (1995). Olfactory bulb glycogen metabolism: noradrenergic modulation in the young rat. *Brain Res.*, **674**, 230–237.

Cornell-Bell, A. H., and Finkbeiner, S. M. (1991). Ca^{2+} waves in astrocytes. *Cell Calcium*, **12**, 185–204.

Cornell-Bell, A. H., Thomas, P. G., and Smith, S. J. (1990). The excitatory neurotransmitter glutamate causes filopodia formation in cultured hippocampal astrocytes. *Glia*, **8**, 322–334.

Cornell-Bell, A. H., Finkbeiner, S. M., Cooper, M. S., and Smith, S. J. (1990). Glutamate induces calcium in cultured astrocytes: long-range glial signaling. *Science*, **247**, 470–473.

Cornell-Bell, A. H., Thomas, P. G., and Caffrey, J. M. (1992). Ca^{2+} and filopodial responses to glutamate in cultured astrocytes and neurons. *Can. J. Physiol. Pharmacol.*, **70**, S206–S218.

Corning, W. C., and Kelly, S. (1973). Platyhelminthes: the turbellarians. In *Invertebrate Learning*, ed. W. C. Corning, J. A. Dyal, and A. O. D. Williams, pp. 171–224. New York: Plenum Press.

Corvalen, V., Cole, R., DeVellis, J., and Hagiwara, S. (1990). Neuronal modulation of calcium channel activity in cultured rat astrocytes. *Proc. Natl Acad. Sci., USA*, **87**, 4345–4348.

Cowley, G., Springen, K., Leonard, E., Robins, K., and Gordon, J. (1990). The promise of Prozac. *Newsweek* March, **26**, 38–41.

Craik, F. I. M., and Lockhart, R. S. (1972). Levels of processing: a framework for memory research. *J. Verb. Learn. Verb. Behav.*, **11**, 671–684.

Cremer, H., Lange, R., Christoph, A., Plomann, M., Vopper, G., Roes, J., Brown, R., Baldwin, S., Kraemer, P., Scheff, S., Barthels, D., Rajewsky, K., and Willie, W. (1994). Inactivation of the N-CAM gene in mice results size reduction of the olfactory bulb and deficits in spatial learning. *Nature*, **367**, 455–459.

Creutzfeldt, O. D., and Houchin, J. (1974). Neural basis of EEG waves. In *Handbook of Electroencephalography and Clinical Neurophysiology*, eds A. Rémond and O. Creutzfeldt, Vol. 2C, pp. 5–55. Amsterdam: Elsevier.

Creutzfeldt, O. D., Watanabe, S., and Lux, H. D. (1966). Relations between EEG phenomena and potentials of single cortical cells. I. Evoked responses after thalamic and epicortical stimulation. *Electroenceph. Clin. Neurophysiol.*, **20**, 1–18.

Crick, F. (1994). *The Astonishing Hypothesis: The Scientific Search for the Soul*, pp. 177–199. New York: Charles Scribner's Sons.

Crowe, S. F., Ng, K. T., and Gibbs, M. E. (1989). Memory formation processes in weakly reinforced learning. *Pharmacol. Biochem. Behav.*, **33**, 881–887.

Crowe, S. F., Ng, K. T., and Gibbs, M. E. (1991a). Possible noradrenergic involvement in training stimulus intensity. *Pharmacol. Biochem. Behav.*, **39**, 717–722.

Crowe, S. F., Ng, K. T., and Gibbs, M. E. (1991b). Forebrain noradrenaline concentration following weakly reinforced training. *Pharmacol. Biochem. Behav.*, **40**, 173–176.

Cserr, H. F., De Pasquale, M., Nicholson, C., Patlak, C., Pettigrew, K. D., and Rice, M. E. (1991). Extracellular volume decreases while cell volume is maintained by ion uptake in rat brain during acute hypernatremia. *J. Physiol. (Lond)*, **442**, 277–295.

Cubbels, J. F., Walkley, S. U., and Makman, M. H. (1988). The effects of gabaculine in vivo on the distribution of GABA-like immunoreactivity in the rat retina. *Brain Res.*, **458**, 82–90.

Cuffin, N. B. and Cohen, D. (1979). Comparison of MEG and EEG. *Electroenceph. Clin. Neurophysiol.*, **47**, 640–644.

Cull-Candy, S. G., Wyllie, D. J. A., and Traynelis, S. F. (1991). Excitatory amino acid-gated channel types in mammalian neurons and glia. In *Excitatory Amino Acids and Synaptic Function*. New York: Academic Press.

Cummins, C. J., Glover, R. A., and Sellinger, O. Z. (1979). Astroglial uptake is modulated by extracellular K$^+$. *J. Neurochem.*, **33**, 779–785.

D'Amelio, F., Eng, L. A., and Gibbs, M.A. (1990). Glutamine synthetase immunoreactivity is present in oligodendroglia of various regions of the central nervous system. *Glia*, **3**, 335–341.

Damen, E. J. P., and Brunia, C. H. M. (1987). Changes in heart rate and slow brain potentials related to motor preparation and stimulus anticipation in a time estimation task. *Psychophysiology*, **24**, 700–713.

Dani, J. W., and Smith, S. J. (1995). The triggering of astrocytic calcium waves by NMDA-induced neuronal activation. *Ciba Found. Symp.*, **188**, 195–209.

Dash, P. K., Hochner, B., and Kandel, E. R. (1990). Injection of the cAMP-responsive element into the nucleus of *Aplysia* in sensory neurons blocks long-term facilitation. *Nature*, **345**, 718–721.

Daum, I., Rockstroh, B., Birbaumer, N., Elbert, T., Canavan, A., and Lutzenberger, W. (1993). Behavioral treatment of slow cortical potentials in intractable epilepsy: neuropsychological predictors of outcome. *J. Neurosurgery Psychiatry*, **56**, 94–97.

Dave, V., and Kimelberg, H. (1994). Na$^+$-dependant, fluoxetine-sensitive serotonin uptake by astrocytes tissue-printed from rat cerebral cortex. *J. Neurosci.*, **14**, 4972–4986.

David, E., Finkenzeller, P., Kallert, S., and Keidel, W. D. (1969). Akustischen Reizen zugeordnete Gleichspannungsänderungen am intakten Schädel des Menschen. *Pflügers Archiv der gesamten Physiologie*, **309**, 362–367.

David, G., Barrett, J. N. and Barrett, E. F. (1992). Evidence that action potentials activate an internodal potassium conductance in lizard myelinated axons. *J. Physiol.*, **445**, 277–301.

Davis, C. W., and Finn, A. L. (1985). Cell volume regulation in frog urinary bladder. *Fed. Proc.*, **44**, 2520–2525.

Davis, L. E., Burnett, A. L., and Haynes, J. F. (1968). Histological and ultrastructural study of the muscular and nervous system in *Hydra* II nervous system. *J. Exp. Zool.*, **167**, 295–332.

Davson, H. (1989). History of the blood–brain barrier concept. In *Implications of the Blood–Brain Barrier and its Manipulation. Vol. 1*, ed. E. A. Neuwelt, pp. 27–52. New York: Plenum.

De Graan, P. N. E., Oestreicher, A. B., Schotman, P., and Schrama, L. H. (1991). Protein kinase C substrate B-50 (GAP-43) and neurotransmitter release. *Prog. Brain Res.*, **89**, 187–207.

Deecher, D. C., Wilcox, B. D., Dave, V., Rossman, P. A., and Kimelberg, H. K. (1993). Detection of 5-hydroxytryptamine$_2$ receptors by radioligand binding, Northern blot analysis, and Ca^{2+} responses in rat primary astrocyte cultures. *J. Neurosci. Res.*, **35**, 246–256.

Deecke, L., Heise, B., Kornhuber, H. H., Lang, M., and Lang, W. (1984). Brain potentials associated with voluntary manual tracking: Bereitschaftspotential, conditioned premotion positivity, directed attention potential, and relaxation potential. In *Brain and Information: Event-Related Potentials,* eds R. Karrer, J. Cohen and P. Tueting, pp. 450–464. Annals of the New York Academy of Sciences, Vol. 425. New York.

Deecke, L., Kornhuber, H.H., Schreiber, H., Lang, M., Lang, W., Kornhuber, A., Heise, B., and Keidel, M. (1986). Bereitschaftspotential associated with writing and drawing. In *Cerebral Psychophysiology: Studies in Event-Related Potentials*, eds W.C. McCallum, R. Zappoli and F. Denoth, pp. 245–247. *Electroenceph. Clin. Neurophysiol.*, Suppl. 38. Amsterdam: Elsevier.

Deecke, L., Uhl, F., Spieth, F., Lang, W., and Lang, M. (1987). Cerebral potentials preceding and accompanying verbal and spatial tasks. In *Current Trends in Event-Related Potential Research,* eds R. J. Johnson, J. W. Rohrbaugh, and R. Parasuraman, pp. 17–23. EEG Suppl: Vol. 40. Amsterdam: Elsevier.

Deitmer, J. W. (1991). Electrogenic sodium-dependent bicarbonate secretion by glial cells of the leech central nervous system. *J. Gen. Physiol.*, **98**, 637–655.

Deitmer, J. W. (1992a). Evidence for glial control of extracellular pH in the leech central nervous system. *Glia*, **5**, 43–47.

Deitmer, J. W. (1992b). Bicarbonate-dependent changes of intracellular sodium and pH in identified leech glial cells. *Pflügers Arch.*, **420**, 584–589.

Deitmer, J. W. (1995). pH regulation. In *Neuroglia*, eds H. Kettenmann and B. R. Ransom, pp. 230–245. New York Oxford: Oxford University Press.

Deitmer, J. W., and Munsch, T. (1992). Kainate/glutamate-induced changes in intracellular calcium and pH in leech glial cells. *NeuroReport*, **3**, 693–696.

Deitmer, J. W., and Munsch, T. (1994). Neuron–glia dialogue in the leech central nervous system: glial cell responses to glutamate and kainate. *Verh. Dtsch. Zool. Ges., 87*, 185–194.

Deitmer, J. W., and Rose, C. R. (1996). pH regulation and proton signalling by glial cells. *Prog. Neurobiol.*, **48**, 73–103.

Deitmer, J. W., and Schlue, W. R. (1987). The regulation of intracellular pH by identified glial cells and neurons in the central nervous system of the leech. *J. Physiol.*, **388**, 261–283.

Deitmer, J. W., and Schlue, W. R. (1989). An inwardly directed electrogenic sodium-bicarbonate co-transport in leech glial cells. *J. Physiol.*, **411**, 179–194.

Deitmer, J. W., and Schneider, H. P. (1995). Voltage-dependent clamp of intracellular pH of identified leech glial cells. *J. Physiol.*, **485**, 157–166.

Deitmer, J.W., and Schneider, H.P. (1997). Intracellular acidification of the leech giant glial cell evoked by glutamate and aspartate. *Glia*, **19**, 111–122.

Deitmer, J.W., and Szatkowski, M. (1990). Membrane potential dependence of intracellular pH regulation by identified glial cells in the leech central nervous system. *J. Physiol.*, **421**, 617–631.

Deitmer, J. W., Schneider, H. P., and Munsch, T. (1993). Independent changes of intracellular calcium and pH in identified leech glial cells. *Glia*, **7**, 299–306.

Deitmer, J. W., Schneider, H. P., Reusch, M., and Munsch, T. (1995). Are kainate/AMPA receptor channels H^+ permeable? *Proc. 23rd Göttingen Neurobiology Conference 1995*, p. 699.

Dekker, L. V., De Graan, P. N. E., Versteeg, D. H. G., Oestreicher, A. B., and Gispen, W. H. (1990). Evidence for a relationship between B-50 (GAP-43) and [^{3}H]-noradrenaline release in rat brain synaptosomes. *Eur. J. Pharmacol.*, **188**, 113–122.

Del Cerro, S., Garcia-Estrada, J., and Garcia-Segura, L. M. (1995). Neuro-active steroids regulate astroglia morphology in hippocampal cultures from adult rats. *Glia*, **14**, 65–71.

Delisle, M., Stuss, D. T., and Picton, T. W. (1986). Event-related potentials to feedback in a concept-formation task. In *Cerebral Psychophysiology: Studies in Event-Related Potentials*, eds W. C. McCallum, R. Zappoli, and F. Denoth, pp. 103–105. Electroencephal. Clin. Neurophysiol. Suppl. 38. Amsterdam: Elsevier.

Denis-Donini, S., Glowinski, J., and Prochiantz, A. (1984). Glial heterogeneity may define the three-dimensional shape of mouse mesencephalic dopaminergic neurons. *Nature*, **307**, 641–643.

Dermietzel, R., and Spray, D. C. (1993). Gap junctions in the brain: where, what type, how many and why? *TINS*, **16**, 186–192.

Dermietzel, R., Hertzberg, E. L., Kessler, J. A., and Spray, D. C. (1991). Gap junctions between cultured astrocytes. *J. Neurosci.*, **11**, 1421–1432.

Derouiche, A., and Rauen, T. (1995). Coincidence of L-glutamate/L-aspartate transporter (GLAST) and glutamine synthetase (GS) immunoreactions in retinal glia: evidence for coupling of GLAST and GS in transmitter clearance. *J. Neurosci. Res.*, **42**, 131–143.

Descarries, L., Seguela, P., and Watkins, K.C. (1991). Nonjunctional relationships of monoamine axon terminals in the cerebral cortex of adult rat. In *Volume Transmission in the Brain: Novel Mechanisms for Neural Transmission*, eds K. Fuxe and L. F. Agnati, pp. 53–62. New York: Raven Press.

Despeyroux, S., Amedee, T., and Coles, J. A. (1994). Axon contact is associated with modified expression of functional potassium channels in mouse Schwann cells. *Proc. R. Soc. Lond.* B, **258**, 255–260.

Diamond, M. C., Law, F., Rhodes, H., Lindner, B., Rosenzweig, N. R., Krech, D., and Bennett, E. L. (1966). Increases in cortical depth and glia numbers in rats subjected to enriched environment. *J. Comp. Neurol.*, **128**, 117–125.

Dienel, G. A., and Cruz, N. F. (1993). Synthesis of deoxyglucose-1–phosphate, deoxyglucose-1,6–biphosphate and other metabolites of 2–deoxy-D-[^{14}C]glucose in rat brain in vivo: influence of time and tissue glucose level. *J. Neurochem.*, **60**, 2217–2231.

Dierig, S. (1994). Extending the neuron doctrine: Carl Ludwig Schleich (1859–1922) and his reflections on neuroglia at the inception of the neural-network concept in 1894. *TINS*, **17**, 449–452.

Dietzel, I., and Heinemann, U. (1983). Extracellular electrolyte changes during enhanced neuronal activity can be explained by spatial glial K$^+$ buffering in addition to small increases in osmotic pressure-possibly induced by increases in metabolic activity. In *Cerebral Blood Flow, Metabolism and Epilepsy*, eds M. Baldy-Moulinier, D.-H. Ingvar, and B. S. Meldrum, pp. 195–201. London: John Libbey.

Dietzel, I., and Heinemann, U. (1986). Dynamic variations of the brain cell microenvironment in relation to neuronal hyperactivity. *Ann. NY Acad. Sci.*, **481**, 72–86.

Dietzel, I., Heinemann, U., Hofmeier, G., and Lux, H.D. (1980). Transient changes in the size of the extracellular space in the sensorymotor cortex of cats in relation to stimulus-induced changes in potassium concentration. *Exp. Brain Res.*, **40**, 432–439.

Dietzel, I., Heinemann, U., and Lux, H. D. (1989). Relations between slow extracellular potential changes, glial potassium buffering, and electrolyte and cellular volume changes during neuronal hyperactivity in cat brain. *Glia*, **2**, 25–44.

Dietzel, I., Heinemann, U., Hofmeier, G., and Lux, H. D. (1989). Relations between slow extracellular potential changes, glial potassium buffering, and electrolyte and cellular volume changes during neural hyperactivity in cat brain. *Glia*, **2**, 25–44.

Dighiero, P., Hauw, J. J., Fillet, A. M., Courtois, Y., and Goureau, O. (1994). Expression of inducible nitric oxide synthase in cytomegalovirus-infected glial cells of retinas from AIDS patients. *Neurosci. Lett.*, **166**, 31–34.

Dixon, R. A., Kobilka, B. K., Strader, D. J., Benovic, J. L., Dohlman, H. G., Frielle, T., Bolanowski, M. A., Bennett, C. D., Rands, E., Diehl, R. E., Mumford, R. A., Slater, E. E., Sigal, I. S., Caron, M. G., Lefkowitz, R. J., and Strader, C. D. (1986). Cloning of the gene and cDNA for mammalian β-adrenergic receptor and homology with rhodopsin. *Nature*, **321**, 75–79.

Djamgoz, M. B. A., and Wagner, H.-J. (1992). Localization and function of dopamine in the adult vertebrate retina. *Neurochem. Int.*, **20**, 139–191.

Doherty P., Cohen J., and Walsh F. S. (1990). Neurite outgrowth in response to transfected N-CAM changes during development and is modulated by polysialic acid. *Neuron*, **5**, 209–219.

Doherty, P., Fruns, M., Seaton, P., Dickson, G., Barton, C. H., Sears, T. A., and Walsh, F. S. (1990). A threshold effect of the major isoforms of NCAM on neurite outgrowth. *Nature*, **343**, 464–466.

Donchin, E., Otto, D., Gerbrandt, L. K., and Pribram, K. H. (1971). While a monkey waits: Electrocortical events recorded during the foreperiod of a reaction time study. *Electroenceph. Clin. Neurophysiol.*, **31**,115–127.

Doucette, R. (1990). Glial influence on axonal growth in the primary olfactory system. *Glia*, **3**, 433–449.

Doyle, E., Nolan, P., Bell, R., and Regan, C. M. (1992a). Hippocampal NCAM180 transiently increases sialylation during the acquisition and consolidation of a passive response in the adult rat. *J. Neurosci. Res.*, **31**, 513–523.

Doyle, E., Nolan, P., Bell, R., and Regan, C. M. (1992b). Intraventricular infusions of anti-neural cell adhesion molecules in a discrete post training period impair consolidation of a passive avoidance response in the rat. *J. Neurochem.*, **59**, 1570–1573.

Doyle, E., Nolan, P. M., Bell, R., and Regan, C. M. (1992c). Neurodevelopmental events underlying information acquisition and storage. *Network*, **3**, 89–94.

Drain, P., Folkers, E., and Quinn, W. C. (1991). cAMP-dependent protein kinase and the disruption of learning in transgenic flies. *Neuron*, **6**, 71–82.

Drapeau, P., and Nachshen, D. A. (1988). Effects of lowering extracellular and cytosolic pH on calcium fluxes, cytosolic calcium levels, and transmitter release in presynaptic nerve terminals isolated from rat brain. *J. Gen. Physiol.*, **91**, 305–315.

Drescher, U., Kremoser, C., Handwerker, C., Löschinger, J., Noda, M., and Bonhoeffer, F. (1995). In vitro guidance of retinal ganglion cell axons by RAGS, a 25 kDa tectal protein related to ligands for Eph receptor tyrosine kinases. *Cell*, **82**, 359–370.

Dreyer, E. B., Leifer, D., Heng, J. E., McConnell, J. E., Gorla, M., Levin, L. A., Barnstable, C. J., and Lipton S. A. (1995). An astrocytic binding site for neuronal Thy-1 and its effect on neurite outgrowth. *Proc. Natl Acad. Sci. USA*, **92**, 11195–11199.

Dringen, R., Gebhardt, R., and Hamprecht, B. (1993a). Glycogen in astrocytes: possible function as lactate supply for neighboring cells. *Brain Res.*, **623**, 208–214.

Dringen, R., Schmoll, D., Cesar, M., and Hamprecht, B. (1993b). Incorporation of radioactivity derived from [^{14}C]lactate into glycogen of cultured mouse astroglial cells: evidence for gluconeogenesis in brain cells. *Physiol. Chem. Hoppe-Seyler*, **374**, 343–347.

Dringen, R., Peters, H., Wiesinger, H., and Hamprecht, B. (1995). Lactate transport in cultured glial cells. *Dev. Neurosci.*, **17**, 63–69.

Duffy, S., and MacVicar, B. A. (1993). Voltage-dependent ionic channels in astrocytes. In *Astrocytes, Pharmacology and Function,* ed. S. Murphy, p. 137. San Diego: Academic Press.

Duffy, S., and MacVicar, B. A. (1995). Adrenergic calcium signaling in astrocyte networks within the hippocampal slice. *J. Neurosci.*, **15**, 5535–5550.

Duffy, S., Fraser, D. D., and MacVicar, B. A. (1995). Potassium channels. In *Neuroglia,* ed. H. Kettenmann and B. R. Ransom, pp. 185–201. New York and Oxford: Oxford University Press.

Dumuis, A., Pin, J. P., and Oomargari, K. (1989). ATP-evoked calcium mobilisation and prostanoid release from astrocytes. *J. Neurochem.*, **52**, 971–977.

Dumuis, A., Pin, J. P., Oomargari, K., Sebben, M., and Bockaert, J. (1990). Arachidonic acid released from striatal neurons by joint stimulation of ionotropic and metabotropic quisqualate receptors. *Nature*, **347**, 182–184.

Duncan, A., Ibrahim, M., Berry, M., and Butt, A. M. (1996). Transfer of horseradish peroxidase from oligodendrocyte to axon in the myelinating neonatal rat optic nerve: artefact or transcellular exhange? *Glia*, **17**, 349–355.

Duncan, I. D., Hammang, J. P., and Gilmore, S. A. (1988). Schwann cell myelination of the myelin deficient rat spinal cord following X-irradiation. *Glia*, **1**, 233–239.

Duncan, I. D., Hammang, J. P., Jackson, K. F., Wood, P. M., Bunge, R. P., and Langford, L. (1988). Transplantation of oligodendrocytes and Schwann cells into the spinal cord of the myelin-deficient rat. *J. Neurocytol.*, **17**, 351–360.

Durkovic, R. O., and Cohen, D. H. (1966). DC potential activity in a nervous system lacking neocortex: the pigeon telencephalon. *Anat. Record.*, **154**, 341.

Durkovic, R. O., and Cohen, D. H. (1968). Spontaneous evoked and defensively conditioned steady potential changes in the pigeon telencephalan. *Electroenceph. Clin. Neurophysiol.*, **24**, 474–481.

Dworkin, B. R., Elbert, T., Rau, H., Birbaumer, N., Pauli, P., Droste, C., and Brunia, C. H. M. (1984). Central effects of baroreceptor activation in humans: attenuation of skeletal reflexes and pain perception. *Proc. Natl Acad. Sci. USA*, **91**, 6329–6333.

Eberhardt, W., and Reichenbach, A. (1987). Spatial buffering of potassium by retinal Müller (glial) cells of various morphologies calculated by a model. *Neuroscience*, **22**, 687–696.

Eccles, J. C. (1953). *The Neurophysiological Basis of Mind*. Oxford: Clarendon.

Eccles, J. C. (1964). *The Physiology of Synapses*. Berlin: Springer-Verlag.

Edwards, C., and Rogers, K. J. (1972). Some factors influencing brain glycogen in the neonate chick. *J. Neurochem.*, **19**, 2759–2766.

Ehinger, B. (1977). Glial and neuronal uptake of GABA, glutamic acid, glutamine, and glutathione in the rabbit retina. *Exp. Eye Res.*, **25**, 221–234.

Elbert, T. (1978). *Biofeedback langsamer kortikaler Potentiale*. Dissertation. Muenchen: Minerva Publikation.

Elbert, T., and Rockstroh, B. (1987). Threshold regulation – a key to the understanding of the combined dynamics of EEG and event-related potentials. *J. Psychophysiol.*, **4**, 317–333.

Elbert, T., Rockstroh, B., Lutzenberger, W., and Birbaumer, N. (1980). Biofeedback of slow cortical potentials. Part I. *Electroencephal. Clin. Neurophysiol.*, **48**, 293–301.

Elbert, T., Lutzenberger, W., Rockstroh, B., and Birbaumer, N. (1983). When regulation of slow brain potentials fails – a contribution to the psychophysiology of perceptual aberration and anhedonia. *Adv. Biol. Psychiat.*, **13**, 98–106.

Elliot, A. S., and Nunez, A. A. (1994). An ultrastructural study of somal appositions in the suprachiasmatic nucleus and anterior hypothalamus of the rat. *Brain Res.*, **662**, 278–282.

Elvin, M., and Koopowitz, H. (1994). Neuroanatomy of the rhabdocoel flatworm *Mesotoma ehrenbergii* (Focke, 1836). I. Neuronal diversity in the brain. *J. Comp. Neurol.*, **343**, 319–331.

Endres, W., Ballanyi, K., Serve, G., and Grafe, P. (1986). Excitatory amino acids and intracellular pH in motoneurons of the isolated spinal cord. *Neurosci. Lett.*, **72**, 54–58.

Eng, L. F., Vanderhaeghen, J. J., Bignami, A., and Gerstl, B. (1971). An acidic protein isolated from fibrous astrocytes. *Brain Res.*, **28**, 351–354.

Engel, A. K., and Müller, C. M. (1989). Postnatal development of vimentin-immunoreactive radial glial cells in the primary visual cortex of the cat. *J. Neurocytol.*, **18**, 437–450.

Enkvist, M. O. K., and McCarthy, K. D. (1994). Astroglial gap junction communication is increased by treatment with either glutamate or high K^+ concentration. *J. Neurochem.*, **62**, 489–495.

Erickson, H. P., and Bourdon, M. A. (1989). Tenascin: an extracellular matrix protein prominent in specialized embryonic tissues and tumors. *Annu. Rev. Cell Biol.*, **5**, 71–92.

Erickson, P. A., Fisher, S. K., Anderson, D. H., Stern, W. H., and Borgulla, G. A. (1983). Retinal detachment in the cat: the outer nuclear and outer plexiform layers. *Invest. Ophthalmol. Vis. Sci.*, **24**, 927–942.

Eriksson, P. S., Nilsson, M., Wagberg, M., Rönnbäck, L., and Hansson, E. (1992). Volume regulation of single astroglial cells in primary culture. *Neurosci. Lett.*, **143**, 195–199.

Evans, P. D., Reale, V., and Villegas, J. (1986). Peptidergic modulation of the membrane potential of the Schwann cell of the squid giant nerve fibre. *J. Physiol.*, **379**, 61–82.

Evans, P. D., Reale, V., Merzon, R. M., and Villegas, J. (1992). N-methyl-D-aspartate (NMDA) and non-NMDA (metabotropic) type glutamate receptors modulate the membrane potential of the Schwann cell of the squid giant nerve fibre. *J. Exp. Biol.*, **173**, 229–249.

Evans, P. D., Reale, V., Merzon, R. M., and Villegas, J. (1995). The pharmacology of receptors present on squid giant axon Schwann cells. In *Cephalopod Neurobiology*, eds N. J. Abbott, R. Williamson and L. Maddock, pp. 213–228. Oxford: Oxford University Press.

Evequoz-Mercier, V., and Tsacopoulos, M. (1991). The light-induced increase of carbohydrate metabolism in glial cells of the honeybee retina is not mediated by K^+ movement nor by cAMP. *J. Gen. Physiol.*, **98**, 497–515.

Ewert, J. P. (1989). The release of visual behaviour in toads: stages of parallel/hierarchical information processing. In *Visuomotor Coordination; Amphibians, Comparisons, Models and Robots,* eds J. P. Ewert and M. A. Arbib, pp. 39–120. New York: Plenum.

Fabricius, M., Jensen, L. H., and Lauritzen, M. (1993). Microdialysis of interstitial amino acids during spreading depression and anoxic depolarization in rat neocortex. *Brain Res.*, **612**, 61–69.

Facchinetti, F., Ciani, E., Dall'Olio, R., Virgili, M., Contestabile, A., and Fonnum, F. (1996). Structural, neurochemical and behavioural consequences of neonatal blockade of NMDA receptor through chronic treatment with CGP 39551 or MK-801. *Dev. Brain Res.*, **74**, 219–224.

Faff-Michalak, L., Reichenbach, A., Dettmer, D., Kellner, M., and Albrecht, J. (1994). K^+-, hypoosmolarity-, and NH_4^+-induced taurine release from cultured rabbit Müller cells: role of Na^+ and Cl^- ions and relation to cell volume changes. *Glia*, **10**, 114–120.

Fahrbach, S. E., Morrell, J. I., and Pfaff, D. W. (1984). Oxytocin induction of short-latency maternal behavior in nulliparous, estrogen-primed female rats. *Horm. Behav.*, **18**, 267–286.

Fahrenbach, W. P. (1976). The brain of the horseshoe crab *Limulus polyphemus*. I. Neuroglia. *Tissue Cell*, **8**, 395–410.

Faissner, A. (1993). Tenascin glycoproteins in neural pattern formation – facets of a complex picture. *Persp. Dev. Neurobiol.*, **1**, 155–164.

Faissner, A., and Schachner, M. (1995). Tenascin and janusin: glial recognition molecules involved in neural development and regeneration. In *Neuroglia*, eds H. Kettenmann and B. R. Ransom, pp. 411–426. New York and Oxford: Oxford University Press.

Farah, M. J., and Peronnet, F. (1989). Event-related potentials in the study of mental imagery. *J. Psychophysiol.*, **3**, 99–109.

Farb, C., Aoki, C., and LeDoux, J. (1995). Differential distribution of AMPA and NMDA receptors in the amygdala: a light and electron microscopic immunocytochemical study. *J. Comp. Neurol.*, **362**, 86–108.

Federoff, S., and Vernadakis, A. (1986). *Astrocytes – Development, Morphology, and Regional Specialization of Astrocytes – Volumes 1–3*. Orlando: Academic Press.

Felts, P. A., and Smith, K. J. (1992). Conduction properties of central nerve fibers remyelinated by Schwann cells. *Brain Res.*, **574**, 178–192.

Ferraro, T. N., and Hare, T. A. (1985). Free and conjugated amino acids in human CSF: influence of age and sex. *Brain Res.*, **338**, 53–60.

Field, K. G., Olsen, G. J., Lane, D. J., Giovannoni, S. J., Ghiselin, M. T., Raff, E. C., Pace, N. R., and Raff, R. A. (1988). Molecular phylogeny of the animal kingdom. *Science*, **239**, 748–753.

Field, K. G., Olsen, G. J., Giovannoni, S. J., Raff, E. C., Pace, N. R., and Raff, R. A. (1989). Phylogeny and molecular data: response. *Science*, **243**, 550–551.

Finkbeiner, S. M. (1992). Calcium waves in astrocytes-filling in the gaps. *Neuron*, **8**, 1101–1108.

Fishman, H. M., Tewari, K. P., and Stein, P. G. (1990). Injury-induced vesiculation and membrane redistribution in the squid gant axon. *Biochimica Biophysica Acta*, **1023**, 412–435.

Fishman, R. B., and Hatten, M. E. (1993). Multiple receptor systems promote CNS neural migration. *J. Neurosci.*, **13**, 3485–3495.

Fleming, L. M., and Johnson, G. V. W. (1995). Modulation of the phosphorylation state of tau in situ: The role of calcium and cyclic AMP. *Biochem. J.*, **309**, 41–47.

Flood, N. B., and Overmier, J. B. (1981). Learning in Teleost fish: role of the telencephalon. In *Brain Mechanisms of Behaviour in Lower Vertebrates,* ed. P. R. Laming, pp. 259–280. Cambridge: Cambridge University Press.

Flott, B., and Seifert, W. (1991). Characterization of glutamate uptake systems in astrocyte primary cultures from rat brain. *Glia*, **4**, 293–304.

Font, E., Garcia-Verdugo, J. M., Desfilis, E., and Pérez-Cañellas, M. (1995). Neuron–glia interrelations during 3-acetylpyridine-induced degeneration and regeneration in the adult lizard brain. In *Neuron–Glia Interrelations During Phylogeny*: II Plasticity and Regeneration, eds A. Vernadakis and B. I. Roots, pp. 275–302. Totowa, N.J.: Humana Press Inc.

Fox, G. B., Kennedy, N., and Regan, C. M. (1995). Polysialylated neural cell adhesion molecule expression by neurons and astroglial processes in the rat dentate gyrus declines dramatically with increasing age. *Int. J. Dev. Neurosci.*, **13**, 663–672.

Fox, G. B., O'Connell, A. W., Murphy, K. J., and Regan, C. M. (1995). Memory consolidation induces a transient and type-dependent increase in the frequency of NCAM polysialylated cells in the adult rat hippocampus. *J. Neurochem.*, **65**, 2796–2799.

Fox, P. T., and Raichle, M. E. (1986). Focal physiological uncoupling of cerebral blood flow and oxidative metabolism during somatosensory stimulation in human subjects. *Proc. Natl Acad. Sci. USA*, **83**, 1140–1144.

Frandsen, A., Quistorff, B., and Schousboe, A. (1990). Phenobarbital protects cerebral cortex neurones against toxicity induced by kainate but not by other excitatory amino acids. *Neurosci. Lett.*, **111**, 233–238.

Franks, J. J., Horn, J. L., Janicki, P. K., and Singh, G. (1995). Halothane, isoflurane, xenon and nitrous oxide inhibit calcium-ATPase pump activity in rat brain synaptic plasma membranes. *Anesthesiol.*, **82**, 108–117.

Fraser, D. D., Duffy, S., Angelides, K. J., Perez-Velazquez, J. L., Kettenmann, H., and MacVicar, B. A. (1995). GABA/Benzodiazepine receptors in acutely isolated hippocampal astrocytes. *J. Neurosci.*, **15**, 2720–2732.

Freude, G., and Ullsperger, P. (1987). Changes in Bereitschaftspotential during fatiguing and non-fatiguing hand movements. *Eur. J. Applied Physiol.*, **56**, 105–108.

Frisch, K. von. (1954). *Life and Senses of the Honeybee*. London: Methuen.

Frishman, L. J., Yamamoto, F., Bogucka, J., and Steinberg, R. H. (1992). Light-evoked changes in $[K^+]_o$ in proximal portion of light-adapted cat retina. *J. Neurophysiol.*, **67**, 1201–1212.

Fukuda, Y., and Loeschke, H. H. (1977). Effect of H^+ on spontaneous neuronal activity in the surface layer of the rat medulla oblongata *in vitro*. *Pflügers Arch.*, **371**, 125–134.

Fukunaga, K., Soderling, T. R., and Miyamoto, E. (1992). Activation of Ca^{2+}/calmodulin-dependent kinase 11 and protein kinase C by glutamate in cultured rat hippocampal neurons. *J. Biol. Chem.*, **267**, 22527–22533.

Fuller, R. W., Wong, D. T., and Robertson, D. W. (1991). Fluoxetine, a selective inhibitor of serotonin uptake. *Med. Res. Rev.*, **11**, 17–34.

Funauchi, M., Haruta, H., and Tsumoto, T. (1994). Effects of an inhibitor for calcium/calmodulin-dependent protein phosphatase, calcineurin, on induction of long-term potentiation in rat visual cortex. *Neurosci. Res.*, **19**, 269–278.

Futamachi, K. J., and Pedley, T. A. (1976). Glial cells and extracellular potassium: their relationship in mammalian cortex. *Brain Res.*, **109**, 311–322.

Fuxe, K., and Agnati, L. F. (1991). *Volume Transmission in the Brain. Novel Mechanisms for Neural Transmission*. New York: Raven Press.

Fuxe, K., Tinner, B., Chadi, G., Harfstrand, A., and Agnati, L. F. (1994). Evidence for a regional distribution of hyaluronic acid in the rat brain using a highly specific hyaluronic acid recognizing protein. *Neurosci. Lett.*, **169**, 25–30.

Galambos, R. (1961). A glial–neuronal theory of brain function. *Proc Natl Acad Sci. USA*, **47**, 129–136.

Galambos, R., Juhász, G., Kékesi, A. K., Nyitrai, G., and Szilágyi, N. (1994). Natural sleep modifies the rat electroretinogram. *Proc. Natl Acad. Sci. USA.*, **91**, 5153–5157.

Garcia-Segura, L. M., Baetens, D., and Naftolin, F. (1986). Synaptic remodelling in arcuate nucleus after injection of estradiol valerate in adult female rats. *Brain Res.*, **366**, 131–136.

Garcia-Segura, L. M., Luquin, S., Parducz, A., and Naftolin, F. (1994). Gonadal hormone regulation of glial fibrillary acidic protein immunoreactivity and glial ultrastructure in the rat neuroendocrine hypothalamus. *Glia*, **10**, 59–69.

Garcia-Segura, L. M., Canas, B., Parducz, A., Rougon, G., Theodosis, D., Naftolon, F., and Torres-Aleman, I. (1995). Estradiol promotion of changes in the morphology of astroglia growing in culture depends on the expression of polysialic acid of neural membranes. *Glia*, **13**, 209–216.

Garcia-Segura, L. M., Chowen, J .A., Duenas, M., Parducz, A., and Naftolin, F. (1996). Gonadal steroids and astroglial plasticity. *Cell. Mol. Neurobiol.*, **16**, 225–237.

Gardiner, K. A., Laming, P. R., and Blumsom, N. L. (1993). Brain amino acid levels are related to seizure propensity in the gerbil *(Meriones unguiculatus)*. *Comp. Biochem. Physiol.*, **106B**, 799–804.

Gardner-Medwin, A. R. (1983a). Analysis of potassium dynamics in mammalian brain tissue. *J. Physiol.*, **336**, 393–426.

Gardner-Medwin, A. R. (1983b). A study of the mechanisms by which potassium moves through brain tissue in the rat. *J. Physiol. (Lond.)*, **335**, 353–374.

Gardner-Medwin, A. R. (1986). A new framework for assessment of potassium-buffering mechanisms. *Ann. NY Acad. Sci.*, **481**, 287–302.

Gardner-Medwin, A. R., and Nicholson, C. (1983). Changes of extracellular potassium activity induced by electric current through brain tissue in the rat. *J. Physiol. (Lond.)*, **335**, 375–392.

Gardner-Medwin, A. R., Coles, J. A., and Tsacopoulos, M. (1981). Clearance of extracellular potassium: evidence for spatial buffering by glial cells in the retina of the drone. *Brain Res.*, **209**, 452–457.

Garner, M. M., and Burg, M. B. (1994). Macromolecular crowding and confinement in cells exposed to hypertonicity. *Am. J. Physiol.*, **266**, C877–C892.

Garthwaite, J. (1991). Glutamate, nitric oxide and cell–cell signalling in the nervous system. *Trends Neurosci.*, **14**, 60–67.

Geddes, L. A. (1972). *Electrodes and the Measurement of Bioelectric Events*. New York. John-Wiley & Sons, Inc.

Gemba, H., Sasaki, K., and Tsujimoto, T. (1986). Cortical field potentials associated with hand movements triggered by warning and imperative stimuli in the monkey. *Electroenceph. Clin. Neurophysiol. Suppl.*, **38**, 351–367.

Ghandour, M. S., Vincendon, G., and Gombos, G. (1980). Astrocyte and oligodendrocyte distribution in adult rat cerebellum – an immunohistological study. *J. Neurocytol.*, **9**, 637–646.

Gianotti, C., Nunzi, M. G., Gispen, W. H., and Corradetti, R. (1992). Phosphorylation of the presynaptic protein B-50 (GAP-43) is increased during electrically induced long-term potentiation. *Neuron*, **8**, 843–848.

Giaume, C., Fromaget, C., El Aoumari, A., Cordier, J., Glowinski, J., and Gros, D. (1991). Gap junctions in cultured astrocytes: single-channel currents and characterization of channel-forming protein. *Neuron*, **6**, 133–143.

Gibbs, M. E. and Ng, K. T. (1977). Psychobiology of memory: towards a model of memory formation. *Biobehav. Rev.*, **1**, 113–136.

Gibbs, M. E., and Ng, K. T. (1979). Behavioural stages in memory formation. *Neurosci. Lett.*, **13**, 279–283.

Gibbs, M. E. and Ng, K. T. (1984). Dual action of cycloheximide on memory formation in day-old chicks. *Behav. Brain Res.*, **12**, 21–27.

Gibbs, M. E., Gibbs, C. L. and Ng, K. T. (1979). The influence of calcium on short-term memory. *Neurosci. Lett.*, **14**, 355–360.

Gibbs, M. E., O'Dowd, B. S., Hertz, L., Robinson, S. R., Sedman, G. R., and Ng, K. T. (1996). Inhibition of glutamine synthetase activity prevents memory consolidation. *Cogn. Brain Res.*, **4**, 57–64.

Gierer, A., and Müller, C. M. (1995). Development of layers, maps and modules. *Curr. Opin. Neurobiol.*, **5**, 91–97.

Gill, R., Foster, A. C., and Woodruff, G. N. (1987). Systemic administration of MK-801 protects against ischemia-induced hippocampal neurodegeneration in the gerbil. *J. Neurosci.*, **7**, 3343–3349.

Gilman, A. G., and Schrier, B. K. (1972). Adenosine cyclic $3',5'$-monophosphate in fetal rat brain cell cultures. *Mol. Pharmacol.*, **8**, 410–416.

Gimpl, G., Walz, W., Ohlemeyer, C., and Kettenmann, H. (1992). Bradykinin receptors in cultured astrocytes from neonatal rat brain are linked to physiological responses. *Neurosci. Lett.*, **144**, 139–142.

Gledhill, R. F., Harrison, B. M., and McDonald, W. I. (1973). Demyelination and remyelination after acute spinal cord compression. *Exp. Neurol.*, **38**, 472–487.

Goff, W. R., Allison, T., and Vaughan, H. G. (1978). The functional neuroanatomy of event-related potentials. In *Event-Related Brain Potentials in Man*, eds E. Callaway, P. Tueting and S. H. Koslow, pp. 1–79. New York: Academic Press.

Gold, P. E., and McGaugh, J. L. (1975). A single-trace, two-process view of memory storage processes. In *Short-Term Memory*, eds D. Deutsch and J. A. Deutsch, pp. 335–378. New York: Academic Press.

Goldman, J. E., and Abramson, B. (1996). Cyclic AMP-induced shape changes of astrocytes are accompanied by rapid depolymerization of actin. *Brain Res.*, **528**, 189–196.

Goldman-Rakic, P. S. (1984). Modular organization of prefrontal cortex. *TINS*, **7**, 419–429.

Goldring, S., O'Leary, J. L., Winter, D. L., and Pearlman, A. L. (1959). Identification of a prolonged post-synaptic potential of cerebral cortex. *Proc. Soc. Exp. Biol. Med.*, **100**, 429–431.

Goldstein, L. E., Rasmusson, A. M., Bunney, B. S., and Roth, R. H. (1994). The NMDA glycine site antagonist (+)-HA-966 selectively regulates conditioned stress-induced metabolic activation of the mesoprefrontal cortical dopamine but not serotonin systems: a behavioral, neuroendocrine, and neurochemical study in the rat. *J. Neurosci.*, **14**, 4937–4950.

Golowasch, J., and Deitmer, J.W. (1993). pH regulation in the stomatogastric ganglion of the crab *Cancer pagurus*. *J. Comp. Physiol. A*, **172**, 573–581.

Golubev, A. I. (1988). Glia and neuroglia relationships in the cerebral nervous system of the Turbellaria (Electron microscopic data). *Forschr. Zool.*, **36**, 31–37.

Gooday, D. J. (1990). Retinal axons in *Xenopus laevis* recognise differences between tectal and diencephalic glial cells *in vitro*. *Cell Tiss. Res.*, **259**, 595–598.

Gottfried, J. A., and Chesler, M. (1994). Endogenous H^+ modulation of NMDA receptor-mediated EPSCs revealed by carbonic anhydrase inhibition in rat hippocampus. *J. Physiol.*, **478**, 373–378.

Gout, O., and Dubois-Dalcq, M. (1993). Directed migration of transplanted glial cells toward a spinal cord demyelinating lesion. *Int. J. Dev. Neurosci.*, **11**, 613–623.

Gray, E. G. (1959). Axo-somatic and axo-dendritic synapses of the cerebral cortex. *J. Anat.*, **93**, 420–433.

Gray, P. T. and Ritchie, J. M. (1985). Ion channels in Schwann cells and glial cells. *TINS*, **8**, 411–415.

Greengaard, P. (1987). Neuronal phosphoproteins – mediators of signal transduction. *Mol. Neurobiol.*, **1**, 81–119.

Greenough, W. T. (1988). The turned-on brain: developmental and adult responses to the demands of information storage. In *From Message To Mind*, eds S. S. Easter, K. F. Barald and B. M. Carlson, pp. 288–302. Sunderland: Sinauer Assoc. Inc.

Greenough, W. T. and Chang, F.-L. F. (1988). Plasticity of synaptic structure in the cerebral cortex. In *Cerebral Cortex*, eds A. Peters and E. G. Jones, pp. 391–439. New York: Plenum.

Greenwood, R. S., Takato, M., and Goldring, S. (1981). Potassium activity and changes in glial and neuronal membrane potentials during initiation and spread of afterdischarge in cerebral cortex of cat. *Brain Res.*, **218**, 279–298.

Grichtenko, J. J., and Chesler, M. (1994a). Depolarization-induced alkalinization of astrocytes in gliotic hippocampal slices. *Neuroscience*, **62**, 1071–1078.

Grichtenko, J. J., and Chesler, M. (1994b). Depolarization-induced acid secretion in gliotic hippocampal slices. *Neuroscience*, **62**, 1057–1070.

Grierson, J. P., Petroski, R. E., Ling, D. S. F., and Geller, H. M. (1990). Astrocyte topography and tenascin/cytotactin expression: correlation with the ability to support neuritic outgrowth. *Dev. Brain Res.*, **55**, 11–19.

Griffith L. C., Verselis, L. M., Aitken, K. M., Kyriacou, C. P., Danho, W., and Greenspan, R. J. (1993). Inhibition of calcium/calmodulin-dependent protein kinase in *Drosophila* disrupts behavioral plasticity. *Neuron*, **10**, 501–509.

Griffiths, R., Greiff, J. M. C., Haycock, J., Elton, C. D., and Rowbotham, D. J. (1995). Inhibition by halothane of potassium stimulated acetylcholine release from rat cortical slices. *Br. J. Pharmacol.*, **116**, 2310–2314.

Grimmelikhuijzen, C. J. P., and Westfall, J. A. (1995). The nervous systems of Cnidarians. In *The Nervous Systems of Invertebrates: An Evolutionary and Comparative Approach*, eds O. Breidbach and W. Kutsch, pp. 7–24. Basel, Switzerland: Birkhäuser Verlag.

Grimmelikhuijzen, C. J. P., Spencer, A. N., and Carré, D. (1986). Organization of the nervous system of physonectid siphonophores. *Cell Tiss. Res.*, **246**, 463–479.

Grossfeld, R. M., Hargittai, P. T., and Lieberman, E. M. (1995). Glutamate-mediated neuron–glia signaling in invertebrates and vertebrates. In *Neuron–Glia Interrelations During Phylogeny*, vol. 2, *Plasticity and Regeneration*, ed. A. Vernadakis and B. I. Roots, pp. 129–159. Totowa, N. J.: Humana Press.

Grossman, R. G. (1972). Alterations in the microphysiology of glial cells and neurons and their environment in injured brain. *Clin. Neurosurg.*, **19**, 69–83.

Groves, A. K., Barnett, S. C., Franklin, R. J. M., Crang, A. J., Mayer, M., Blakemore, W. F., and Noble, M. (1993). Repair of demyelinated lesions by transplantation of purified O–2A progenitor cells. *Nature*, **362**, 453–456.

Grözinger, B., Kornhuber, H. H., Kriebel, J., and Murata, K. (1972). Menschliche Hirnpotentiale vor dem Sprechen. *Pflügers Archiv der gesamten Physiologie, Suppl.*, **332**, R100.

Grumet, M., Hoffman, S., Crossin, K. L., and Edelman, G. M. (1985). Cytotactin, an extracellular matrix protein of neural and non-neural tissues that mediates glia–neuron interaction. *Proc. Natl Acad. Sci. USA*, **82**, 8075–8079.

Grünewald, G., Grünewald-Zuberbier, E., Netz, J., Homberg, V., and Sander, G. (1979). Relationship between the late component of the contingent negative variation and the Bereitschaftspotential. *Electroencephal. Clin. Neurophysiol.*, **46**, 583–645.

Gruol, D. L., Baker, J. L., Mae Huang, L. Y., MacDonald, J. F., and Smith, T. G. (1980). Hydrogen ions have multiple effects on the excitability of cultured mammalian neurons. *Brain Res.*, **193**, 247–252.

Gu, Q., and Singer, W. (1995). Involvement of serotonin in developmental plasticity of kitten visual cortex. *Eur. J. Neurosci.*, **7**, 1146–1153.

Guillery, R. W. (1969). The organization of synaptic interconnections in the laminae of the dorsal lateral geniculate nucleus of the cat. *Z. Zellforsch.*, **96**, 1–38.

Guillery, R. W., Mason, C. A., and Taylor, J. S. H. (1995). Developmental determinants at the mammalian optic chiasm. *J. Neurosci.*, **15**, 4727–4737.

Guizzetti, M., Costa, P., Peters, J., and Costa, L. G. (1996). Acetylcholine as a mitogen: Muscarinic receptor-mediated proliferation of rat astrocytes and human astrocytoma cells. *Eur. J. Pharmacol.*, **297**, 265–273.

Gumnit, R. J. (1961). The distribution of direct current responses evoked by sounds in the auditory cortex of the cat. *Electroenceph. Clin. Neurophysiol.*, **13**, 889–895.

Gutnick, M. J., Connors, B. W., and Ransom, B. R. (1981). Dye coupling between glial cells in the guinea pig neocortical slice. *Brain Res.*, **213**, 486–492

Gwyn, D. G., Nicholson, G. P., and Flumerfelt, B. A. (1977). The inferior olivary nucleus of the rat: a light and electron microscopic study. *J. Comp. Neurol.*, **174**, 489–520.

Haag, G., Larbig, W., and Birbaumer, N. (1981). Differentielle Psychotherapieindikation bei psychosomatischen Störungen: Ergebnisse einer klinisch-experimentellen Studie [Differential Indication of Psychotherapy for Psychosomatic Disorders. Results of a Clinical Experimental Study]. In *Experimentelle Forschungsergebnisse in der Psychosomatischen Medizin [Results of Experimental Research in Psychosomatic Medicine]*, ed. W. Zander, pp.73–76. Göttingen: Vandenhoeck and Ruprecht.

Hablitz, J. J., and Heinemann, U. (1989). Alterations in the microenvironment during spreading depression associated with epileptiform activity in the immature neocortex. *Dev. Brain Res.*, **46**, 243–252.

Hajek, I., Subbarao, K. V., and Hertz, L. (1996). Acute and chronic effects of potassium and noradrenaline on Na^+-ATPase activity in cultured mouse neurons and astrocytes. *Neurochem. Int.*, **28**, 335–342.

Haley, J. E., and Schuman, E. M. (1994). Involvement of nitric oxide in synaptic plasticity and learning. *Semin. Neurosci.*, **6**, 11–20.

Hámori, J., and Horridge, G. A. (1966a). The lobster optic lamina. I. General organization. *J. Cell Sci.*, **1**, 249–256.

Hámori, J., and Horridge, G. A. (1966b). The lobster optic lamina. IV. Glial cells. *J. Cell Sci.*, **1**, 275–280.

Hamprecht, B., and Dringen, R. (1994). On the role of glycogen and pyruvate uptake in astroglial-neuronal interaction. In *Pharmacology of Cerebral Ischemia*, ed. H. Oberpichler-Schwenk, pp. 191–202. Stuttgart: Wissenschaftlische Verlagsgesellschaft.

Hamprecht, B., and Dringen, R. (1995). Energy metabolism. In *Neuroglia*, ed. H. Kettenmann and B. R. Ransom, pp. 473–487. New York and Oxford: Oxford University Press.

Hamprecht, B., Dringen, R., Pfeiffer, B., and Kurz, G. (1993). The possible roles of astrocytes in energy metabolism of the brain. In *Biological and Pathological Astrocyte–Neuron Interactions*, eds Federoff *et al.*, pp. 83–91. Plenum Press: New York.

Hansen, J. C., and Hillyard, S. A. (1983). Selective attention to multidimensional auditory stimuli. *J. Exp. Psychol.*, **9**, 1–19.

Hansson, E. (1994). Metabotropic glutamate receptor activation induces astroglial swelling. *J. Biol. Chem.*, **269**, 21955–21961.

Hansson, E., and Rönnbäck, L. (1991). Receptor regulation of the glutamate, GABA and taurine high-affinity uptake into astrocytes in primary culture. *Brain Res.*, **548**, 215–221.

Hansson, E., and Rönnbäck, L. (1992). Adrenergic receptor regulation of amino acid neurotransmitter uptake in astrocytes. *Brain Res. Bull.*, **29**, 297–301.

Hansson, E., and Rönnbäck, L. (1995). Astrocytes in glutamate neurotransmission. *FASEB J.*, **9**, 343–350.

Hansson, E., Eriksson, P., and Nilsson, M. (1985). Amino acid and monoamine transport in primary astroglial cultures from defined brain regions. *Neurochem. Res.*, **10**, 1335–1341.

Harrison, B. M., and McDonald, W. I. (1977). Remyelination after transient experimental compression of the spinal cord. *Ann. Neurol.*, **1**, 542–551.

Harrison, N. L., and Gibbons, S. J. (1994). Zn^{2+}: an endogeneous modulator of ligand- and voltage-gated ion channels. *Neuropharmacol.*, **33**, 935–952.

Härtig, W., Grosche, J., Distler, C., Grimm, D., El-Hifnawi, E., and Reichenbach, A. (1995). Alterations of Müller (glial) cells in dystrophic retinae of RCS rats. *J. Neurocytol.*, **24**, 507–517.

Hartley, Z., and Dubinsky, J. M. (1993). Changes in intracellular pH associated with glutamate excitotoxicity. *J. Neurosci.*, **13**, 4690–4699.

Hashimoto, S., Gemba, H., and Sasaki, K. (1979). Analysis of slow cortical potentials preceding self-paced hand movements in the monkey. *Exp. Neurol.*, **65**, 218–229.

Hassel, B., and Sonnewald, U. (1995). Glial formation of pyruvate and lactate from TCA cycle intermediates: implications for the inactivation of transmitter amino acids. *J. Neurochem.*, **65**, 2227–2234.

Hassel, B., Sonnewald, U., Unsgard, G., and Fonnum, F. (1994). NMR spectroscopy of cultured astrocytes: effects of glutamine and the gliotoxin fluorocitrate. *J. Neurochem.*, **62**, 2187–2194.

Hassinger, T. D., Atkinson, P. B., Strecker, G. J., Whalen, L. R., Dudek, F. E., Kossel, A. H., and Kater, S. B. (1995). Evidence for glutamate-mediated activation of hippocampal neurons by glial calcium waves. *J. Neurobiol.*, **28**, 159–170.

Hatten, M. E. (1990). Riding the glial monorail: a common mechanism for glial-guided neuronal migration in different regions of the developing mammalian brain. *TINS*, **13**, 179–184.

Hatten, M. E., Liem, R. K. H., and Mason, C. A. (1986). Weaver mouse cerebellar granule neurons fail to migrate on wild-type astroglial processes, in vitro. *J. Neurosci.*, **6**, 2676–2683.

Hatten, M. E., Lynch, M., Rydel, R. E., Sanchez, J., Josepph-Silverstein, J., Moscatelli, D., and Rifkin, D. B. (1988). In vitro neurite extension by granulle neurons is dependent upon astroglial-derived fibroblast growth factor. *Dev. Biol.*, **125**, 280–289.

Hatton, G. I. (1990). Emerging concepts of structure–function dynamics in adult brain: the hypothalamo-neurohypophysial system. *Prog. Neurobiol.*, **34**, 437–504.

Hatton, G. I. (1997). Function-related plasticity in hypothalamus. *Annu. Rev. Neurosci.*, **20**, 375–397.

Hatton, G. I., and Tweedle, C. D. (1982). Magnocellular neuropeptidergic neurons in hypothalamus: increases in membrane apposition and number of specialized synapses from pregnancy to lactation. *Brain Res. Bull.*, **8**, 197–204.

Hatton, G. I., Perlmutter, L. S., Salm, A. K., and Tweedle, C. D. (1984). Dynamic neuronal–glial interactions in hypothalamus and pituitary: implications for control of hormone synthesis and release. *Peptides*, **5**, 121–138.

Hatton, G. I., Yang, Q. Z., and Cobbett, P. (1987). Dye coupling among immunocytochemically identified neurons in the supraoptic nucleus: increased incidence in lactating rats. *Neuroscience*, **21**, 923–930.

Hawrylak, N., and Greenough, W. T. (1995). Monocular deprivation alters the morphology of glial fibrillary acidic protein-immunoreactive astrocytes in the rat visual cortex. *Brain Res.*, **683**, 187–199.

Hawrylak, N., Chang, F-L., and Greenough, W. T. (1993). Synaptic and astrocytic response to kindling in hippocampal subfield CA1. II. Synaptogenesis and astrocytic processes increases to in vivo kindling. *Brain Res.*, **603**, 309–316.

Hawrylak, N., Fleming, J., and Salm, A. K. (1995). Dehydration and rehydration reversibly alter glial fibrillary acidic protein in the rat supraoptic nucleus. *Glia*, **22**, 260–271.

Hebb, D. O. (1947). The effects of early experience on problem solving at maturity. *Am. Psych.*, **2**, 306–307.

Hebb, D. O. (1949). *The Organization of Behavior*. New York:Wiley.

Heil, M., Rösler, F., and Hennighausen, E. (1994). Dynamics of activation in long-term memory: the retrieval of verbal, pictorial, spatial, and color information. *J. Exp. Psychol.*, **20**, 185–200.

Heil, M., Rösler, F., and Hennighausen, E. (1996). Topographically distinct cortical activation in episodic long-term memory: The retrieval of spatial versus verbal information. *Mem. Cognit.*, **24**, 777–795.

Heinemann, U., and Dietzel, I. (1984). Extracellular potassium concentration in chronic alumina cream foci of cats. *J. Neurophysiol.*, **52**, 421–434.

Heinemann, U., and Lux, H. D. (1975). Undershoots following stimulus-induced rises of extracellular potassium concentration in cerebral cortex of cat. *Brain Res.*, **93**, 63–76.

Heinemann, U., and Lux, H. D. (1977). Ceiling of stimulus induced rises in extracellular potassium concentration in the cerebral cortex of cat. *Brain Res.*, **120**, 231–249.

Heinemann, U., and Pumain, R. (1979). Changes in extracellular free Ca^{++} activity induced by iontophoresis of excitatory substances in the sensorimotor cortex of cats. *Pflügers Arch. Ges. Physiol.*, **379**, Suppl., R183.

Heinemann, U., Lux, H. D., and Gutnick, M. J. (1977). Extracellular free calcium and potassium during paroxysmal activity in the cerebral cortex of the cat. *Exp. Brain Res.*, **27**, 237–243.

Heinemann, U., Lux, H. D., Marciani, M. G., and Holmeier, G. (1979). Slow potentials in relation to changes in extracellular potassium activity in the cortex of cats. In *Origin of Cerebral Field Potentials*, eds E. J. Speckman and H. Caspers, pp. 33–48. Stuttgart: George Thieme.

Heinemann, U., Neuhaus, S., and Dietzel, I. (1983). Aspects of potassium regulation in normal and gliotic brain tissue. In *Current Problems in Epilepsy/Cerebral Blood Flow, Metabolism and Epilepsy*, eds M. Baldy-Moulinier, D.-H. Ingvar, and B. S. Meldrum, pp. 271–277. London, Paris: John Libbey EUROTEXT.

Heinemann, U., Albrecht, D., and Ficker, E. (1990). Epileptogenicity and cellular currents in rat hippocampus during ontogenesis. *J. Basic Clin. Physiol. Pharmacol.*, **1**, 49–56.

Heiple, J. M., and Taylor, D. L. (1982). An optical technique for measurement of intracellular pH in single living cells. In *Intracellular pH: Its Measurement, Regulation and Utilization in Cellular Functions*, eds R. Nucitelli and D.W. Deamer, pp. 22–54. New York: Alan R Liss.

Hemmer, W., and Wallimann, T. (1993). Functional aspects of creatine kinase in brain. *Dev. Neurosci.*, **15**, 249–260.

Henshel, D. S., and Miller, R. F. (1992). Catecholamine effects on dissociated tiger salamander Müller (glial) cells. *Brain Res.*, **575**, 208–214.

Herkenham, M. (1987). Mismatches between neurotransmitter and receptor localizations in brain: observations and implications. *Neuroscience*, **23**, 1–38.

Herrick, C. J. (1942). Optic and postoptic systems in the brain of *Ambystoma tigrinum*. *J. Comp. Neurol.*, **77**, 191–353.

Herrington, J., Stern, R. C., Evers, A. S., and Lingle, C. J. (1991). Halothane inhibits two components of calcium current in clonal (GH3) pituitary cells. *J. Neurosci.*, **11**, 2226–2240.

Hertz, L. (1965). Possible role of neuroglia: a potassium-mediated neuronal–neuroglial–neuronal impulse transmission system. *Nature*, **4989**, 1091–1094.

Hertz, L. (1979). Functional interactions between neurons and astrocytes. 1. Turnover and metabolism of putative amino acid transmitters. *Prog. Neurobiol.*, **13**, 277–323.

Hertz, L. (1982). Astrocytes. In *Handbook of Neurochemistry, vol.1.*, ed. A. Lajtha, pp. 319–355. New York: Plenum Press.

Hertz, L. (1989). Is Alzheimer's disease an anterograde degeneration, originating in the brainstem, and disrupting metabolic interactions between neurons and glial cells? *Brain Res. Rev.*, **14**, 335–353.

Hertz, L. (1992). Autonomic control of neuronal-astrocytic interactions regulating metabolic activities and ion fluxes in the CNS. *Brain Res. Bull.*, **29**, 303–313.

Hertz, L., and Peng, L. (1992a). Energy metabolism at the cellular level of the CNS. *Can. J. Physiol. Pharmacol.*, **70**, S145–S157.

Hertz, L., and Peng, L. (1992b). The effects of monoamine transmitters on neurons and astrocytes. Correlation between energy metabolism and intracellular messengers. *Prog. Brain Res.*, **94**, 283–301.

Hertz, L., and Richardson, J. S. (1984). Is neuropharmacology merely the pharmacology of neurons – or are astrocytes important too? *Trends Pharmacol. Sci.*, July, 272–276.

Hertz, L., Drejer, J., and Schousboe, A. (1988). Energy metabolism in glutamatergic neurons, GABAergic neurons and astrocytes in primary culture. *Neurochem. Res.*, **13**, 605–610.

Hertz, L., McFarlin, D. E., and Waksman, B. H. (1990). Astrocytes: auxiliary cells for immune responses in the central nervous system. *Immunology Today*, **11**, 265–268.

Hertz, L., Peng, L., Westergaard, N., Yudkoff, M., and Schousboe, A. (1992). Neuronal-astrocytic interactions in metabolism of transmitter amino acids of the glutamate family. In *Drug Research Related to Neuroactive Amino Acids*, eds A. Schousboe, N. H. Diemer, and H. Kofod, pp. 30–50. Alfred Benzon Symposium 32, Munksgaard, Copenhagen.

Hertz, L., O'Dowd, B., and Ocherashvilli, E. (1994). Glial cells. In *Encyclopedia of Human Behavior*, ed. V. S. Ramachandran, pp. 429–439. Orlando, FL.: Academic Press.

Hertz, L., Gibbs, M. E., O'Dowd, B. S., Sedman, G. L., Robinson, S. R., Peng, L., Huang, R., Hertz, E., Hajek, I., Syková, E., and Ng, K. T. (1996). Astrocyte-neuron interaction during one-trial aversive learning in the neonate chick. *Neurosci. Behav. Rev.*, **20**, 537–551.

Hildebrand, C., and Waxman, S. G. (1983). Regional node-like membrane specializations in non-myelinated axons of rat retinal nerve fibre layer. *Brain Res.*, **258**, 23–32.

Hillis, D. M., and Moritz, C. (1990). An overview of applications of molecular systematics. In *Molecular Systematics*, eds D. M. Hillis and C. Moritz. Sunderland, MA: Sinauer Associates.

Hinde, R. A. (1962). Some aspects of the imprinting problem. *Symp. Zool. Soc Lond.*, **8**, 129–138.

Hines, M., and Shrager, P. (1991). A computational test of the requirements for conduction in demyelinated axons. *Restor. Neurol. Neurosci.*, **3**, 81–93.

Hirst, W. D., Rattray, M. A. N., Price, G. W., and Wilkin, G. P. (1994). Expression of 5-HT_{1A}, 5-HT_{2A} and 5-HT_{2C} receptors on astrocytes. *Soc. Neurosc. Abstr.*, **20**, 1547.

Hochachka, P. W., and Mommsen, T. P. (1983). Protons and anaerobiosis. *Science*, **219**, 1391–1397.

Hodgkin, A. L. and Huxley, A. F. (1952). A quantitative description of membrane current and its application to conduction and excitation in nerve. *J. Physiol. (Lond.)*, **117**, 500–544.

Hof, P. R., Pascale, E., and Magistretti, P. J. (1988). K^+ at concentrations reached in the extracellular space during neuronal activity promotes a Ca^{2+}-dependent glycogen hydrolysis in mouse cerebral cortex. *J. Neurosci.*, **8**, 1922–1928.

Hoffman, E. K., and Simonsen, L. O. (1989). Membrane mechanisms in volume and pH regulation in vertebrate cells. *Physiol. Rev.*, **69**, 315–382.

Hogstad, S., Svenneby, G., Torgner, I. Aa., Kvamme, E., Hertz, L., and Schousboe, A. (1988). Glutaminase in neurons and astrocytes cultured from mouse brain: kinetic properties and effects of phosphate, glutamate and ammonia. *Neurochem. Res.*, **13**, 383–388.

Holscher, C. (1994). Inhibitors of metabotropic glutamate receptors produce amnesic effects in chicks. *NeuroReport*, **5**, 1037–1040.

Honda, S., Yamamoto, M., and Saito, N. (1995). Immunocytochemical localization of three subtypes of GABA transporter in rat retina. *Mol. Brain Res.*, **33**, 319–325.

Honmou, O., Felts, P. A., Waxman, S. G., and Kocsis, J. D. (1996). Restoration of normal conduction properties in demyelinated spinal cord axons in the adult rat by transplantation of exogenous Schwann cells. *J. Neurosci.*, **16**, 3199–3210.

Hoppe, D., Lux, H.-D., Schachner, M., and Kettenmann, H. (1989). Activation of K^+ currents in cultured Schwann cells is controlled by extracellular pH. *Pflügers Arch.*, **415**, 22–28.

Hoppe, D., Chvatal, A., Kettenmann, H., Orkand, R. K., and Ransom, B. R. (1991). Characteristics of activity-dependent potassium accumulation in mammalian peripheral nerve in vitro. *Brain Res.*, **552**, 106–112.

Horst, R. L., Ruchkin, D. S., and Munson, R. C. (1987). Event-related potential processing negativities related to workload. In *Current Trends in Event-Related Potential Research,* eds R. Johnson, J. W. Rohrbaugh, and R. Parasuraman, pp. 186–190. EEG Suppl., Vol. 40. Amsterdam: Elsevier.

Hösli, E., and Hösli, J. (1993). Receptors for neurotransmitters on astrocytes in the mammalian central nervous system. *Prog. Neurobiol.*, **40**, 477–506.

Hounsgaard, J., and Nicholson, C. (1983). Potassium accumulation around individual purkinje cells in cerebellar slices from guinea-pig. *J. Physiol.*, **340**, 359–388.

Howd, A. G., Hornby, M. F., Kirvell, S. L., and Butt, A. M. (1995). GABA-mediated changes in extracellular potassium: a developmental study in the isolated rat optic nerve. *J. Physiol.*, **489**, 76P.

Howd, A. G., Kirvall, S. L., and Butt, A. M. (1996). GABA-mediated changes in extracellular potassium in the developing rat optic nerve. *J. Physiol.*, **494**, 89P.

Hoyenga, K. B., and Hoyenga, K. T. (1988). *Psychobiology: The Neuron and Behavior.* Pacific Grove, Calif.: Brooks/Cole.

Hoyle, G. (1953). Potassium ions and insect nerve. *J. Exp. Biol.*, **30**, 121–135.

Huang, R., and Hertz, L. (1994). Clonidine enhances astrocytic glutamine uptake by authentic α_2-adrenoceptor stimulation. *NeuroReport*, 5, 632–634.

Huang, R., Shuaib, A., and Hertz, L. (1994). Glutamate uptake and glutamate content in primary cultures of mouse astrocytes during anoxia, substrate deprivation and simulated ischaemia under normothermic and hypothermic conditions. *Brain Res.*, 618, 346–351.

Huang, R., Kala, G., Murthy, Ch. R. K., and Hertz, L. (1994a). Effects of chronic exposure to ammonia on glutamate and glutamine interconversion and compartmentation in homogenous primary cultures of mouse astrocytes. *Neurochem. Res.*, 19, 257–265.

Huang, R., Peng, L., Chen, Y., Hajek, I., Zhao, Z., and Hertz, L. (1994b). Signalling effect of monoamines and of elevated potassium concentrations on brain energy metabolism at the cellular level. *Dev. Neurosci.*, 16, 337–351.

Hudson, L. D., Puckett, C., Berndt, J., Chan, J., and Gencic, S. (1989). Mutation of the proteolipid protein gene PLP in a human X chromosome-linked myelin disorder. *Proc. Natl Acad. Sci.*, 86, 8128–8131.

Hutchins, J. B., and Casagrande, V. A. (1990). Development of the lateral geniculate nucleus: interactions between retinal afferent, cytoarchitectonic, and glial cell process lamination in ferret and tree shrews. *J. Comp. Neurol.*, 298, 113–128.

Huxley, A. F., and Stämpfli, R. (1949). Evidence for saltatory conduction in peripheral myelinated nerve fibres. *J. Physiol. (Lond.)*, 108, 315–339.

Huxlin, K. R. (1995). NADPH-diaphorase expression in neurons and glia of the normal adult rat retina. *Brain Res.*, 692, 195–206.

Ikeda, T., and Puro, D. G. (1995). Regulation of retinal glial cell proliferation by antiproliferation molecules. *Exp. Eye Res.*, 60, 435–444.

Immel, J., and Steinberg, R. H. (1986). Spatial buffering of K^+ by the retinal pigment epithelium in frog. *J. Neurosci.*, 6, 3197–3204.

Inoue, I., Tsutsui, I., and Brown, E. R. (1997). K^+ accumulation and K^+ conductance inactivation during action potential trains in giant axons of the squid, *Sepioeuthis*. *J. Physiol. (Lond.)*, 500, 355–366.

Inoue, S. (1989). *Biology of Sleep Substances*. Boca Raton: CRC Press.

Inoue, S. (1993). Sleep promoting substance (SPS) and physiological sleep regulation. *Zool. Science*, 10, 557–576.

Irwin, D. A., and Rebert, C. S. (1970). Slow potential changes in cat brain during classical appetitive conditioning of jaw movements using two levels of reward. *Electroenceph. Clin. Neurophysiol.*, 28, 119–126.

Irwin, R. P., Lin, S. Z., Long, R. T., and Paul, S. M. (1994). N-methyl-D-aspartate induces a rapid, reversible, and calcium-dependent intracellular acidosis in cultured fetal rat hippocampal neurons. *J. Neurosci.*, 14, 1352–1357.

Izumi, Y., Benz, A. M., Zorumski, C. F., and Olney, J. W. (1994). Effects of lactate and pyruvate on glucose deprivation in rat hippocampal slices. *NeuroReport*, 5, 617–620.

Jabs, R., Paterson, I. A., and Walz, W. (1996). Down-regulation of glial voltage gated sodium channels after reactive gliosis in situ. *Soc. Neurosci. Abstr.*, 22, (1969).

Jahromi, B. S., Robitaille, R., and Charlton, M. P. (1992). Transmitter release increases intracellular calcium in perisynaptic Schwann cells in situ. *Neuron*, 8, 1069–1077.

Jansen, J. K. S., and Nicholls, J. G. (1973). Conductance changes, an electrogenic pump and the hyperpolarization of leech neurones following impulses. *J. Physiol.*, 229, 635–655.

Jarolimek, W., Misgeld, U., and Lux, H. D. (1989). Activity dependent alkaline and acid transients in guinea pig hippocampal slices. *Brain Res.*, 505, 225–232.

Jarolimek, W., Misgeld, U., and Lux, H. D. (1990). Neurons sensitive to pH in slices of the rat ventral medulla oblongata. *Pflügers Arch.*, **416**, 247–253.

Jasper, H. H. (1958). The ten-twenty electrode system of the International Federation. *Electroenceph. Clin. Neurophysiol.*, **20**, 371–375.

Jasper, H., Khan, R. T., and Elliot, K. A. C. (1965). Amino acids released from the cerebral cortex in relation to its state of activation. *Science*, **147**, 1448–1449.

Jean, T., Frelin, C., Vigne, P., and Lazdunski, M. (1986). The Na^+/H^+ exchange system in glial cell lines. Properties and activation by an hyperosmotic shock. *Eur. J. Biochem.*, **160**, 211–219.

Jendelová, P., and Syková, E. (1991). Role of glia in K^+ and pH-homeostasis in the neonatal rat spinal cord. *Glia*, **4**, 56–63.

Jendelová, P., Chvátal, A., Šimonová, Z., and Syková, E. (1994). Effect of excitatory amino acids on extracellular pH in isolated rat spinal cord. *Abstracts, 17th Ann. Meeting ENA*, p. 199.

Jensen, A. M., and Chiu, S. (1993). Interactions between astrocytes and other cells in the central nervous system. In *Astrocytes: Pharmacology and Function*, ed. S. Murphy, pp. 309–330. San Diego: Academic Press, Inc.

Jeserich, G., Stratmann, A., and Strelau, J. (1995). A cellular and molecular approach to myelinogenesis in the CNS of trout. In *Neuron–Glia Interrelations During Phylogeny: I. Phylogeny and Ontogeny of Glial Cells*, eds A. Vernadakis and B. I. Roots, pp. 249–269. Totowa, NJ: Humana Press Inc.

Johnson, R. Jr. (1986). A triarchic model of P300 amplitude. *Psychophysiology*, **23**, 367–384.

Johnston, A. R., and Gooday, D. J. (1991). *Xenopus* temporal retinal axons collapse on contact with glial cells from caudal tectum in vitro. *Development*, **113**, 409–417.

Johnston, B. M., Patuzzi, R., Syka, J., and Syková, E. (1989). Stimulus-related potassium changes in organ of Corti of guinea-pig. *J. Physiol. (Lond)*, **408**, 77–92.

Johnston, G. A. R., Kennedy, S. M. E., and Twitchin, B. (1979). Action of the neurotoxin kainic acid on high affinity uptake of L-glutamatic acid in rat brain slices. *J. Neurochem.*, **32**, 121–127.

Johnston, T. D. (1988). Developmental explanation and the ontogeny of bird song: nature/nurture redux. *Behav. Brain Sci.*, **11**, 617–663.

Jonas, P. (1993). Glutamate receptors in the central nervous system. *Ann. NY Acad. Sci.*, **707**, 126–135.

Jones, R. S. G., and Heinemann, U. (1987). Abolition of the orthodromically evoked IPSP of CA1 pyramidal cells before the EPSP during washout of calcium from hippocampal slices. *Exp. Brain Res.*, **65**, 676–680.

Jones, T., and Greenough, W. T. (1996). Ultrastructural evidence for increased contact between astrocytes and synapses in rats reared in a complex environment. *Neurobiol. Mem. Learn*, **65**, 45–56.

Jucker, M., Mondadori, C., Mohajeri, H., Bartsch, U., and Schachner, M. (1995). Transient upregulation of NCAM mRNA in astrocytes in response to entorhinal cortex lesions and ischaemia. *Mol. Brain Res.*, **28**, 149–156.

Juurlink, B. H. J., and Hertz, L. (1985). Plasticity of astrocytes in primary cultures: an experimental tool and a reason for methodological caution. *Dev. Neurosci.*, **7**, 263–277.

Juurlink, B. H. J., and Hertz, L. (1992). Astrocytes. In *Neuromethods: vol. 23, Cell Cultures*, eds A. A. Boulton, G. B. Baker and W. Walz, pp. 269–321. New York: Humana Clifton Press.

Juurlink, B. H. J., and Hertz, L. (1993). Ischemia-induced death of astrocytes and neurones in primary culture: pitfalls in quantifying neuronal cell death. *Dev. Brain Res.*, **71**, 239–246.

Kadekaro, M., Crane, A. M., and Sokoloff, L. (1985). Differential effects of electrical stimulation of sciatic nerve on metabolic activity in spinal cord and dorsal root ganglion in the rat. *Proc. Natl Acad. Sci. USA*, **82**, 6010–6013.

Kahneman, D. (1973). *Attention and Effort*. Englewood Cliffs, NJ: Prentice-Hall.

Kai-Kai, M. A., and Pentreath, V. W. (1981). The structure, distribution and quantitative relationships of the glia in the abdominal ganglia of the horse leech, *Haemopis sanguisuga*. *J. Comp. Neurol.*, **202**, 193–210.

Kaila, K. (1994). Ionic basis of GABA(A) receptor channel function in the nervous system. *Prog. Neurobiol.*, **42**, 489–537.

Kaila, K., and Voipio, J. (1987). Postsynaptic fall in intracellular pH induced by GABA-activated bicarbonate conductance. *Nature*, **330**, 163–165.

Kaila, K., Saarikoski, J., and Voipio, J. (1990). Mechanism of action of GABA on intracellular pH and on surface pH in crayfish muscle fibres. *J. Physiol.*, **427**, 241–260.

Kaila, K., Panula, P., Karhunen, T., and Heinonen, E. (1991). Fall in intracellular pH mediated by GABA$_A$ receptors in cultured rat astrocytes. *Neurosci. Lett.*, **126**, 9–12.

Kaila, K., Paalasmaa, P., Taira, T., and Voipio, J. (1992). pH transients due to monosynaptic activation of GABA$_A$ receptors in rat hippocampal slices. *NeuroReport*, **3**, 105–108.

Kalat, J. W. (1992). *Biological Psychology*. Belmont, Calif.: Wadsworth.

Kanai, Y., and Hediger, M. A. (1992). Primary structure and functional characterization of high-affinity glutamate transporter. *Nature*, **360**, 467–471.

Kanai, Y., Bhide, P. G., DiFiglia, M., and Hediger, M. A. (1995). Neuronal high-affinity glutamate transport in the rat central nervous system. *NeuroReport*, **6**, 2357–2362.

Kandel, E. R. (1983). From metapsychology to molecular biology: explorations into the nature of anxiety. *Am. J. Psychiatry*, **140**, 1277–1293.

Kandel, E. R., Schwartz, J. H. and Jessell, T. M. (1991). *Principles of Neuroscience*, 3rd edition. New York: Elsevier.

Kanner, B. I., and Schuldiner, S. (1987). Mechanism of transport and storage of neurotransmitters. *CRC Crit. Rev. Biochem.*, **22**, 1–38.

Kapfhammer, J. P., and Schwab, M. E. (1992). Modulators of neuronal migration and neurite growth. *Curr. Opin. Cell Biol.*, **4**, 863–868.

Kapfhammer, J. P., and Schwab, M. E. (1994). Inverse patterns off myelination and GAP-43 expression in the adult CNS: neurite growth inhibitors as regulators of neuronal plasticity. *J. Comp. Neurol.*, **340**, 194–206.

Karahashi, Y., and Goldring, S. (1966). Intracellular potentials from 'idle' cells in cerebral cortex of cat. *Electroenceph. Clin. Neurophysiol.*, **20**, 600–607.

Karwoski, C. J., and Proenza, L. M. (1977). Relationship between Müller cell responses, a local transretinal potential, and potassium flux. *J. Neurophysiol.*, **40**, 244–259.

Karwoski, C. J., Frambach, D. A., and Proenza, L. M. (1985). Laminar profile of resistivity in frog retina. *J. Neurophysiol.*, **54**, 1607–1619.

Karwoski, C. J., Coles, J. A., Lu, H., and Huang, B. (1989). Current-evoked transcellular K$^+$ flux in frog retina. *J. Neurophysiol.*, **61**, 939–952.

Kasamatsu, T. (1991). Adrenergic regulation of visuocortical plasticity: a role of the locus coeruleus system. In *Progress in Brain Research. Neurobiology of the Locus Coeruleus*, Vol. 88, eds C. D. Barnes and O. Pompeiano, pp. 599–616. Amsterdam: Elsevier.

Kastritsis, C. H. C., Salm, A. K., and McCarthy, K. D. (1992). Stimulation of the P_{2Y} purinergic receptor on type 1 astroglia results in inositol phosphate formation and calcium mobilization. *J. Neurochem.*, **58**, 1277–1284.

Kato, S., Ishita, S., Sugawara, K., and Mawatari, K. (1993). Cystine/glutamate antiporter expression in retinal Müller glial cells: implications for DL-alpha-aminoadipate toxicity. *Neuroscience*, **57**, 473–482.

Kaufman, E. E., and Driscoll, B. F. (1992). CO_2 fixation in neuronal and glial cells in culture. *J. Neurochem.*, **58**, 258–262.

Kauppinen, R. A., Enkvist, K., Holopainen, I., and Akerman, K. E. (1988). Glucose deprivation depolarizes plasma membrane of cultured astrocytes and collapses transmembrane potassium and glutamate gradients. *Neuroscience*, **26**, 283–289.

Kawamura, H., and Sawyer, C. H. (1964). DC potential changes in rabbit brain during slow wave and paradoxical sleep in the rabbit. *Am. J. Physiol.*, **207**, 1379–1386.

Keifer, J. C., Baghdoyan, H. A., Becker, L., and Lydic, R. (1994). Halothane decreases pontine acetylcholine release and increases EEG spindles. *NeuroReport*, **5**, 577–580.

Keirstead, S. A., and Miller, R. F. (1995). Calcium waves in dissociated retinal glial (Müller) cells are evoked by release of calcium from intracellular stores. *Glia*, **14**, 14–22.

Kelly, J. P., and Van Essen, D.C. (1974). Cell structure and function in the visual cortex of the cat. *J. Physiol.*, **238**, 515–547.

Kelly, J. S., Krnjevic, K., Morris, M. E., and Yirn, G. K. W. (1969). Anionic permeability of cortical neurons. *Exp. Brain. Res.*, **7**, 11–31.

Kemper, H., and Dohring (1967). *Die sozialen Faltenwespen Mitteleuropas*. Berlin: Paul Parey.

Kempski, O., Gross, U., and Baethmann, A. (1982). An in vitro model of cytotoxic brain edema: cell volume and metabolism of cultivated glial- and nerve-cells. *Adv. Neurosurg.*, **10**, 254–258.

Kempski, O., Von Rosen, S., Weigt, H., Staub, F., Peters, J., and Baethmann, A. (1991). Glial ion transport and volume control. *Ann. NY Acad. Sci.*, **633**, 306–317.

Kettenmann, H. (1987). Oligodendrocytes control extracellular potassium by active uptake and spatial buffering. In *Biochemistry of Glial Cells*, eds T. Grisar et al. Oxford, New York: Pergamon Press.

Kettenmann, H., and Ransom, B. R. (1988). Electrical coupling between astrocytes and between oligodendrocytes studied in mammalian cell cultures. *Glia*, **6**, 64–73.

Kettenmann, H., and Ransom, B. R., eds (1995). *Neuroglia*. New York and Oxford: Oxford University Press.

Kettenmann, H., and Schlue, W. R. (1988). Intracellular pH regulation in cultured mouse oligodendrocytes. *J. Physiol.*, **406**, 147–162.

Kettenmann, H., Sonnhof, U., and Schachner, M. (1983). Exclusive potassium dependence of the membrane potential in cultured mouse oligodendrocytes. *J. Neurosci.*, **3**, 500–505.

Kettenmann, H., Ransom, B. R., and Schlue, W. R. (1990). Intracellular pH shifts capable of uncoupling cultured oligodendrocytes are seen only in low HCO_3^- solution. *Glia*, **3**, 110–117.

Kettenmann, H., Backus, K. H., and Schachner, M. (1984). Aspartate, glutamate and gamma-aminobutyric acid depolarize cultured astrocytes. *Neurosci. Lett.*, **52**, 25–29.

Kety, S. S. (1972). Brain catecholamines, affective states and memory. In *Chemistry of Mood, Motivation and Memory,* ed. J. L. McGaugh. New York: Plenum.

Keyser, D. O., and Pellmar, T. C. (1994). Synaptic transmission in the hippocampus: critical role for glial cells. *Glia*, **10**, 237–243.

Khalsa, S. B. S., Ralph, M. R., and Block, G. D. (1991). Does low intracellular pH stop the motion of the bulla circadian pacemaker. *J. Neurosci.*, **11**, 2672–2679.

Kim, W. T., Rioult, M. G., and Cornell-Bell, A. H. (1994). Glutamate-induced calcium signaling in astrocytes. *Glia*, **11**, 173–184.

Kimelberg, H. K. (1983). Primary astrocyte cultures – a key to astrocyte function. *Cell. Mol. Neurobiol.*, **3**, 1–16.

Kimelberg, H. K. (1988). *Glial Cell Receptors*. New York: Raven Press.

Kimelberg, H. K. (1989). Excitatory amino-acid stimulated uptake of ^{22}Na$^+$ in primary astrocyte cultures. *J. Neurosci.*, **9**, 1141–1149.

Kimelberg, H. K. (1991). Swelling and volume control in brain astroglial cells. In *Advances in Comparative and Environmental Physiology*, eds R. Gilles et al., vol. 9, pp 81–117. Berlin, Heidelberg: Springer-Verlag.

Kimelberg, H. K. (1995). Receptors on astrocytes – what possible functions. *Neurochem. Intl.*, **26**, 27–40.

Kimelberg, H. K., and Aschner, M. (1994). Astrocytes and their functions, past and present. In *Alcohol and Glial Cells*, ed. F. E. Lancaster, pp. 1–40. Bethesda: NIH, NIAAA.

Kimelberg, H. K., and Norenberg, M. D. (1989). Astrocytes. *Sci. Am.*, **260**, 66–76.

Kimelberg, H. K., and O'Connor, E. R. (1988). Swelling-induced depolarization of astrocyte potentials. *Glia*, **1**, 219–224.

Kimelberg, H. K., Goderie, S. K., Higman S., Pang, S., and Waniewski, R. A. (1990). Swelling-induced release of glutamate, aspartate, and taurine from astrocyte cultures. *J. Neurosci.*, **10**, 1583–1591.

Kimelberg, H. K., Goderie, S. K., Conley, P. A., Higman, S., Goldschmidt, R., and Amundson, R. H. (1992). Uptake of [^{3}H]serotonin and [^{3}H]glutamate by primary astrocyte cultures I. Effects of different sera and time in culture. *Glia*, **6**, 1–8.

Kimelberg, H. K., Jalonen, T., and Walz, W. (1993). Regulation of the brain microenvironment: transmitters and ions. In *Astrocytes: Pharmacology and Function*, ed. S. Murphy, pp. 193–228. New York: Academic Press.

Kimelberg, H. K., Cai, Z., Rastogi, P., Goderie, S., and Charniga, C. (1995a). Serum-dependent up-regulation of transmitter stimulated Ca^{2+} responses in acutely isolated astrocytes. *Soc. Neurosci. Abstr.*, **21**, 581.

Kimelberg, H. K., Rutledge, E., Goderie, S., and Charniga, C. (1995b). Astrocytic swelling due to hypotonic or high K$^+$ medium causes inhibition of glutamate and aspartate uptake and increases their release. *J. Cereb. Blood Flow Metab.*, **15**, 409–416.

Kimelberg, H. K., Cai, Z., Rastogi, P., Charniga, C. J., Goderie, S., Dave, V., and Jalonen, T. O. (1997). Transmitter-induced calcium responses differ in astrocytes acutely isolated from rat brain and in culture. *J. Neurochem.*, **68**, 1088–1098.

King, J.C., Ronsheim, P.M. and Rubin, B.S. (1995). Dynamic relationships between LHRH neuronal terminals and the end-feet of tanycytes in cycling rats revealed by confocal microscopy. *Soc. Neurosci. Abstr.*, **21**, 265.

Kirchhoff, F., Mülhardt, C., Pastor, A., Becker, C.-M., and Kettenmann, H. (1996). Expression of glycine receptor subunits in glial cells of the rat spinal cord. *J. Neurochem.*, **66**, 1383–1390.

Kiss, J.Z., Wang, C. and Rougon, G. (1993). Nerve-dependent expression of high polysialic acid neural cell adhesion molecule in neurohypophysial astrocytes of adult rats. *Neuroscience*, **53**, 213–221.

Klee, C. B., Draetta, G. F. and Hubbard, M. J. (1988). Calcineurin. *Adv. Enzymol.*, **61**, 149–200.

Klintsova, A., Levy, W. and Desmond, N. (1995). Astrocytic volume fluctuates in the hippocampal CA1 region across the estrous cycle. *Brain. Res.*, **690**, 269–274.

Knapp, P.E., Booth, C.S., and Skoff, R.P. (1993). The pH of jimpy glia is increased: intracellular measurements using fluorescent laser cytometry. *Int. J. Dev. Neurosci.*, **11**, 215–226.

Kocsis, J. D. and Waxman, S. G. (1980). Absence of potassium conductance in central myelinated axons. *Nature*, **287**, 348–349.

Kocsis, J. D. and Waxman, S. G. (1983). Long-term regenerated nerve fibres retain sensitivity to potassium channel blocking agents. *Nature*, **304**, 640–642.

Kocsis, J. D., Malenka, R. C. and Waxman, S. G. (1983). Effects of extracellular potassium concentration on the excitability of the parallel fibres of the rat cerebellum. *J. Physiol. (Lond.)*, **334**, 225–244.

Koh, S.-W. M., Kyritsis, A., and Chader, G. J. (1984). Interaction of neuropeptides and cultured glial (Müller) cells of the chick retina: elevation of intracellular cyclic AMP by vasoactive intestinal peptide and glucagon. *J. Neurochem.*, **43**, 199–203.

Kohama, S. G., Goss, J. R., McNeill, T. H., and Finch, C. E. (1995). Glial fibrillary acidic protein mRNA increases at proestrus in the arcuate nucleus of mice. *Neurosci. Lett.*, **183**, 164–166.

Konishi, T. (1990a). Dye coupling between mouse Schwann cells. *Brain Res.*, **508**, 85–92.

Konishi, T. (1990b). Voltage-gated potassium currents in myelinated Schwann cells in the mouse. *J. Physiol.*, **431**, 123–139.

Konishi, T. (1991). Potassium channel-dependent changes in the volume of developing mouse Schwann cells. *Brain Res.*, **565**, 57–66.

Konnerth, A., Lux, H. D., and Morad, M. (1987). Proton-induced transformation of calcium channel in chick dorsal root ganglion cells. *J. Physiol.*, **386**, 603–633.

Koopowitz, H., and Chien, P. (1975). Ultrastructure of nerve plexus in flatworms. II. Sites of synaptic interactions. *Cell Tissue Res.*, **157**, 207–216.

Korf, J., de Boer, J., Baarsma, R., Venema, K., and Okken, A. (1993). Monitoring of glucose and lactate using microdialysis: application in neonates and rat brain. *Dev. Neurosci.*, **15**, 240–246.

Kornack, D. R., and Rakic, P. (1995). Radial and horizontal deployment of clonally related cells in the primate neocortex: relationship to distinct mitotic lineages. *Neuron*, **15**, 311–321.

Kornhuber, H. H., and Deecke, L. (1964). Hirnpotentialänderungen beim Menschen vor und nach Willkürbewegungen, dargestellt mit Magnetbandspeicherung und Rückwärtsanalyse. *Pflügers Archiv der gesamten Physiologie*, **281**, 52.

Kornhuber, H. H., and Deecke, L. (1965). Hirnpotentialänderungen bei Willkürbewegungen und passiven Bewegungen des Menschen: Bereitschaftspotentiale und Reafferente Potentiale. *Pfluegers Archiv fuer die gesamte Physiologie*, **284**, 1–17.

Korte, G. E., and Rosenbluth, J. (1981). Ependymal astrocytes in the frog cerebellum. *Anat. Rec.*, **199**, 267–279.

Korunka, C., Bauer, H., Wolek, A., and Leodolter, M. (1990). The brain triggered oddball CNV. In *Psychophysiological Brain Research*, eds C. H. M. Brunia, A. W. K. Gaillard and A. Kok, Vol. 2, pp. 55–59. Tilburg: University Press.

Kosslyn, S. M. (1987). Seeing and imagining in the cerebral hemispheres: a computational approach. *Psychol. Rev.*, **94**, 148–175.

Kosslyn, S. M., and Koenig, O. (1992). *Wet Mind.* New York: Free Press.

Kotchoubey, B., Schleichert, H., Lutzenberger, W., and Birbaumer, N. (1997). A new method for rhythmic self-regulation of slow cortical potentials in two dimensions. *Appl. Psychophysiol. Biofeedback*, **22**, 77–93.

Kraig, R. P., Ferreira-Filho, C. R., and Nicholson, C. (1983). Alkaline and acid transients in cerebellar micro-environment. *J. Neurophysiol.*, **49**, 831–850.

Kressin, K., Kuprijanova, E., Jabs, R., Seifert, G., and Steinhäuser, C. (1995). Developmental regulation of Na^+ and K^+ conductances in glial cells of mouse hippocampal brain slices. *Glia*, **15**, 173–187.

Kriegler, S., and Chiu, S. Y. (1993). Calcium signaling of glial cells along mammalian axons. *J. Neurosci.*, **13**, 4229–4245.

Kristeva, R. (1977). Study of the motor potential during voluntary recurrent movement. *Electroenceph. Clin. Neurophysiol.*, **42**, 588.

Kristeva, R. (1984). Bereitschaftspotential of pianists. In *Brain and Information: Event-Related Potentials*, eds R. Karrer, J. Cohen and P. Tueting, pp. 477–482. Annals of the New York Academy of Sciences (Vol. 425). The New York Academy of Sciences, New York.

Kristeva, R., and Cheyne, D. (1990). Similarities between attentional and preparatory states. *Behav. Brain Sci.*, **13**, 247.

Kristeva, R., and Kornhuber, H. H. (1980). Cerebral potentials related to the smallest human finger movement. In *Multidisciplinary Perspectives in Event-Related Brain Potential Research*, ed. D. A. Otto, pp. 177–182. Washington, DC: U.S. Environmental Protection Agency.

Kříž, N., Syková, E., and Vyklický, L. (1975). Extracellular potassium changes in the spinal cord of the cat and their relation to slow potentials, active transport and impulse transmission. *J. Physiol. (Lond.)*, **249**, 167–182.

Krizaj, D., Rice, M. E., Wardle, R. A., and Nicholson, C. (1996). Water compartmentalization and extracellular tortuosity after osmotic changes in cerebellum of *Trachemys scripta*. *J. Physiol. (Lond.)*, **492**, 887–896.

Krnjevic, K., and Schwartz, S. (1967). Some properties of unresponsive cells in the cerebral cortex. *Exp. Brain Res.*, **3**, 306–319.

Kruger, L., and Maxwell, D. S. (1967). Comparative fine structure of vertebrate neuroglia: teleosts and reptiles. *J. Comp. Neurol.*, **129**, 115–142.

Krull, C. E., Morton, D. B., Faissner, A., Schachner, M., and Tolbert, L. P. (1993). Spatiotemporal pattern of expression of tenascin-like molecules in a developing insect olfactory system. *J. Neurobiol.*, **25**, 515–534.

Kuffler, S. W., and Nicholls, J. G. (1964). Glial cells in the central nervous system of the leech; their membrane potential and potassium content. *Arch. Exp. Path. Pharmakol.*, **248**, 216–222.

Kuffler, S. W., and Nicholls, J. G. (1966). The physiology of neuroglial cells. *Ergebn. Physiol.*, **57**, 1–90.

Kuffler, S. W., and Nicholls, J. G. (1976). *From Neuron to Brain*. Sunderland, MA: Sinauer Assoc.

Kuffler, S. W., and Potter, D. D. (1964). Glia in the leech central nervous system: physiological properties and neuron–glia relationship. *J. Neurophysiol.*, **27**, 290–320.

Kuffler, S. W., Nicholls, J. G., and Orkand, R. K. (1966). Physiological properties of glial cells in the central nervous system of amphibia. *J. Neurophysiol.*, **29**, 768–787.

Kulkarni, R. S., Zorn, L. J., Anantharam, V., and Bayley, H. (1996). Inhibitory effects of Ketamine and halothane on recombinant potassium channels from mammalian brain. *Anesthesiology*, **84**, 900–909.

Kurz, G. M., Wiesinger, H., and Hamprecht, B. (1993). Purification of cytosolic malic enzyme from bovine brain, generation of monoclonal antibodies, and immunocytochemical localization of the enzyme in glia of neural primary cultures. *J. Neurochem.*, **60**, 1467–1474.

Kuwabara, T., and Cogan, D. G. (1961). Retinal glycogen. *Arch. Ophthalmol.*, **66**, 94–104.

Kvamme, E. (1983). Glutamine. In *Handbook of Neurochemistry* 2nd edn, Vol. 3, ed. A. Lajtha, pp. 405–422. New York: Plenum.

Kvamme, E., Svenneby, G., Hertz, L., and Schousboe, A. (1982). Properties of phosphate activated glutaminase in astrocytes cultured from mouse brain. *Neurochem. Res.*, **7**, 761–770.

Laake, J. H., Slyngstad, T. A., Haug, F.-M. S., and Ottersen, O. P. (1995). Glutamine from glial cells is essential for the maintenance of the nerve terminal pool of glutamate: Immunogold evidence from hippocampal slice cultures. *J. Neurochem.*, **65**, 871–881.

Laboritt, H., and Zerbib, R. (1987). Phorbol esters antagonize scopolamine-induced amnesia of a passive avoidance learning. *Res. Commun. Psychol. Psychiatr. Behav.*, **12**, 105–117.

Labourdette, G., and Sensenbrenner, M. (1995). Growth factors and their receptors in the central nervous system. In *Neuroglia*, eds H. Kettenmann and B. R. Ransom, pp. 441–459. New York and Oxford: Oxford University Press.

Lachapelle, F., Duhamel-Clerin, E., Gansmuller, A., Baron-Van Evercooren, A., Villarroya, H., and Gumpel, M. (1994). Transplanted transgenically marked oligodendrocytes survive, migrate and myelinate in the normal mouse brain as they do in the shiverer mouse brain. *Eur. J. Neurosci.*, **6**, 814–824.

Lafarga, M., Berciano, M. T., Del Olmo, E., Andres, M. A., and Pazos, A. (1992). Osmotic stimulation induces changes in the expression of β-adrenergic receptors and nuclear volume of astrocytes in supraoptic nucleus of the rat. *Brain Res.*, **588**, 311–316.

Lambert, J. D. C., and Heinemann, U. (1986). Aspects of the action of excitatory amino acids on hippocampal CA1 neurons. In *Calcium Electrogenesis and Neuronal Functioning*, eds U. Heinemann, M. Klee, E., Neher, and W. Singer, pp. 279–290. Heidelberg: Springer-Verlag.

Laming P. R., ed. (1981a). *Brain Mechanisms of Behaviour in Lower Vertebrates*. Cambridge: Cambridge University Press.

Laming, P. R. (1981b). The physiological basis for alert behaviour in fish. In *Brain Mechanisms of Behaviour in Lower Vertebrates*, ed. P. R. Laming, pp. 203–224. Cambridge: Cambridge University Press.

Laming, P. R. (1989a). Central representation of arousal. In *Visuomotor Coordination: Amphibians, Comparisons, Models and Robots*, eds J.-P. Ewert and M. A. Arbib, pp. 693–727. New York: Plenum Press.

Laming, P. R. (1989b). Do glia contribute to behaviour? A neuromodulatory review. *J.Comp. Biochem. Physiol.*, **94A**, 555–568.

Laming, P. R. (1992). Information processing and neuromodulation in the visual system of frogs and toads. *Network*, **3**, 71–88.

Laming, P. R. (1993). Modelling membrane potentials is more flexible than spikes. In *Neural Computing Research and Applications*, ed. G. Orchard, pp. 29–41. Bristol: Institute of Physics Press.

Laming, P. R., and Brooks, M. (1985). Effects of visual, chemical and tactile stimuli on the auditory evoked response of the teleost, *Rutilus rutilus*. *Comp. Biochem. Physiol.*, **82A**, 667–673.

Laming, P. R, and Bullock, T. H. (1991). Changes in early acoustic-evoked potentials by mildly arousing priming stimuli in carp *(Cyprinus carpio)*. *J. Comp. Biochem. Physiol.*, **99A**, 567–575.

Laming, P. R., and Ennis, P. (1981). Habituation of fright and arousal responses in the teleosts *Carassius auratus* and *Rutilus rutilus. J. Comp. Physiol. Psychol.*, **96**, 460–466.

Laming, P. R., and Ewert, J. P. (1983). The effects of pretectal lesions on neuronal, sustained potential shift and electroencephalagraphic responses of the toad tectum to presentation of a visual stimulus. *J. Comp. Biochem. Physiol.*, **154**, 89–101.

Laming, P. R., and Ewert, J. P. (1984). Visual unit, EEG and sustained potential shift responses to biologically significant stimuli in the brain of toads *(Bufo bufo). J. Comp. Physiol.*, **154**, 89–101.

Laming, P. R., and Hornby, P. (1981). The effects of unilateral telencephalic lesions on behavioural arousal and its habituation in the roach, *Rutilus rutilus. Behav. Neural Biol.*, **33**, 59–65.

Laming, P. R., and Lenke, R. (1991). Glutamate, not GABA causes prolonged elevation of cardiac arousal responses in goldfish. *Comp. Biochem. Physiol.*, **99C**, 101–103.

Laming, P. R., and McKee, M. (1981). Deficits in habituation of cardiac arousal responses incurred by telencephalic ablation in Goldfish (*Carassius auratus*) and their relation to other telencephalic functions. *J. Comp. Physiol. Psychol.*, **95**, 460–467.

Laming, P. R., and Savage, G. E. (1980). Physiological changes observed in the goldfish (*Carassius auratus*) during behavioural arousal and fright. *Behav. Neural Biol.*, **29**, 255–275.

Laming, P. R., Borchers, H. W., and Ewert, J. P. (1984). Visual unit, EEG and sustained potential shift responses in the brain of toads (*Bufo bufo*) during alert and defensive behaviour. *Physiol. Behav.*, **32**, 463–468.

Laming, P. R., Ewert, J. P., and Borchers, H. W. (1984). The effects of telencephalic ablation on unit, EEG and sustained potential shift responses of the toad tectum to a visual stimulus. *Behav. Neurosci.*, **98**, 118–124.

Laming, P. R., Rooney, D. J., and Ferguson, Judy (1987). Epileptogenesis is associated with heightened arousal responses in fish. *Physiol. Behav.*, **40**, 617–624.

Laming, P. R., Cosby, S. L., and O'Neill, J. K. (1989). Seizures in the Mongolian gerbil are related to a deficiency in cerebral glutamine synthetase. *J. Comp. Biochem.Physiol.*, **94C**, 399–404.

Laming, P. R., Elwood, R. W., and Best, P. M. (1989). Epileptic tendencies in relation to behavioural responses to a novel environment in the Mongolian gerbil. *Behav. Neural Biol.*, **51**, 92–101.

Laming, P. R., Bullock, T. H., and McClune, M. (1991a). Changes in EEG power, acoustic evoked potentials and heart rate after mildly arousing non-acoustic priming stimulus in the carp, *(Cyprinus carpio). J. Comp. Biochem. Physiol.*, **100A**, 81–93.

Laming, P. R., Bullock, T. H., and McClune, M. (1991b). Sustained potential shifts and changes in acoustic evoked potentials after presentation of a non-acoustic stimulus to carp *(Cyprinus carpio). J. Comp. Biochem. Physiol.*, **100A**, 95–104.

Laming, P. R., Rooney, D. J., and Szabo, T. (1991). Arousal and epileptogenesis in the electric fish *(Gnathonemus petersii). J. Comp. Biochem. Physiol.*, **99A**, 405–409.

Laming, P. R., Ocherashvili, I. V., and Nicol, A. U. (1992). Dendritic and sustained shifts in potential to electrical stimulation of the anuran tectal surface. *J. Comp. Biochem. Physiol.*, **101A**, 91–96.

Laming, P. R., Ocherashvili, I. V., Nicol, A. U., Roughan, J. V., and Laming, B. A. (1995). Sustained potential shifts in the toad tectum reflect prey catching and avoidance behaviour. *Behav. Neurosci.*, **109**, 150–160.

Landau, E. M., Gavish, B., Nashen, D. A., and Latan, I. (1981). pH dependence of acetylcholine receptor channel. *J. Gen. Physiol.*, **77**, 647–666.

Lane, N. J. (1972). Fine structure of a lepidopteran nervous system and its accessibility to peroidase and lanthanum. *Z. Zellforsch. Mikroskop Anat.*, **131**, 205–222.

Lang, D. M., Rubin, B. P., Schwab, M. E., and Stuermer, C. A. O. (1995). CNS myelin and oligodendrocytes of the *Xenopus* spinal cord – but not optic nerve – are nonpermissive for axon growth. *J. Neurosci.*, **15**, 99–109.

Lang, M., Lang, W., Goldenberg, G., Podreka, I., and Deecke, L. (1987a). EEG and rCBF evidence for left fronto-cortical activation when memorizing verbal material. In *Current Trends in Event-Related Potential Research,* eds R. Johnson, J. W. Rohrbaugh, and R. Parasuraman, pp. 328–334. Amsterdam: Elsevier.

Lang, M., Lang, W., Uhl, F., Kornhuber, A., Deecke, L., and Kornhuber, H. H. (1987b). Slow negative potential shifts indicating verbal cognitive learning in a concept formation task. *Hum. Neurobiol.*, **6**, 183–190.

Lang, M., Lang, W., Podreka, I., Steiner, M., Uhl, F., Suess, E., Mueller, C., and Deecke, L. (1988). DC-potential shifts and regional cerebral blood flow reveal frontal cortex involvement in human visuomotor learning. *Exp. Brain Res.*, **71**, 353–364.

Lang, W., Lang, M., Uhl, F., Koska, Ch., Kornhuber, A., and Deecke, L. (1988). Negative DC shifts of supplementary and motor cortex preceding and accompanying simultaneous and sequential bimanual finger movements. *Exp. Brain Res.*, **71**, 579–587.

Lang, W., Zilch, O., Koska, C., Lindinger, G., and Deecke, L. (1989). Negative cortical DC shifts preceding and accompanying simple and complex sequential movements. *Exp. Brain Res.*, **74**, 99–104.

Lara, J. M., Alonso, J. R., Vecino, E., Coveñas, R., and Aijon, J. (1989). Neuroglia in the optic tectum of teleosts. *J. Hirnforsch.*, **30**, 465–472.

Larrabee, M. G. (1992). Extracellular intermediates of glucose metabolism: fluxes of endogenous lactate and alanine through extracellular pools in embryonic sympathetic ganglia. *J. Neurochem.*, **59**, 1041–1052.

Larrabee, M. G. (1995). Lactate metabolism and its effects on glucose metabolism in an excised neural tissue. *J. Neurochem.*, **64**, 1734–1741.

Larrabee, M. G., and Horowicz, P. (1956). Glucose and oxygen utilization in sympathetic ganglia I. Effects of anesthetics. II Substrates for oxidation at rest and in activity. In: Molecular structure and functional activity of nerve cells. *Publication No. 1 of Amer. Inst. Biol. Sci.*

Laurent, T. C., Preston, B. N., Pertoft, H., Gustafsson, B., and McCabe, M. (1975). Diffusion of linear polymers in hyaluronate solutions. *Eur. J. Biochem.*, **53**, 129–136.

Lavialle, M., and Serviere, J. (1993). Circadian fluctuations in GFAP distribution in the Syrian hamster suprachiasmatic nucleus. *NeuroReport*, **4**, 1243–1246.

Lavialle, M., and Serviere, J. (1995). Developmental study in the circadian clock of the golden hamster: a putative role of astrocytes. *Dev. Brain Res.*, **86**, 264–282.

Le Gal La Salle G., Rougon, G., and Valin, A. (1992). Embryonic form of NCAM in rat hippocampus: its re-expression on glial cells following kainic acid-induced status epilepticus. *J. Neurosci.*, **12**, 872–882.

Lee, K. S., Schottler, F., Oliver, M., and Lynch, G. (1980). Brief bursts of high-frequency stimulation produce two types of structural change in the hippocampus. *J. Neurophysiol.*, **44**, 247–258.

Leghissa, S. (1955). La struttura microscopica e la citoarchitettonica del tetto ottico dei pesci teleostei. *Z. Anat. Entwickl. Gesch.*, **118**, 427–463.

Lehmann, J. C., Kapkov, D., and Shank, R. P. (1993). Kinetics of 20-oxoglutarate uptake by synaptosomes from bovine and rat retina and cerebral cortex and regulation by glutamate and glutamine. *Dev. Neurosci.*, **15**, 330–335.

Lehmenkühler, A., Caspers, H., Speckmann, E.-J., Bingmann, D., Lipinski, H. G., and Kersting, U. (1988). Neurons, glia and ions in hypoxia, hypercapnia and acidosis. In *Mechanisms of Cerebral Hypoxia and Stroke*, ed. G. Somjen, pp. 153–164. New York: Plenum.

Lehmenkühler, A., Speckmann, E.-J., Walden, J., and Caspers, H. (1993a). Generation of cortical DC potentials under seizure conditions. In *Functions of Neuroglia. Proceedings of the International Symposium*, eds A. I. Roitbak, and E. V. Ocherashvili, pp. 177–182. Moscow: The Publishing House 'Kabur'.

Lehmenkühler, A., Syková, E., Svoboda, J., Zilles, K., and Nicholson, C. (1993b). Extracellular space parameters in the rat neocortex and subcortical white matter during postnatal development determined by diffusion analysis. *Neuroscience*, **55**, 339–351.

Lehre, K. P., Levy, L. M., Ottersen, O. P., Storm-Mathisen, J., and Danbolt, N. C. (1995). Differential expression of two glial glutamate transporters in the rat brain: quantitative and immunocytochemical observations. *J. Neurosci.*, **15**, 1835–1853.

Leibowitz, D. H. (1992). The glial spike theory. 1. On an active role of neuroglia in spreading depression and migraine. *Proc. Roy. Soc. Lond. B.*, **250**, 287–295.

Leng, G., Shibuki, K., and Way, S. A. (1988). Effects of raised extracellular potassium on the excitability of, and hormone release from, the isolated rat neurohypophysis. *J. Physiol.*, **399**, 591–605.

Lenhoff, H. M., and Schneiderman, H. A. (1959). The chemical control of feeding in the Portuguese man-of-war, *Physalia physalis*, and its bearing on the evolution of the Cnidaria. *Biol. Bull. Woods Hole*, **116**, 452–460.

Lentz, T. L., and Barrnett, R. J. (1965). Fine structure of the nervous system of *Hydra*. *Am. Zool.*, **5**, 341–356.

Lester, D., and Alkon, D. L. (1991). Activation of protein kinase C phosphorylation pathways: A role for storage of associative memory. *Prog. Brain Res.*, **89**, 235–248.

Lester, R. A. J., and Jahr, C. E. (1990). Quisqualate receptor-mediated depression of calcium currents in hippocampal neurons. *Neuron*, **4**, 741–749.

Lev-Ram, V., and Grinvald, A. (1986). Ca^{2+}- and K^+-dependent communication between central nervous system myelinated axons and oligodendrocytes revealed by voltage-sensitive dyes. *Proc. Natl Acad. Sci. USA*, **83**, 6651–6655.

Levi, G., and Gallo, V. (1995). Release of neuroactive amino acids from glia. In *Neuroglia*, ed. H. Kettenmann and B. R. Ransom, pp. 815–826. New York and Oxford: Oxford University Press.

Levy, L. M., Lehre, K. P., Rolstad, B., and Danbolt, N. C. (1993). A monoclonal antibody raised against an $[Na^+ + K^+]$coupled L-glutamate transporter purified from rat brain confirms glial cell localisation. *FEBS Lett.*, **317**, 79–84.

Libri, V., Giglio, A., and Nisticò, G. (1993). Evidence that nitric oxide modulates learning processes and memory in mice. *Pharmacol. Commun.*, **3**, 81–88.

Lickey, M. E., and Fox, S. S. (1966). Localisation and habituation of sensory evoked DC responses in cat cortex. *Exp. Neurol.*, **15**, 437–454.

Lieberman, E. M., Abbott, N. J., and Hassan, S. (1989). Evidence that glutamate mediates axon-to-Schwann cell signaling in the squid. *Glia*, **2**, 94–102.

Lieberman, E. M., Hargittani, P. T., and Grossfeld, R. M. (1994). Electrophysiological and metabolic interactions between axons and glia in crayfish and squid. *Progr. Neurobiol.*, **44**, 333–376.

Liepe, B. A., Stone, C., Koistinaho, J., and Copenhagen, D. R. (1994). Nitric oxide synthase in Müller cells and neurons of salamander and fish retina. *J. Neurosci.*, **14**, 7641–7654.

Linden, D. J. (1994). Long-term synaptic depression in the mammalian brain. *Neuron*, **12**, 457–472.

Liu, Y., Jia, W., Strosberg, A. D., and Cynader, M. (1993). Development and regulation of β-adrenergic receptors in kitten visual cortex: an immunocytochemical and autoradiographic study. *Brain Res.*, **632**, 274–286.

Livsey, C. T., Huang, B., Xu, J., and Karwoski, C. J. (1990). Light-evoked changes in extracellular calcium concentration in frog retina. *Vision Res.*, **30**, 853–861.

Lo, W. D., Wolny, A. C., Shin, D., and Hinkle G. H. (1993). Blood-brain barrier permeability and the brain extracellular space in acute cerebral inflammation. *J. Neurol. Sci.*, **118**, 188–193.

Lomneth, R., Medrano, S., and Gruenstein, E. I. (1990). The role of transmembrane pH gradients in the lactic acid induced swelling of astrocytes. *Brain Res.*, **523**, 69–77.

Longoni, B., Demontis, G. C., and Olsen, R. W. (1993). Enhancement of gamma aminobutyric acid receptor function and binding by the volatile anaesthetic halothane. *J. Pharmacol. Exp. Ther.*, **266**, 153–159.

Looren de Jong, H., Kok, A., and van Rooy, J. C. G. M. (1987). Electrophysiological indices of visual selection and memory search in young and old subjects. In *Current Trends in Event-Related Potential Research,* eds R. Johnson, J. W. Rohrbaugh, and R. Parasuraman, pp. 341–349. EEG Suppl., Vol. 40. Amsterdam: Elsevier.

López, T., López-Colomé, A. M., and Ortega, A. (1994). AMPA/KA receptor expression in radial glia. *NeuroReport*, **5**, 504–506.

López-Colomé, A. M., Murbartián, J., and Ortega, A. (1995). Excitatory amino acid-induced AP-1 DNA binding activity in Müller glia. *J. Neurosci. Res.*, **41**, 179–184.

Loskota, J. J., and Lomax, P. (1975). The Mongolian gerbil *(Meriones unguiculatus)* as a model for the study of the epilepsies: EEG records of seizures. *Electroenceph. Clin. Neurophysiol.*, **38**, 597–603.

Lothman, E. W., and Somjen, G.G. (1975). Extracellular potassium activity, intracellular and extracellular potential responses in the spinal cord. *J. Physiol.*, **252**, 115–136.

Loveless, N. E. and Sanford, A. J. (1973). The CNV baseline: Considerations of internal consistency of data. In *Event-Related Slow Potentials of the Brain: Their Relations to Behaviour,* eds W. C. McCallum and J. A. Knott, pp. 19–23. Electroenceph. Clin. Neurophysiol., Suppl. 33. Amsterdam: Elsevier.

Loveless, N. E, and Sanford, A. J. (1974). Slow potential correlates of preparatory set. *Biol. Psychol.*, **1**, 303–314.

Lu, J., Moreira, L. F., Hansen, E. L., Darrow, J. M., and Menaker, M. (1996). Morphological changes in CSN glial cells during the estrous cycle may affect phase shifts to light pulses. *Soc. Res. Biol. Rhythms Abstr.* 116.

Lundbaek, J. A., and Hansen, A. J. (1992). Brain interstitial volume fraction and tortuosity in anoxia. Evaluation of the ion-selective microelectrode method. *Acta Physiol. Scand.*, **146**, 473–484.

Luthi, A., Laurent, J. P., Figurov, A., Muller, D., and Schachner, M. (1994). Hippocampal long-term potentiation and neural cell adhesion molecules L1 and NCAM. *Nature,* **372**, 777–779.

Lutzenberger, W., Elbert, T., Rockstroh, B., and Birbaumer, N. (1979). The effects of self-regulation of slow cortical potentials on performance in a signal detection task. *Int. J. Neurosci.*, **9**, 175–183.

Lutzenberger, W., Birbaumer, N., Elbert, T., Rockstroh, B., Bippus, W., and Breidt, R. (1980). Self-regulation of slow cortical potentials in normal subjects and in patients with frontal lobe lesions. In *Motivation, Motor and Sensory Processes of the Brain:*

Electrical Potentials, Behavior and Clinical Use, eds H. H. Kornhuber and L. Deecke, pp. 427–430. Amsterdam: Elsevier.

Lutzenberger, W., Elbert, T., and Rockstroh, B. (1987). A brief tutorial on the implications of volume conduction for the interpretation of the EEG. *J. Psychophysiol.*, **1**, 81–89.

Lux, H. D., and Neher, E. (1973). The equilibration time course of $[K^+]_e$ in cat cortex. *Exp. Brain Res.*, **17**, 190–205.

Lux, H. D., Heinemann, U., and Dietzel, I. (1986). Ionic changes and alterations in the size of the extracellular space during epileptic activity. In *Advances in Neurology Vol.44. Basic Mechanisms of the Epilepsies: Molecular and Cellular Approaches*, eds A. V. Delgado-Escueta, A. A. Ward, D. M. Woodbury, and R. J. Porter, pp. 619–639. New York: Raven Press.

Lynn, R. (1966). *Attention, Arousal and the Orientation Reaction*. Oxford: Pergamon Press.

Lyons, S. A., Morell, P., and McCarthy, K. D. (1994). Schwann cells exhibit P(2Y) purinergic receptors that regulate intracellular calcium and are up-regulated by cyclic AMP analogues. *J. Neurochem.*, **63**, 552–560.

Lyons, S. M., Morrell, P., and McCarthy, K. D. (1995). Schwann cell ATP-mediated calcium increase in vivo and in situ are dependent on contact with neurons. *Glia*, **13**, 27–38.

Mackenzie, M. L., Ghabriel, M. N., and Allt, G. (1984). Nodes of Ranvier and Schmidt-Lanterman incisures: an in vivo lanthanum tracer study. *J. Neurocytol.*, **13**, 1043–1055.

MacVicar, B. A., and Tse, F. W. Y. (1988). Norepinephrine and cyclic adenosine $3':5'$-cyclic monophosphate enhance a nifedipine-sensitive calcium current in cultured rat astrocytes. *Glia*, **1**, 359–365.

MacVicar, B. A., Tse, F. W. Y., Crichton, S. A., and Kettenmann, H. (1989). GABA-activated C_l- channels in astrocytes in hippocampal slices. *J. Neurosci.*, **9**, 3577–3583.

MacVicar, W. C. (1985). Voltage-dependent calcium channels in glial cells. *Science*, **226**, 1345–1347.

Maggs, A., and Scholes, J. (1990). Reticular astrocytes in the fish optic nerve: macroglia with epithelial characteristics form an axially repeated lacework pattern, to which nodes of Ranvier are apposed. *J. Neurosci.*, **10**, 1600–1614.

Magistretti, P. J., and Pellerin, L. (1996). Cellular bases of brain energy metabolism and their relevance to functional brain imaging: evidence for a prominent role of astrocytes. *Cereb. Cortex*, **6**, 50–61.

Magistretti, P. J., Sorg, O., and Martin, J. L. (1993). Regulation of glycogen metabolism in astrocytes: physiological, pharmacological, and pathological aspects. In *Astrocytes: Pharmacology and Function*, ed. S. Murphy, pp. 243–265. San Diego: Academic Press.

Magistretti, P. J., Sorg, O., Yu, N., Martin, J.-L. and Pellerin, L. (1993). Neurotransmitters regulate energy metabolism in astrocytes: implications for the metabolic trafficking between neural cells. *Dev. Neurosci.*, **15**, 306–312.

Magistretti, P. J., Pellerin, L., and Martin, J.-L. (1995). An integrated cellular perspective. In *Psychopharmacology: The Fourth Generation of Progress*, eds F. E. Bloom and D. J. Kupfer, pp. 657–670. New York: Raven Press.

Mahowald, M., and Douglas, R. (1991). A silicon neuron. *Nature*, **354**, 515–518.

Majkowski, I., and Donadio, M. (1984). Electro-clinical studies of epileptic seizures in Mongolian gerbils. *Electroenceph. Clin. Neurophysiol.*, **57**, 369–377.

Malchow, R. P., Qian, H., and Ripps, H. (1989). γ-Aminobutyric acid (GABA)-induced currents of skate Müller (glial) cells are mediated by neuronal-like GABA$_A$ receptors. *Proc. Natl Acad. Sci. USA*, **86**, 4326–4330.

Malenka, R. C., Kauer, J. A., Perkel, D. J., Mauk, M. D., Kelly, P. T., Nicoll, R. A., and Waxham, M. N. (1989). An essential role for postsynaptic calmodulin and protein kinase activity in long-term potentiation. *Nature*, **340**, 554–557.

Malhotra, S. K., Shnitka, T. K., and Elbrink, J. (1990). Reactive astrocytes – review. *Cytobios.*, **61**, 133–160.

Manger, T. M., and Koeppen, B. M. (1992). Characterization of acidbase transporters in cultured outer medullary collecting duct cells. *Am. J. Physiol.*, **263**, F996–F1003.

Mann, R., Mulligan, R. C., and Baltimore, D. (1983). Construction of a retrovirus packaging mutant and its use to produce helper-free defective retrovirus. *Cell*, **33**, 153–159.

Maragos, W. F., Penny, J. B., and Young, A. B. (1988). Anatomic correlation of NMDA and ^{3}H-TCP-labeled receptors in rat brain. *J. Neurosci.*, **8**, 493–501.

Marcus, R. C., Blazeski, R., Godement, P., and Mason, C. A. (1995). Retinal axon divergence within the optic chiasm: uncrossed axons diverge from crossed fibers within a midline glial specialization. *J. Neurosci.*, **15**, 3716–3729.

Margolis, R. U., Aquino, D. A., Klinger, M. M., Ripellino, J. A., and Margolis, R. K. (1986). Structure and localization of nervous tissue proteoglycans. *Ann. NY Acad. Sci.*, **481**, 46–54.

Margraf, R. R., Wielt, D. B., Charniga, C. J., Linne, M. L., Kimelberg, H. K., and Jalonen, T. O. (1995). Serotonin affects sK$^+$$_{Ca}$ channel activity in rat cortical astrocytes. *Soc. Neurosci. Abstr.*, **21**, 1365.

Marrero, H., Astion, M. L., Coles, J. A., and Orkand R. K. (1989). Facilitation of voltage-gated ion channels in frog neuroglia by nerve impulses. *Nature*, **339**, 378–380.

Marshall, K. C., and Engberg, J. (1980). The effects of hydrogen ions on spinal neurons. *Can. J. Physiol. Pharmacol.*, **58**, 650–655.

Martin, A., Haxby, J. V., Lalonde, F. M., Wiggs, C. L., and Ungerleider, L. G. (1995). Discrete cortical regions associated with knowledge of color and knowledge of action. *Science*, **270**, 102–105.

Matthies, H. (1989). In search of cellular mechanisms of memory. *Prog. Neurobiol.*, **32**, 277–349.

Matthies, H. G., and Reymann, K. G. (1993). Protein kinase A inhibitors prevent the maintenance of hippocampal long-term potentiation. *NeuroReport*, **4**, 712–714.

Matute, C., and Miledi, R. (1993). Neurotransmitter receptors and voltage-dependent Ca^{2+} channels encoded by mRNA from the adult corpus callosum. *Proc. Natl Acad. Sci. USA*, **90**, 3270–3274.

Mayer, M. L., and Miller, R. J. (1990). Excitatory amino acid receptors, second messengers and regulation of intracellular Ca^{2+} in mammalian neurons. *TIPS*, **11**, 254–260.

Mazel, T., Roitbak, T., Šimonová, Z., Brichová, H., Harvey, A., and Syková, E. (1996). Morphology and diffusion parameters in rat brain during ageing. *Abstracts, Second Eur. Meeting on Glial Cell Function in Health and Disease*, p. 61.

McBain, C. J., Traynelis, S. F., and Dingledine, R. (1990). Regional variation of extracellular space in the hippocampus. *Science*, **249**, 674–677.

McCallum, W. C. (1988). Potentials related to expectancy, preparation and motor activity. In *Handbook of Electroencephalography and Clinical Neurophysiology, Vol. 3. Human Event-Related Potentials*, ed. T. W. Picton, pp. 427–534. Amsterdam: Elsevier.

McCallum, W. C., Cooper, R., and Pocock, P. V. (1988). Brain slow potential and ERP changes associated with operator load in a visual tracking task. *Electroenceph. Clin. Neurophysiol.*, **69**, 453–468.

McCarthy, K. D., and de Vellis, J. (1978). Alpha-adrenergic receptor modulation of beta-adrenergic, adenosine and prostaglandin E increased adenosine 3':5'-cyclic monophosphate levels in primary cultures of glia. *J. Cyclic Nucleotide Res.*, **4**, 15–26.

McCarthy, K. D., and de Vellis, J. (1980). Preparation of separate astroglial and oligodendroglial cell cultures from rat cerebral tissue. *J. Cell Biol.*, **85**, 890–902.

McCarthy, K. D., and Salm, A. K. (1991). Pharmacologically-distinct subsets of astroglia can be identified by their calcium response to neuroligands. *Neuroscience*, **41**, 325–333.

McCarthy, K. D., Prime, J., Harmon, T., and Pollenz, R. (1985). Receptor-mediated phosphorylation of astroglial intermediate filament proteins in cultured astroglia. *J. Neurochem.*, **44**, 723–730.

McCarthy, K. D., Enkvist, K., and Shao, Y. (1995). Astroglial adrenergic receptors: expression and function. In *Neuroglia*, eds H. Kettenmann and B.R. Ransom, pp. 354–366. New York, Oxford: Oxford University Press.

McCarthy, N. A., and O'Neil, R. G. (1992). Calcium signaling in cell volume regulation. *Physiol. Rev.*, **72**, 1037–1061.

McFarlane, C., Warner, D. S., and Dexter, F. (1995). Interactions between NMDA and AMPA glutamate receptor antagonists during halothane anaesthesia in the rat. *Neuropharmacology*, **34**, 659–663.

McGaugh, J. L. (1966). Time-dependent processes in memory storage. *Science*, **153**, 1351–1358.

McGaugh, J. L. (1990). Significance and remembrance: the role of neuromodulatory systems. *Psychol. Sci.*, **1**, 15–25.

McKenna, M. C., Tildon, J. T., Stevenson, J. H., and Kingwell, K. (1993). Regulation of astrocyte malic enzyme by metabolites. *Trans. Am. Soc. Neurochem.*, **24**, A54.

McKeon, R. J., and Silver, J. (1995). Functional significance of glial-derived matrix during development and regeneration. In *Neuroglia*, eds H. Kettenmann and B. R. Ransom, pp. 398–410. New York and Oxford: Oxford University Press.

McNeill, T. H., and Sladek, J. R., Jr. (1980). Simultaneous monoamine histofluorescence and neuropeptide immunocytochemistry: II. Correlative distribution of catecholamine varicosities and magnocellular neurosecretory neurons in the rat supraoptic and paraventricular nuclei. *J. Comp. Neurol.*, **193**, 1023–1033.

Mennerick, S., and Zorumski, C. F. (1994). Glial contributions to excitatory neurotransmission in cultured hippocampal cells. *Nature*, **368**, 59–62.

Merzenich, M. M., Kaas, J. H., Wall, J. T., Nelson, R. J., Sur, M., and Felleman, D. J. (1983). Topographic reorganization of somatosensory cortical areas 3b and 1 in adult monkeys following restricted deafferentation. *Neuroscience*, **8**, 3–55.

Meshul, C. K., and Seil, F. J. (1988). Transplanted astrocytes reduce synaptic density in the neuropil of cerebellar neurons. *Brain Res.*, **441**, 23–32.

Meshul, C. K., Seil, F. J., and Herndon, R. M. (1987). Astrocytes play a role in regulation of synaptic density. *Brain Res.*, **402**, 139–145.

Meucci, O., Fatatis, A , Holzwarth, J. A., and Miller, R. J. (1996). Developmental regulation of the toxin sensitivity of Ca^{2+}-permeable AMPA receptors in cortical glia. *J. Neurosci.*, **16**, 519–530.

Meyer, M. R., Reddy, G. R., and Edwards, J. S. (1987). Immunological probes reveal spa⁺ᴵ ᴵ ᴵ.ᴵᴵ developmental diversity in insect neuroglia. *J. Neurosci.*, **7**, 512–521.

Mi, H., Deerinck, T. J., Ellisman, M. H., and Schwarz, T. L. (1995). Differential distribution of closely related potassium channels in rat Schwann cells. *J. Neurosci.*, **15**, 3761–3774.

Mi, H., Deerinck, T. J., Jones, M., Ellisman, M. H., and Schwarz, T. L. (1996). Inwardly rectifying K^+ channels that may participate in K^+ buffering are localized in microvilli of Schwann cells. *J. Neurosci.*, **16**, 2421–2429.

Miller, J. D. (1993). On the nature of the circadian clock in mammals. *Am. J. Physiol.*, **264**, R821–R832.

Miller, P. D., Styren, S. D., Lagenaur, C. F., and DeKosky, S. T. (1994). Embryonic neural cell adhesion molecule (N-CAM) is elevated in the denervated rat dentate gyrus. *J. Neurosci.*, **14**, 4217–4225.

Miller, S., Bridges, R. J., and Cotman, C. W. (1993). Stimulation of phosphoinsitide hydrolysis by trans-(+/−)-ACPD is greatly enhanced when astrocytes are cultured in a serum-free defined medium. *Brain Res.*, **618**, 175–178.

Miller, S., Kesslak, J. P., Romano, C., and Cotman, C. W. (1995). Roles of metabotropic glutamate receptors in brain plasticity and pathology. *Ann. NY Acad. Sci.*, **757**, 460–474.

Minton, A. P., Colclasure, G. C., and Parker, J. C. (1992). Model for the role of macromolecular crowding in regulation of cellular volume. *Proc. Natl Acad. Sci. USA*, **89**, 10504–10506.

Minturn, J. E., Sontheimer, H., Black, J. A., Ransom, B. R., and Waxman, S. G. (1992). Sodium channel expression in optic nerve astrocytes chronically-deprived of axonal contact. *Glia*, **6**, 19–29.

Mitzdorf, U. (1985). Current source-density method and application in cat cerebral cortex: investigation of evoked potentials and EEG phenomena. *Physiol. Rev.*, **65**, 37–100.

Miyano, K., Tanifuji, Y., and Eger, E. (1993). The effect of halothane dose on striatal dopamine – An in vivo microdialysis study. *Brain Res.*, **605**, 342–344.

Mollace, V., Salvemini, D., Anggard, E., and Vane, J. (1990). Cultured astrocytoma cells inhibit platelet aggregation by releasing a nitric oxide-like factor. *Biochem. Biophys. Res. Commun.*, **172**, 564–569.

Monaghan, D. T., and Cotman, C. W. (1985). Distribution of N-methyl-D-aspartate-sensitive L-[3H]-glutamate-binding sites in rat brain. *J. Neurosci.*, **5**, 2909–2919.

Montgomery, D. L. (1994). Astrocytes: form, functions, and roles in disease. *Vet. Path.*, **31**, 145–167.

Moore, J. W., Joyner, R. W., Brill, M. H., Waxman, S. G., and Najar-Joa, M. (1978). Simulations of conduction in uniform myelinated fibres: relative sensitivity to changes in nodal and internodal parameters. *Biophys. J.*, **21**, 147–161.

Morga, E., and Heuschling, P. (1996). Interleukin-4 down-regulates MHC class II antigens on cultured rat astrocytes. *Glia*, **17**, 175–179.

Morita, M., and Best, J. B. (1966). Electron microscopic studies of planaria. III. Some observations on the fine structure of planarian nervous tissue. *J. Exp. Zool.*, **161**, 391–413.

Moscona, A. A. (1983). On glutamine synthetase, carbonic anhydrase and Müller glia in the retina. *Prog. Retinal Res.*, **2**, 111–35.

Movshon, J. A., and Van Sluyters, R. C. (1981). Visual neural development. *Annu. Rev. Psych.*, **32**, 477–522.

Mudrick-Donnan, L. A., Williams, P. J., Pittman, Q. P., and MacVicar, B.A. (1993). Postsynaptic potentials mediated by GABA and dopamine evoked in stellate glial cells of the pituitary pars intermedia. *J. Neurosci.*, **13**, 4660–4666.

Müller, C. M. (1990). Dark-rearing retards the maturation of astrocytes in restricted layers of cat visual cortex. *Glia*, **3**, 487–494.

Müller, C. M. (1992a). A role for glial cells in activity-dependent central nervous plasticity? Review and hypothesis. *Int. Rev. Neurobiol.*, **34**, 215–281.

Müller, C. M. (1992b). Astrocytes in cat visual cortex studied by GFAP and S-100 immunocytochemistry during postnatal development. *J. Comp. Neurol.*, **317**, 309–323.

Müller, C. M., and Best, J. (1989). Ocular dominance plasticity in adult cat visual cortex after transplantation of cultured astrocytes. *Nature*, **342**, 427–430.

Müller, C. M., Akhavan, A. C., and Bette, M. (1993). Possible role of S-100 in glia-neuronal signalling involved in activity-dependent plasticity in developing mammalian cortex. *J. Chem. Neuroanat.*, **6**, 215–227.

Müller, C. M., Faissner, A., and Altrogge, S. (1995). Transient tenascin immunoreactive boundaries during the development of functional layers in ferret lateral geniculate nucleus. *Soc. Neurosc. Abstr.*, **21**, 1796.

Müller, H. (1851). Zur Histologie der Netzhaut. *Z. Wissensch. Zool.*, **3**, 234–237.

Müller, T., Grosche, J., Ohlemeyer, C., and Kettenmann, H. (1993). NMDA activated currents in Bergmann glial cells from the mouse cerebellar slice hint to a distinct NMDA receptor. *NeuroReport*, **4**, 671–674.

Müller, T., Moller, T., Berger, T., Schnitzer, J., and Kettenmann, H. (1992). Calcium entry through kainate receptors and resulting potassium-channel blockade in Bergmann glial cells. *Science*, **256**, 1563–1566.

Munsch, T., and Deitmer, J. W. (1991). Intracellular pH modulates the input resistance of neuropile glial cells in the leech central nervous system. In *Synapse, Transmission, Modulation*, eds N. Elsner and H. Penzlin, p. 385. Stuttgart: Thieme Verlag.

Munsch, T., and Deitmer, J. W. (1992). Calcium transients in identified leech glial cells in situ evoked by high potassium concentrations and 5–hydroxytryptamine. *J. Exp. Biol.*, **167**, 251–265.

Munsch, T., and Deitmer, J. W. (1994). Sodium-bicarbonate cotransport current in identified leech glial cells. *J. Physiol.*, **474**, 43–53.

Muntz, K. H., Calianos, T. A., Buja, M., Willerson, J. T., Bernatowicz, M., Homcy, C. J., and Graham, R. M. (1988). Electron microscopic localization of the β-adrenergic receptor using a ferritim-alprenolol probe. *Mol. Pharmacol.*, **34**, 444–451.

Muresan, Z., and Besharse, J. C. (1993). D2–like dopamine receptors in amphibian retina: localization with fluorescent ligands. *J. Comp. Neurol.*, **331**, 149–160.

Murphy, K. J., O'Connell, A. W., and Regan, C. M. (1996). Repetitive and transient increases in hippocampal neural cell adhesion molecule polysialylation state following multi-trial spatial training. *J. Neurochem.*, **66**, S2–S17.

Murphy, S. (1993). *Astrocytes, Pharmacology and Function.* San Diego: Academic Press, Inc.

Murphy, S., and Pearce, B. (1987). Functional receptors for neurotransmitters on astroglial cells. *Neuroscience*, **22**, 381–394.

Murray, M. (1968). Effects of dehydration on the rate of proliferation of hypothalamic neuroglia cells. *Exp. Neurol.*, **20**, 460–468.

Murugaiyan, P., and Salm, A. K. (1995). Dehydration-induced proliferation of identifed pituicytes in fully adult rats. *Glia*, **15**, 65–76.

Naftolin, F., Leranth, C., Perez, J., and Garcia-Segura, L. M. (1993). Estrogen induces synaptic plasticity in adult primate neurons. *Neuroendocrinology.*, **57**, 935–939.

Nakamura, M., Ozawa, N., Shinba, T., and Yamamoto, K. (1993). CNV-like potentials on the cortical surface associated with conditioning in head-restrained rats. *Electroenceph. Clin. Neurophysiol.*, **88**, 155–162.

Nakhoul, N. L., Abdulnour, N., Akhoul, S., Khuri, R. N., Lieberman, E. M., and Hargittai, P. T. (1994). Intracellular pH regulation in rat Schwann cells. *Glia*, **10**, 155–164.

Narumi, S., Kimelberg, H. K., and Bourke, R. S. (1978). Effects of norepinephrine on the morphology and some enzyme activities of primary monolayer cultures from rat brain. *J. Neurochem.*, **31**, 1479–1490.

Naujoks-Manteuffel, C., and Roth, G. (1995). Neuroglia in adult amphibians. In *Neuron–Glia Interrelations During Phylogeny: II Plasticity and Regeneration*, eds A. Vernadakis and B. I. Roots, pp. 391–437. Totowa, NJ: Humana Press Inc.

Nauman, D. J. (1968). Open field behaviour of the Mongolian gerbil. *Psychonom. Sci.*, **10**, 163–164.

Neal, M. J., Cunningham, J. R., Shah, M. A., and Yazulla, S. (1972). Immunocytochemical evidence that vigabatrin in rat causes GABA accumulation in glial cells of the retina. *Neurosci. Lett.*, **98**, 29–32.

Neary, J. T., Rathbone, M. P., Cattabeni, F., Abbracchio, M. P., and Burnstock, G. (1996). Trophic actions of extracellular nucleotides and nucleosides on glial and neuronal cells. *TINS*, **19**, 13–18.

Nedergaard, M. (1994). Direct signalling from astrocytes to neurons in cultures of mammalian brain cells. *Science*, **263**, 1768–1771.

Newman, E. A. (1984). Regional specialization of retinal glial cell membrane. *Nature*, **309**, 155–157.

Newman, E. A. (1985a). Membrane physiology of retinal glial (Müller) cells. *J. Neurosci.*, **5**, 2225–2239.

Newman, E. A. (1985b). Voltage-dependent calcium and potassium channels in retinal glial cells. *Nature*, **317**, 809–11.

Newman, E. A. (1986a). High potassium conductance in astrocyte endfeet. *Science*, **233**, 453–454.

Newman, E. A. (1986b). Regional specialization of the membrane of retinal glial cells and its importance to K^+ spatial buffering. *Ann. NY Acad. Sci.*, **481**, 273–286.

Newman, E. A. (1986c). The Müller cell. In *Astrocytes, Vol.1*, eds S. Fedoroff and A. Vernadakis, pp. 149–171. New York: Academic Press Inc.

Newman, E. A. (1987). Distribution of potassium conductance in mammalian Müller (glial) cells. A comparative study. *J. Neurosci.*, **7**, 2423–2432.

Newman, E. A. (1991). Sodium-bicarbonate cotransport in retinal Müller (glial) cells of the salamander. *J. Neurosci.*, **11**, 3972–3983.

Newman, E. A. (1993). Inward-rectifying potassium channels in retinal glial (Müller) cells. *J. Neurosci.*, **13**, 3333–3345.

Newman, E. A. (1994). A physiological measure of carbonic anhydrase in Müller cells. *Glia*, **11**, 291–299.

Newman, E. A. (1995). Glial cell regulation of extracellular potassium. In *Neuroglia*, eds H. Kettenmann and B. R. Ransom, pp. 717–731. New York and Oxford: Oxford University Press.

Newman, E. A. (1996a). Acid efflux from retinal glial cells generated by sodium bicarbonate cotransport. *J. Neurosci.*, **16**, 159–168.

Newman, E. A. (1996b). Regulation of extracellular potassium and pH by polarized ion fluxes in glial cells: the retinal Müller cell. *The Neuroscientist*, **2**, 110–119.

Newman, E. A., and Astion, M. L. (1991). Localization and stoichiometry of electrogenic sodium bicarbonate cotransport in retinal glial cells. *Glia*, **4**, 424–8.

Newman, E. A., and Odette, L. L. (1984). Model of electroretinogram b-wave generation: a test of the K^+ hypothesis. *J. Neurophysiol.*, **51**, 164–182.

Newman, E. A., Frambach, D. A., and Odette, L. L. (1984). Control of extracellular potassium levels by retinal glial cell K^+ siphoning. *Science*, **225**, 1174–1175.

Ng, K. T., and Gibbs, M. E. (1991). Stages in memory formation: a review. In *Neural and Behavioural Plasticity: The Use of the Domestic Chick as a Model*, ed. R. J. Andrew, pp. 351–369. Oxford: Oxford University Press.

Ng, K. T., Gibbs, M. E., Crowe, S. F., Sedman, G. L., Hua F., Zhao, W., O'Dowd B. O., Rickard, N., Gibbs, C. L., Syková, E., Svoboda J., and Jendelová, P. (1991). Molecular mechanisms of memory formation. *Mol. Neurobiol.*, **5**, 333–350.

Ng, K. T., O'Dowd, B. S., Rickard, N. S., Robinson, S. R., Gibbs, M. E., Rainey, C., Zhao, W-Q., Sedman, G. L., and Hertz, L. (1997). Complex roles of glutamate in the Gibbs-Ng model of aversive learning in the new-born chick. *Neurosci. Bio–Behav. Rev.*, **21**, 45–54.

Nicholls, D., and Attwell, D. (1990). The release and uptake of excitatory amino acids. *TIPS*, **11**, 462–468.

Nicholls, J. G., and Kuffler, S. W. (1964). Extracellular space as a pathway for exchange between blood and neurons in the central nervous system of the leech: ionic composition of glial cells and neurons. *J. Neurophysiol.*, **27**, 645–673.

Nicholls, J. G., and Kuffler, S. W. (1965). Na and K content of glial cells and neurons determined by flame photometry in the central nervous system of the leech. *J. Neurophysiol.*, **28**, 519–525.

Nichols, R. A., Chilcote, T. J., Czernik, A. J., and Greengard, P. (1992). Synapsin I regulates glutamate release from rat brain synaptosomes. *J. Neurochem.*, **58**, 783–785.

Nicholson, C. (1980). Dynamics of the brain cell microenvironment. *Neurosci. Res. Prog. Bull.*, **18**, 177–322.

Nicholson, C. (1983). Regulation of the ion microenvironment and neuronal excitability. In *Basic Mechanisms of Neuronal Hyperexcitability*, eds H. M. Jasper and N. M. van Gelder, pp. 185–216. New York: Alan R. Liss, Inc.

Nicholson, C. (1985). Diffusion from an injected volume of a substance in brain tissue with arbitrary volume fraction and tortuosity. *Brain Res.*, **333**, 325–329.

Nicholson, C. (1992). Quantitative analysis of extracellular space using the method of TMA^+ iontophoresis and the issue of TMA^+ uptake. *Can. J. Physiol. Pharmacol.*, **70**, S314–S322.

Nicholson, C. (1993). Ion-selective microelectrodes and diffusion measurements as tools to explore the brain cell microenvironment. *J. Neurosci. Meth.*, **48**, 199–213.

Nicholson, C. (1995). Interaction between diffusion and Michaelis–Menten uptake of dopamine following iontophoresis in striatum. *Biophys. J.*, **68**, 1699–1715.

Nicholson, C., and Hounsgaard, J. (1983). Diffusion in the slice microenvironment and implications for physiological studies. *Fed. Proc.*, **42**, 2865–2868.

Nicholson, C., and Kraig, R. P. (1981). The behavior of extracellular ions during spreading depression. In *The Application of Ion-Selective Microelectrodes*, ed. T. Zeuthen, pp 217 238. Research Monographs in Cell and Tissue Physiology, 4. Amsterdam: Elsevier/North Holland.

Nicholson, C., and Phillips, J. M. (1981). Ion diffusion modified by tortuosity and volume fraction in the extracellular microenvironment of the rat cerebellum. *J. Physiol.*, **321**, 225–257.

Nicholson, C., and Tao, L. (1993). Hindered diffusion of high molecular weight compounds in brain extracellular microenvironment measured with integrative optical imaging. *Biophys. J.*, **65**, 2277–2290.

Nicholson, C., Ten Bruggencate, G., Steinberg, R., and Stöckle, H. (1977). Calcium modulation in brain extracellular microenvironment demonstrated with ion-selective micropipette. *Proc. Natl Acad. Sci. USA*, **74**, 1287–1290.

Nicholson, C., Phillips, J. M., and Gardner-Medwin, A. R. (1979). Diffusion from an iontophoretic point source in the brain. *Brain Res.*, **169**, 580–584.

Nicol, A. U., and Laming, P. R. (1992). Sustained potential shift responses and their relationship to the ECG response during arousal in the goldfish *(Carassius auratus)*. *J. Comp. Biochem. Physiol.*, **101A**, 517–532.

Nicol, A. U., and Laming, P. R. (1993). Sustained potential shifts, alterations in acoustic evoked potential amplitude and bradycardic responses to onset of illumination in the goldfish *(Carassius auratus)*. *J. Comp. Physiol.*, **173A**, 353–362.

Nicol, A. U., Savage, U. and Laming, P. R. (1993). The depth profile of electrically induced tectal SPS responses in the goldfish, *(Carassius auratus)*. *Behav. Neural Biol.*, **59**, 58–161.

Niedermeyer, E. (1982). Epileptic seizure disorders. In *Electroencephalography*, eds E. Niedermeyer and F. Lopes da Silva, pp. 339–428. Baltimore: Urban and Schwartzenburg.

Nielsen, C. (1995). *Animal Evolution: Interrelationships of the Living Phyla*. New York: Oxford University Press.

Nilius, B., and Reichenbach, A. (1988). Efficient K^+ buffering by mammalian retinal glial cells is due to cooperation of specialized ion channels. *Pflügers Arch.*, **411**, 654–660.

Nilsson, M., Hansson, E., and Ronnback, L. (1991). Adrenergic and $5-HT_2$ receptors on the same astroglial cell. A microspectrofluorimetric study on cytosolic Ca^{2+} responses in single cells in primary culture. *Dev. Brain Res.*, **63**, 33–41.

Nixdorf-Bergweiler, B. E., Albrecht, D., and Heinemann, U. (1994). Developmental changes in the number, size and orientation of GFAP-positive cells in the CA1 region of rat hippocampus. *Glia*, **12**, 180–195.

Noel, J., and Pouysségur, J. (1995). Hormonal regulation, pharmacology, and membrane sorting of vertebrate Na^+/H^+ exchanger isoforms. *Am. J. Physiol.*, **268**, C283–C296.

Norenberg, M. D., and Martinez-Hernandez, A. (1979). Fine structural localisation of glutamine synthetase in astrocytes of rat brain. *Brain Res.*, **161**, 303–310.

Northcutt, R. G., and Kaas, J. H. (1995). The emergence and evolution of mammalian neocortex. *TINS*, **18**, 373–379.

Nosten-Bertrand, M., Errington, M. L., Murphy, K. P. S. J., Tokugawa, Y., Barboni, E., Kozlova, E., Michalovich, D., Morris, R. G. M., Silver, J., Stewart, C. L., Bliss, T. V. P., and Morris, R. J. (1996). Normal spatial learning despite regional inhibition of LTP in mice lacking Thy-1. *Nature*, **379**, 826–829.

O'Connor, E. R., and Kimelberg, H. K. (1993). Role of calcium in astrocyte volume regulation and in the release of ions and amino acids. *J. Neurosci.*, **13**, 2638–2650.

O'Dowd, B. S. (1995). *Metabolic Activity in Astrocytes Essential for the Consolidation of One-Trial Passive Avoidance Memory in the Day-Old Chick*. Doctoral Dissertation. La Trobe University, Australia.

O'Dowd, B. S., Gibbs, M. E., Ng, K. T., Hertz, E. and Hertz, L. (1994a). Astrocytic glycogenolysis energizes intermediate memory processes in neonate chicks. *Dev. Brain Res.*, **78**, 137–141.

O'Dowd, B., Gibbs, M., Sedman, G., and Ng, K. T. (1994b). Astrocytes implicated in the energizing of intermediate memory processes in neonate chicks. *Cog. Brain Res.*, **2**, 93–102.

O'Dowd, B. S., Barrington, J., Ng, K. T., Hertz, E., and Hertz, L. (1995). Glycogenolytic response of primary chick and mouse cultures of astrocytes to noradrenaline across development. *Dev. Brain. Res.*, **88**, 220–223.

O'Leary, J. L., and Goldring, S. (1964). DC potentials in the brain. *Physiol. Rev.*, **44**, 91–125.

O'Rourke, N. A., Sullivan, D. P., Kaznowski, C. E., Jacobs, A. A., and McConnell, S. K. (1995). Tangential migration of neurons in the developing cerebral cortex. *Development*, **121**, 2165–2176.

Oakley, B. II., Katz, B. J., Xu, Z., and Zheng, J. B. (1992). Spatial buffering of extracellular potassium by Müller (glial) cells in the toad retina. *Exp. Eye Res.*, **55**, 539–550.

Obenchain, F. D. (1974). Structure and anatomical relationships of the synganglion in the American dog tick, *Dermacentor variabilis* (Acari: Ixodidae). *J. Morph.*, **142**, 205–223.

Ocherashvili, E., and Roitbak, A. (1992). Relationships between electrically induced slow negative potentials and changes in extracellular potassium concentrations in cerebral cortex of the cat. *Neurosci. Lett.*, **136**, 72–74.

Odette, L. L., and Newman, E. A. (1988). Model of potassium dynamics in the central nervous system. *Glia*, **1**, 198–210.

Ogston, A. G., and Sherman, T. F. (1961). Effects of hyaluronic acid upon diffusion of solutes and flow of solvent. *J. Physiol. (Lond.)*, **156**, 67–74.

Oland, L. A., and Tolbert, L. P. (1989). Patterns of glial proliferation during formation of olfactory glomeruli in an insect. *Glia*, **2**, 10–24.

Oland, L. A., Tolbert, L. P., and Mossman, K. L. (1988). Radiation-induced reduction of the glial population during development disrupts the formation of olfactory glomeruli in an insect. *J. Neurosci.*, **8**, 353–367.

Oland, L. A., Krull, C. E., and Tolbert, L. P. (1995). Glial cells play a key role in the construction of insect olfactory glomeruli. In *Neuron–Glia Interrelations During Phylogeny: II Plasticity and Regeneration*, eds A. Vernadakis and B. I. Roots, pp. 25–48. Totowa, NJ: Humana Press Inc.

Olds, J. L., Anderson, M. L, McPhie, D. L., Staten, L. D., and Alkon, D. L. (1989). Imaging of memory-specific changes in the distribution of protein kinase C in the hippocampus. *Science*, **245**, 866–869.

Oliet, S. H. R., and Bourque, C. W. (1994). Osmoreception in magnocellular neurosecretory cells: from single channels to secretion. *TINS*, **17**, 340–344.

Olmos, G., Naftolin, F., Perez, J., Tranque, P. A. and Garcia-Segura, L. M. (1989). Synaptic remodeling in the rat arcuate nucleus during the estrous cycle. *Neuroscience*, **32**, 663–667.

Onodera, K., and Takeuchi, A. (1979). An analysis of the inhibitory post-synaptic current in the voltage-clamped crayfish muscle. *J. Physiol.*, **286**, 265–282.

Onozuka, M., Kishii, K., Imai, S., and Ozono, S. (1987). Modification of the Na^+, K^+-pump of glial cells within cobalt-induced epileptogenic cortex of rat. *Brain Res.*, **420**, 259–267.

Orkand, P. M., Bracho, H., and Orkand, R. K. (1973). Glial metabolism: alteration by potassium levels comparable to those during neural activity. *Brain Res.*, **54**, 467–471.

Orkand, R. K. (1995). Effects of nerve impulses on glial membranes. In *Neuroglia*, eds H. Kettenmann and B. R. Ransom, pp. 460–470. New York and Oxford: Oxford University Press.

Orkand, R. K., Nicholls, J. G., and Kuffler, S. W. (1966). The effect of nerve impulses on the membrane potential of glial cells in the central nervous system of amphibia. *J. Neurophysiol.*, **29**, 788–806.

Osborne, N. N. (1993). Neuromediators and their receptors (adrenergic and endothelin types) in the eye. *Therapie*, **48**, 549–558.

Osborne, N. N., and Ghazi, H. (1989). The effect of substance P and other tachykinins on inositol phospholipid hydrolysis in rabbit retina, superior colliculus and retinal cultures. *Vision Res.*, **29**, 757–764.

Osborne, N. N., and Ghazi, H. (1990). Agonist-stimulated inositol phospholipid hydrolysis in the mammalian retina. *Prog. Retinal Res.*, **9**, 101–134.

Osorio, D. (1991). Patterns of function and evolution in the arthropod optic lobe. In *Evolution of the Eye and Visual System*, eds J. R. Cronly-Dillon and R. L. Gregory, pp. 203–228. London: Macmillan.

Otori, Y., Shimada, S., Tanaka, K., Ishimoto, I., Tano, Y., and Tohyama, M. (1994). Marked increase in glutamate-aspartate transporter (GLAST/GluT-1) mRNA following transient retinal ischemia. *Mol. Brain Res.*, **27**, 310–314.

Ottersen, O. P. (1989). Quantitative electron microscopic immunocytochemistry of neuroactive amino acids. *Anat. Embryol.*, **180**, 1–15.

Paalasmaa, P., Taira, T., Voipio, J., and Kaila, K. (1994). Extracellular alkaline transients mediated by glutamate receptors in the rat hippocampal slice are not due to a proton conductance. *J. Neurophysiol.*, **72**, 2031–2033.

Pannicke, T., Stabel, J., Heinemann, U., and Reichelt, W. (1994). Alpha-aminoadipic acid blocks the Na^+-dependent glutamate transport into acutely isolated Müller glial cells from guinea pig retina. *Pflügers Arch.*, **429**, 140–142.

Pannicke, T., Francke, M., Biedermann, B., Wiedemann, P., Faude, F., and Reichelt, W. (1995). Electrophysiological features of Müller glial cells from healthy and pathological human retina. *Soc. Neurosci. Abstr.*, **21**, 1071.

Pape, L., and Katzman, R. (1970). Effects of hydration on blood and cerebrospinal fluid osmolarities. *Proc. Soc. Exp. Biol. Med.*, **134**, 430–433.

Pappas, C. A., and Ransom, B. R. (1993). A depolarization-stimulated bafilomycin-inhibitable H^+ pump in hippocampal astrocytes. *Glia*, **9**, 280–291.

Pappas, C. A., and Ransom, B. (1994). Depolarization-induced alkalinization (DIA) in rat hippocampal astrocytes. *J. Neurophysiol.*, **72**, 2816–2826.

Pasternack, M., Bountra, C., Voipio, J., and Kaila, K. (1992). Influence of extracellular and intracellular pH to GABA-gated chloride conductance in crayfish muscle fibres. *Neuroscience*, **47**, 921–929.

Pastor, A., Chvátal, A., Syková, E., and Kettenmann, H. (1995). Glycine- and GABA-activated currents in identified glial cells of the developing rat spinal cord slice. *Eur. J. Neurosci.*, **7**, 1188–1198.

Paterson, J. A. and LeBlond, C. P. (1977). Increased proliferation of neuroglia and endothelial cells in the supraoptic nucleus and hypophysial neural lobe of young rats drinking hypertonic sodium chloride solution. *J. Comp. Neurol.*, **175**, 373–390.

Patterson, T. A., Elvarado, M. C., Warner, I. T., Bennett, E. L., and Rosenzweig, M. R. (1986). Memory stages and brain symmetry in chick learning. *Behav. Neurosci.*, **100**, 856–865.

Paylor, R., Rudy, J. W., and Wehner, J. M. (1991). Acute phorbol ester treatment improves spatial learning performance in rats. *Behav. Brain Res.*, **45**, 189–193.

Pearce, B. (1993). Amino acid receptors. In *Astrocytes. Pharmacology and Function*, ed. S. Murphy, pp. 47–66. Academic Press.

Pearce, B., and Murphy, S. (1993). Protein kinase C down-regulation in astrocytes: differential effects on agonist-stimulated inositol phosphate accumulation. *Neurochem. Int.*, **23**, 407–412.

Pearse, J. S., and Pearse, V. B. (1978). Vision in cubomedusan jellyfishes. *Science*, **199**, 458.

Pellerin, L., and Magistretti, P. J. (1994). Glutamate uptake into astrocytes stimulates aerobic glycolysis: a mechanism coupling neuronal activity to glucose utilization. *Proc. Natl Acad. Sci. USA*, **91**, 10625–10629.

Peng, L., and Hertz, L. (1993). Potassium induced stimulation of oxidative metabolism of glucose in cultures of intact cerebellar granule cells but not in corresponding cells with dendritic degeneration. *Brain Res.*, **629**, 331–334.

Peng, L., Juurlink, B. H. J., and Hertz, L. (1991). Differences in transmitter release, morphology and ischemia-induced cell injury between cerebellar granule cell cultures developing in the presence and in the absence of a depolarizing potassium concentration. *Dev. Brain Res.*, **63**, 1–12.

Peng, L., Schousboe, A., and Hertz, L. (1991). Utilization of α-ketoglutarate as a precursor for transmitter glutamate in cultured cerebellar granule cells. *Neurochem. Res.*, **16**, 29–34.

Peng, L., Hertz, L., Huang, R., Sonnewald, U., Petersen, S. B., Westergaard, N., Larsson, O, and Schousboe, A. (1993). Utilization of glutamine and of TCA cycle constituents as precursors for transmitter glutamate and GABA. *Dev. Neurosci.*, **15**, 367–377.

Peng, L., Zhang, X., and Hertz, L. (1994). High extracellular potassium concentrations stimulate oxidative metabolism in a glutamatergic neuronal culture and glycolysis in cultured astrocytes, but have no stimulatory effect in a GABAergic neuronal culture. *Brain Res.*, **663**, 168–172.

Peng, L., Juurlink, B. H. J., and Hertz, L. (1996). Pharmacological and developmental evidence that the potassium-induced stimulation of deoxyglucose uptake in astrocytes is a metabolic manifestation of increased Na^+, K^+-ATPase activity. *Dev. Neurosci.*, **18**, 357–359.

Peng, Y.-W., Blackstone, C. D., Huganir, R. L., and Yau, K.-W. (1995). Distribution of glutamate receptor subtypes in the vertebrate retina. *Neuroscience*, **66**, 483–497.

Pentreath, V. W. (1982). Potassium signalling of metabolic interactions between neurons and glia. *TINS*, **10**, 339–345.

Pentreath, V. W., Radojcic, T., Seal, L. H., and Winstanley, E. K. (1985). The glial cells and glia-neuron relations in the buccal ganglia of *Planorbis corneus* (L.): cytological, qualitative and quantitative changes during growth and ageing. *Phil. Trans. Roy. Soc. Lond. B*, **307**, 399–455.

Pentreath, V.W., Pennington, A. J., Seal, L. H., and Swift, K. (1987). Modulation by neuronal signals of energy substrate in the glial cells of the leech segmental ganglia. In *Glial–Neuronal Communication in Development and Regeneration*, eds H. H. Althaus and W. Seifert, pp. 211–229. *NATO ASJ. Ser.*, Ser. H 2.

Pérez-Pinzon, M. A., Tao, L., and Nicholson, C. (1995). Extracellular potassium, volume fraction, and tortuosity in rat hippocampal CA1, CA3 and cortical slices during ischemia. *J. Neurophysiol.*, **74**, 565–573.

Perkel, D. H., and Bullock, T. H. (1981). Neural coding. *Neuroscience Research Program Bulletin*, **6**, 221–348.

Perlmutter, L. S., Tweedle, C. D., and Hatton, G. I. (1984). Neuronal/glial plasticity in the supraoptic dendritic zone: dendritic bundling and double synapse formation at parturition. *Neuroscience*, **13**, 769–779.

Perlmutter, L. S., Tweedle, C. D., and Hatton, G. I. (1985). Neuronal/glial plasticity in the supraoptic dendritic zone in response to acute and chronic dehydration. *Brain. Res.*, **361**, 225–232.

Perouansky, M., Baranov, D., Salman, M., and Yaari, Y. (1995). Effects of halothane on glutamate receptor-mediated excitatory postsynaptic currents – a patch-clamp study in adult mouse hippocampal slices. *J. Anaesthesiol.*, **83**, 109–119.

Peters, A. (1966). The node of Ranvier in the central nervous system. *Q. J. Exp. Physiol.*, **51**, 229–236.

Peters, A., Palay, S. L., and Webster, H. deF. (1976). *The Fine Structure of the Nervous System. Neurons and Their Supporting Cells.* 3rd edition. New York, Oxford: Oxford University Press.

Peterson, G. M., and Ribak, C. E. (1987). Hippocampus of the seizure-sensitive gerbil is a specific site for anatomical changes in the GABAergic system. *J. Comp. Neurol.*, **261**, 405–422.

Peterson, G. M., Ribak, C. E., and Oertel, W. H. (1985). A regional increase in the number of hippacampal GABAergic neurons and terminals in the seizure sensitive gerbil. *Brain Res.*, **340**, 384–389.

Peyrethon, J. (1968). *Sommeil et evolution. Etude polygraphique des etats de sommeil chez les poissons et les reptiles,* pp. 1–102. Lyon: Tixier.

Pfeiffer, B., Grosche, J., Reichenbach, A., and Hamprecht, B. (1994). Immunocytochemical demonstration of glycogen phosphorylase in Müller (glial) cells in the mammalian retina. *Glia*, **12**, 62–67.

Pichon, Y., Abbott, N. J., Brown, E. R., Inoue, I., and Revest, P. A. (1995). Periaxonal ion regulation in the squid. In *Cephalopod Neurobiology*, eds N. J. Abbott, R. Williamson and L. Maddock, pp. 229–251. Oxford: Oxford University Press.

Pines, G., Danbolt, N. C., Björas, M., Zhang, Y., Bendahan, A., Eide, L., Koepsel, H., Storm-Mathisen, J., Seeberg, E., and Kanner, B. I. (1992). Cloning and expression of a rat brain L-glutamate transporter. *Nature*, **360**, 464–467.

Pini, A. (1993). Chemorepulsion of axons in the developing mammalian central nervous system. *Science*, **261**, 95–98.

Pirch, J. H. (1977). Amphetamine effects on brain slow potentials associated with discrimination in the rat. *Pharmacol. Biochem. Behav.*, **6**, 697–700.

Pirch, J. H. (1980). Effects of dextroamphetamine on event-related slow potentials in rat cortex during a reaction task. *Neuropharmacology*, **19**, 365–370.

Pirch, J. H., and Corbus, M. J. (1985). Conditioned cortical slow potential responses in urethane anaesthetised rats. *Int. J. Neurosci.*, **25**, 207–218.

Pirch, J. H., Corbus, M. J., and Rigdon, G. C. (1983). Single-unit and slow potential responses from rat frontal cortex during associative conditioning. *Exp. Neurol.*, **82**, 118–130.

Pirch, J. T., Turco, K., and Rucker, H. K. (1992). A role for acetylcholine in conditioning-related responses of rat frontal cortex neurons: microiontophoretic evidence. *Brain Res.*, **586**, 19–26.

Pirttilä, T. R. M., and Kauppinen, R. A. (1993). Extracellular pH and buffering power determine intracellular pH in cortical brain slices during and following hypoxia. *NeuroReport*, **5**, 213–216.

Pocock, G., and Richards, C. D. (1991). Cellular mechanisms in general anaesthesia. *Br. J. Anaesth.*, **66**, 116–128.

Poitry-Yamate, C. L., Poitry, S., and Tsacopoulos, M. (1995). Lactate released by Müller glia is metabolized by photoreceptors from mammalian retina. *Neuroscience*, **15**, 5179–5191.

Poitry-Yamate, C., and Tsacopoulos, M. (1991). Glial (Müller) cells take up and phosphorylate [^{3}H] 2-deoxy-D-glucose in a mammalian brain. *Neurosci. Lett.*, **122**, 241–244.

Porter, J. T., and McCarthy, K. D. (1995a). GFAP-positive hippocampal astrocytes in situ respond to glutamatergic neuroligands with increases in [Ca^{2+}]$_i$. *Glia*, **13**, 101–102.

Porter, J. T., and McCarthy, K. D. (1995b). Adenosine receptors modulate [Ca^{2+}]$_i$ in hippocampal astrocytes in situ. *J. Neurochem.*, **65**, 1515–1523.

Porter, J. T., and McCarthy, K. D. (1996). Hippocampal astrocytes in situ respond to glutamate released from synaptic terminal. *J. Neurosci.*, **16**, 5073–5081.

Porter, S., Blairclark, M., Glaser, L., and Bunge, R. P. (1986). Schwann cells stimulated to proliferate in the absence of neurons retain full functional capability. *J. Neurol. Science*, **6**, 3070–3078.

Potter, H. D. (1969). Structural characteristics of cell and fiber populations in the optic tectum of the frog (*Rana catesbeiana*). *J. Comp. Neurol.*, **136**, 203–232.

Potter, H. D. (1971). The distribution of neurofibrils coextensive with microtubules and neurofilaments in dendrites and axons of the tectum, cerebellum and pallium of the frog. *J. Comp. Neurol.*, **43**, 385–410.

Pow, D. V., and Crook, D. K. (1996). Direct immunocytochemical evidence for the transfer of glutamate from glial cells to neurons: use of specific antibodies directed against the D-stereoisomers of glutamate and glutamine. *Neuroscience*, **70**, 295–302.

Pow, D. V., and Morris, J. F. (1989). Dendrites of hypothalamic magnocellular neurons release neurohypophyseal peptides by exocytosis. *Neuroscience*, **32**, 435–439.

Pow, D. V., and Robinson, S. R. (1994). Glutamate in some retinal neurons is derived solely from glia. *Neuroscience*, **60**, 355–366.

Price, J., Turner, D., and Cepko, C. (1987). Lineage analysis in the vertebrate nervous system by retrovirus-mediated gene transfer. *Proc. Natl Acad. Sci. USA*, **84**, 156–160.

Prokopová, Š., Voříšek, I., and Syková, E. (1996). Diffusion parameters in myelinated and unmyelinated tissue. *Abstracts, Second European Meeting on Glial Cell Function in Health and Disease*, pp. 74–75.

Pullen, R. G., DePasquale, M., and Cserr, H. F. (1987). Bulk flow of cerebrospinal fluid into brain in response to acute hyperosmolality. *Am. J. Physiol.*, **253**, F538–F545.

Pumain, R., Menini, C., Heinemann, U., Lowel, J., and Silva-Barreat, C. (1985). Chemical synaptic transmission is not necessary for epileptic seizures to persist in the baboon (*Papio papio*). *Exp. Neurol.*, **89**, 250–258.

Puro, D. G. (1995). Growth factors and Müller cells. *Prog. Retinal Eye Res.* **15**, 89–101.

Puro, D. G., and Stuenkel, E. L. (1995). Thrombin-induced inhibition of potassium currents in human retinal glial (Müller) cells. *J. Physiol. (Lond.)*, **485**, 337–248.

Puro, D. G., Yuan, J. P., and Sucher, N. J. (1996). Activation of NMDA receptor-channels in human retinal Müller glial cells inhibits inward-rectifying potassium currents. *Visual Neurosci.*, **13**, 319–326.

Puro, D. G., Hwang, J.-J., Kwon, O.-J., and Chin, H. (1996). Characterization of an L-type calcium channel expressed by human retinal Müller (glial) cells. *Mol. Brain Res.*, **37**, 41–48.

Pysh, J. J. (1969). The development of the extracellular space in neonatal rat inferior colliculus: an electron microscopic study. *Am. J. Anat.*, **124**, 411–430.

Qian, H., Malchow, R. P., and Ripps, H. (1993). The effects of lowered extracellular sodium on γ-aminobutyric acid (GABA)-induced currents of Müller (glial) cells of the skate retina. *Cell. Mol. Neurobiol.*, **13**, 147–58.

Quastoff, S., Strupp, M., and Grafe, P. (1992). High conductance anion channel in Schwann cell vesicles from rat spinal roots. *Glia*, **5**, 17–24.

Quick, I. A., and Laming, P. R. (1990). Relationship between ECG, EEG and SPS responses during arousal in the goldfish *(Carassius auratus)*. *J. Comp. Biochem. Physiol.*, **95A**, 459–471.

Radojcic, T., and Pentreath, V. W. (1979). Invertebrate glia. *Prog. Neurobiol.*, **12**, 115–179.

Raff, M. C., Abney, E. R., Cohen, J., Lindsay, R., and Noble, M. (1983). Two types of astrocytes in cultures of developing rat white matter: differences in morphology, surface gangliosides, and growth characteristics. *J. Neurosci.*, **3**, 1289–1300.

Raff, R. A., Field, G. J., Olsen, S. J., Giovannoni, D. J., Lane, M. T., Ghiselin, M. T., Pace, N. R., and Raff, E. C. (1989). Metazoan phylogeny based on analysis of 18S ribosomal RNA. In *The Hierarchy of Life. Molecules and Morphology in Phylogenetic Analysis*, eds B. Fernholm, K. Brener, and H. Jörnvall, pp. 247–260. Amsterdam: Excerpta Medica/Elsevier.

Rakic, P. (1971a). Guidance of neurons migrating to the fetal monkey neocortex. *Brain Res.*, **33**, 471–476.

Rakic, P. (1971b). Neuron–glia relationship during granule cell migration in developing cerebellar cortex. A Golgi and electron microscopic study in *Macacus rhesus*. *J. Comp. Neurol.*, **141**, 283–312.

Ramakers, G. M., De Graan, P. N., Urban, I. J., Kraay, D., Tang, T., Pasinelli, P., Oestreicher, A. B., and Gispen, W. H. (1995). Temporal differences in the phosphorylation state of pre- and postsynaptic protein kinase C substrates B-50/ GAP-43 and neurogranin during long-term potentiation. *J. Biol. Chem.*, **270**, 13892–13898.

Ramcharan, E. J., and Matthews, M. R. (1996). Autoradiographic localization of functional muscarinic receptors in the rat superior cervical sympathetic ganglion reveals an extensive distribution over non-synaptic surfaces of neuronal somata, dendrites and nerve endings. *Neuroscience*, **71**, 797–832.

Ramon y Cajal, S. (1909). *Histologie du systeme nerveaux de l'homme et des vertebres*. Vol. 1. Paris: Maloine.

Ramon y Cajal, S. (1911). *Histologie du systeme nerveaux de l'homme et des vertebres*. Vol. 2. Paris: Maloine.

Ransom, B. R. (1992). Glial modulation of neural excitability mediated by extracellular pH: a hypothesis. In *Neuronal–Astrocytic Interactions*, eds A. C. H. Yu, L. Hertz , M. D. Noremberg, E. Syková, and S. Waxman. *Prog. Brain Res.*, **94**, 37–46.

Ransom, B. R. (1995). Gap junctions. In *Neuroglia*, eds H. Kettenmann and B. R. Ransom, pp. 299–318. New York and Oxford: Oxford University Press.

Ransom, B. R. and Carlini, W. J. (1986). Electrophysiological properties of astrocytes. In *Astrocytes*, Vol 2, *Biochemistry, Physiology and Pharmacology of Astrocytes*, eds S. Fedoroff and A. Vernadakis, pp. 1–49. Orlando: Academic Press.

Ransom, B. R., and Goldring, S. (1973a). Slow depolarisation in cells presumed to be glia in cerebral cortex of cat. *J. Neurophysiol.*, **36**, 879–892.

Ransom, B. R., and Goldring, S. (1973b). Ionic determinants of membrane potentials presumed to be glia in cerebral cortex of cat. *J. Neurophysiol.*, **36**, 855–868.

Ransom, B. R., Carlini, W. G., and Connors, B. (1986). Brain extracellular space: developmental studies in rat optic nerve. *Ann. NY Acad. Sci.*, **481**, 78–105.

Ransom, B. R., Greenwood, R. S., Goldring, S., and Letcher, F. S. (1977). The effect of barbiturate and procaine on glial and neuronal contributions to evoked cortical steady potential shifts. *Brain Res.*, **134**, 479–499.

Rebert, C. S. (1985). Components of cerebral systems mediating preparatory set and response to rare events. *Electroenceph. Clin. Neurophysiol.*, **61**, 78–79.

Rebert, C. S., Diehl, J. J., and Matteucci, M. J. (1993). The distribution and detection of brain slow potentials and their relationship to neuroglial activities and higher mental functions. In *Slow Potential Changes in the Human Brain*, eds W. C. McCallum and S. H. Curry, pp. 275–291. New York: Plenum Press.

Redburn, D. A., and Madtes, P. Jr. (1986). Postnatal development of ^{3}H-GABA-accumulating cells in rabbit retina. *J. Comp. Neurol.*, **243**, 41–57.

Reichelt, W., Dettmer, D., Brückner, G., Brust, P., Eberhardt, W., and Reichenbach, A. (1989). Potassium as a signal for both proliferation and differentiation of rabbit retinal (Müller) glia growing in cell culture. *Cell. Signaling*, 1, 187–194.

Reichelt, W., Hernandez, M., Damian, R. T., Kisaalita, W. S., and Jordan, B. L. (1996). GABA$_A$ receptor currents recorded from Müller glial cells of the baboon (*Papio cynocephalus*) retina. *Neurosci. Lett.*, **203**, 159–162.

Reichenbach, A. (1989). Glia: neuron index: review and hypothesis to account for different values in various mammals. *Glia*, **2**, 71–77.

Reichenbach, A. (1991). Glial K$^+$ permeability and CNS K$^+$ clearance by diffusion and spatial buffering. *Ann. NY Acad. Sci.*, **633**, 272–286.

Reichenbach, A., and Eberhardt, W. (1988). Cytotopographical specialization of enzymatically isolated rabbit retinal Müller (glial) cells: K$^+$ conductivity of the cell membrane. *Glia*, 1, 191–197.

Reichenbach, A., and Robinson, S. R. (1995a). Ependymoglia and ependymoglia-like cells. In *Neuroglia*, eds B. Ransom and H. Kettenmann, pp.58–84. New York – Oxford: Oxford University Press.

Reichenbach, A., and Robinson, S. R. (1995b). The involvement of Müller cells in the outer retina. In *Neurobiology and Clinical Aspects of the Outer Retina*, eds M. B. A. Djamgoz, S. N. Archer and S. Vallerga, pp. 395–416. London: Chapman and Hall.

Reichenbach, A., Hagen, E., Schippel, K., and Eberhardt, W. (1988). Quantitative electron microscopy of rabbit Müller (glial) cells in dependence on retinal topography. *Z. mikrosk.-anat. Forsch.*, **102**, 721–755.

Reichenbach, A., Schneider, H., Leibnitz, L., Reichelt, W., Schaaf, P., and Schümann, R. (1989). The structure of rabbit retinal Müller (glial) cells is adapted to the surrounding retinal layers. *Anat. Embryol.*, **180**, 71–79.

Reichenbach, A., Henke, A., Eberhardt, W., Reichelt, W., and Dettmer, D. (1992). K$^+$ regulation in retina. *Can. J. Physiol. Pharmacol.* **70** (Suppl.), S239–247.

Reichenbach, A., Stolzenburg, J.-U., Eberhardt, W., Chao, T. I., Dettmer, D., and Hertz, L. (1993). What do retinal Müller (glial) cells do for their neuronal 'small siblings'? *J. Chem. Neuroanat.*, **6**, 201–13.

Reichenbach, A., Fuchs, U., Kasper, M., El-Hifnawi, E., and Eckstein, A.-K. (1995). Hepatic retinopathy: morphological features of retinal (Müller) cells accompanying hepatic failure. *Acta Neuropathol.*, **90**, 273–281.

Reid, C. B., Liang, I., and Walsh, C. (1995). Systematic widespread clonal organization in cerebral cortex. *Neuron*, **15**, 299–310.

Reinecke, M. (1975). Die Gliazellen der Cerebralganglien von *Helix pomatia* L. (Gastropoda: Pulmonata). I Ultrastructur und Organisation. *Zoomorphologie*, **82**, 105–136.

Reist, N. E., and Smith, S. J. (1992). Neurally evoked calcium transients in terminal Schwann cells at the neuromuscular junction. *Proc. Natl Acad. Sci. USA*, **89**, 7625–7629.

Rentsch, F. J. (1979). Preretinal proliferation of glial cells after mechanical injury of the rabbit retina. *Albr. v. Graefe's Arch. klin. exp. Ophthalmol.*, **188**, 79–84.

Reuter, M., and Gustafsson, M. K. S. (1995). The flatworm nervous system: pattern and phylogeny. In *The Nervous Systems of Invertebrates: An Evolutionary and Comparative Approach*, eds O. Breidbach, and W. Kutsch, pp. 25–59. Basel, Switzerland: Birkhauser Verlag.

Reuter, M., Wikgren, M., and Palmberg, I. (1980). The nervous system of *Microstomum lineare* (Turbellaria, Macrostomida). I. A fluorescence and electron microscopic study. *Cell Tiss. Res.*, **211**, 31–40.

Rice, M. E., and Nicholson, C. (1995). Diffusion and ion shifts in the brain extracellular microenvironment and their reference for voltametric measurements. In *Neuromethods 27: Volumetric Methods in Brain Systems*, eds A. A. Boulton, G. B. Baker and R.N. Adams, pp. 27–79. Totowa, NJ: Humana Press.

Rice, M. E., Okada, Y., and Nicholson, C. (1993). Anisotropic and heterogeneous diffusion in the turtle cerebellum. *J. Neurophysiol.*, **70**, 2035–2044.

Richerson, G. B. (1995). Response to CO_2 of neurons in the rostral ventral medulla *in vitro*. *J. Neurophysiol.*, **73**, 933–944.

Richter, F., Wicher, C., Schmidt, D., Leichsenring, A., and Haschke, W. (1992). Activation state of the cortex could be changed by reinforcement of low-amplitude visual evoked potentials in rabbits. *Neurosci. Lett.*, **135**, 133–135

Rickard, N. S., and Ng, K. T. (1995). Blockade of metabotropic glutamate receptors prevents long-term memory consolidation. *Brain Res. Bull.*, **36**, 355–359.

Rickard, N. S., Ng, K. T., and Gibbs, M. E. (1994). A nitric oxide agonist stimulates consolidation of long-term memory in the 1–day old chick. *Behav. Neurosci.*, **108**, 640–644.

Rieger, R. M., Tyler, S., Smith III, J. P. S., and Rieger, G. (1991). Platyhelminthes: Turbellaria. In *Microscopic Anatomy of Invertebrates 3: Platyhelminthes and Nemertinea*, eds F. W. Harrison and B. J. Bogitsh, pp. 7–140. New York: Wiley-Liss Inc.

Rink, T. J., Tsien, R. Y., and Pozzan, T. (1982). Cytoplasmic pH and free Mg^{2+} in lymphocytes. *J. Cell Biol.*, **96**, 189–196.

Ritchie, J. M., and Rogart, R. B. (1977). The density of sodium channels in mammalian myelinated nerve fibers and the nature of the axonal membrane under the myelin sheath. *Proc. Natl Acad. Sci. USA*, **74**, 211–215.

Robert, A., and Jirounek, P. (1994). Uptake of potassium by nonmyelinating Schwann cells induced by axonal activity. *J. Neurophysiol.*, **72**, 2570–2579.

Robinson, I. C. A. F., and Coombes, J. E. (1993). Neurohypophysial peptides in cerebrospinal fluid: an update. *Ann. NY Acad. Sci.*, **689**, 269–284.

Robinson, S. R., Hampson, E. C. G. M., Munro, M. N., and Vaney, D. I. (1993). Unidirectional coupling of gap junctions between neuroglia. *Science*, **262**, 1072–1074.

Robinson, S. R., Lee, K. M., Rosa, M. G. P., Schmid, L. M., and Vaney, D. I. (1994). Selective blockade of Müller cell glutamine in cat retina causes ocular dominance shifts in visual cortex. *Abstr. Soc. Neurosci.*, **20**, 1575.

Robson, J. A., and Geisert, E. E. Jr. (1994). Expression of a keratin sulfate proteoglycan during development of the dorsal lateral geniculate nucleus in the ferret. *J. Comp. Neurol.*, **340**, 349–360.

Rockstroh, B., Lutzenberger, W., Elbert, T., and Birbaumer, N. (1988). Bilateral electrodermal and electrocortical activity in anticipating of sensorimotor tasks. *Psychophysiol.*, **9**, 185–192.

Rockstroh, B., Elbert, T., Canavan, A., Lutzenberger, W. and Birbaumer, N. (1989). *Slow Brain Potentials and Behavior* II. (2nd Edition). Baltimore: Urban and Schwarzenberg.

Rockstroh, B., Elbert, T., Birbaumer, N., and Lutzenberger, W. (1990). Biofeedback produced hemispheric asymmetry of slow cortical potentials and its behavioural effects. *Int. J. Psychophysiol.*, **9**, 151–165.

Rockstroh, B., Elbert, T., Birbaumer, N., Wolf, P., Düchting-Röth, A., Reker, M., Daum, I., Lutzenberger, W., and Dichgans, J. (1993). Cortical self-regulation in patients with epilepsies. *Epilepsy Res.*, **14**, 63–72.

Röder, B., Rösler, F., and Hennighausen, E. (1997). Different cortical activation patterns in blind and sighted human subjects during encoding and transformation of haptic images. *Psychophysiol.*, **34**, 292–307.

Röder, B., Rösler, F., Hennighausen, E., and Necker, F. (1996). Event-related potentials during auditory and somatosensory discrimination in sighted and blind human subjects. *Cog. Brain Res.*, **4**, 77–93.

Rodieck, R. W. (1988). The primate retina. In *Comparative Primate Biology, Vol. 4: Neurosciences*, pp. 203–278. New York: Alan R. Liss, Inc.

Roettger, V. R., and Goldfinger, M. D. (1991). HPLC-EC determination of free primary amino acid concentrations in cat cisternal cerebrospinal fluid. *J. Neurosci Meth.*, **39**, 263–270.

Rohde, K. (1970). Nerve sheath in *Multicotyle purvisi* Dawes. *Naturwissenschaften*, **57**, 502–503.

Rohde, K., and Webb, R. (1986). Ultrastructure of neuroglia in the peripheral nervous system of *Temnocephala* sp. (Turbellaria, Temnocephalida). *Zool. Anz.*, **216**, 53–57.

Roitbak, A. I. (1965). Slow negative potentials of the cortex and neuroglia (in Russian). In *The Modern Problems of the Physiology and Pathology of the Nervous System*, ed. V.V. Parin, pp. 68–93. Moscow: Meditsina.

Roitbak, A. I. (1983). *Neuroglia: Eigenschaften, Funktionen, Bedeutung*. Jena: Gustav Fischer Verlag.

Roitbak, A. I. (1988). Neuroglia: properties, functions and significance in nervous activity. *Sov. Sci. Rev.F. Physiol. Gen. Biol.*, **2**, 355–402.

Roitbak, A. I. (1993). *Glia and Its Role in Nervous Activity* (In Russian). Moscow: Nauka.

Roitbak, A. I., and Fanardjian, V. V. (1973). Intracellular potentials of cortical glial cells during electrical stimulation of the cortex. *Dokl. Akad. Nauk SSSR*, **211**, 748–751.

Roitbak, A. I., and Fanardjian, V. V. (1981). Depolarization of cortical glial cells in response to electrical stimulation of the cortical surface. *Neuroscience*, **6**, 2529–2537.

Roitbak, A. I., Fanardjian, V. V., Melkonyan, D. S., and Melkonyan, A. A. (1987). Contribution of glia and neurons to the surface-negative potentials of the cerebral cortex during its electrical stimulation. *Neuroscience*, **20**, 1057–1067.

Roitbak, A. I., Ocherashvili, I. V., Laming, P. R., and Roitbak, T. A. (1992). Stimulus-evoked sustained potential shifts and changes in $[K^+]$: of the frog optic tectum. *J. Comp. Physiol.*, **170A**, 327–333.

Ronn, L. C. B., Bock, E., Linnemann, D., and Jahnsen, H. (1995). NCAM-antibodies modulate induction of long-term potentiation in rat hippocampal CA1. *Brain Res.*, **677**, 145–151.

Ronnevi, L. O. (1978). Origin of glial processes responsible for the spontaneous postnatal phagocytosis of boutons on cat spinal motoneurons. *Cell Tiss. Res.*, **189**, 203–217.

Rooney, D. J., and Laming, P. R. (1986). Localisation of telencephalic regions concerned with habituation of cardiac and ventilatory resonses associated with arousal in the goldfish, *(Carassius auratus)*. *Behav. Neurosci.*, **100**, 45–50.

Rooney, D. J., and Laming, P. R. (1988). Effects of ablation of the goldfish telencephalon on short-term (within session) and long-term (between session) habituation of arousal responses. *Behav. Neural Biol.*, **49**, 83–96.

Roos, A., and Boron, W. F. (1981). Intracellular pH. *Physiol. Rev.*, **61**, 296–434.

Roots, B. I. (1978). A phylogenetic approach to the anatomy of glia. In *Dynamic Properties of Glia Cells*, eds E. Schofeniels, B. Franck, L. Hertz and D. B. Towers, pp. 45–54. New York: Pergamon Press.

Roots, B. I. (1984). Evolutional aspects of the structure and function of the nodes of Ranvier. In *The Node of Ranvier*, eds J. C. Zagoren, and S. Fedoroff, pp. 1–29. Orlando, FL: Academic Press.

Roots, B. I. (1986). Phylogenetic development of astrocytes. In *Astrocytes. Development, Morphology and Regional Specialization of Astrocytes,* Vol I, eds S. Fedoroff, and A. Vernadakis, pp. 1–34. Orlando, FL: Academic Press Inc.

Roots, B. I. (1993). The evolution of myelin. In *Advances in Neural Sciences*, Vol 1, ed. S. Malhotra, pp. 187–213. Greenwich: JAI Press Inc.

Roots, B. I. (1995). The evolution of myelinating cells. In *Neuron–Glia Interrelations During Phylogeny*, vol. 1, *Phylogeny and Ontogeny of Glial Cells*, eds A. Vernadakis and B. I. Roots, pp. 223–248. Totowa, N.J.: Humana Press.

Rose, C. R. (1993). Reizinduzierte extra- und intrazelluläre pH-Veränderungen im Zentralnervensystem des Blutegels *Hirudo medicinalis*. Dissertation, Universität Kaiserslautern, Germany.

Rose, C. R., and Deitmer, J. W. (1994). Evidence that glial cells modulate extracellular pH transients induced by neuronal activity in the leech central nervous system. *J. Physiol.*, **481**, 1–5.

Rose, C. R., and Deitmer, J. W. (1995a). Stimulus-evoked changes of extra- and intracellular pH in the leech central nervous system. I. Bicarbonate dependence. *J. Neurophysiol.*, **73**, 125–131.

Rose, C. R., and Deitmer, J. W. (1995b). Stimulus-evoked changes of extra- and intracellular pH in the leech central nervous system. II. Mechanisms and maintenance of pH homeostasis. *J. Neurophysiol.*, **73**, 132–140.

Rose, C. R., and Ransom, B. R. (1996a). Intracellular sodium homeostasis in rat hippocampal astrocytes. *J. Physiol.*, **491**, 291–305.

Rose, C. R., and Ransom, B. R. (1996b). Mechanisms of H^+ and Na^+ changes induced by glutamate, kainate, and D-aspartate in rat hippocampal astrocytes. *J. Neurosci.*, **16**, 5393–5404.

Rose, S. P. R. (1991). How chicks make memories, the cellular cascade from c-fos to dendritic remodelling. *TINS*, **14**, 390–397.

Rose, S. P. R., and Csillag, A. (1985). Passive avoidance training results in lasting changes in deoxyglucose metabolism in left hemisphere regions of chick brain. *Behav. Neural Biol.*, **44**, 315–325.

Rosenbluth, J. (1995). Glial membranes and axoglial junctions. In *Neuroglia*, eds H. Kettenmann and B. R. Ransom, pp. 613–633. New York and Oxford: Oxford University Press.

Rosenbluth, J., Hasegawa, M., Shirasaki, N., Rosen, C. L. and Liu, Z. (1990). Myelin formation following transplantation of normal fetal glia into myelin-deficient rat spinal cord. *J. Neurocytol.*, **19**, 718–730.

Rosenthal, K., and Sick, T. L. (1992). Glycolytic and oxidative metabolic contributions to potassium ion transport in rat cerebral cortex. *Can. J. Physiol. Pharmacol.*, **70**, 165–169.

Rosenzweig, M. R., Bennett, E. L., and Diamond, M. C. (1972). Chemical and anatomical plasticity in brain, replications and extensions. In *Macromolecules and Behavior*, ed. J. Gaito, pp. 205–278. New York: Appleton-Century-Crofts.

Rosewater, K., and Sontheimer, H. (1994). Fibrous and protoplasmic astrocytes express GABA$_A$ receptors that differ in benzodiazepine pharmacology. *Brain Res.*, **636**, 73–80.

Rosin, D. L., Zeng, D., Stornetta, R. L., Norton, F. R., Riley, T., Okusa, M. D., Guyenet, P. G., and Lynch, K. R. (1996). Immunohistochemical localization of alpha$_{2A}$-adrenergic receptors in catecholaminergic and other brainstem neurons in the rat. *Neuroscience*, **56**, 139–155.

Rösler, F., and Heil, M. (1991). A negative slow wave related to conceptual load which vanishes if the amount of load is increased? A reply to Ruchkin and Johnson. *Psychophysiology*, **28**, 363–364.

Rösler, F., Schumacher, G., and Sojka, B. (1990). What the brain reveals when it thinks. Event-related potentials during mental rotation and mental arithmetic. *German J. Psychol.*, **14**, 185–203.

Rösler, F., Heil, M., and Glowalla, U. (1993). Monitoring retrieval from long-term memory by slow event-related brain potentials. *Psychophysiology*, **30**, 170–182.

Rösler, F., Röder, B., Heil, M., and Hennighausen, E. (1993). Topographic differences of slow event-related brain potentials in blind and sighted adult human subjects during haptic mental rotation. *Cog. Brain Res.*, **1**, 145–159.

Rösler, F., Heil, M., and Hennighausen, E. (1995a). Distinct cortical activation patterns during long-term memory retrieval of verbal, spatial and color information. *J. Cog. Neurosci.*, **7**, 51–65.

Rösler, F., Heil, M., and Hennighausen, E. (1995b). Exploring memory functions by means of brain electrical topography, a review. *Brain Topogr.*, **7**, 301–313.

Rösler, F., Heil, M., Bajric, J., Pauls, A. C., and Hennighausen, E. (1995). Patterns of cerebral activation while mental images are rotated and changed in size. *Psychophysiology*, **32**, 135–150.

Ross, D. M., and Pantin, C. F. A. (1940). Factors influencing facilitation in Actinozoa. The action of certain ions. *J. Exp. Biol.*, **17**, 61–73.

Rothstein, J. D., Martin, L., Levey, A. I., Dykes-Hoberg, M., Jin, L., Wu, D., Nash, N., and Kuncl, R. W. (1994). Localization of neuronal and glial glutamate transporters. *Neuron*, **13**, 713–725.

Rothstein, J. D., Dykes-Hoberg, M., Pardo, C. A., Bristol, L. A., Jin, L., Kuncl, R. W., Kanai, Y., Hediger, M. A., Wang, Y. F., Schielke, J. P., and Welty, D. F. (1996). Knockout of glutamate transporters reveals a major role for astroglial transport in excitotoxicity and clearance of glutamate. *Neuron*, **16**, 675–686.

Roughan, J. V., and Laming, P. R. (1998). Epicortical slow potential shifts and sensory evoked potentials are related to seizure propensity in gerbils. *J. Comp. Physiol.*, in press.

Rougon, G. (1993). Structure, metabolism and cell biology of polysialic acids. *Eur. J. Cell Biol.*, **61**, 197–207.

Rousselet, A., Autillo-Touati, A., Araud, D., and Prochiantz, A. (1990). In vitro regulation of neuronal morphogenesis and polarity by astrocyte-derived factors. *Dev. Biol.*, **137**, 33–45.

Rowland, V. (1968). Cortical steady potential (direct current potential) in reinforcement and learning. In *Progress in Physiological Psychology*, eds E. Stellar and J. M. Sprague, pp 1–77. New York: Academic Press.

Rowland, V., Bradley, H., School, P., and Deutschman, D. (1967). Cortical steady potential shifts in conditioning. *Cond. Reflex.*, **2**, 3–22.

Rowland, V., Gluck, H., Sumergrad, S., and Dines, G. (1985). Slow and multiple unit potentials in trace and temporal conditioning controlled by electrical reward in the rat. *Electroenceph. Clin. Neurophysiol.*, **61**, 559–568.

Roy, M. L., and Sontheimer, H. (1995). β-adrenergic modulation of glial inwardly rectifying potassium channels. *J. Neurochem.*, **64**, 1576–1584.

Ruchkin, D. S., Johnson, R., Mahaffey, D., and Sutton, S. (1988). Toward a functional categorization of slow waves. *Psychophysiol.*, **25**, 339–353.

Rucker, H. K., Corbus, M. J., and Pirch, J. H. (1986). Discriminative conditioning-related slow potential and single-unit responses in the frontal cortex of urethane-anaesthetised rats. *Brain Res.*, **376**, 368–372.

Saint Marie, R. L., and Carlson, S. D. (1983). Glial membrane specializations and the compartmentalization of the lamina ganglionaris of the housefly compound eye. *J. Neurocytol.*, **12**, 243–275.

Saint Marie, R. L., Carlson, S. D., and Chi, C. (1984). The glial cells of insects. In *Insect Ultrastructure*, Vol. 2, eds R. C. King, and H. Akai. New York: Plenum Publishing Corp.

Sakatani, K., Black, J. A., and Kocsis, J. D. (1992). Transient presence and functional interaction of endogenous GABA and GABA$_A$ receptors in developing rat optic nerve. *Proc. Roy. Soc. Lond. B*, **247**, 155–161.

Sakatani, K., Hassan, Z., and Chesler, M. (1994). Effects of GABA on axonal conduction and extracellular potassium activity in the neonatal rat optic nerve. *Exp. Neurol.*, **127**, 291–297.

Salem, R. D., Hammerschlag, R., Bracho, H., and Orkand, R. K. (1975). Influence of potassium ions on accumulation and metabolism of ^{14}C-glucose by glial cells. *Brain Res.*, **86**, 499–503.

Salm, A. K., and McCarthy, K. D. (1989). Expression of beta-adrenergic receptors by astrocytes isolated from adult rat cortex. *Glia*, **2**, 346–352.

Salm, A. K., and McCarthy, K. D. (1992). The evidence for astrocytes as a target for central noradrenergic activity, expression of adrenergic receptors. *Brain Res. Bull.*, **29**, 265–275.

Salm, A. K., Modney, B. K., and Hatton, G. I. (1988). Alterations in supraoptic nucleus ultrastructure of maternally behaving virgin rats. *Brain Res. Bull.*, **21**, 685–691.

Salm, A. K., Smithson, K. G., and Hatton, G. I. (1995). Lactation associated redistribution of the glial fibrillary acidic protein within the supraoptic nucleus. *Cell Tissue Res.*, **242**, 9–15.

Sanderson, M. J., Charles, A. C., Boitano, S., and Dirksen, E. (1994). Mechanisms and function of intracellular calcium signaling. *Mol. Cell Endocrinol.*, **98**, 178–187.

Sapirstein, V. S., Strocchi, P., and Gilbert, J. M. (1984). Properties and function of brain carbonic anhydrase. *Ann. N.Y. Acad. Sci.*, **429**, 481–493.

Sarantis, M., and Attwell, D. (1990). Glutamate uptake in mammalian retinal glia is voltage- and potassium-dependent. *Brain Res.*, **516**, 322–325.

Sarantis, M., and Mobbs, P. (1992). The spatial relationship between Müller cell processes and the photoreceptor output synapse. *Brain Res.*, **584**, 299–304.

Sarthy, P. V. (1982). The uptake of (^{3}H) γ-aminobutyric acid by isolated glial (Müller) cells from the mouse retina. *J. Neurosci. Methods*, **5**, 77–82.

Sarthy, P. V. (1983). Release of (^{3}H) γ-aminobutyric acid from glial (Müller) cells of the rat retina, effects of K +, veratridine, and ethylenediamine. *J. Neurosci.*, **3**, 2494–2503.

Sarthy, P. V. and Lam, D. M. K. (1978). Biochemical studies of isolated glial (Müller) cells from the turtle retina. *J. Cell Biol.*, **78**, 675–684.

Saubermann, A. J., Castiglia, C. M., and Foster, M. C. (1992). Preferential uptake of rubidium from extracellular space by glial cells compared to neurons in leech ganglia. *Brain Res.*, **577**, 64–72.

Schell, M. J., Molliver, M. E., and Snyder, S. H. (1995). D-Serine, an endogeneous synaptic modulator, localization to astrocytes and glutamate stimulated release. *Proc. Natl Acad. Sci. USA*, **92**, 3948–3952.

Scherer, J., and Schnitzer, J. (1989). The rabbit retina, a suitable mammalian tissue for obtaining astroglia-free Müller cell cultures. *Neurosci. Lett.*, **97**, 51–56.

Schlaggar, B. L., and O'Leary, D. D. M. (1991). Potential of visual cortex to develop an array of functional units unique to somatosensory cortex. *Science*, **252**, 1556–1560.

Schmitt, F. O., and Samson, F. E. (1969). The brain cell microenvironment. *Neurosci. Res. Prog. Bull.*, **7**, 277–417.

Schmoll, D., Fuhrmann, E., Gebhardt, R., and Hamprecht, B. (1995a). Significant amounts of glycogen are synthesized from 3–carbon compounds in astroglial primary cultures from mice with participation of the mitochondrial phosphoenolpyruvate carboxykinase isoenzyme. *Eur. J. Biochem.*, **227**, 308–315.

Schmoll, D., Cesar, M., Fuhrmann, E., and Hamprecht, B. (1995b). Colocalization of fructose-1,6–biphosphatase and glial fibrillary acidic protein in rat brain. *Brain Res.*, **677**, 341–344.

Schneider, G.-H., Baethmann, A., and Kempski, O. (1992). Mechanisms of glial swelling induced by glutamate. *Can. J. Physiol. Pharmacol.*, **70**, S334–S343.

Schneider, F., Rockstroh, B., Heimann, H., Lutzenberger, W., Mattes, R., Elbert, T., Birbaumer, N., and Bartels, M. (1992a). Self-regulation of slow cortical potentials in psychiatric patients: depression. *Biofeedback Self-Reg.*, **17**, 277–292.

Schneider, F., Heimann, H., Mattes, R., Lutzenberger, W., and Birbaumer, N. (1992b). Self-regulation of slow cortical potentials in psychiatric patients: depression. *Biofeedback Self-Reg.*, **17**, 203–214.

Schneider, F., Elbert, T., Heimann, H., Welker, A., Stetter, F., Mattes, R., Birbaumer, N., and Mann, K. (1993). Self-regulation of slow cortical potentials in psychiatric patients, alcohol dependency. *Biofeedback Self-Reg.*, **18**, 23–32.

Schoepp, D. D., Bockaert, J., and Sladeczek, F. (1990). Pharmacological and functional characteristics of metabotropic excitatory amino acid receptors. *TIPS*, **11**, 508–515.

Schoepp, D. D., Johnson, B. G., and Monn, J. A. (1992). Inhibition of cyclic AMP formation by a selective metabotropic glutamate receptor agonist. *J. Neurochem.*, **58**, 1184–1186.

Schousboe, A. (1980). Primary cultures of astrocytes from mammalian brain as a tool in neurochemical research. *Cell. Mol. Neurobiol.*, **26**, 505–513.

Schousboe, A. (1981). Transport and metabolism of glutamate and GABA in neurons and glial cells. *Int. Rev. Neurobiol.*, **22**, 1–45.

Schousboe, A., Drejer, J., and Hertz, L. (1988). Uptake and release of glutamate and glutamine in neurones and astrocytes in primary cultures. In *Glutamine and Glutamate in Mammals*, Vol. 2, ed. E. Kvamme, pp. 21–38. Boca Raton: CRC Press.

Schousboe, A., Westgaard, N., Sonnewald, U., Petersen, S. B., Yu, A. C. H., and Hertz, L. (1992). Regulatory role of astrocytes for neuronal biosynthesis and homeostasis of glutamate and GABA. *Prog. Brain Res.*, **94**, 199–211.

Schousboe, A., Westergaard, N., Sonnewald, U., Petersen, S., Huang, R., and Hertz, L. (1993). Glutamate and glutamine metabolism and compartmentation in astrocytes. *Dev. Neurosci.*, **15**, 359–366.

Schurr, A., West, C.A., and Rigor, B. M. (1988). Lactate-supported synaptic function in the rat hippocampal slice preparation. *Science*, **240**, 1326–1328.

Schwab, M. E. (1995). Oligodendrocyte inhibition of nerve fiber growth and regeneration in the mammalian central nervous system. In *Neuroglia*, eds H. Kettenmann and B. R. Ransom, pp. 859–868. New York and Oxford: Oxford University Press.

Schwab, M. E., and Schnell, L. (1991). Channeling of developing rat corticospinal tract axons by myelin-associated neurite growth inhibitors. *J. Neurosci.*, **11**, 709–721.

Schwaninger, M., Blume, R., Oetjen, E., Lux, G., and Knepel, W. (1993). Inhibition of cAMP-responsive element-mediated gene transcription by cyclosporin A and FK506 after membrane depolarisation. *J. Biol. Chem.*, **268**, 23111–23115.

Schwartz, E. A. (1993). L-Glutamate conditionally modulates the K^+ current of Müller glial cells. *Neuron*, **10**, 1141–1149.

Schwartz, E. A., and Tachibana, M. (1990). Electrophysiology of glutamate and sodium co-transport in a glial cell of the salamander retina. *J. Physiol. (Lond.)*, **426**, 43–80.

Schwartz, J. P., and Nishiyama, N. (1994). Neurotrophic factor gene expression in astrocytes during development and following injury. *Brain Res. Bull.*, **35**, 403–407.

Schwiening, C. J., Kennedy, H. J., and Thomas, R. C. (1993). Calcium-hydrogen exchange by the plasma membrane Ca-ATPase of voltage-clamped snail neurons. *Proc. R. Soc. Lond. B*, **283**, 285–289.

Sedman, G., O'Dowd, B., Rickard, N., Gibbs, M. E., and Ng, K. T. (1992). Brain metabolic activity associated with long term memory consolidation. *Mol. Neurobiol.*, **5**, 351–354.

Seeburg, P. H. (1993). The molecular biology of mammalian glutamate receptor channels. *TINS*, **16**, 359–364.

Seil, F. J., Eckenstein, F. P., and Reier, P. J. (1992). Induction of dendritic spine proliferation by an astrocyte secreted factor. *Exp. Neurol.*, **117**, 85–89.

Seil, F., Meshul, C., and Herndon, R. (1988). Synapse regulation by transplanted astrocytes, a tissue culture study. *Prog. Brain Res.*, **78**, 395–399.

Sendtner, M. (1995). Growth factors and their receptors in the peripheral nervous system. In *Neuroglia*, ed. H. Kettenmann and B. R. Ransom, pp. 427–440. New York and Oxford: Oxford University Press.

Serafini, T., Kennedy, T. E., Galko, M. J., Mirzayan, C., Jessell, T. M., and Tessier-Lavigne, M. (1994). The netrins define a family of axon outgrowth-promoting proteins homologous to *C. elegans* UNC-6. *Cell*, **78**, 409–424.

Servit, Z. (1977). Phylogenesis and ontogenesis of the epileptic seizure. *World Neurol.*, **3**, 259–272.

Sesack, S. R., Aoki, C., and Pickel, V. M. (1994). Ultrastructural localization of D_2 receptor-like immunoreactivity in midbrain dopamine neurons and their striatal targets. *J. Neurosci.*, **14**, 88–106.

Shaefor, P. J., and Rowland, V. (1974). Dissociation of cortical steady potential shifts from mass action potentials in cats awaiting food rewards. *Physiol. Psychol.*, **2**, 471–480.

Shain, W., Forman, D. S., Madelian, V., and Turner, J. N. (1987). Morphology of astroglial cells is controlled by beta-adrenergic receptors. *J. Cell Biol.*, **105**, 2307–2314.

Shank, R. P., Bennett, G. S., Freytag, S. O., and Campbell, G. L. (1985). Pyruvate carboxylase, an astrocyte-specific enzyme implicated in the replenishment of amino acid neurotransmitter pools. *Brain Res.*, **329**, 64–367.

Shao, Y., and McCarthy, K. D. (1993). Regulation of astroglial responsiveness to neurogliands in primary culture. *Neuroscience*, **55**, 991–1001.

Shao, Y., Enkvist, K., and McCarthy, K. (1993). Astroglial adrenergic receptors. In *Astrocytes, Pharmacology and Function*, ed. S. Murphy, pp. 25–46. San Diego, New York, Boston, London, Sydney, Tokyo, Toronto: Academic Press, Harcourt Brace Jovanovich, Publishers.

Sheller, R. A., and Bittner, G. D. (1992). Maintenance and synthesis of proteins for an anucleate axon. *Brain Res.*, **580**, 68–80.

Sheller, R. A., Tytell, M., Smyers, M., and Bittner, G. D. (1995). Glia-to-axon communication: enrichment of glial proteins transferred to the squid giant axon. *J. Neurosci. Res.*, **41**, 324–334.

Shepard, R. N., and Cooper, L. A. (eds) (1982). *Mental Images and Their Transformations*. Cambridge, MA: MIT Press.

Shepherd, G. M. (1981). The nerve impulse and the nature of nervous function. In *Neurons Without Impulses*, eds A. Roberts and B. M. H. Bush, pp. 1–27. Cambridge, London: Cambridge University Press.

Sherrington, C. S. (1906). *The Integrative Action of the Nervous System*. New Haven: Yale University Press.

Sheu, F. S., McCabe, B. J., Horn, G., and Routtenberg, A. (1993). Learning selectively increases protein kinase C substrate phosphorylation in specific regions of the chick brain. *Proc. Natl Acad. Sci. USA*, **90**, 2705–2709.

Shibuki, K., Gomi, H., Lu, C., Bao, S., Kim, J., Wakatsuki, H., Fujisanki, T., Fujimoto, K., Katoh, A., Ikeda, T., Chen, C., Thompson, R., and Itohara, S. (1996). Deficient cerebellar long-term depression, impaired eye-blink conditioning, and normal motor coordination in GFAP mutant mice. *Neuron*, **16**, 587–599.

Shrager, P. (1989). Sodium channels in single demyelinated mammalian axons. *Brain Res.*, **483**, 149–154.

Shrode, L. D., and Putnam, R.W. (1994). Intracellular pH regulation in primary rat astrocytes and C6 glioma cells. *Glia*, **12**, 196–210.

Siesjö, B. K. (1978). *Brain Energy Metabolism*. New York: John Wiley.

Siesjö, B. K. (1985). Acid–base homeostasis in the brain: physiology, chemistry, and neurochemical pathology. In *Progress in Brain Research*, Vol. 63, eds K. Kogure, K. A. Hossman, B. K. Siesjo, and F. A. Welsh, pp. 121–154. Amsterdam: Elsevier.

Sillito, A. M. (1984). Functional considerations of the operation of GABAergic inhibitory processes in the visual cortex. In *Cerebral Cortex*, eds E. G. Jones and A. Peters, pp. 91–117. New York: Plenum Press.

Silver, J., and Robb, R. (1979). Studies on the development of the eye cup and optic nerves in normal mice and in mutants with congenital optic nerve aplasia. *Dev. Biol.*, **68**, 175–190.

Šimonová, Z., Svoboda, J., Orkand, P., Bernard, C. A., Lassmann, H., and Syková, E. (1996). Changes of extracellular space volume and tortuosity in the spinal cord of Lewis rats with experimental autoimmune encephalomyelitis. *Physiol. Res.*, **45**, 11–22.

Simons, R., and Riordan, J. R. (1990). Single base substitution in codon 74 of the *md* rat myelin proteolipid gene. *Ann. New York Acad. Sci.*, **605**, 146–154.

Sims, T. J., Gilmore, S. A., Waxman, S. G., and Klinge, E. (1985a). Dorsal–ventral differences in the glia limitans of the spinal cord: an ultrastructural study in developing normal and irradiated rats. *J. Neuropath. Exp. Neurol.*, **44**, 415–430.

Sims, T. J., Waxman, S. G., Black, J. A., and Gilmore, S. A. (1985b). Perinodal astrocytic processes at nodes of Ranvier in developing normal and glial cell deficient rat spinal cord. *Brain Res.*, **337**, 321–333.

Singer, W., and Lux, H. D. (1975). Extracellular potassium gradients and visual receptive fields in the cat striate cortex. *Brain Res.*, **96**, 378–383.

Singh, G., Janicki, P. K., Horn, J. L., Janson, V. E., and Franks, J. J. (1995). Inhibition of plasma- membrane Ca^{2+} ATPase pump activity in cultured C6 glioma cells by halothane and Xenon. *Life Sci.*, **56**, 219–224.

Singla, C. L. (1978). Fine structure of the neuromuscular system of *Polyorchis pencillatus* (Hydromedusae, Cnidaria). *Cell Tiss. Res.*, **193**, 163–174.

Singleton, P. A., and Salm, A. K. (1996). Differential expression of tenascin by astrocytes associated with the supraoptic nucleus (SON) of hydrated and dehydrated adult rats. *J. Comp. Neurol.*, **373**, 186–199.

Sirevaag, A. M., and Greenough, W. T. (1987). Differential rearing affects on rat visual cortex synapses. III. Neuronal and glial nuclei, boutons dendrites and capillaries. *Brain Res.*, **424**, 320–332.

Sirevaag, A. M., and Greenough, W. T. (1991). Plasticity of GFAP-immunoreactive astrocyte size and number in visual cortex of rats reared in complex environments. *Brain Res.*, **540**, 273–278.

Skatchkov, S. N., Vyklický, L., and Orkand, R. K. (1995). Potassium currents in endfeet of isolated Müller cells from the frog retina. *Glia*, **15**, 54–64.

Skatchkov, S. N., Vyklický, L., Clasen, T., and Orkand, R. K. (1996). Effect of cutting the optic nerve on K^+ currents in endfeet of Müller cells isolated from frog retina. *Neurosci. Lett.*, **208**, 81–84.

Skinner, J. E. (1978). A neurophysiological model for regulation of sensory input to cerebral cortex. In *Multidisciplinary Perspectives in Event-Related Brain Potential Research*, ed. D. A. Otto, pp. 616–625. Washington, DC: U.S. Environmental Protection Agency.

Skinner, J. E. (1984). Central gating mechanisms that regulate event-related potentials and behavior. In *Self-Regulation of the Brain and Behavior*, eds T. Elbert, B. Rockstroh, W. Lutzenberger and N. Birbaumer, pp. 42–55. Heidelberg: Springer.

Skinner, J. E., Reed, J. C., Welch, K. M. A., and Nell, J. H. (1978). Cutaneous shock produces correlated shifts in slow potential amplitude and cyclic 3'5'-adenosine monophosphate level in the parietal cortex of the conscious rat. *J. Neurochem.*, **30**, 699–704.

Smith, K. J., Blakemore, W. F., and McDonald, W. I. (1981). The restoration of conduction by central remyelination. *Brain*, **104**, 383–404.

Smith, K. J., Blakemore, W. F., and McDonald, W. I. (1983). Central remyelination restores secure conduction. *Nature*, **280**, 395–396.

Smith, S. E., Gottfried, J. A., Chen, J. C. T., and Chesler, M. (1994). Calcium dependence of glutamate receptor-evoked alkaline shifts in hippocampus. *NeuroReport*, **5**, 2441–2445.

Smith, S. J. (1992). Do astrocytes process neural information? In *Neuronal–Astrocytic Interactions*, eds A. C. H. Yu, L. Hertz , M. D. Norenberg, E. Syková, and S. Waxman. *Prog. Brain Res.*, **94**, 37–46.

Smithson, K. G., Suarez, I., and Hatton, G. I. (1990). Beta-adrenergic stimulation decreases glial and increases neural contact with the basal lamina in rat neurointermediate lobes incubated in vitro. *J. Neuroendocrinol.*, **2**, 693–699.

Sochocka, E., Juurlink, B. H., Code, W. E., Hertz, V., Peng, L., and Hertz, L. (1994). Cell death in primary cultures of mouse neurons and astrocytes during exposure to and 'recovery' from hypoxia, substrate deprivation and simulated ischaemia. *Brain Res.*, **638**, 21–28.

Sohal, R. S., Sharma, S. P., and Couch, E. F. (1972). Fine structure of the neural sheath, glia and neurons in the brain of the housefly, *Musca domestica. Z. Zellforsch. Mikrosk. Anat.*, **135**, 449–459.

Sokoloff, L. (1992). The brain as a chemical machine. In *Progress in Brain Research*, eds A. C. H. Yu, L. Hertz, M. D. Norenberg, E. Syková, and S. G. Waxman, pp. 94, 19–33, Amsterdam: Elsevier Science.

Sokoloff, L., Reivich, M., Kennedy, C., des Rosiers, M. H., Patlak, C. S., and Pettigrew, K. D., Sakurada, O., and Shinohara, M. (1977). The [^{14}C]deoxyglucose method for the measurement of local cerebral glucose utilization: theory, procedure, and normal values in the conscious and anesthetized albino rat. *J. Neurochem.*, **28**, 897–916.

Sokolov, E. N. (1963). Higher nervous functions: the orienting reflex. *Annu. Rev. Physiol.*, **25**, 545–580.

Somjen, G. G. (1967). Effects of general anaesthetics on spinal cord of mammals. *Anaesthesiology*, **28**, 135–143.

Somjen, G. G. (1973). Electrogenesis of sustained potentials. *Prog. Neurobiol.*, **1**, 199–237.

Somjen, G. G. (1975). Electrophysiology of neuroglia. *Annu. Rev. Physiol.*, **37**, 163–190.

Somjen, G. G. (1984). Interstitial ion concentration and the role of neuroglia in seizures. In *Electrophysiology of Epilepsy*, eds H. V. Wheal and P. A. Schwartzkran, pp. 301–341. New York: Academic Press.

Somjen, G. G. (1988). Nervenkitt: notes on the history of the concept of neuroglia. *Glia*, **1**, 2–9.

Somjen, G. G. (1993). Nervenkitt; Notes on the history of the concept of neuroglia. In *Functions of Neuroglia*, eds A. I. Roitbak and E. V. Ocherashvili, pp. 7–20. Moscow: Kabur.

Somjen, G. G. (1995). Electrophysiology of mammalian glial cells in situ. In *Neuroglia*, eds H. Kettenmann and B. R. Ransom, pp. 319–331. New York and Oxford: Oxford University Press.

Somjen, G. G., and Trachtenberg, M. (1979). Neuroglia as generators of extracellular current. In *Origin of Cerebral Field Potentials*, eds E.-J. Speckmann and H. Caspers, pp. 21–32. Stuttgart: George Thieme.

Somjen, G. G., Aitken, P. G., Giacchino, J. L., and McNamara, J. O. (1986). Interstitial ion concentrations and paroxysmal discharges in hippocampal formation and spinal cord. In *Advances in Neurology, Vol. 44.*, eds A. V. Delgado-Escueta, A. A. Ward, D. M. Woodbury and R. J. Porter, pp. 663–680. New York: Raven Press.

Sonnewald, U., Westergaard, N., Hassel, B., Muller, T. B., Unsgard, G., Fonnum, F., Hertz, L., Schousboe, A., and Petersen, S. B. (1993). NMR spectroscopic studies of ^{13}C-acetate and ^{13}C-glucose metabolism in neocortical astrocytes: evidence for mitochondrial heterogeneity. *Dev. Neurosci.*, **15**, 351–357.

Sontheimer, H. (1992). Astrocytes, as well as neurons, express a diversity of ion channels. *Can. J. Physiol. Pharmacol.*, **70** (Suppl.), S223–S238.

Sontheimer, H. (1995). Glial influences on neuronal signaling. *Neuroscientist*, **1**, 123–126.

Sontheimer, H., and Ritchie, J. M. (1995). Voltage-dependent sodium and calcium channels. In *Neuroglia*, eds H. Kettenmann and B. R. Ransom, pp. 202–220. New York and Oxford: Oxford University Press.

Sontheimer, H., Kettenmann, H., Backus, K. II., and Schachner, M. (1988). Glutamate opens Na$^+$/K$^+$ channels in cultured astrocytes. *Glia*, **1**, 328–336.

Sontheimer, H., Perouansky, M., Hoppe, D., Lux, H. D., Grantyn, R., and Kettenmann, H. (1989a). Glial cells of the oligodendrocyte lineage express proton-activated Na$^+$ channels. *J. Neurosci. Res.*, **24**, 496–500.

Sontheimer, H., Trotter, J., Schachner, M., and Kettenmann, H. (1989b). Channel expression correlates with differentiation stage during the development of oligodendrocytes from their precursor cells in culture. *Neuron*, **2**, 1135–1145.

Sontheimer, H., Black, J. A., and Waxman, S. G. (1996). Voltage-gated Na$^+$ channels in glia: properties and possible functions. *TINS*, **19**, 325–331.

Sorg, O., and Magistretti, P. J. (1991). Characterisation of the glycogenolysis elicited by vasoactive intestinal peptide, noradrenaline and adenosine in cultures of mouse cerebral cortex astrocytes. *Brain Res.*, **563**, 227–233.

Sorg, O., and Magistretti, P. J. (1992). Vasoactive intestinal peptide and noradrenaline exert long-term control on glycogen levels in astrocytes: blockade by protein synthesis inhibition. *J. Neurosci.*, **12**, 4923–4931.

Sotelo, C., and Palay, S. L. (1971). Altered axons and axon terminals in the lateral vestibular nucleus of the rat. Possible example of axonal remodelling. *Lab. Invest.*, **25**, 653–671.

Sotelo, C., Llinás, R., and Baker, R. (1974). Structural study of inferior olivary nucleus of the cat: morphological correlates of electrotonic coupling. *J. Neurophysiol.*, **37**, 541–559.

Soury, J. (1899). *Le Système Nerveux Central. Structure et Fonctions. Histoire Critique et des Doctrines*, 2 Vols. Paris: Carré et Naud.

Speckmann, E.-J., Caspers, H., and Elger, C. E. (1984). Neuronal mechanisms underlying the generation of field potentials. In *Self-Regulation of the Brain and Behavior,* eds T. Elbert, B. Rockstroh, W. Lutzenberger and N. Birbaumer, pp. 9–25. Berlin: Springer-Verlag.

Speckmann, E.-J., Caspers, H., and Janzen, R. W. C. (1972). Relations between cortical DC shifts and membrane potential changes of cortical neurons asosciated with seizure activity. In *Synchronization of EEG activity in Epilepsies,* ed. H. Petsche, pp. 93–111. New York: M.A.B. Brazier Springer.

Sperry, R. W. (1948). Orderly patterning of synaptic associations in regeneration of intracerebral fiber tracts mediating visuomotor coordination. *Anat. Rec.*, **102**, 63–75.

Squire, L. R. (1987). *Memory and Brain*. New York: Oxford Press.

Sretavan, D.W., and Shatz, C. J. (1986). Prenatal development of retinal ganglion cell axons: segregation into eye-specific layers within the cat's lateral geniculate nucleus. *J. Neurosci.*, **6**, 234–251.

Stamm, J. (1979). The monkey's prefrontal cortex functions in motoric programming. *Acta Neurobiol. Exp.*, **36**, 683–705.

Stamm, J. (1984). Performance enhancements with cortical negative slow potential shifts in monkey and man. In *Self-Regulation of the Brain and Behavior*, eds T. Elbert, B. Rockstroh, W. Lutzenberger and N. Birbaumer, pp. 199–215. Heidelberg: Springer.

Stamm, J., Birbaumer, N., Lutzenberger, W., Elbert, T., Rockstroh, B., and Schlottke, P. F. (1982). Event-related potentials during a continuous performance test vary with attentive capacities. In *Event Related Potentials in Children: Basic Concepts and Clinical Application*, ed. A. Rothenberger, pp. 273–294. Amsterdam: Elsevier.

Staub, F., Baethmann, A., Peters, J., Weigt, H., and Kempski, O. (1990). Effects of lactacidosis on glial cell volume and viability. *J. Cereb. Blood Flow Metab.*, **10**, 866–876.

Steinberg, R. H., Oakley, B., II, and Niemeyer, G. (1980). Light-evoked changes in $[K^+]_o$ in retina of intact cat eye. *J. Neurophysiol.*, **44**, 897–921.

Steindler, D. A., and Cooper, N. G. F. (1987). Glial and glycoconjugate boundaries during postnatal development of the central nervous system. *Dev. Brain Res.*, **36**, 27–38.

Steindler, D. A., Cooper, N. G. F., Faissner, A., and Schachner, M. (1989). Boundaries defined by adhesion molecules during development of the cerebral cortex: the J1/tenascin glycoprotein in the mouse somatosensory cortical barrel field. *Dev. Biol.*, **131**, 243–260.

Steinhäuser, C. (1993). Electrophysiologic characteristics of glial cells. *Hippocampus*, **3**, 113–124.

Steinhäuser, C., and Gallo, V. (1996). News on glutamate receptors in glial cells. *TINS*, **19**, 339–345.

Steinhäuser, C., Berger, T., Frotscher, M., and Kettenmann, H. (1992). Heterogeneity in the membrane current pattern of identified glial cells in the hippocampal slice. *Eur. J. Neurosci.*, **4**, 472–484.

Steinhäuser, C., Jabs, R., and Kettenmann, H. (1994). Properties of GABA and glutamate responses in identified glial cells of the mouse hippocampal slice. *Hippocampus*, **4**, 19–36.

Steinhäuser, C., Kressin, K., Kuprijanova, E., Weber, M., and Seifert, G. (1994). Properties of voltage-activated Na^+ and K^+ currents in mouse hippocampal glial cells in situ and after acute isolation. *Pflügers Arch.*, **428**, 610–620.

Stent, G. S. (1973). A physiological mechanism for Hebb's postulate of learning. *Proc. Natl Acad. Sci. USA*, **70**, 997–1001.

Stephens, G. J., Djamgoz, M. B., and Wilkin, G. P. (1993). A patch clamp study of excitatory amino acid effects on cortical astrocyte subtypes in culture. *Receptors Channels*, **1**, 39–52.

Stephenson, R. M., and Andrew, R. J. (1981). Amnesia due to β-antagonists in a passive avoidance task in the chick. *Pharmacol. Biochem. Behav.*, **15**, 597–604.

Steward, M. S., Bourne, R. C., and Gabbott, P. L. A. (1986). Decreased levels of the astrocytic marker, glial fibrillary acidic protein, in the visual cortex of dark-reared rats: measurements by enzyme-linked immunosorbent assay. *Neurosci. Lett.*, **63**, 147–152.

Stichel, C. C., Müller, C. M., and Zilles, K. (1991). Distribution of glial fibrillary acidic protein and vimentin immunoreactivity during rat visual cortex development. *J. Neurocytol.*, **20**, 97–108.

Stone, E. A., and Ariano, M. A. (1989). Are glial cells targets of the central noradrenergic system? A review of the evidence. *Brain Res. Rev.*, **14**, 297–309.

Stone, E. A., Bing, G., John, S. M., and Zhang, Y. (1992a). Cellular localisation of responses to catecholamines in brain tissue. *Brain Res.*, **94**, 303–307.

Stone, E. A., John, S. M., Bing, G., and Zhang, Y. (1992b). Studies on the cellular localization of biochemical responses to catecholamines in the brain. *Brain Res. Bull.*, **29**, 285–288.

Stone, E. A., Sessler, F. M., and Weimin, L. (1990). Glial localization of adenylate-cyclase-coupled β-adrenoceptors in rat forebrain slices. *Brain Res.*, **530**, 295–300.

Stone, S. E., and Colbjornsen, C. M. (1989). Effects of the glial toxin, fluorocitrate (FC), on the β-arenergic and dopaminergic cyclic AMP responses in rat brain. *FASEB J.*, **3**, A1201.

Strader, C. D., Pickel, V. M., Joh, T. H., Strohsacker, M. W., Shorr, R. G. L., Lefkowitz, R. J., and Caron, M. G. (1983). Antibodies to the β-adrenergic receptor: attenuation of catecholamine-sensitive adenylate cyclase and demonstration of postsynaptic receptor localization in brain. *Proc. Natl Acad. Sci. USA*, **80**, 1840–1844.

Strader, C. D., Sigal, I. S., Blake, A. D., Cheung, A. H., Register, R. B., Rands, E., Zerncik, B. A., Candelore, M. R., and Dixon, R. A. (1987). The carboxyl terminus of the hamster β-adrenergic receptor expressed in mouse L cells is not required for receptor sequestration. *Cell*, **49**, 855–863.

Strettoi, E., Raviola, E., and Dacheux, R. F. (1992). Synaptic connections of the narrow-field, bistratified rod amacrine cell (AII) in the rabbit retina. *J. Comp. Neurol.*, **325**, 152–168.

Stuermer, C. A. O. (1995). Glial cells and axonal regeneration in the central nervous system. In *Neuroglia*, ed. H. Kettenmann and B. R. Ransom, pp. 905–915. New York and Oxford: Oxford University Press.

Subbarao, K. V., and Hertz, L. (1990a). Effects of adrenergic agonists on glycogenolysis in primary cultures of astrocytes. *Brain Res.*, **536**, 220–226.

Subbarao, K. V., and Hertz, L. (1990b). Noradrenaline induced stimulation of oxidative metabolism in astrocytes but not in neurones in primary cultures. *Brain Res.*, **527**, 346–349.

Subbarao, K. V., and Hertz, L. (1991). Stimulation of energy metabolism by β-adrenergic agonists in primary cultures of astrocytes. *J. Neurosci. Res.*, **28**, 399–405.

Subbarao, K. V., Stolzenburg, J. U., and Hertz, L. (1995). Pharmacological characteristics of potassium-induced glycogenolysis in astrocytes. *Neurosci Lett.*, **196**, 45–48.

Sukhdeo, S. C., Sukhdeo, M. V. K., and Mettrick, D. F. (1988). Neurocytology of the cerebral ganglion of *Fasciola hepatica* (Platyhelminthes). *J. Comp. Neurol.*, **278**, 337–343.

Summy-Long, J. Y., Neumann, I., Terrell, M. L., Koehler, E., Mantz, S., Landgraf, R., and Kadekaro, M. (1994). Metabolic crosstalk in hypothalamic magnocellular nuclei during osmotic stimulation of one SON. *Brain Res. Bull.*, **33**, 645–654.

Suzuki, J., and Nakamota, Y. (1978). Sensory precipitatory epilepsy focus in El mice and Mongolian gerbils. *Folia Psychiatr. Neurol. Japan*, **32**, 349–353.

Suzuki, M., and Raisman, G. (1992). The glial framework of central white matter tracts: segmented rows of contiguous interfascicular oligodendrocytes and solitary astrocytes give rise to a continuous meshwork of transverse and longitudinal processes in the adult rat fimbria. *Glia*, **6**, 222–235.

Svoboda, J., and Syková, E. (1991). Extracellular space volume changes in the rat spinal cord produced by nerve stimulation and peripheral injury. *Brain Res.*, **560**, 216–224.

Svoboda, J., Motin, V., Hájek, I., and Syková, E. (1988). Increase in extracellular potassium level in rat spinal dorsal horn induced by noxious stimulation and peripheral injury. *Brain Res.*, **458**, 97–105.

Swann, J. W., and Brady, R. J. (1983). Penicillin-induced epileptogenesis in immature rat CA3 hippocampal pyramidal cells. *Dev. Brain Res.*, **12**, 243–254.

Swanson, R. A. (1992). Physiological coupling of glial glycogen metabolism to neuronal activity in brain. *Can. J. Physiol. Pharmacol.*, **70**, S138–S144.

Swanson, R. A., and Graham, S. H. (1994). Fluorocitrate and fluoroacetate effects on astrocyte metabolism in vitro. *Brain Res.*, **664**, 94–100.

Swanson, R. A., Morton, M. T., Sagar, S. M., and Sharp, F. R. (1992). Sensory stimulation induces local cerebral glycogenolysis: Demonstration by autoradiography. *Neuroscience*, **51**, 451–461.

Sweadner, K. J. (1992). Overlapping and diverse distribution of Na-K ATPase isozymes in neurons and glia. *Can. J. Physiol. Pharmacol.*, **70**, S255–S259.

Sweadner, K. J. (1995). Na,K-ATPase and its isoforms. In *Neuroglia*, ed. H. Kettenmann and B. R. Ransom, pp. 259–272. New York and Oxford: Oxford University Press.

Syková, E. (1983). Extracellular K^+ accumulation in the central nervous system. *Prog. Biophys. Mol. Biol.*, **42**, 135–189.

Syková, E. (1987). Modulation of spinal chord transmission by changes in extracellular K^+ activity and extracellular volume. *Can. J. Physiol. Pharmacol.*, **65**, 1058–1066.

Syková, E. (1992a). Ion-selective electrodes. In *Monitoring Neuronal Activity: A Practical Approach*, ed. J. Stamford, pp. 261–282. New York: Oxford University Press.

Syková, E. (1992b). Ionic and volume changes in the microenvironment of nerve and receptor cells. In *Progress in Sensory Physiology* 13, eds H. Autrum, D. Ottoson, E. R. Perl, R. F. Schmidt, H. Shimazu and W. D. Willis, pp. 1–167. New York: Springer-Verlag.

Syková, E. (1997). The extracellular space in CNS: its regulation, volume and geometry in normal and pathological neuronal function. *The Neuroscientist*, **3**, 334–347.

Syková, E., and Chvátal, A. (1993). Extracellular ionic and volume changes: the role of glia–neuron interaction. *J. Chem. Neuroanat.*, **6**, 247–260.

Syková, E., and Svoboda, J. (1990). Extracellular alkaline–acid–alkaline transients in the rat spinal cord evoked by peripheral stimulation. *Brain Res.*, **512**, 181–189.

Syková, E., Rothenberg, S., and Krekule, I. (1974). Changes of extracellular potassium concentration during spontaneous activity in the mesencephalic reticular formation of the rat. *Brain Res.*, **79**, 333–337.

Syková, E., Hník. P, and Vyklický, L. (1981). *Ion-Selective Microelectrodes and Their Use in Excitable Tissues*. New York and London: Plenum Press.

Syková, E., Jendelová, P., Svoboda, J., Sedman, G., and Ng, K. T. (1990). Activity-related rise in extracellular potassium concentration in the brain of 1–3-day-old chicks. *Brain Res. Bull.*, **24**, 569–575.

Syková, E., Jendelová, P., Šimonová, Z., and Chvátal A. (1992). K$^+$ and pH homeostasis in the developing rat spinal cord is impaired by early postnatal X-irradiation. *Brain Res.*, **594**, 19–30.

Syková, E., Šimonová, Z., and Svoboda, J. (1994). Increase of the extracellular volume fraction in spinal cord of rats with autoimmune encephalomyelitis. *Abstracts, 17th Ann. Meeting ENA, Vienna* 56.

Syková, E., Svoboda, J., Polák, J., and Chvátal, A. (1994a). Extracellular volume fraction and diffusion characteristics during progressive ischemia and terminal anoxia in the spinal cord of the rat. *J. Cereb. Blood Flow Metab.*, **14**, 301–311.

Syková, E., Lehmenkühler, A., Voříšek, I., Vargová, L., Škobisová, E., Kauder, C., and Nicholson, C. (1994b). Ischemic changes in [K$^+$]$_e$ and diffusion properties of neonatal and adult rat cortex. *Abstracts Society for Neurocience Meeting, Florida*, 20, p. 223.

Syková, E., Vargová, L., Šimonová, Z., and Nicholson, C. (1995). Effects of K$^+$, hypotonic solution, glutamate, AMPA and NMDA on diffusion parameters in isolated rat spinal cord during development. *Abstracts Society for Neuroscience Meeting*, 21, San Diego, p. 222.

Syková, E., Mazel, T., and Roitbak, T. (1996). Extracellular space diffusion parameters in the rat brain during ageing. *Abstracts Society for Neuroscience, Washington*, **22**, 1495.

Syková, E., Svoboda, J., Šimonová, Z., Lehmenkühler, A., and Lassmann, H. (1996). X-irradiation-induced changes in the diffusion parameters of the developing rat brain. *Neuroscience*, **70**, 597–612.

Szatkowski, M., and Attwell, D. (1994). Triggering and execution of neuronal death in brain ischaemia: two phases of glutamate release by different mechanisms. *TINS*, **17**, 359–365.

Szatkowski, M., and Schlue, W. R. (1994). Chloride-dependent pH regulation in connective glial cells of the leech nervous system. *Brain Res.*, **665**, 1–4.

Szatkowski, M., Barbour, B., and Attwell, D. (1990). Non-vesicular release of glutamate from glial cells by reversed electrogenic glutamate uptake. *Nature*, **348**, 443–446.

Szeligo, F., and LeBlond, C. P. (1977). Response of the three main types of glial cells of cortex and corpus callosum in rats handled during suckling or exposed to enriched control and impoverished environments following weaning. *J. Comp. Neurol.*, **172**, 247–264.

Szuchet, S. (1995). The morphology and ultrastructure of oligodendrocytes and their functional implications. In *Neuroglia*, eds H. Kettenmann and B. R. Ransom, pp. 23–43. New York and Oxford: Oxford University Press.

Taira, T., Smirnov, S., Voipio, J., and Kaila, K. (1993). Intrinsic proton modulation of excitatory transmission in rat hippocampal slices. *NeuroReport*, **4**, 93–96.

Takahashi, K. I., and Copenhagen, D. R. (1996). Modulation of neuronal function by intracellular pH. *Neurosci. Res.*, **24**, 109–116.

Takahashi, S., Driscoll, B. F., Law, M. J., and Sokoloff, L. (1995). Role of sodium and potassium ions in regulation of glucose metabolism in cultured astroglia. *Proc. Natl Acad. Sci. USA*, **92**, 4616–4620.

Takato, M., and Goldring, S. (1979). Intracellular marking with lucifer yellow CH and horseradish peroxidase of cells electrophysiologically characterized as glia in the cerebral cortex of the cat. *J. Comp. Neurol.*, **186**, 173–188.

Takenoshita, M. and Steinbach, J. H. (1991). Halothane blocks low-voltage-activated calcium current in rat sensory neurons. *J. Neurosci,* **11**, 1404–1412.

Takeuchi, A., and Takeuchi, N. (1967). Anion permeability of the inhibitory postsynaptic membrane of the crayfish neuromuscular junction. *J. Physiol.*, **205**, 377–391.

Tanabe, Y., Masu, M., Ishii, T., Shigemoto, R., and Nakanishi, S. (1992). A family of metabotropic glutamate receptors. *Neuron*, **8**, 169–179.

Tang, C. M., Dichter, M., and Morad, M. (1990). Modulation of the N-methyl-D-aspartate channel by extracellular H^+. *Proc. Natl Acad. Sci. USA*, **87**, 6445–6449.

Tang, C. M., Orkand, P.M., and Orkand, R.K. (1985). Coupling and uncoupling of amphibian neuroglia. *Neurosci. Lett.*, **54**, 237–242.

Tang, J., Landmesser, L., and Rutishauser, U. (1992). Polysialic acid influences specific pathfinding by avian motoneurons. *Neuron*, **8**, 1031–1044.

Tansey, F. A., Farooq, M., and Cammer, W. (1991). Glutamine synthetase in oligodendrocytes and astrocytes: new biochemical and immunocytochemical evidence. *J. Neurochem.*, **56**, 266–272.

Tao, L., and Nicholson, C. (1995). The three dimensional point spread functions of a microscope objective in image and object space. *J. Microsc.*, **178**, 267–271.

Tao, L., and Nicholson, C. (1996). Diffusion of albumins in rat cortical slices and relevance to volume transmission. *Neuroscience*, **75**, 839–847.

Tao, L., Vořišek, I., Lehmenkühler, A., Syková, E., and Nicholson, C. (1995). Comparison of extracellular tortuosity derived from diffusion of 3kDa dextran and TMA^+ in rat cortical slices. *Abstracts Society for Neuroscience, San Diego*, **21**, 604.

Tayler, M. J. (1978). Bereitschaftspotential during the acquisition of a skilled motor task. *Electroenceph. Clin. Neurophysiol.*, **45**, 568–576.

Teichberg, V. I. (1991). Glial glutamate receptors: likely actors in brain signalling. *FASEB J.*, **5**, 3086–3091.

Teresawa, S., and Timiras, P. (1968). Electrical activity during the estrous cycle of the rat: cyclic changes in limbic structures. *Endocrinology*, **83**, 207–216.

Theodosis, D. T., and Poulain, D. A. (1984). Evidence for structural plasticity in the supraoptic nucleus of the rat hypothalamus in relation to gestation and lactation. *Neuroscience*, **11**, 183–193.

Theodosis, D. T., and Poulain, D.A. (1993). Activity-dependent neuronal–glial and synaptic plasticity in the adult mammalian hypothalamus. *Neuroscience*, **57**, 501–535.

Theodosis, D. T., Poulain, D. A., and Vincent, J.-D. (1981). Possible morphological bases for synchronisation of neuronal firing in the rat supraoptic nucleus during lactation. *Neuroscience*, **6**, 919–929.

Theodosis, D. T., Rougon, G., and Poulain, D. A. (1991). Retention of embryonic features by an adult neuronal system capable of plasticity: polysialylated neural cell adhesion molecule in the hypothalamo-neurohypophysial system. *Proc. Natl Acad. Sci.*, **88**, 5494–5498.

Therianos, S., Leuzinger, S., Hirth, F., Goodman, C. S., and Reichert, H. (1995). Embryonic development of the *Drosophila* brain: formation of commissural and descending pathways. *Development*, **212**, 3849–3860.

Thiessen, D. D., Lindzey, G., and Friend, H. C. (1968). Spontaneous seizures in the Mongolian gerbil. *Psychonom. Sci.*, **11**, 227–228.

Thio, C. L., Waxman, S. G., and Sontheimer, H. (1993). Ion channels in spinal cord astrocytes in situ. III. Modulation of channel expression by co-culture with neurons and neuron-conditioned medium. *J. Neurophysiol.*, **69**, 819–831.

Thomas, R. C. (1984). Experimental displacement of intracellular pH and the mechanism of its subsequent recovery. *J. Physiol.*, **354**, 3P-22P.

Thomas, R. C., Coles, J. A., and Deitmer, J. W. (1991). Homeostatic muffling. *Nature*, **350**, 564.

Thompson, R. F., and Spencer, W. A. (1966). Habituation: a model phenomenon for the study of neural substrates of behaviour. *Psychol. Rev.*, **73**, 16–43.

Thomsen, C., Kristensen, P., Mulvihill, E., Haldeman, B., and Suzdak, P. D. (1992). L-2-Amino-4-phosphonobutyrate (L-AP4) is an agonist at the type IV metabotropic glutamate receptor which is negatively coupled to adenylate cyclase. *Eur. J. Pharmacol. Mol. Pharmacol. Sect.*, **227**, 361–362.

Tildon, J. T. (1993). Introduction. *Dev. Neurosci.*, **15**, 154–155.

Tildon, J. T., McKenna, M. C., Stevenson, J. H., and Couto, R. (1993). Transport of L-lactate by cultured rat brain astrocytes. *Neurochem. Res.*, **18**, 177–184.

Tinbergen, N. (1954). The origin and evolution of courtship and threat display. In *Evolution as a Process*, eds J. S. Huxley, A. C. Hardy and E. B. Ford, pp. 233–250. London: Allen and Unwin.

Ting. Y.L.-T., and Degani, H. (1993). Energetics and glucose metabolism in hippocampal slices during depolarization: ^{31}P and ^{13}C NMR studies. *Brain Res.*, **610**, 16–23.

Tiveron, M-C., Barboni, E., Rivero, E. B. P., Gormley, A. M., Seeley, P. J., Grosveld, F., and Morris, R. (1992). Selective inhibition of neurite outgrowth on mature astrocytes by Thy-1 glycoprotein. *Nature*, **355**, 745–748.

Tolbert, L. P., and Hildebrand, J. G. (1981). Organization and synaptic ultrastructure of glomeruli in the antennal lobes of the moth *Manduca sexta*: a study using thin sections and freeze-fracture. *Proc. R. Soc. Lond. B.*, **213**, 279–301.

Tolbert, L. P., and Oland, L. A. (1989). A role for glia in the development of organized neuropilar structures. *TINS*, **12**, 70–75.

Tolbert, L. P. and Oland, L. A. (1990). Glial cells form boundaries for developing insect olfactory glomeruli. *Exp. Neurol.*, **109**: 19–28.

Torp, R., Andine, P., Hagberg, H., Karagulle, T., Blackstad, T. W., and Ottersen, O. P. (1991). Cellular and subcellular redistribution of glutamate-, glutamine- and taurine-like immunoreactivities during forebrain ischemia: a semiquantitative electron microscopic study in rat hippocampus. *Neuroscience*, **41**, 433–447.

Tower, D. B. (1992). A century of neuronal and neuroglial interactions, and their pathological implications: an overview. In *Neuronal–Astrocytic Interactions*.

Implications for Normal and Pathological CNS Function, eds A. C. H. Yu, L. Hertz, M. D. Norenberg, E. Sykova, and S. G. Waxman, pp. 3–17. Amsterdam: Elsevier.

Tranque, P., Suarez, I., Olmos, G., Fernandez, B. and Garcia-Segura, L. (1987). Estradiol-induced redistribution of glial fibrillary acidic protein immunoreactivity in the rat brain. *Brain Res.*, **406**, 348–351.

Traynelis, S. F., and Cull-Candy, S. G. (1990). Proton inhibition of *N*-methyl-D-aspartate receptors in cerebellar neurons. *Nature*, **345**, 347–350.

Traynelis, S. F., and Cull-Candy, S. G. (1991). Pharmacological properties and H$^+$ sensitivity of excitatory amino acid receptor channels in rat cerebellar granule neurons. *J. Physiol.*, **433**, 727–763.

Traynelis, S. F., Hartley, M., and Heinemann, S. F. (1995). Control of proton sensitivity of the NMDA receptor by RNA splicing and polyamines. *Science*, **268**, 873–876.

Treherne, J. E., and Pichon, Y. (1972). The insect blood–brain barrier. *Adv. Insect Physiol.*, **9**, 257–313.

Trimmel, M., Streicher, F., Groll-Knapp, E., and Haider, M. (1989). Brain DC potentials during and following cued, sustained motor activity (muscle tension). *J. Psychophysiol.*, **3**, 349–359.

Trombley, P. Q., and Westbrook, G. L. (1992). L-AP4 inhibits calcium currents and synaptic transmission via a G-protein coupled glutamate receptor. *J. Neurosci.*, **12**, 2043–2050.

Tsacopoulos, H., Veuthey, A. L., Saravelos, S. G., Perrottet, P., and Tsoupras, G. (1994). Glial cells transform glucose to alanine which fuels the neurons in the honeybee retina. *J. Neurosci.*, **14**, 1339–1352.

Tsacopoulos, M. (1995). Metabolic exchanges and signal trafficking between glial cells and photoreceptor-neurons in the honey bee retina. *Verh. Dtsch. Zool. Ges.*, **88**, 53–59.

Tsacopoulos, M., and Magistretti, P. J. (1996). Metabolic coupling between glia and neurons. *J. Neurosci.*, **16**, 877–885.

Tsacopoulos, M., and Poitry, S. (1995). Metabolite exchanges and signal trafficking between glial cells and neurones in the insect retina. In *Neuron-Glial Relations During Phylogeny: II Plasticity and Regeneration*, eds A. Vernadakis and B. Roots, pp. 79–94. Totowa: Humana Press.

Tsacopoulos, M., Coles, J. A., and Van de Werve G. (1987). The supply of metabolic substrates from glia to photoreceptors in the retina of the honeybee drone. *J. Physiol. (Paris)*, **82**, 279–287.

Tsacopoulos, M., Evequoz-Mercier, V., Perrottet, P., and Buchner, E. (1988). Honeybee retinal glial cells transform glucose and supply the neurons with metabolic substrate. *Proc. Natl Acad. Sci. USA*, **85**, 8727–8731.

Tsumoto, T. (1990). Excitatory amino acid transmitters and their receptors in neural circuits of the cerebral cortex. *Neurosci. Res.*, **9**, 79–102.

Turner, A. M., and Greenough W. T. (1985). Differential rearing effects on rat visual cortex synapses. I. Synaptic and neuronal density and synapse per neuron. *Brain Res.*, **329**, 195–203.

Tweedle, C. D., and Hatton, G. I. (1976). Ultrastructural comparisons of neurons of supraoptic and circularis nuclei in normal and dehydrated rats. *Brain Res. Bull.*, **1**, 103–121.

Tweedle, C. D., and Hatton, G. I. (1977). Ultrastructural changes in rat hypothalamic neurosecretory cells and their associative glia during minimal dehydration and rehydration. *Cell Tissue Res.*, **181**, 59–72.

Tweedle, C. D., and Hatton, G. I. (1980). Evidence for dynamic interactions between pituicytes and neurosecretory axons in the rat. *Neuroscience*, **5**, 661–667.

Uchihori, Y., and Puro, D. G. (1993). Glutamate as a neuron-to-glial signal for mitogenesis – role of glial *N*-methyl-D-aspartate receptors. *Brain Res.*, **613**, 212–220.

Uga, S., and Smelser, G. K. (1973). Comparative study of the fine structure of retinal Müller cells in various vertebrates. *Invest. Ophthalmol.*, **12**, 434–448.

Uhl, F., Lang, W., Lang, M., Kornhuber, A., and Deecke, L. (1990). DC potential evidence for bilateral symmetrical frontal activation in non-verbal associative learning. *J. Psychophysiol.*, **4**, 241–248.

Utzschneider, D., Black, J. A., and Kocsis, J. D. (1992). Conduction properties of spinal cord axons in the myelin-deficient rat mutant. *Neuroscience*, **49**, 221–228.

Utzschneider, D. A., Archer, D. R., Duncan, I. R., Waxman, S. G. and Kocsis, J. D. (1994). Transplantation of myelin-forming cells enhances impulse conduction in amyelinated spinal cord axons in the myelin-deficient rat. *Proc. Natl Acad. Sci.*, **91**, 53–57.

Uyeda, C. T., Eng, L. F., and Bignami, A. (1972). Immunological study of the glial fibrillary acidic protein. *Brain Res.*, **37**, 81–89.

Van Calker, D., and Hamprecht, B. (1980). Effects of neurohormones on glial cells. In *Advances in Cellular Neurobiology*, eds S. Fedoroff and L. Hertz, pp. 31–67. New York: Academic Press.

Van Calker, D., Muller, M., and Hamprecht, B. (1979). Adenosine regulates via two different types of receptors, the accumulation of cyclic AMP in cultured brain cells. *J. Neurochem.*, **33**, 999–1005.

Van den Pol, A. N. (1980). The hypothalamic suprachiasmatic nucleus of rat: intrinsic anatomy. *J. Comp. Neurol.*, **191**, 661–702.

Van den Pol, A. N., and Dudek, F. E. (1993). Cellular communication in the circadian clock, the suprachiasmatic nucleus. *Neuroscience*, **56**, 793–811.

Van den Pol, A. N., Finkbeiner, S., and Cornell-Bell, A. H. (1992). Calcium excitability and oscillations in suprachiasmatic nucleus neurons and glia in vitro. *J. Neurosci.*, **12**, 2648–2664.

Van den Pol, A. N., Romano, C., and Ghosh, P. (1995). Metabotropic glutamate receptor mGluR5 subcellular distribution and developmental expression in hypothalamus. *J. Comp. Neurol.*, **362**, 134–150.

Van der Toorn, A., Syková, E., Dijkhuisen, R. M., Voříšek I., Vargová, L., Škobisová, E., van Lookeren Campagne, M., Reese, T., and Nicolay, K. (1996). Dynamic changes in water ADC, energy metabolism, extracellular space volume and tortuosity in neonatal rat brain during terminal anoxia. *Magnetic Resonance in Medicine*, **36**, 52–60.

Van der Zee, E. A., De Jong, G. I., Strosberg, A. D., and Luiten, P. G. M. (1993). Muscarinic acetylcholine receptor-expression in astrocytes in the cortex of young and aged rats. *Glia*, **8**, 42–50.

Van Harreveld, A., Crowell, J., and Malhotra, S. K. (1965). A study of extracellular space in the central nervous system. *J. Cell Biol.*, **25**, 117–137.

Vargová, L., and Syková, E. (1995). Effects of K$^+$, hypotonic solution and excitatory amino acids on diffusion parameters in the isolated rat spinal cord. *Abstracts, Ann. Meeting ENA*, p. 176.

Vartanian, T., Sprinkle, T. J., Dawson, G., and Szuchet, S. (1988). Oligodendrocyte substratum adhesion modulates expression of adenylate cyclase-linked receptors. *Proc. Natl Acad. Sci. USA*, **85**, 939–943.

Vaughan, Jr., H. G., and Arezzo, J. C. (1988). The neural bases of event-related potentials. In *Human Event-Related Potentials*, ed. T. Picton, pp. 45–96. Amsterdam: Elsevier.

Verkhratsky, A., and Kettenmann, H. (1996). Calcium signalling in glial cells. *TINS*, 19, 346–352.

Vignais, L., Nait Oumesmar, B., Mellouk, F., Gout, O., Labourdette, G., Baron-Van Evercooren, A., and Gumpel, M. (1993). Transplantation of oligodendrocyte precursors in the adult demyelinated spinal cord: migration and remyelination. *Intl. J. Dev. Neurosci.*, 11, 603–612.

Villegas, G. M., and Fernández, J. (1966). Permeability to thorium dioxide of the intercellular spaces of the frog cerebral hemisphere. *Exp. Neurol.*, 15, 18–36.

Villegas, J. (1995). Learning from the axon-Schwann cell relationships of the giant nerve fiber of the squid. In *Neuron–Glia Interrelations During Phylogeny*, vol. 2, *Plasticity and Regeneration*, eds A. Vernadakis and B. I. Roots, pp. 95–127. Totowa, N. J.: Humana Press.

Virchow, R. (1856). *Gesammelte Abhandlungen zur wissenschaftichen*. Frankfurt am Main: Medizin. Hamm.

Vitouch, O, Bauer, H., Gittler, G., Leodolter, M., and Leodolter, U. (1997). Cortical activity during spatial and verbal processing studied with slow cortical potential topography. *Int. J. Psychophysiol*, 27, 183–200.

Vizi, E. S., Gyires, K., Somogyi, G. T., and Ungvary, G (1983). Evidence that transmitter can be released from regions of the nerve cell other than presynaptic axon terminal: axonal release of acetylcholine without modulation. *Neuroscience*, 10, 967–972.

Voigt, T. (1989). Development of glial cells in the cerebral wall of ferrets: direct tracing of their transformation from radial glia into astrocytes. *J. Comp. Neurol.*, 289, 74–88.

Voipio, J., and Kaila, K. (1993). Interstitial PCO_2 and pH in rat hippocampal slices measured by means of a novel fast CO_2/H^+-sensitive microelectrode based on a PVC-gelled membrane. *Pflügers Arch.*, 423, 193–201.

Voipio, J., Pasternack, M., Rydqvist, B., and Kaila, K. (1991). Effect of γ-aminobutyric acid on intracellular pH in the crayfish stretchreceptor neuron. *J. Exp. Biol.*, 156, 349–361.

Von Boxberg, Y., Deiss, S., and Schwarz, U. (1993). Guidance and topographic stabilization of nasal chick retinal axons on target-derived components, in vitro. *Neuron*, 10, 345–357.

Voříšek, I., and Syková, E. (1997). Ischemia-induced changes in the extracellular space diffusion parameters, K^+ and pH in the developing rat cortex and corpus callosum. *J. Cereb. Blood Flow Metabol.*, 17, 191–203.

Vrba, R. (1962). Glucose metabolism in rat brain in vivo. *Nature*, 195, 663–665.

Vyklický, L. (1978). Transient changes in extracellular potassium and presynaptic inhibition. In *Iontophoresis and Transmitter Mechanisms in the Mammalian Central Nervous System*, eds R. W. Ryall and J. S. Kelly, pp. 284–286. Amsterdam: Elsevier.

Vyklický, L., Vlachová, V., and Kruse, K. J. (1990). The effect of external pH changes of responses to excitatory amino acids in mouse hippocampal neurons. *J. Physiol.*, 430, 497–517.

Vyskočil, F., Kříž, N., and Bureš, J. (1972). Potassium-selective microelectrodes used for measuring the extracellular brain potassium during spreading depression and anoxic depolarization. *Brain Res.*, 39, 255–259.

Wagner, H.-J., Pilgrim, Ch. and Brandl, J. (1974). Penetration and removal of horseradish peroxidase injected into the cerebrospinal fluid: role of cerebral perivascular spaces, endothelium and microglia. *Acta Neuropathol. (Berl.)*, 27, 299–315.

Wakakura, M., and Yamamoto, N. (1994). Cytosolic calcium transient increase through the AMPA/kainate receptor in cultured Müller cells. *Vision Res.*, 34, 1105–1109.

Wallace, C., Hawrylak, N., and Greenough, W. T. (1991). Studies of synaptic structural modifications after long-term potentiation and kindling: context for a molecular morphology. In *Long-Term Potentiation: A Debate of Current Issues*, eds M. Baudry and J. Davis, pp. 189–232. Cambridge: MIT Press.

Walter, W. G., Cooper, R., Aldridge, V. J., McCallum, W. C., and Winter, A. L. (1964). Contingent negative variation: an electric sign of sensorimotor association and expectancy in the human brain. *Nature*, **203**, 380–384.

Walz, W. (1988). Brain but not retinal glial cells have carbonic anhydrase activity in the honeybee drone. *Neurosci. Lett.*, **85**, 47–50.

Walz, W. (1989). Role of glial cells in the regulation of the brain ion microenvironment. *Prog. Neurobiol.*, **33**, 309–333.

Walz, W., and Hertz, L. (1983). Functional interactions between neurons and astrocytes – II. Potassium homeostasis at the cellular level. *Prog. Neurobiol.*, **20**, 133–183.

Walz, W., and Hinks, E. C. (1986). A trans-membrane sodium cycle in astrocytes. *Brain Res.*, **368**, 226–232.

Walz, W., and Kimelberg, H. K. (1985). Differences in cation transport properties of primary astrocyte cultures from mouse and rat brain. *Brain Res.*, **340**, 333–340.

Walz, W., and MacVicar, B. A. (1988). Electrophysiological properties of glial cells. Comparison of brain slices with primary cultures. *Brain Res.*, **443**, 321–324.

Walz, W., and Mukerji, S. (1988). Lactate release from cultured astrocytes and neurones: a comparison. *Glia*, **1**, 366–370.

Walz, W., and Schlue, W. R. (1982). Ionic mechanism of a hyperpolarizing 5-hydroxytryptamine effect on leech neuropile glial cells. *Brain Res.*, **250**, 111–121.

Walz, W., and Wuttke, W.A. (1989). Resistance of astrocyte electrical membrane properties to acidosis changes in the presence of lactate. *Brain Res.*, **504**, 82–86.

Walz, W., Klimazsevski, A., Paterson, A. I. (1993). Glial swelling in ischemia: a hypothesis. *Dev. Neurosci.*, **15**, 216–225.

Walz, W., Paterson, I. A., and Wuttke, W. A. (1996). Potassium accumulation in reactive glial cells in situ. *Soc. Neurosci. Abstr.*, **22**, 1497.

Warren, S., Humphreys, A., Juraska, J., and Greenough, W. (1995). LTP varies across the estrous cycle: enhanced synaptic plasticity in proestrus rats. *Brain. Res.*, **703**, 26–30.

Watanabe, K., Arai, T., Aoki, M., Mori, H., and Mori, K. (1993). Effects of halothane on the synthesis of neurotransmitter amino acids in mouse brain. *Acta Anaesthesiol. Scand.*, **37**, 706–709.

Waxman, S. G. (1977). Conduction in myelinated, unmyelinated, and demyelinated fibers. *Arch. Neurol.*, **34**, 585–590.

Waxman, S. G. (1993). Peripheral nerve abnormalities in multiple sclerosis. *Muscle Nerve*, **16**, 1–5.

Waxman, S. G., and Bennett, M. V. L. (1972). Relative conduction velocities of small myelinated and non-myelinated fibers in the central nervous system. *Nature New Biol.*, **238**, 217–219.

Waxman, S. G., and Black, J. A. (1995). Axoglial interactions of the cellular and molecular levels in central nervous system myelinated fibers. In *Neuroglia*, ed. H. Kettenmann and B. R. Ransom, pp. 587–610. New York and Oxford: Oxford University Press.

Waxman, S. G., and Brill, M. H. (1978). Conduction through demyelinated plaques in multiple sclerosis: computer simulations of facilitation by short internodes. *J. Neurol. Neurosurg. Psychiatry*, **41**, 408–417.

Waxman, S. G., and Foster, R. E. (1980). Development of the axon membrane during differentiation of myelinated fibres in spinal nerve roots. *Proc. R. Soc. (Lond.) B*, **209**, 441–446.

Waxman, S. G., Black, J. A., Duncan, I. D., and Ransom, B. R. (1990). Macromolecular structure of axon membrane and action potential conduction in myelin deficient heterozygote rat optic nerves. *J. Neurocytol.*, **19**, 11–27.

Wells, M. J. (1962). *Brain and Behaviour in Cephalopods*. London: Heinemann.

Wenzel, J., Lammert, G., Meyer, U., and Krug, M. (1991). The influence of long-term potentiation on the spatial relationship between astrocytic processes and potentiated synapses in the dentate gyrus neuropil of the rat brain. *Brain Res.*, **560**, 122–131.

Westergaard, N., Varming, T., Peng, L., Sonnewald, U., Hertz, L., and Schousboe, A. (1993). Uptake, release and metabolism of alanine in neurones and astrocytes in primary cultures. *J. Neurosci. Res.*, **35**, 540–545.

Westergaard, N., Sonnewald, U., and Schousboe, A. (1994). Release of a-ketoglutarate, malate and succinate from cultured astrocytes: possible role in amino acid transmitter homeostasis. *Neurosci. Lett.*, **176**, 105–109.

Westergaard, N., Sonnewald, U., Unsgard, G., Peng, L., Hertz, L., and Schousboe, A. (1994). Uptake, release and metabolism of citrate in neurones and astrocytes in primary cultures. *J. Neurochem.*, **62**, 1727–1733.

Whitaker-Azmitia, P. M., Murphy, R., and Azmitia, E. C. (1990). Stimulation of astroglial 5–HT 1A receptors releases the serotonergic growth factor, protein S-100, and alters astroglial morphology. *Brain Res.*, **528**, 155–158.

Whitaker-Azmitia, P. M., Clarke, C., and Azmitia, E. C. (1993). Localization of 5–HT$_{1A}$ receptors to astroglial cells in adult rats: implications for neuronal–glial interactions and psychoactive drug mechanism of action. *Synapse*, **14**, 201–205.

Wicht, H., Derouiche, A., and Korf, H. W. (1994). An immunocytochemical investigation of glial morphology in the Pacific hagfish: radial and astrocyte-like glia have the same phylogenetic age. *J. Neurocytol.*, **23**, 565–576.

Wijers, A. A., Mulder, G., Okita, T., and Mulder, L. J. M. (1989a). Event-related potentials during memory search and selective attention to letter size and conjunctions of letter size and color. *Psychophysiology*, **26**, 529–547.

Wijers, A. A., Mulder, G., Okita, T., Mulder, L. J. M. (1989b). Attention to color: an analysis of selection, controlled search, and motor activation, using event-related potentials. *Psychophysiology*, **26**, 89–109.

Wijers, A. A., Otten, L. J., Feenstra, S., Mulder, G., and Mulder, L. J. M. (1989c). Brain potentials during selective attention, memory search, and mental rotation. *Psychophysiology*, **26**, 452–467.

Wiley-Livingston, C. A., and Ellisman, M. H. (1980). Development of axonal membrane specializations defines nodes of Ranvier and precedes Schwann cell myelin elaboration. *Dev. Biol.*, **79**, 334–355.

Wilkin, G.P., Marriott, D.R., and Cholewinski, A.J. (1990). Astrocyte heterogeneity. *TINS*, **13**, 43–46.

Williams, J. H., Errington, M. L., Lynch, M. A., Bliss, T. V. P. (1989). Arachidonic acid induces a long term activity-dependent enhancement of synaptic transmission in the hippocampus. *Nature*, **341**, 739–742.

Willinger, M., Margolis, D. M., and Sidman, R. L. (1981). Neuronal differentiation in cultures of weaver mutant mouse cerebellum. *Supermolec. Struct.*, **17**, 79–86.

Wilson, G. F., and Chiu, S. Y. (1990a). Regulation of potassium channels in Schwann cells during early developmental myelinogenesis. *J. Neurosci.*, **10**, 1615–1625.

Wilson, G. F., and Chiu, S. Y. (1990b). Ion channels in axon and Schwann cell membranes at paranodes of mammalian myelinated fibres studied with patch clamp. *J. Neurosci.*, **10**, 63–3274.

Winder, D. G., and Conn, P. J. (1992). Activation of metabotropic glutamate receptors in the hippocampus increases cyclic AMP accumulation. *J. Neurochem.*, **59**, 375–378.

Winslow, J. W., Moran, P., Valverde, J., Shih, A., Yuan, J. Q., Wong, S. C., Tsai, S. P., Goddard, A., Henzel, W. J., Hefti, F., Beck, K. D., and Caras, I. W. (1995). Cloning of AL-1, a ligand for an Eph-related tyrosine kinase receptor involved in axon bundle formation. *Neuron*, **14**, 973–981.

Witkin, J., Ferin, M., Popilskis, S., and Silverman, A-J. (1991). Effects of gonadal steroids on the ultrastructure of GnRH neurons in the Rhesus monkey: synaptic input and glial apposition. *Endocrinology*, **129**, 1083–1092.

Witzenmann, A., Thanos, S., Boxberg, Y. V., and Bonhoeffer, F. (1993). Differential reactions of crossing and non-crossing rat retinal axons on crude membrane preparations from the chiasm midline: an in vitro study. *Development*, **117**, 725–735.

Wofchuk, S. T., and Rodnight, R. (1994). Glutamate stimulates the phosphorylation of glial fibrillary acidic protein in slices of immature rat hippocampus via a metabotropic receptor. *Neurochem. Int.*, **24**, 517–523.

Wolburg, H., and Berg, K. (1988). Distribution of orthogonal arrays of particles in the Müller cell membrane of the mouse retina. *Glia*, **1**, 246–252.

Wolff, J. R. (1970). Quantitative aspects of astroglia. In *Proceedings of the 6th International Congress of Neuropathology*, pp. 327–336. Paris: Masson Cie.

Woolley, C. and McEwen, B. (1992). Estradiol mediates fluctuation in hippocampal synapse density during the estrous cycle in the adult rat. *J. Neurosci.*, **12**: 2549–2554.

Woolley, C., Gould, E., Frankfurt, M. and McEwen, B. (1990). Naturally occurring fluctuation in dendritic spine density on adult hippocampal pyramidal neurons. *J. Neurosci.*, **10**, 4035–4039.

Würdig, S., and Kugler, P. (1991). Histochemistry of glutamate metabolising enzymes in the rat cerebellar cortex. *Neurosci. Lett.*, **130**, 165–168.

Wurtz, C. C., and Ellisman, M. H. (1986). Alterations in the ultrastructure of peripheral nodes of Ranvier associated with repetitive action potential propagation. *J. Neurosci.*, **6**, 3133–3143.

Wurtz, R. H. (1965). Steady potential shifts in the rat during desynchronised sleep. *Electroenceph. Clin. Neurophysiol.*, **19**, 521–523.

Wuttke, W. A. (1990). Mechanism of potassium uptake in neuropil glial cells in the central nervous system of the leech. *J. Neurophysiol.*, **63**, 1089–1097.

Wuttke, W., and Walz, W. (1990). Sodium- and bicarbonate-independent regulation of intracellular pH in cultured mouse astrocytes. *Neurosci. Lett.*, **117**, 105–110.

Wyllie, D. J. A., and Cull-Candy, S. G. (1994). A comparison of non-NMDA receptor channels in type-2 astrocytes and granule cells from rat cerebellum. *J. Physiol.*, **475**, 95–114.

Wyllie, D. J. A., Mathie, A., Symonds, C. J., and Cull-Candy, S. G. (1991). Activation of glutamate receptors and glutamate uptake in identified macroglial cells in rat cerebellar cultures. *J. Physiol. (Lond.)*, **432**, 235–258.

Xie, Y., Zacharias, E., Hoff, P., and Tegtmeier, F. (1995). Ion channel involvement in anoxic depolarisation induced by cardiac arrest in rat brain. *J. Cereb. Blood Flow Metab.*, **15**, 587–594.

Yamamura, T., Stevens, W. C., Okamura, A., Harada, K. and Kemmotsu, O. (1993). Correlative study of behavior and synaptic events during halothane anaesthesia in the lamprey. *J. Anaesth. Analg.*, **76**, 342–347.

Yin, J. C., Del Vecchio, M., Zhou, H., and Tully, T. (1995). CREB as a memory modulator: induced expression of a dCREB2 activator isoform enhances long-term memory in Drosophila. *Cell*, **81**, 107–115.

Yoder, E. J., Tamir, H., and Ellisman, M. H. (1996). 5-hydroxytryptamine$_{2A}$ receptors on cultured rat Schwann cells. *Glia*, **17**, 15–27.

Young, J. Z. (1961). Learning and discrimination in the octopus. *Biol. Rev.*, **36**, 32–96.

Young, J. Z. (1967). Some comparisons between the nervous systems of cephalopods and mammals. In *Invertebrate Nervous Systems. Their Significance for Mammalian Neurophysiology*, ed. C. A. G. Wiersema, pp. 353–362. Chicago: The University of Chicago Press.

Young, J. Z. (1971). *The Anatomy of the Nervous System of Octopus Vulgaris*. Oxford: Clarendon Press.

Yu, A. C. H., Drejer, J., Hertz, L., and Schousboe, A. (1983). Pyruvate carboxylase activity in primary cultures of astrocytes and neurones. *J. Neurochem.*, **41**, 1484–1487.

Yu, N., Martin, J.-L., Stella, N., and Magistretti, P. J. (1993). Arachidonic acid stimulates glucose uptake in cerebral cortical astrocytes. *Proc. Natl Acad. Sci. USA*, **90**, 4042–4046.

Yudkoff, M., Nissim, I., Hertz, L., Pleasure, D., and Erecinska, M. (1992). Nitrogen metabolism. Neuronal–astroglial relationships. *Prog. Brain Res.*, **94**, 213–224.

Yulis, C. R., Peruzzo, B., and Rodriguez, E. M. (1984). Immuncytochemistry and unltrastructure of the neuropil located ventral to the rat supraoptic nucleus. *Cell Tissue Res.*, **236**, 171–180.

Zeller, N. K., Dubois-Dalcq, M., and Lazzarini, R. A. (1989). Myelin protein expression in the myelin-deficient rat brain and cultured oligodendrocytes. *J. Mol. Neurosci.*, **1**, 139–149.

Zemcik, B. A., and Strader, C. D. (1988). Fluorescent localization of the β-adrenergic receptor on DDT-1 cells. *Biochemistry*, **251**, 333–339.

Zhao, W.-Q., Bennett, P., and Ng, K. T. (1995). The impairment of long-term memory formation by the phosphatase inhibitor okadaic acid. *Brain Res. Bull.*, **36**, 557–561.

Zhao, W.-Q., Ng, K. T., and Sedman, G. L. (1995). Passive avoidance learning induced change in GAP43 phosphorylation in day-old chicks. *Brain Res. Bull.*, **36**, 11–17.

Zhao, W.-Q., Sedman, G. L., Gibbs, M. E., and Ng, K. T. (1994a). Effect of PKC inhibitors and activators on memory. *Behav. Brain Res.*, **60**, 151–160.

Zhao, W.-Q., Sedman, G., Gibbs, M.. and Ng, K. T. (1994b). Phosphorylation changes following weakly-reinforced learning and ACTH-induced memory consolidation for a weak learning experience. *Brain Res. Bull.*, **36**, 161–168.

Zhao, W.-Q., Polya, G. M., Wang, B. H., Gibbs, M. E., Sedman, G. L., and Ng, K. T. (1995). Inhibition of cAMP-dependent protein kinase impairs long-term memory formation in day-old chicks. *Neurobiol. Learn. Mem.*, **64**, 106–118.

Zhao, W.-Q., Bennett, P., Rickard, N., Sedman, G. L., and Ng, K. T. (1996). The involvement of CA^{2+}/calmodulin-dependent protein kinase in memory formation in day-old chicks. *Neurobiol. Learn. Mem.*, **66**, 24–35.

Zimmerman, S. B., and Minton, A. P. (1993). Macromolecular crowding – biochemical, biophysical, and physiological consequences. *Annu. Rev. Biophys. Biomol. Str.*, **22**, 27–65.

Zorn, L., Kulkarni, R., Anatharum, V., Bayley, H., and Treistman, S. N. (1993). Halothane acts on many potassium channels, including a minimal potassium channel. *Neurosci. Letts.* **161**, 81–84.

Index

Full names are given here; for abbreviations found in the text please consult pages xiii–xvi